FORENSIC MEDICINE – FROM OLD PROBLEMS TO NEW CHALLENGES

Edited by **Duarte Nuno Vieira**

Forensic Medicine – From Old Problems to New Challenges
Edited by Duarte Nuno Vieira

Published by InTech

Janeza Trdine 9, 51000 Rijeka, Croatia

Publishing Process Manager Davor Vidic

Technical Editor Teodora Smiljanic

Cover Designer InTech Design Team

Additional hard copies can be obtained from orders@intechopen.com

Forensic Medicine – From Old Problems to New Challenges, Edited by Duarte Nuno Vieira
p. cm.
ISBN 978-953-307-262-3

For EU product safety concerns:
IN TECH d.o.o., Prolaz Marije Krucifikse Kozulić 3, 51000 Rijeka, Croatia,
info@intechopen.com or visit our website at intechopen.com.

Meet the editor

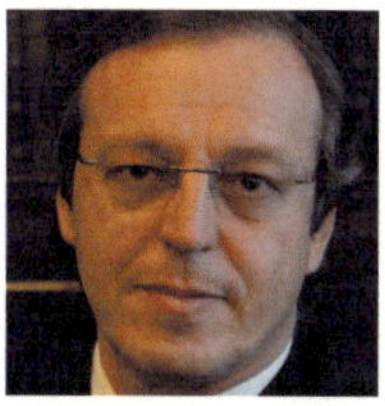

Dr. Duarte Nuno Vieira is a Full Professor of Forensic Medicine and Forensic Sciences and of Ethics and Medical Law at the University of Coimbra. He is Chief Forensic Pathologist and National Director of the Portuguese National Institute of Forensic Medicine, President of the Portuguese Medico-Legal Council and Member of the Portuguese National Council of Ethics for Life Sciences. Professor Vieira is the current President of the International Academy of Legal Medicine, International Association of Forensic Sciences, World Police Medical Officers and European Council of Legal Medicine. He is past-President of the Mediterranean Academy of Forensic Sciences and of the Latin-American Association of Medical Law. He works actively in the field of human rights, as Forensic Expert of the International Rehabilitation Council for Torture Victims, Forensic Adviser of the International Committee of Red Cross and Temporary Forensic Consultant of the UN High Commissioner of Humans Rights. Professor Vieira has attended more than 450 conferences as keynote invited speaker in Europe, North, Central and South-America, Asia, Australasia, Africa and Middle-East, and has been awarded 11 scientific prizes and 12 honorary fellowship from governments and scientific associations from European, Asian, African and central and south-American countries. He has published more than 300 scientific papers and is the editor or co-editor of 5 books in Portuguese, French and English languages.

Contents

Preface

Forensic medicine has attracted considerable attention from the media and general public in recent years, largely due to the impact of successful television series dealing with the subject and to certain high-profile cases (involving crime, natural disasters or technological accidents) in which it played a significant part.

Forensic medicine is a continuously evolving science that is constantly being updated and improved, not only as a result of technological and scientific advances (which bring almost immediate repercussions) but also because of developments in the social and legal spheres.

We are undoubtedly living in a period of constant rapid change. Thus, if forensic medicine departments are to fulfil their role as centres of training, expertise and research, the professionals working in them need to be attentive to those changes by being prepared to constantly update their knowledge and skills. One of the most important ways of keeping in touch with new developments in the field is through reading, which enables us to share in the reflections and experiences of other professionals and brings us into contact with different realities and perspectives.

A great many books have been published about forensic medicine in recent years. However, most are very similar in structure, with chapters that review the various areas of expert intervention; indeed, the only differences between them tend to concern certain concepts and/or the geographical background of their author(s). All continue to give priority to the traditional paper format, which, despite its many advantages, also brings limitations, conditioning access to contents (particularly amongst professionals from poorer countries) and restricting dissemination and circulation.

This book does not follow this usual publication policy, and in that respect, it is not simply new, it is (if I may dare to say so) radically new. It contains innovative perspectives and approaches to classic topics and problems in forensic medicine, offering reflections about the potential and limits of emerging areas in forensic expert research; it transmits the experience of some countries in the domain of cutting-edge expert intervention, and shows how research in other fields of knowledge may have very relevant implications for this practice.

There are chapters on the potential of pharmacogenetics and forensic microbiology, chapters offering different perspectives on perennial themes such as the diagnosis of death by drowning or anaphylactic shock, others reflecting on the particular experience of some countries in areas as problematic as child abuse, and some that apparently have little or nothing to do with forensic medicine at all (such as the chapter about research into cerebral vascularisation), but whose results ultimately have a huge relevance for expert practice in forensic pathology.

This book is thus a miscellany of different approaches to various aspects of forensic medical practice, all of which are extremely interesting. Precisely because it is a miscellany, there seemed little sense in grouping the texts into different chapters or areas; hence, they have been ordered thematically.

When I was contacted by InTech to edit this work, I initially hesitated, wary of reviewing and pronouncing upon texts by authors that had not been selected by me and which had been submitted somewhat randomly without any prior guidance or structuring. But InTech is one of the biggest Open Access publishers of scientific books today, with high-quality publications, worldwide readership and no copyright transfer, and it was that which ultimately prompted me to accept the invitation. For this is an entirely new posture in the world of publishing. Indeed, my decision to participate as editor was strengthened when I discovered amongst the authors some of the world's leading authorities in the field of forensic medicine whose work I have long admired and respected, alongside some newer names, people who were taking their first steps in international scientific publications and producing articles of a very promising quality.

All in all, this has proved to be a particularly interesting experience, from which I have derived great pleasure and benefit, and I truly hope that the reader will find in the book the same opportunities for professional enrichment as I have done.

Finally, some acknowledgements are due. Firstly, my thanks go to InTech for having invited me to participate in this work as editor, and to Davor Vidic, publishing process manager of this book, for the support, professionalism and efficiency with which he responded to my multiple requests, as well as for his endless patience with regard to my own systematic delays in responding to him. But above all, I would like to thank the authors for having taken the time to write the chapters contained in this book (thereby generously sharing their knowledge, experiences, reflections, expert practice and research with the international forensic medicine community) and for having contributed economically to the publication of this work, particularly as most of them could easily have published their texts in any other scientific journal or book. With this gesture, they have thus made possible the publication of an Open Access book that is free to professionals around the world and only a click away, thereby demonstrating a highly-developed social conscience as regards the growing imperative to openly share information. Indeed, it is my opinion that those that have achieved a particular status, professional or academic, in the world of forensic medicine have a moral duty to ensure that their knowledge and experience reach those who, for economic or geographical reasons, may have difficulty in accessing scientific literature. This is what the various authors of this book have done. To all, my heartfelt thanks!

Duarte Nuno Vieira, MD, MSc, PhD
President of IALM (2006-12), IAFS (2008-11),
WPMO (2008-11), ECLM (2009.) and MAFS (2005-07)
Full Professor of Forensic Medicine and Forensic Sciences,
Head of the National Institute of Forensic Medicine of Portugal
University of Coimbra,
Portugal

1

Avoiding Errors and Pitfalls in Evidence Sampling for Forensic Genetics

B. Ludes and C. Keyser
Laboratoire d'anthropologie moléculaire, Institut de médicine légale, Université de Strasbourg France

1. Introduction

DNA fingerprinting or DNA profiling (as it is now known) was first developed by Alec Jeffreys in 1985 (Jeffreys et al., 1985), who found that in the human genome, some regions contained DNA sequences that were repeated over and over again, next to each other. He also discovered that the number of repeated unit could differ from individual to individual allowing human identity testing. Since that time, DNA typing methods has been commonly used in criminal cases (to identify a suspect or a victim or to absolve an innocent individual) as well as in the identification of missing persons or in paternity testing. Today, the most commonly used DNA repeat regions used are microsatellites also known as Short Tandem Repeats (STR). These loci in which the repeat unit is at least two bases but no more than seven in length, are amplified by PCR (Polymerase Chain Reaction) in a multiplex fashion (multiple primers) reducing sample consumption. Today, for the majority of forensic cases where DNA of preserved quality is available, the identification procedures of biological samples are performed by commercially well-validated kits incorporating 15-16 highly variable STR loci (plus amelogenin) such as PowerPlex^R (Promega) and AmpF*l*STR^R(Applied Biosystems). With highly automated equipment, STR profiling can process hundreds of samples each day and became the cornerstone of forensic DNA testing, including national DNA databases with STR-profiles of convicted felons. Nevertheless, it is of great importance to make the distinction between the samples containing large quantities of high quality DNA and those containing minute amounts of DNA and/or poor quality molecules. If for the first type of samples, the occurrences of errors or pitfall are rare, in the second type, the interpretation of the allelic profiles should be done with care and caution.
In this article, the authors will focus on the analysis of challenging samples, in other words, samples containing either (i) minute amount of DNA or (ii) degraded DNA or (iii) mixture of DNA or (iv) DNA polymerase inhibitors or (v) contaminating DNA molecules. Indeed, DNA is stable and remains intact when stored in a dry or frozen state but will be degraded when stored under inappropriate or bacterially contaminated conditions. Two types of damage are mainly likely to affect DNA over time: hydrolytic and oxidative damage. Hydrolytic damage results in deamination of bases and in depurination and depyrimidination, whereas oxidative damage results in modified bases (Lindahl, 1993). Both mechanisms reduce the number as well as the size of the fragments that can be amplified by PCR. Failure to amplify DNA may also result from the presence of inhibitors that interfere

with the PCR such as low-molecular-weight compounds, supposedly derived from the crime scene environment, which coextract with the target DNA molecules and potently inhibit the activity of the DNA polymerase (Keyser-Tracqui C. and Ludes B., 2005). Contamination by DNA coming from outside the case represents one of the major limitations to DNA analysis. The authors will describe the strategies developed to overcome the difficulties which begin with the biological sample collection.

2. Biological sample collection

2.1 Samples

Various kinds of samples can be typed with the PCR-based methodologies such as:

- Blood samples and blood stains
- Cigarette buts (Hochmeister et al., 1991)
- Human hairs with a special mention of the possibility of analysis of single hair (Higuchi et al., 1991)
- Urine samples and urine stains (Brinkmann et al., 1992)
- Fingernail scraping (Wiegand et al., 1993)
- Bite marks (Sweet et al., 1997)
- All kinds of touched objects (Van Oorschot and Jones, 1997) such as tools, clothing, firearms, parts of vehicle, food, condoms, glass, bottles, lip cosmetics, wallets, jewellery, paper, cables, stones and construction material (Van Hoofstat et al., 1999; Webb et al., 2001; Wickenheiser, 2002; Rutty, 2002; Polley et al., 2006; Petricevic et al. 2006; Sewell et al., 2008; Horsman-Hall et al., 2009)
- FTA cards can be used to collect blood or saliva in order to assure a better preservation of the DNA molecules by the specific fixation on the treated card paper
- Teeth and bone tissues as well as burnt tissues

Touched objects provide a wide scope for revealing the offender's DNA profile in investigations of offences including theft, burglary, vehicle crimes, street robbery, drug cases, homicide, rape and sex offences, clandestine laboratories, armed robbery, assaults, crime. The positive DNA identification from those samples allowed the creation of national offender databases (Harbison et al., 2001; Gunn, 2003; Walsh and Buckleton, 2005; Gill et al., 2000; Whitaker et al. 2001) to identify serial offenders and criminals.

2.2 Collecting methodologies

One of the best methods to collect trace samples is the use of swabs after having identified as precisely as possible the areas to target. The first step is to swab the hole defined surface by one or several moistened swab multiple times with some pressure and rotation given to the swabs. The second step is to complete the swabbing by the application of dry swabs to recapture the moisture containing hydrated cells. Co-extraction of these swabs to enhance overall retrieval of DNA is recommended (Castella and Mangin, 2008; Sweet et al., 1997; Pang and Cheung, 2007).

The moistening agent can be sterile water, 0, 01% sodium dodecyl sulphate (Wickenheiser, 2002) or isopropanol (Hansson et al., 2009). The quantities of cellules retrieved depend also of the physical characteristics of the surface (Wickenheiser, 2002) and the use of different moistening agents for different surfaces may facilitate collection. The quality of the swabs is also important, the quality should be DNA-free; cotton swabs are the most frequently used but other types such as foam may also be considered (Wickenheiser, 2002; Hansson et al.,

2009; 57, 111, 112). It has been shown that the yield of DNA from moist or frozen swabs are higher that from dried swabs. After collecting the biological material from a surface it is recommended to process the swab in the laboratory. If these conditions are not available, the swabs must be frozen immediately after collection.

According to some authors, tape is the best way to retrieve DNA containing material from worn clothing or from touched surfaces without collecting in the same time inhibitory factors present on this material (staining chemicals and/or color denim). By pressing a strip of tape multiple times over a target area, the most recently deposited material , with fewer inhibitory factors, are collected. In our experience, this method is not often used and should be replaced by a easiest way to collect DNA such as cutting away stain fragment samples.

To isolate relevant target cells from other over-whelming cell types, laser microdissection techniques were used. The different cell types can be recognized by morphological characteristics, various chemical staining or fluorescence labeling techniques. These methods allow to establish a clear DNA profile from few cells present in a mixture samples that otherwise had not be detected while swabbed by the major component and not detectable in the profile (Elliott et al., 2003; Anslinger et al., 2005; Anoruo et al., 2007 ; Sanders et al., 2006). With laser micro dissection techniques (Anslinger et al., 2007; Vandewoestyne et al., 2009), it has been shown that cells derived from a male contributor can be analyzed separately from those derived from a female contributor after morphological or fluorescent labeling identification. For this method, coated glass slides are required and a sample must be transferred from the collection material to the slide. As cells could be lost during this transfer, it would be preferable to use actually laser microdissection methodology is directly used on the initial collection material.

3. DNA analyses

3.1 DNA extraction

The classical ways of DNA extraction from forensic routine case work were the organic methods and sometimes the use of resin like Chelex 100R Bio-Rad (Walsh et al., 1991) which may induce the molecule degradation during long storage periods. Actually, in cases of degraded samples or when only minute amounts of DNA are available, the use of silica-coated magnetic beads to capture the molecules from the rest of the lysed cells is recommended. These extraction procedures are also performed in some laboratories by robotic systems (Greenspoon et al, 2004; Frégeau et al., 2010). The loss of DNA during the extraction step could be linked to the substrate sustaining the sample. Nevertheless, this loss is principally linked to the used methodologies namely the organic extraction techniques. The majority of samples submitted for analyses contain relatively large amounts of DNA, above the 0.1-0.5ng minimum required by most common STR profiling systems. Below this amount, specific methods like those used by molecular anthropologists on ancient DNA samples must be developed.

The optimization of the extraction methods involves:

- The extraction of all the available DNA;
- To remove all amplification inhibiting elements without the loss of DNA;
- To amplify all the extracted molecules with adding the amplification reagents to the device containing the DNA rather to add the DNA to the amplification tube and to loose molecules in pipette tips or on the tube walls ;

3.2 DNA quantitation

It seems not necessary to quantitate all the samples in particular highly degraded samples or trace samples given the expected low concentration of DNA. The only advantage lay in having an indication of the approximate quantity present in order to prevent repeat analyses of over-amplified samples and when interpreting the profile. It must be emphasized that a negative quantitation result should not prevent to process the samples. With the real-time quantitation method applied on low template samples, the results should be taken as an indication of the concentration and not as an absolute measurement as with higher DNA amounts. In criminal cases, it is of common practice to retain a certain amount of the samples for the future further typing by a second laboratory as a cross examination.

3.3 DNA amplification

For samples containing enough DNA of high molecular weight, the classical technics of DNA extraction can be performed without pitfall, appropriate technologies were developed to increase the chance to obtain useful profiles from very minute DNA samples such as the low copy number (LCN) procedure with extra cycles or low template DNA (LTDNA) methods. Minute samples or trace DNA refers to samples where only 100pg to 200pg of DNA could be extracted according to different authors. These methods increased the possibility to amplify successfully DNA from trace scene samples (McCartney, 2009; Budowle et al., 2009). Difficulties can be raised in the interpretation of those profiles where the peak heights may be below a validated threshold level.

During this step, the exponential amplification of DNA results in the production of billions of copies of the template molecule. So every DNA contamination will be also amplified and can false the result and on the other hand the excess of DNA produced by the PCR will be present either on the machines used but also in the surrounding environment such as the air and the work surfaces. To avoid these contaminations, all the steps of the analyses (pre-PCR, PCR itself, post-PCR) must be performed in physically separated laboratories.

The step of amplification is a very critical one and was optimized for low level template amounts. Amplification is the main field where the biologists must have control of the quality of the molecule. To enhance the success of trace DNA amplification, it was proposed to increase the number of cycles (Gill et al., 2000). The number of cycles used during the PCR of the STR loci is increased to 34 compared to the standard 28 cycle reactions. In molecular anthropology and in ancient DNA work, the number of cycles could be increased up to 60 in order to maximize the success of amplification (Rameckers et al., 1997). Numerous authors have described the efficacy of increasing cycle numbers ((Gill et al., 2000; Whitaker et al., 2001; Kloosterman et Kersbergen, 2003). Complete profiles with substantial increases in peak heights have been described (Gill et al., 2000) but contaminating DNA may also be amplified through enhancing the number of cycles. When the sensitivity is increased, more sporadic contamination will be detected and the laboratories must enhance the stringency of contamination prevention. "Mini-STR" kits were developed containing redesigned primers which had significantly higher success rates with degraded DNA due to smaller amplicons. The minifiler STR kit^{R} produced by Applied Biosystem showed a higher success rate with degraded or inhibited DNA than the classical kits and requires also a lower template input approximately 0.125 ng compared to 0.5ng (Mulero et al., 2008). The optimization of the multiplex with the increased priming and amplification efficiency of the new primers can explain the better sensitivity of the amplification.

The efficiency of the amplification reaction can also be increased by the addition of chemical adjuvants such as bovine serum albumin (BSA). BSA is known to prevent the inhibition of the activity of Taq polymerase by sequestering phenolic compounds which otherwise scavenge the polymerase (Kreader, 1996).

3.4 Detection of amplified product

To increase the detection of amplified product , methods have been developed to purify the PCR amplicons, to remove salts, ions and unused dNTPs and primers from the reaction by using filtration (Microcon filter columns), silica gel membranes (Quiagen MinElute) or enzyme hydrolysis (ExoSAP-IT) (Forster et al., 2008; Petricevic et al., 2010; Smith and Ballantyne, 2007)). This purification step is performed to remove negative ions such as Cl- which prevents inter-molecular competition occurring during electrokinetic injection allowing a maximum amount of DNA to be injected into the capillary of the sequencer. To enhance the quantity of DNA available for the detection, it is also possible to concentrate the PCR product during the purification process.

3.5 Difficulties of the typing of trace DNA

The side effect of increasing the ability to amplify the DNA molecule and in particular minutes amounts of material is the increased likelihood of contamination being detected and of artifacts of the amplification process due to stochastic effects.
Four major cases of interpretation difficulties can be summarized:

- Allele drop-out is due to a preferential amplification of one allele at one or more heterozygous loci. This kind of pitfall is relatively frequent when very low quantities of DNA are amplified (Whitaker et al., 2001; Gill et al., 2000; Gill et al., 2005; Lucy et al., 2007). The interpretation of profiles obtained from minutes amounts of DNA must in each case take in account the possibility of an allele drop out.
- Allele drop in, this occurrence is due to amplification artifacts such as stutter. This artifact may be also frequently seen in the analyses of trace DNA amounts (Whitaker et al., 2001). When stutter alleles are present in a STR profile it is rather difficult or impossible to characterize the number of individuals having their DNA in the sample and assigning of alleles within a mixture.
- Allele drop is due to sporadic contamination occurring from various origins such as crime scene, sampling, non DNA free material or at the laboratory work.
- A decreased heterozygote allele balance within a locus and between loci. In this feature, the peak height imbalance within and between loci are due to the same amplification effects that cause drop-out. In those cases, the evaluation of the zygosity at a particular loci may be extremely difficult.

No methods can actually eliminate completely artifact product during the amplification step in particular when the DNA is degraded or present in minute amounts but their occurrence should be statistically evaluated. To be able to develop such an approach it is of importance to understand the factors that may cause each type of artifact and the accurate data regarding the frequency and scale of their occurrence. Benschop et al. (2010) present one of the first large-scale efforts to characterize artifacts generated by different trace DNA amplifications. These authors showed also their investigations to highlight an effective method to generate a useful consensus profile.

3.6 Pitfall at the interpretation step

For each profile interpretation, the sampling of biological material found at the crime scene must be replaced into context and the possibility of pitfalls should be taken into account such as the possibilities of material transfer, the difficulties of the amplification process and the possibility of artifacts affecting the true result. This interpretation carefulness is of particular importance when the analyses are performed on degraded or very low quantities of DNA and has to consider imperatively the four most common features which can occur in those cases: allele drop-out, allele drop-in, stutter bands, contamination and decreased heterozygote balance. Strict interpretation guidelines can give reliable and robust result and minimize these pitfalls.

The introduction of detection thresholds may give a reliability of DNA profiles interpretations in particular for degraded DNA or minutes amounts of DNA. The background noise is generally eliminated by the establishing a threshold of 50 RFU. In order to avoid false homozygote by allelic drop-out , separate thresholds were established referred to as the low-template DNA threshold *T*, the match interpretation threshold (Budowle et al., 2009), the limit of quantitation (Gilder et al., 2007) is set at 150-200 RFU. The allele peaks should be above this limit to be sure that it is a true homozygous but even the respect of this limit may not prevent allele drop-out in all cases. Other authors (Gill and Buckleton, 2010) have recommended that instead of thresholds, a more continuous measure should be used which is modeled on the risk of dropout based on peak heights.

One of the most used methods to eliminate incorrect genotypes is to replicate the amplifications reactions and to generate consensus profiles (Whitaker et al., 2001; Gill et al., 2000; Benschop et al. , 2010; Taberlet et al., 1996). But currently, no consensus has been found on either the minimum number of replicates needed or how frequently one needs to observe an allele within the number of replicates conducted to be sure that the found allele is a true one. Benschop et al., (2010) consider that four replicates for degraded or very low amounts of DNA may be the most appropriate rules for considering a profile as a true one.

Gill et al. (2000) proposed a statistical model, mentioned by other authors (Balding and Buckleton, 2009; Gill and Buckleton, 2010; Curran, 2005), which provides the necessary probabilistic methods where the probability of observing the evidence profile can be combined with prior knowledge regarding dropout, the number of potential contributors, the possibility of contamination and other factors (Van Oorschot et al., 2010).

3.7 Mixture interpretation

A particular mention must be made for DNA mixture interpretation. In fact mixed samples are by definition composed of one or more major contributors with high quantities of DNA and with a minor contributor present only at trace levels, in other cases, the contributors are all present at trace levels. A profile can be falsely identified as a false mixed samples when high stutter peaks are present indicating that the DNA is coming from multiple individuals although it truly derive from a single source. In mixed samples, the high probability of drop-in, drop-out and increased stutter bands avoid the precise determination of the number of contributors and the separation of the genotypes at any given locus. This is frequently the case in degraded DNA or when the DNA is present in very few amounts (Walsh et al., 1996; LeClair et al., 2004; Gibb et Huell, 2009).

In such cases, the amplification reaction is also source of bias and pitfalls in over-amplification of some alleles and allowing a dropping-out of minor contributor's alleles at some loci.

Recommendations were published by the International Society of Forensic Genetics on mixture sample interpretation (Gill et al, 2006). A likelihood ratio (LR) approach was proposed for the interpretation for low template level mixture with the incorporation of an assessment of the probability of allele drop-in and drop-out in such cases.
Bright et al. (2010) proposed the use of the heterozygote balance and average peak heights at each locus to calculate the mixture ratio and distinguish among the contributors' genotypes (Van Oorschot et al., 2010).
For all these reasons, interpretation of mixture samples must be done very carefully particularly in cases where DNA is degraded or present in few quantities.

4. Contaminations issues

Contaminations are the major pitfall in the analyses of DNA in the forensic field either in producing valuable profiles or in accurate interpretation of the results. This is a major issue when the samples are degraded or when the DNA molecules are present in minute amounts. Contaminations may appear in every step of the analysis process from the sampling on the crime scene to the laboratory work. Rutty and Graham (2005) highlight that the contaminations can occur on the body itself or during the sampling of the evidences, at the scene of the crime, during the transportation of the body to the mortuary, at the autopsy room and after, of course, during the laboratory procedures.
At the crime scene, one of the more frequent situation where contaminations of the crime scene can occur if the individuals who entered the scene speak or caught and handle evidences over the corps before the arrival of the forensic investigative team. Rutty and Graham (2005) described airborne DNA contamination in mortuaries.
Methods were described in order to avoid the possibility of contaminations:

- To perform analyses about the persistence of DNA on different kinds of surfaces in various environmental conditions (Toothman et al., 2008; Rutty et al., 2003; Cook et Dixon, 2007);
- To improve and standardize the sample collection methodologies in order to improve the targeting of the samples and to decrease unwanted underlying DNA;
- To collect the profiles of all the persons involved in the collecting and laboratory steps to recognize a contamination coming from these professionals;
- Some laboratories require samples from the area immediately adjacent to the target area to have a so called "blank sample".

The operating procedures on the crime scene must be precisely fixed to minimize the possibility of contaminations (Rutty et al., 2003):

- To avoid breathing, talking and of course coughing during the sampling step in restricting the access of non specialist investigators to the scene;
- The use full-body scene suit (to avoid contamination by cell shedding coming from exposed areas of skin), hood, hair net, gloves and mouth masks by all the investigators in charge of the sampling step;
- To avoid direct touching of the evidences containing the DNA and changing gloves and masks regularly at the crime scene and obviously in the laboratories;
- All the results are compared against the database containing the DNA profiles of all the persons who were involved in all the steps of the sampling and laboratory processing of the evidences in order to detect contaminations coming from them;

- To use DNA-free disposable equipment to collect the DNA on the target surfaces (Van Oorschot et al., 2005), and to systematically decontaminate thoroughly all the devices which would be in physical contact with the sample.
- For victims taken to a hospital in attempt to seek treatment, the different surfaces (stretcher, hospital beds, tables), the instruments which will be used (scissors to cut away the clothing, electrocardiogram leads, other medical equipment).

Methods to minimize the possibility of contamination in the laboratory have been largely developed. Some of the guidelines are:

- Use of DNA-free plastic ware and consumables, recommendations for manufacturers and laboratories were made by several scientific societies (Gill et al., 2010), Scientific Working Group on DNA Analysis Methods [SWGDAM], European Network of Forensic Science Institutes [ENFSI], Biology Specialist Advisory Group [BSAG];
- Shortwave (254 nm) UV exposition of the working surfaces when nobody is working and frequent and thorough cleaning of work areas within laboratories. The top of doors of each room are also equipped with UV source. All appliances, containers, pipets, racks, laboratory coats and work areas (laminar airflow surfaces, PCR box) are cleaned and irradiated by UV during the non-working hours (Keyser-Tracqui et Ludes, 2005).
- Periodic assessment of the level and location of DNA within the work place and on relevant tools;
- All the different steps of the analysis process going from the sample examination step to the extraction procedure, the DNA amplification reaction and at the end, the interpretation of the profiles must be conducted in dedicated laboratory rooms. The analyses of traces samples are also performed a part of the high DNA quality and quantity DNA samples. A "one-way traffic" rule is also observed in the laboratory, once the technician has entered the PCR or the post-PCR rooms, they are not allowed to return to the extraction or pre-PCR rooms until the next day or a complete cloth changing in order to prevent contamination by aerosol particles. All general equipment and apparatus, pipets as well as reagents are dedicated to the analysis area (Extraction, pre-PCR, post-PCR rooms) ;
- Cross comparison of results obtained from different cases (having recorded at which locations the analyses were performed by whom and at what time) to detect unexpected contaminations;
- Analysis of reference samples and extraction (blank) as well as amplification controls at each step of the procedure are a major help to highlight inter-case contamination. The extraction control checks the purity of the extraction reagents and the amplification control indicates the purity of the PCR reagents with no DNA added.

The possibility of the presence of contaminations should be taken in mind at every profile interpretations in particular in cases of degraded DNA or if the molecule is present in very few quantities. As described before the difficulty of the interpretation of a mixed sample must be emphasized, in fact the profile can contain background DNA, crime-related DNA, post-crime contamination.

5. Conclusions

Since the method of DNA fingerprints has been described two majors goals have been followed, first to obtain highly discriminating genetic profiles from minute amounts of DNA and for highly degraded samples, second to avoid the possibility of contaminations due to the crime scene work, the sampling step or the laboratories procedures.

Swabbing and taping a touched area for retrieval of DNA seems simple but experience in case works showed how easy it is to get wrong. The scene crime technicians should be trained and wear appropriate scene clothing to protect the crime scene and its environment. The interpretation of the results should take in account these contamination possibilities by a LR framework incorporating the criminal aspects of DNA evidence (Raymond et al., 2008).

6. References

Anoruo B, van Oorschot R, Mitchell J, Howells D: Isolating cells from non-sperm cellular mictures using the PALM microlaser micro dissection system. *Forensic Sci Int* 2007, 173:93-96.

Anslinger K, Bayer B, Mack B, Eisenmenger W: Sex-specific fluorescent labelling of cells for laser microdissection and DNA profiling. *Int J Legal Med* 2007, 121:54-56.

Anslinger K, Mack B, Bayer B, Rolf B, Eisenmenger W: Digoxigenin labelling and laser capture microdissection of male cells. *Int J Legal Med* 2005, 119:374-377.

Balding DJ, Buckleton J: Interpreting low template DNA profiles. *Forensic Sci Int Genet* 2009, 4:1-10.

Barash M, Reshef A, Brauner P: The use of adhesive tape for recovery of DNA from crime scene items. *J Forensic Sci* 2010, 55:1058-1064.

Benschop CCG, van der Beek CP, Meiland HC, van Gorp AGM, Westen AA, Sijen T: Low template STR typing: Effect of replication number and consensus method on genotyping reliability and DNA database search results. *Forensic Sci Int Genet., 2010.*

Bright JA, Turkington J, Buckleton J: Examination of the variability in mixed DNA profile parameters for the Identifiler multiplex. *Forensic Sci Int Genet* 2010, 4:111-114.

Brinkmann B, Rand S, Bajanowski T: Forensic identification of urine samples. *Int J Leg Med* 1992, 105:59-61.

Budowle B, Eisenberg AJ, van Daal A: Low copy number has yet to achieve general acceptance. *Forensic Sci Int Genet Suppl Ser* 2009, 2:551-552.

Budowle B, Onorato AJ, Callaghan TF, Della Manna A, Gross AM, Guerrieri RA, Luttman JC, McClure DL: Mixture interpretation: defining the relevant features for guidelines for the assessment of mixed DNA profiles in forensic casework. *J Forensic Sci* 2009, 54:810-821

Castella V, Mangin P: DNA profiling success and relevance of 1739 contact stains from casework. *Forensic Sci Int Genet Suppl Ser* 2008, 1:405-407.

Coble M, Butler J: Characterization of new miniSTR loci to aid analysis of degraded DNA. *J Forensic Sci* 2005, 50:43-53.

Cook O, Dixon L: The prevalence of mixed DNA profiles in fingernail samples taken from individuals in the general population. *Forensic Sci Int Genet* 2007, 1:62-68.

Curran JM, Gill P, Bill MR: Interpretation of repeat measurement DNA evidence allowing for multiple contributors and population substructure. *Forensic Sci Int* 2005, 148:47-55.

Elliott K, Hill DS, Lambert C, Burroughes TR, Gill P: Use of laser microdissection greatly improves the recovery of DNA from sperm on microscope slides. *Forensic Sci Int* 2003, 137:28-36.

Forster L, Thomson J, Kutranov S: Direct comparison of post-28-cycle PCR purification and modified capillary electrophoresis methods with the 34-cycle 'low-copy-number' (LCN) method for analysis of trace forensic DNA samples. *Forensic Sci Int* Genet 2008, 2:318-328.

Frégeau CJ, Lett CM, Fourney RM: Validation of a DNA IQ™-based extraction method for TECAN robotic liquid handling workstations for processing casework. *Forensic Sci Int Genet* 2010, 4:292-304.

Gibb AJ, Huell A, Simmons MC, Brown RM: Characterisation of forward stutter in the AmpFlSTR SGM Plus PCR. *Sci Justice* 2009, 49:24-31.

Gilder JR, Doom TE, Inman K, Krane DE: Run-specific limits of detection and quantitation for STR-based DNA testing. *J Forensic Sci* 2007, 52:97-101.

Gill P, Brenner CH, Buckleton JS, Carracedo A, Krawczak M, Mayr WR, Morling N, Prinz M, Schneider PM, Weir BS, DNA commission of the International Society of Forensic Genetics: DNA commission of the International Society of Forensic Genetics: Recommendations on the interpretations of mixtures. *Forensic Sci Int* 2006, 160:90-101.

Gill P, Buckleton J: A universal strategy to interpret DNA profiles that does not require a definition of low-copy-number. *Forensic Sci Int Genet* 2010, 4:221-227.

Gill P, Curran J, Elliot K: A graphical simulation model of the entire DNA process associated with the analysis of short tandem repeat loci. *Nucl Acid Res* 2005, 33:632-643.

Gill P, Rowlands D, Tully GG, Bastisch I, Staples T, Scott P: Manufacturer contamination of disposable plastic-ware and other reagents - an agreed position statement by ENFSI, SWGDAM and BSAG. *Forensic Sci Int Genet 2010,* 4:269-270.

Gill P, Whitaker J, Flaxman C, Brown N, Buckleton J: An investigation of the rigor of interpretation rules for STRs derived from less than 100 pg of DNA. *Forensic Sci Int* 2000, 112:17-40.

Greenspoon SA, Ban JD, Sykes K, Ballard EJ, Edler SS, Baisden M, Covington BL: Application of the BioMek 2000 Laboratory Automation Workstation and the DNA IQ System to the extraction of forensic casework samples. *J Forensic Sci* 2004, 49:29-39.

Gunn B: An intelligence-led approach to policing in England and Wales and the impact of developments in forensic science. *Australian J Forensic Sci* 2003, 35:149-160.

Harbison SA, Hamilton JF, Walsh SJ: The New Zealand DNA databank: its development and significance as a crime solving tool. Sci Justice 2001, 41: 33-37.

Hansson O, Finnebraaten M, Knutsen Heitmann I, Ramse M, Bouzga M: Trace DNA collection - performance of minitape and three different swabs. *Forensic Sci Int Genet Suppl Ser* 2009, 2:189-190.

Higuchi R, von Beroldingen CH, Sensabaugh GF, Erlich HA: DNA typing from single hairs. *Nature 1988*, 332:543-546.

Hochmeister MN, Budowle B, Jung J, Borer UV, Corney CT, Dirnhofer R : PCR- based typing of DNA extracted from cigarette butts,Int *J leg Med 1991,* 104:229-233.

Horsman-Hall KM, Orihuela Y, Karczynski SL, Davis AL, Ban JD, Greenspoon SA: Development of STR profiles from firearms and fired cartridge cases. *Forensic Sci Int Genet* 2009, 3:242-250.

Jeffreys AJ, Wilson V, Thein SL: Individual-specific fingerprints of human DNA. Nature, 1985, 316: 76-79.

Keyser-Tracqui C, Ludes B: Methods for the study of ancient DNA. In Methods in Molecular Biology, vol 297 : Forensic DNA typing protocols, A. Carracedo ed., Human Press Inc., 2005.

Kloosterman AD, Kersbergen P: Efficacy and limits of genotyping low copy number (LCN) DNA samples by multiplex PCR of STR loci. *J Soc Biol* 2003, 197:351-359.

Kreader CA: Relief of amplification inhibition in PCR with bovine serum albumin or T4 gene 32 protein. *Appl Environ Microbiol* 1996, 62:1102-1106.

LeClair B, Frégeau CJ, Bowen KL, Fourney RM: Systematic analysis of stutter percentages and allele peak height and peak area ratios at heterozygous STR loci for forensic casework and database samples. *J Forensic Sci* 2004, 49:968-80.

Lindahl T: Instability and decay of the primary structure of DNA. Nature 1993, 362: 709-715;

Lucy D, Curran JM, Pirie AA, Gill P: The probability of achieving full allelic representation for LCN-STR profiling of haploid cells. *Sci Justice* 2007, 47:168-171.

McCartney C: LCN DNA: proof beyond reasonable doubt? *Nat Rev Genet* 2009, 9:325.

Mulero JJ, Chang CW, Lagacé RE, Wang DY, Bas JL, McMahon TP, Hennessy LK: Development and validation of the AmpFlSTR MiniFiler PCR amplification kit: a miniSTR multiplex for the analysis of degraded and/or PCR inhibited DNA. *J Forensic Sci* 2008, 53:838-852.

Pang BCM, Cheung BKK: Double swab technique for collecting touched evidence. *Legal Med* 2007, 9:181-184.

Parsons TJ, Huel R, Davoren J, Katzmarzyk C, Milos A, Selmanović A, Smajlović L, Coble MD, Rizvić A: Application of novel 'mini-amplicon' STR multiplexes to high volume casework on degraded skeletal remains. *Forensic Sci Int Genet* 2007, 1:175-179.

Petricevic SF, Bright JA, Cockerton SL: DNA profiling of trace DNA recovered from bedding. *Forensic Sci Int* 2006, 159:21-26.

Petricevic S, Whitaker J, Buckleton J, Vintiner S, Patel J, Simon P, Ferraby H, Hermiz W, Russell A: Validation and development of interpretation guidelines for low copy number (LCN) DNA profiling in New Zealand using the AmpFlSTR SGM Plus multiplex. *Forensic Sci Int* Genet 2010, 4:305-310.

Polley D, Mickiewicz P, Vaughn M, Miller T, Warburton R, Komonski D, Kantautas C, Reid B, Frappier R, Newman J: Investigation of DNA recovery from firearms and cartridge cases. *J Canadian Soc Forensic Sci* 2006, 39:217-228.

Rameckers J, Hummel S, Hermann B: How many cycles does a PCR need? Determinations of cycle numbers depending on the number of targets and the reaction efficiency factor. Naturwissenschaften 1997, 84: 259-262.

Raymond JJ, van Oorschot RA, Walsh SJ, Roux C: Trace DNA analysis: do you know what your neighbour is doing? A multi-jurisdictional survey. *Forensic Sci Int Genet* 2008, 2:19-28.

Rutty GN: An investigation into the transference and survivability of human DNA following simulated manual strangulation with consideration of the problem of third party contamination. *Int J Leg Med* 2002, 116:170-173.

Rutty GN, Hopwood A, Tucker V: The effectiveness of protective clothing in the reduction of potential DNA contamination of the scene crime. *Int J Leg Med 2003*, 117:170-174.

Rutty GN, Graham EAM: Risk of contamination in: Encyclopedia of Forensic and Legal Medicine. Payne-James J, Byard RW, Corey TS, Henderson C eds, Elsevier Academic Press, 2005.

Sanchez JJ, Phillips C, Børsting C, Balogh K, Bogus M, Fondevila M, Harrison CD, Musgrave-Brown E, Salas A, Syndercombe-Court D, et al.: A multiplex assay with 52 single nucleotide polymorphisms for human identification. *Electrophoresis* 2006, 27:1713-1724.

Sanders CT, Sanchez N, Ballantyne J, Peterson DA: Laser microdissection separation of pure spermatozoa from epithelial cells for short tandem repeat analysis. *J Forensic Sci* 2006, 51:748-757.

Sewell J, Quinones I, Ames C, Multaney B, Curtis S, Seeboruth H, Moore S, Daniel B: Recovery of DNA and fingerprints from touched documents. *Forensic Sci Int Genet* 2008, 2:281-285.

Smith PJ, Ballantyne J: Simplified low-copy-number DNA analysis by post-PCR purification. *J Forensic Sci* 2007, 52:820-829.

Sweet D, Lorente JA, Valenzuela A, Lorente M, Villaneuva E: PCR-based DNA typing of saliva stains recovered from human skin. *J Forensic Sci* 1997, 42:447-451.

Sweet D, Lorente M, Lorente JA, Valenzuela A, Villaneuva E: An improved method to recover saliva from human skin: the double swab technique. *J Forensic Sci* 1997, 42:320-322.

Taberlet P, Griffin S, Goossens B, Questiau S, Manceau V, Escaravage N, Waits LP, Bouvet J: Reliable genotyping of samples with very low DNA quantities using PCR. *Nucl Acids Res* 1996, 24:3189-3194.

Toothman MH, Kester KM, Champagne J, Cruz TD, Street WS, Brown BL: Characterisation of human DNA in environmental samples. *Forensic Sci Int* 2008, 178:7-15.

Vandewoestyne M, van Hoofstat D, van Nieuwerburgh F, Deforce D: Suspension fluorescence in situ hybridization (S-FISH) combined with automatic detection and laser microdissection for STR profiling of male cells in male/female mixtures. *Int J Legal Med* 2009, 123:441-447.

Van Hoofstat DE, Deforce DL, Hubert De Pauw IP, Van den Eeckhout EG: DNA typing of fingerprints using capillary electrophoresis: effect of dactyloscopic powders. *Electrophoresis* 1999, 20:2870-2876.

Van Oorschot RAH, Jones MK: DNA fingerprints from fingerprints. *Nature* 1997, 387:767.

Van Oorschot RAH, Treadwell S, Beaurepaire J, Holding NL, Mitchell RJ: Beware of the possibility of fingerprinting techniques transferring DNA. *J Forensic Sci 2005*, 50:1417-1422.

Van Oorshot RAH, Ballantyne KN, Mitchell RJ: Forensic trace DNA: a review. Investigative Genetics 2010,1, 14: 1-17.

Walsh PS, Fildes NJ, Reynolds R: Sequence analysis and characterisation of stutter products at the tetranucleotide repeat locus vWA. *Nucl Acids Res* 1996, 24:2807-2812.

Walsh PS, Metzger DA, Higuchi R: Chelex 100 as a medium for simple extraction of DNA for PCR-based typing from forensic material. *Biotechniques* 1991, 10:506-513.

Walsh SJ, Buckleton J: DNA Intelligence databases. In *Forensic DNA Evidence Interpretation.* Edited by Buckleton J, Triggs CM, Walsh SJ. Florida: CRC Press; 2005:439-469.

Webb LG, Egan SE, Turbett GR: Recovery of DNA for forensic analysis from lip cosmetics. *J Forensic Sci* 2001, 46:1474-1479.

Welch L, Gill P, Tucker VC, Schneider PM, Parson W, Mogensen HS, Morling N: A comparison of mini-STRs versus standard STRs - Results of a collaborative European (EDNAP) exercise. *Forensic Sci Int Genet* 2010.

Whitaker JP, Cotton EA, Gill P: A comparison of the characteristics of profiles produced with the AmpFlSTR SGM Plus multiplex system for both standard and low copy number (LCN) STR DNA analysis. *Forensic Sci Int* 2001, 123:215-223.

Wickenheiser RA: Trace DNA: a review, discussion of theory, and application of the transfer of trace quantities of DNA through skin contact. *J Forensic Sci* 2002, 47:442-450.

Wiegand P, Bajanowski T, Brinkmann B: DNA typing of debris from fingernails. *Int J Leg Med* 1993, 106:81-83.

2

Death Scene Investigation from the Viewpoint of Forensic Medicine Expert

Serafettin Demirci and Kamil Hakan Dogan
Selcuk University,
Turkey

1. Introduction

Medical expertise is crucial in death investigations. It begins with body examination and evidence collection at the scene and proceeds through history, physical examination, laboratory tests, and diagnosis - in short, the broad ingredients of a doctor's treatment of a living patient. The key goal is to provide objective evidence of cause, timing, and manner of death for adjudication by the criminal justice system. Death investigation has been performed for centuries in all societies, although not always by medical professionals (Committee, 2003). The association of law and medicine dates back to the Egyptian culture as early as 3000 B.C. The English coroner system was mentioned in documentations around the 12th century B.C. (Spitz, 2006).

Although the primary goal of a death investigation is to establish the cause and manner of death, the role of the death investigation extends much further than simply answering these two questions. A common question asked is, "Why does it matter? The person is dead." While it is true that the dead cannot benefit, the value in death investigation is to benefit the living and future generations. In a culture that values life, explaining the death in a public forum (the meaning of "forensic") is crucial for many reasons. And this interest goes beyond simple curiosity (Wagner, 2009).

In homicide, suspected homicide, and other suspicious or obscure cases, the forensic medicine expert should visit the scene of the death before the body is removed. Local practice varies but any doctor claiming to be a forensic medicine expert should always make himself available to accompany the police to the locus of the death. This duty is often formalized and made part of a contract of service for those forensic medicine experts who are either full-time or substantially involved in assisting the police, in England and Wales, the 'Home Office Pathologists' are permanently on call for such visits and in many other jurisdictions, such as the medical examiner systems in the USA, and the European State and University Institutes of Forensic Medicine, there is usually a prearranged duty roster for attendance at scenes of death (Saukko & Knight, 2004). In many cases, the scene investigation is more important than the autopsy. A thorough and complete investigation commonly leads to the proper diagnosis of the cause and manner of death prior to an autopsy (Avis, 1993; Dix & Ernst, 1999).

Why go to the scene? The purpose of having the forensic medicine expert attend the death scene is severalfold. By viewing the body in the context of its surroundings, the forensic medicine expert is better able to interpret certain findings at the autopsy such as a patterned imprint across the neck from collapsing onto an open vegetable drawer in a refrigerator. The forensic medicine expert is also able to advise the investigative agency about the nature of the death, whether to confirm a homicide by a specific means, evaluate the circumstances to be consistent with an apparent natural death, or interpret the blood loss from a deceased person as being more likely due to natural disease than to injury. This preliminary information helps the investigative agency to define its perimeter, structure its approach, organize its manpower, secure potentially important evidence, and streamline its efforts. Nonattendance at death scenes has been regarded as one of the classical mistakes in forensic pathology. Hospital pathologists performing forensic autopsies who are not trained to, or able to, attend death scenes should be provided with information on how, when, and where the body was found, by whom, and under what circumstances. In some deaths, the immediate environment does not contribute to death, such as in cases of metastatic breast carcinoma. In other cases, the environment plays a role although it does not cause the death; for example, consider a case in which a person with marked coronary atherosclerosis collapses with a dysrhythmia while shoveling snow. On the other hand, the scene description and scene photographs are critical in documenting that the physical circumstances and body posture are indicative of death due to positional asphyxia because the autopsy in these cases may yield very few findings. The most meticulous autopsy in all academia will provide only a speculative cause and manner of death in a 30-year-old man with a negative history, negative toxicology, and autopsy findings of visceral congestion. Yet at the scene, a screwdriver is next to an uncovered electrical outlet on a rain-soaked patio at the decedent's house, which is undergoing renovation. The cause and manner of death are provided by the scene (Lew & Matshes, 2005).

The examination of a death scene and subsequent collection of potential evidential material requires special skill, knowledge, aptitude, and attitude. The manner in which a death scene investigation is conducted may be a critical factor in determining the success of an investigation. The thorough examination of a death scene requires a disciplined and systematic approach to recording the various observations made and collection of potential evidential material. This must be combined with the analysis of various observations and the interrelationship of potential evidentiary material (Horswell, 2005a).

If resources are sufficient and the circumstances of death so dictate, it is ideal for a forensic medicine expert to perform a scene investigation. This is particularly relevant if the body remains at the scene of death, and has not been transported to the hospital during attempts at resuscitation; however, a scene investigation can be vitally important and provide valuable information even if the body has been transported to the hospital. If a body is pronounced dead at the scene (as opposed to after transport to the hospital), many death investigation systems require a scene investigation. Others have various protocols as to which case types absolutely require a scene investigation (whether or not the body is present at the scene). Case types that should always have a scene investigation include all confirmed or suspected homicides, suicides, accidents, child deaths, traffic-related deaths, in-custody deaths, and workplace-related deaths (Prahlow, 2010).

Death scene investigation may include a combination of the following types of incidents and examinations:

- Accidental deaths, which include a multitude of circumstances, including misadventure
- Suicidal deaths, which include a multitude of circumstances
- Homicidal deaths, which include a multitude of circumstances
- Sudden deaths, with or without suspicious circumstances
- Difficult victim identification, which includes mummification and putrefaction
- Disaster victim identification dealing with multiple casualties (Horswell, 2005a)

This chapter will focus on the steps of death scene investigation and some real cases will be analyzed.

2. Crime scene & death scene

In some "incidents," it may be readily apparent that a crime has indeed been committed and it is a "crime scene."

The *primary crime scene* is an area, place, or thing where the incident occurred or where the majority or a high concentration of physical evidence will be found, for example, where there has been a sudden suspicious death.

Secondary crime scene(s) are areas, places, or things where physical evidence relating to the incident may be found. The potential physical evidence will usually be transported away from the primary crime scene.

Some examples include: The deceased, the get-away vehicle in crimes of armed robbery, the suspect, the suspect's environment, the suspect's vehicle, the weapon used in the crime (Horswell, 2005a). This classification does not infer any priority or importance to the scene, but is simply a designation of sequence of locations (Miller, 2003).

If a deceased person is at the scene we call it the *death scene*. One of the initial and primary tasks is to determine whether a crime has been committed at the death scene.

Every death scene is a potential crime scene. It is important to carefully examine the scene for evidence or unusual circumstances that may indicate the death of the person is other than by natural causes (Moldovan, 2008).

3. Investigative tools and equipment

The forensic medicine expert should always have appropriate equipment ready to take to a scene investigation at a moment's notice. Further equipment may be carried if autopsies have to be carried out in places where good mortuary facilities are not available. Most forensic medicine experts carry a 'murder bag' in their car and though every expert has his own choice of equipment, the following is a reasonable inventory:

- Waterproof apron and rubber gloves.
- Writing implements (pens, pencils, markers).
- Disposable (paper) jumpsuits, hair covers, face shield, etc.
- Thermometer, syringes and needles, sterile swabs.
- Autopsy dissection set, including hand-saw.
- Cutting needles and twine for body closure.
- Swabs and containers for blood and body fluids.
- Formalin jars for histological samples.
- Plastic bags, envelopes, paper, spare pen and pencil.
- Printed body charts for recording external injuries.
- Hand lens, electric torch, mini-tape recorder.
- Foul-weather gear (raincoat, umbrella, etc.).
- Personal comfort supplies (insect spray, sun screen, hat, etc.).
- Camera, usually 35 mm single-lens reflex with electronic flash (with extra battery). The recent advent of compact digital cameras or digital video cameras with the facility to take still pictures has made instant reviewing possible.

The thermometer can be either a long chemical mercury type, reading from 0 to 50°C, or the more modern electronic digital variety with a probe carrying a thermocouple. The amount of equipment varies with the facilities likely to be available. In developed countries there are likely to be good mortuary facilities available in a hospital or municipal mortuary and the police forces will have extensive scenes-of-crime expertise with photography, specimen containers and so on. In developing countries and the more remote areas of other states, the forensic medicine expert may have to be virtually self-sufficient in respect of both crime investigation and the subsequent autopsy.

In addition to medical kit, the experienced forensic medicine expert will always have appropriate clothing such as rubber boots and rain or snow-wear ready to hand for any call (Clark, 1999; Saukko & Knight, 2004).

4. Steps of death scene investigation

The deceased is the most valuable piece of potential evidence at any death scene. Hence, a systematic and thorough examination of the deceased should be undertaken at every death scene. Blood spillage or spatter should be noted and will remain after the removal of the body. Weather conditions, location, and poor lighting may mask some faint injuries and trace evidence on the body, therefore the death-scene investigator should document in writing, by sketch, and by photography all information about the body that can be gathered at the scene (Horswell, 2005b). The forensic medicine expert should focus on the physical condition of a body at a scene. Without a scene investigation, much initial, valuable body information can be lost. The following points will serve as a guide.

4.1 Pre-planning the death scene investigation

When initially notified, a forensic medicine expert should determine as much information as possible from the caller. Approximate age and gender places a subject in a certain "medical category." An attempt should be made to ascertain if there is any evidence of foul play or if any instruments are available that might have played a role in the subject's death. By gathering these data, a forensic medicine expert is able to anticipate additional infonnation that may be needed upon arrival at a scene (Dix et al., 1999). The first rule in performing a death scene investigation is to make certain that the scene is safe and secure. Usually, this requires police involvement but in some instances, it will require other professionals, such as fire department personnel or utility workers. The second rule is to not contaminate or disturb the scene. At the very least, death investigators should wear disposable examination gloves and it is also advisable to wear shoe covers and hair nets. Occasionally, full body covering is desirable. When touching items at a scene, examination gloves should always be worn and care should be taken not to sit on furniture or lean against or brush against walls or furniture (Prahlow, 2010). The death-scene investigator must seek answers to the following questions: is trace evidence at the scene consistent with the death having occurred at this location? Does the body contain any trace evidence that is unusual for this location, for example, mud on soles of shoes, grass, or seed material embedded in or found on the clothing when the deceased was located inside a building? Is the death one that can be attributed to natural causes? Are there any external signs of violence? Is there anything amiss or out of the ordinary regarding the scene? (Horswell, 2005b).

4.2 Cooperation among investigators

A successful death investigation, involving more than one individual, requires cooperation and coordination. Any potential conflicts should be worked out (Dix et al., 1999). The opportunity to meet at the scene initiates the collegial working relationship between the forensic medicine expert and the detective/investigator, and promotes interagency rapport as both professionals strive to solve the medical mystery of why that particular person died at that particular time, under those particular circumstances. This is not melodrama, just intellectual satisfaction for exploring an extremely important, educational, and fascinating aspect of death investigation. After all, a gunshot wound is a gunshot wound: it is the circumstances behind that gunshot wound that are frequently so compelling and always so instructive about human nature (Lew & Matshes, 2005).

4.3 Documentation of the scene

All death scenes should be secured and recorded photographically and diagrammatically. If the information to hand, backed by the postmortem, suggests that the death was due to natural causes then the scene should not be processed any further. However, if there are signs at the scene, and other information suggests that the deceased died in suspicious circumstances, and this is reinforced by signs of a struggle or anything unusual, further processing for latent impressions and trace evidence should take place (Horswell, 2005b).

The four major tasks of documentation are note taking, videography, photography, and sketching. All four are necessary and none is an adequate substitute for another. For example, notes are not substitutes for photography.

Documentation, in all its various forms, begins with the initial involvement of the investigator. The documentation never stops; it may slow down, but the need for documentation remains constant. Death scene documentation will be discussed below in the sequence it should follow at a death scene. The systematic process presented will maintain the organized nature of scientific death scene investigation.

4.3.1 Taking notes at the death scene

Effective notes as part of an investigation provide a written record of all of the crime scene activities. The notes are taken as the activities are completed to prevent possible memory loss if notes are made at a later time. Accurate crime scene note taking is crucial at sider the who, what, when, why, and how, and specifically include:

- *Notification information.* Date and time, method of notification, and information received.
- *Arrival information.* Means of transportation, date and time, personnel present at the scene, and any notifications to be made.
- *Scene description.* Weather, location type and condition, major structures, identification of transient and conditional evidence (especially points of entry), containers holding evidence of recent activities (ashtrays, trash cans, etc.), clothing, furniture, and weapons present.
- *Victim description.* Position, lividity, wounds, clothing, jewelry, and identification (presence or absence).
- *Crime scene team.* Assignments to team members, walk-through information, the beginning and ending times, and the evidence-handling results (Miller, 2003).

The forensic medicine expert should observe a great deal, but do very little. He or she should note the position of the body in relation to nearby objects and establish the plan of the premises if indoors. A sketch or his own photograph is sometimes useful, and some forensic medicine experts use a Polaroid, digital or video camera for instant recording of the death scene.

Any obvious cause of death should be observed, and any blood pools or splashes noted in relation to the position of the corpse. The shape of such splashes should be observed, as blood striking perpendicularly to a surface leaves a circular mark, whilst that landing obliquely is pear-shaped, with the sharper end towards the direction of flight. If the scene is one of apparent violence then the blood flow patterns may indicate the type of weapon and how it was used (Horswell, 2005b; Saukko & Knight, 2004). Both natural and unnatural deaths can produce abundant blood at a scene. Traumatic deaths that involve arterial or venous bleeding, such as stabbing, can produce abundant blood at the scene with spattering. Gunshot wounds can cause extensive external bleeding, but some wounds can cause minimal external bleeding and massive internal bleeding. In short, the amount of blood perceived at a scene does not indicate the severity of the trauma (Wagner, 2009).

4.3.2 Videotaping the death scene

Videotaping a death scene has become a routine documentation procedure. Its acceptance is widespread, due to the three-dimensional portrayal of the scene and increased availability of affordable equipment with user friendly features like zoom lens and compact size. Jury acceptability and expectation have also added to the recognized use of videography in death scene investigations.

Videography of the crime scene should follow the scene survey. The videotaping of death scenes is an orientation format. The operator should remain objective in recording the death scene. Videotaping of death scenes is a valuable tool that allows clear perception that is often not possible with the other documentation tasks. It is not an adequate substitute for any of the other tasks (Miller, 2003).

4.3.3 Photographing the death scene

The purpose of still photography documentation of the death scene is to provide a true and accurate pictorial record of the death scene and physical evidence present. Still photography records the initial condition of the scene. It provides investigators and others with a record that can be analyzed or examined subsequent to the scene investigation, and serves as a permanent record for legal concerns. Photography of a death scene is normally done immediately following the videography of the scene or after the preliminary scene survey. A systematic, organized method for recording the death scene and pertinent physical evidence is best achieved by proceeding from the general to specific guideline. Adherence to this guideline allows orientation of the entire death scene, orientation of the evidence within the scene, and provide; examination quality photographs of specific items of evidence that may be used for analysis away from the scene. The number of photographs that should be taken at a death scene cannot be predetermined or limited (Miller, 2003). Information such as body location and unique circumstances at the death scene may help a forensic medicine expert. It is important to keep in mind the legal implications of the photographs. Will the photographs be subpoenaed? (Dix et al., 1999). The scene and body are photographed before anything is moved or removed. Treat the body with respect. Never remove the clothing in full view of onlookers. If it is not feasible to move the body to a secure area of the scene, police officers may hold up sheets around the body, mobile panels may be used, or police vehicles may be used to block visibility from the public (Lew & Matshes, 2005).

4.3.4 Sketching the death scene

The final task in documentation of a death scene is sketching. All of the previous tasks for documentation record the death scene without regard to the size or measurement of the scene and its physical evidence. Sketching the death scene is the assignment of units of measurement or correct perspective to the overall scene and the relevant physical evidence identified within the scene (Miller, 2003). The deceased's location relative to other objects and structures within the scene is very important. The position of the deceased is plotted: the head and groin of the deceased are good points on the body to use for plotting its position. Accurate measurements should be noted to place the items within the scene in the sketch in the same locations as they appear in the scene (Horswell, 2005b).

4.4 Identification of the deceased

Positive identification of the decedent is crucial in all death inquiries. The family should be notified. Information such as medical history, work, and social history can only be obtained after an identification is established. Care must be taken to insure that the identification is absolutely correct (Dix et al., 1999).

4.5 Examination of the body

A systematic, thorough inspection and evaluation of the decedent should be performed by a forensic medicine expert. If he/she always begins at the top of a subject's body and moves toward the feet, the possibility of missing important injuries or evidence is lessened (Dix et al., 1999). The body should be prone (face up) during the examination, if possible. Photos of the original position of the body must be taken before the body is moved. One begins with a general assessment and progresses from head to toe, pushing clothing aside but not removing it. Some find it easier to assess rigor, livor, and algor mortis initially. The purpose of the assessment of the body at the scene is to provide some insight into the nature of the case and a working cause of death (Wagner, 2009).
One of the most important questions that needs answering is: did death occur at this location? The position in which the deceased was discovered is of particular importance as it will provide an indication as to whether the deceased was moved or not before being discovered. The presence or absence of rigor mortis or stiffness of the body, whether absent, minimal, moderate, advanced or complete, will help the death-scene investigator determine if the person died at that locus in the position as found. Some death-scene investigators with relevant training and experience may feel they are in a position to evaluate rigor mortis and hypostasis. A pink-purple discoloration is usually present at the lowest point of the body. This is due to the settling of the blood by gravitation and the location and state of fixation should be noted and photographed. For example, unfixed livor blanches white when moderate pressure is applied, as opposed to fixed livor mortis, which remains the same color when pressure is applied. If livor mortis is noted on the deceased in areas not consistent with forming in the lowest parts of the body then the death-scene investigator should consider the possibility that the deceased was moved after death (Horswell, 2005b).
Victims may be found in contorted or apparently uncomfortable positions on the floor, commonly the bedroom or bathroom. Generally, the more contorted the body, the more sudden the death. The person appears to have "fallen in his tracks." However, this does not mean the decedent lying apparently comfortably in bed did not also die suddenly. Bodies found in awkward positions that compromise breathing can die of positional asphyxia. The chest wall must be able to rise and fall for respiration to occur. If one is wedged too tightly in a position, the chest wall cannot rise and fall (Wagner, 2009) (Fig. 1) .
Many inexperienced investigators focus on a major injury and neglect to evaluate the rest of the individual. This can lead to important oversights such as fingernail marks, bruises, and

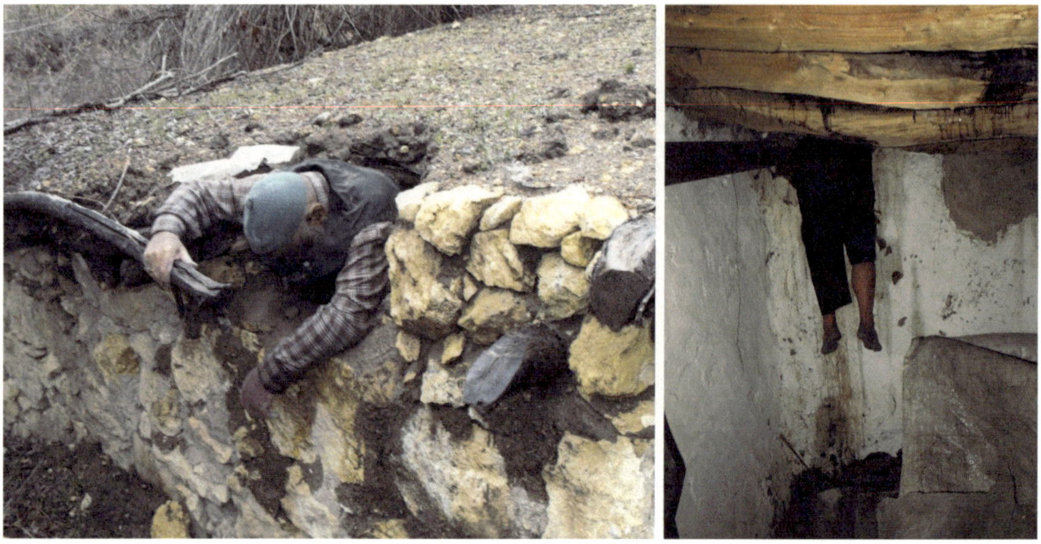

Fig. 1. Seventy two-year-old man had lost the key of the door of his house in his vineyard and he tried to go in from a small hole which he made on the roof. He was stuck and found dead in the hole due to positional asphyxia.

abrasions. Documentation of this inspection should be made noting the presence and absence of unusual markings or abnormalities. Descriptions of the state of rigor and livor mortis as well as the body temperature of a subject helps a forensic medicine expert to estimate the time interval since death. Environmental assessment, including temperature, heating or cooling systems, moisture, and wind conditions must be made at a death scene so that the environmental influence on a decedent can be determined. The assessment should also include the types of clothing and jewelry. This information may be needed to assist in determinating the time a subject was last seen alive. Clothing should be appropriate for the weather and location found. If not, it needs to be explained. One should also determine if the clothing fits an individual. If a subject is decomposing, then clothing may appear too small due to body swelling. If the clothing is the incorrect size, one must determine why. Was the person wearing someone else's when death occurred? Or, was the decedent redressed by another person after death? Note the cleanliness of the clothing. A variance in the clothing or body cleanliness may indicate that he was handled by another individual after death (Dix et al., 1999). General uncleanliness such as lack of bathing, very dirty clothes, urine -or feces- stained clothes, long and dirty nails, and poor oral hygiene may be due to alcoholism, drug abuse, or a mental disorder (Wagner, 2009). Is the clothing worn properly? Are buttons fastened and zippers closed? It is common to find opened zippers in intoxicated males or some elderly persons living alone. If the clothing is inconsistent with normal dressing techniques, consider whether a subject had a disability contributing to this behavior. Jewelry should be carefully noted and reported as to its type, style, color and body location. All jewelry must be listed, regardless of its apparent value. Obvious "missing" jewelry should also be noted, such as only one pierced earring, or no wedding ring on a married individual. Currency and credit cards should be handled as valuable items. Currency should be counted in the presence of another and credit card details noted. If an investigator decides that these items may be given to the next-of-kin at the death scene, he must be certain that the relative has the legal right to such items. No analyses should be performed on a decedent's body at a scene, such as gunshot residue or fingerprinting, without the expressed consent of the forensic medicine expert responsible for the postmortem examination. Clothing should not be removed, a body should not be cleansed, and liquids or powders should not be placed on the deceased as these might interfere with radiographs or chemical testing. If more than one hour has elapsed since the initial body assessment and the decedent is still at the scene, a second assessment should be recorded. A thorough body visualization by a forensic medicine expert gives him/her the capability to differentiate between injuries noted at a scene and any bodily injuries sustained during conveyance to the morgue (Dix et al., 1999).

A common misconception among laypeople is that a "painful" expression on the face or a contorted position means the person suffered during the process of dying. Generally, there is no correlation between facial expressions, body positions, and suffering. Pain and suffering can be assessed before and during the dying process, but it is done carefully and generally by the forensic medicine expert after evaluating the autopsy and investigative information. This information can be useful to the family, and can become arguable in civil court cases (Wagner, 2009).

4.6 Other scene information collection

An investigator must also gather information that relates to cause and manner of death. Each type of death requires specific scene information. For instance, questions to be asked in a motor vehicle fatality would not be the same as those asked in an autoerotic asphyxia death. Since different questions need to be asked, an investigational guide for each specific type of death can be very useful. For example, it is critical in suicides resulting from a handgun that investigators determine the handedness of a subject (Dix et al., 1999). The scene should be searched for a medical history in nearly all death investigations. This search may be as simple as finding an inhaler for asthma nearby a gunshot wound victim or as complicated as going through cabinets full of medication at a residence. The deceased's physician can always be called and the hospital records will be available tomorrow, but one has only a single chance to explore the scene to find out what is really going on with the person's diseases and treatment. Many people do not take the treatments the doctor ordered and reject advice given at the hospital. Only interviewing witnesses and searching the scene will reveal this information (Wagner, 2009).

4.7 Determining what information has already been developed

Prior to a forensic medicine expert's arrival, law enforcement officers, paramedics, and other support personnel probably have communicated with individuals or witnesses at the scene. A forensic medicine expert needs to know this initial information so that he can compare it with the decedent's body data and determine if there are any discrepancies. It is better to ask the question twice and get the same answer, than to accept as fact information that has been checked by one source. A forensic medicine expert needs to determine, for instance, if the body data (rigor, livor, temperature, clothing, injuries, etc.) are different from the witness information (Dix et al., 1999).

4.8 Collecting evidences which may be found at the death scene

Forensic medicine experts and law enforcement agents work cooperatively in a team effort. Although the medical expert has jurisdiction over the body, law enforcement has jurisdiction over the entire scene. The forensic medicine expert is invited to the scene and, as a guest, must comply with house rules. In Britain, for example, several teams converge on a scene of crime, including photographers and video operators, and Scene of Crime Officers (SOCOs) whose function is to collect trace evidence. Scientists from the nearest forensic laboratory often attend with their police liaison officers, as well as fingerprint officers and, of course, the investigating officers from the Criminal Investigation Department. The lead detective will walk the forensic medicine expert through the scene, relaying information and pointing out salient features. The forensic medicine expert should realize that the area within the perimeter of the scene is one giant piece of evidence, and restrict his or her physical contact to the body and items immediately touching the body (Lew & Matshes, 2005; Saukko & Knight, 2004).

Where no such backup is available, the forensic medicine expert must try to collect trace evidence himself, but he should remain within the limits of his own expertise. The forensic medicine expert should accept the instructions of police officers in relation to the approach to the body so as to preserve the immediate environment as much as possible. Out-of-doors access is often limited to a single pathway marked by tapes, and in a building a track to the corpse is usually pointed out by the detective in charge. The doctor should not touch anything unnecessarily and certainly not smoke or leave any object or debris of his or her own. Increasingly, those visiting the scene of a crime are given disposable overalls and overshoes to wear, so that fibers, hairs and so on from the visitor are not spuriously transferred to the scene (Saukko & Knight, 2004). The Locard Exchange Principle states that whenever two objects come into contact, a mutual exchange of matter will take place between them. Linking suspects to victims is the most important and common type of linkage accomplished by physical evidence in criminal investigations. Linking victims and suspects to objects and scenes can also be accomplished by use of the physical evidence (Miller, 2003) (Fig. 2).

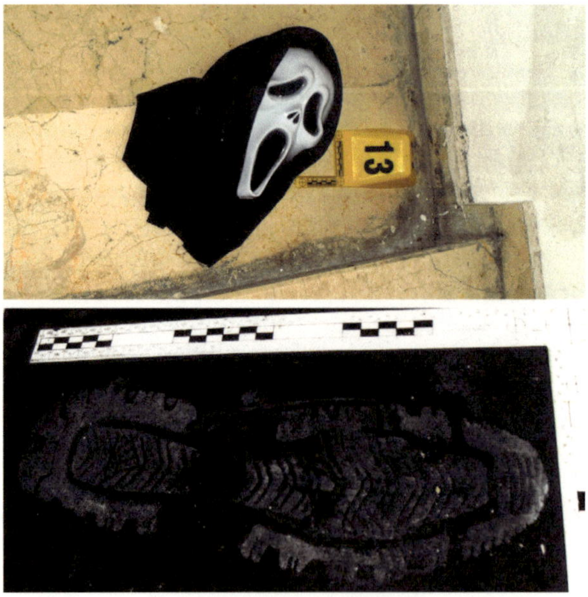

Fig. 2. The 18-year-old murderer killed his employer in his workplace as he did not pay his salary. On the death scene investigation, a horror mask (on the top) and footprints of sports shoes of the murderer (on the bottom) were found. These evidences were used to determine the murderer.

After surveying the overall death scene, it should be easy to recognize the sequence in which evidence is to be collected and areas to be searched and in what order. The collection and search should be systematic, ensuring absolutely nothing is overlooked.

Priority in collection should be given to:

- any items that are in danger of being removed or destroyed by wind, rain, vehicles, animals, tides, and the movement of individuals at the scene
- the collection of any evidence which will enable access to the deceased or any critical area of the death scene, such as along entry and exit paths
- those critical areas of the crime scene which may render the most evidence, or once processed, enable the removal of a body, or the remainder of the examination to be carried out
- areas which may give a quick indication as to the identity of any suspect(s)
- areas which when processed will permit the release of scene guards and other resources
- the general examination of the remainder of the death scene for potential evidence.

In establishing the manner and sequence of collecting potential evidence by death scene investigators, consideration must be given to the possible destruction of evidence and which approach will yield the best result in terms of useful information (Horswell, 2005b).

Clues about the cause and manner of a death and who committed a crime may be found at a scene. The following list includes different types of evidence and how they are usually collected and preserved.

Blood - Dried particles should be scraped into a drycontainer. Some dried areas may be sampled with a wet swab. A specimen should be dried before sealing it in a container. Articles of clothing or other objects containing blood may be submitted to a laboratory for sample removal by a technician.

Semen - An article of clothing containing semen should be collected or the specimen on the clothing can be lifted with water or saline.

Fingerprints - Soft objects that leave an impression may be collected in their entirety. Prints on hard objects like glass or furniture should be lifted at the scene.

Firearms and other weapons - These should be submitted to a lab without special treatment at a scene. A technician must ensure proper handling so that fingerprints are not smudged or ruined.

Bullets and cartridges - These should not be grasped with metal forceps because points of comparison may be damaged.

Hairs and fibers - These should be placed in separate containers and should not be crushed with hard objects such as metal tweezers.

Suspicious foods and pills - Each item should be placed in separate containers or bags to prevent contamination.

Footprints and tire marks - At the scene, casts should be made and close-up photographs should be taken.

Tool marks - There should be close-up photographs of the marks made by tools and, if possible, the damaged material should be removed for analysis by a lab technician.

Blood spatters - These should be photographed and described for analysis as to distance and angle of spatter. Samples may be removed for testing and preservation.

Other - Glass, soil, documents, cigarette butts, tobacco, and all items thought to be involved in arson should be collected and submitted to a lab.

Each item submitted to a lab should be referenced by either a photograph or written description as to its location in the scene. All containers with items submitted to the lab must be labeled on the lid and side of the container, with a case number, date, time, type of specimen, and name of the person who collected the specimen. A "chain of custody" begins at this point and continues until a disposition of the specimen is completed (Dix et al., 1999). Methods of searching critical areas include grids that are larger in less critical areas and smaller in critical areas, or searching in a clockwise or counterclockwise direction from a fixed point, or conducting a line strip search. All these form part of conducting a professional systematic search of a death scene. A systematic approach to the searching of death scenes reduces stress and fatigue and ensures a more comprehensive search and recovery operation, minimizing the chance of losing potentially valuable evidentiary material (Horswell, 2005b). Any weapon or other item possibly related to the death and found at a scene should be brought to the morgue for analysis by a forensic medicine expert. Often, substances are the causative agent in the death. All medication and alcoholic beverage containers should be confiscated as these will be invaluable to the toxicologists. Note the location where each item was found. Studies have shown that a fatal intoxicant is likely to be found in the same location as a decedent. Any drug paraphernalia, notes, or any unusual item that might have been used by the subject should be confiscated (Dix et al., 1999).

4.9 Interviewing persons regarding the death

Interviews should include basic information such as the subject's identification, clothing, time, date, state of health, date and time the body was discovered, and medical, employment, and social history. Any recent events that may have a bearing on the death are also important. A death investigator should always ask if a decedent had recently been involved in any potential harmful situations. This information may be extremely helpful if later attempts are made to make a prior incident a contributing factor in the death. If suicide is suspected, it is preferable to interview family members and close friends as soon as possible after the death is discovered. This may preclude guilt-related, subconscious, erroneous statements made by loved ones several days later (Dix et al., 1999).

4.10 Estimating the post-mortem interval at the scene

The general warmth or coolness of the hands and face can be assessed by touch, and the degree of rigor mortis felt by gently testing the limbs. The ambient (environmental) temperature must be taken as soon as possible after the discovery of the body, preferably by police scene of crime officers who usually arrive at the locus before the forensic medicine expert. The ambient temperature should be taken as near to the body as possible, as microenvironments can exist, even inside buildings or rooms. Information should be sought as to how much disturbance of the ambient temperature might have occurred, such as opening doors and windows, or turning fires or central heating on or off, so that some idea of post-discovery distortions of temperature can be estimated later. The insertion of a thermometer into the rectum at this stage in the investigation, as advocated by some textbooks, is controversial.

At a scene of death, this usually means either pulling down trousers or pants, and otherwise disturbing clothing, often in cramped and ill-lit places, frequently out in the open. It also risks contaminating the rectum and perineum, by introducing seminal fluid from the anal margin into the rectum, making subsequent examination of that area (and taking swabs for semen) of reduced value. As so many violent crimes now have sexual or homosexual overtones, the practice of taking rectal temperatures at the scene should be performed only if the forensic scientists or police scene of crime officers are satisfied that trace evidence from the clothing, swabs from the vulva, vagina and anus, etc., can be obtained satisfactorily before rectal thermometry is performed.

In other words, a cost-benefit analysis must be made at the scene, to decide if the difficulties of taking a rectal temperature are worth the small potential advantage of an earlier measurement. In many cases, where the body has obviously been there long enough for the core temperature to have reached ambient - or where other circumstantial evidence has indicated that the time of death is known to a greater degree of accuracy that can be hoped for by thermometry - then nothing is lost by postponing the procedure until the body arrives at the mortuary for autopsy, which, in British practice, is usually directly after the body is moved from the scene.

If the autopsy is to be delayed for many hours owing to difficulties with transport or lack of facilities, then much more must be done at the scene and temperature measurements are justified.

An alternative is to use a place other than the rectum. The axilla and mouth give low readings, which cannot reliably be correlated with the deep temperature because of variable exposure to the air temperature. More useful is the auditory meatus or nostril, the thermometer or thermocouple probe being inserted as deeply as possible. Reliable, reproducible readings can be obtained from these sites, which have the great advantage of being easily accessible without moving clothing, as well as not being required for swabbing to investigate possible sexual assaults (Saukko & Knight, 2004).

Using scene markers to determine when an individual died, though unscientific, is often more accurate than determinations made by scientific means. This is especially true in badly decomposed bodies. Scene markers include:

- Uncollected mail or newspapers.
- Whether the lights are on or off.
- A TV schedule opened to a time and date.
- How the individual is dressed.
- Any food that is out or dirty dishes in the sink.
- Sales receipts or dated slips of paper in the deceased's pockets.
- When the neighbors last saw the individual or observed a change in his habits. Thus, if he typically went for a walk every evening and suddenly is no longer seen, then one might conclude that death occurred on or about the day he failed to take his walk (DiMaio & DiMaio, 2001). Different clues from a scene also must not be overlooked: Was food being prepared? Was a major appliance on? Were there indicators as to a decedent's activities just prior to or at the time of death? A forensic medicine expert may use the answers to such questions to arrive at an estimation of the time of death (Dix et al., 1999).

4.11 Ending the death scene investigation

When the forensic medicine expert has made the best examination possible in the circumstances, his next function is to ensure that the corpse is removed to the mortuary for autopsy with the least disturbance and loss of evidence. He should supervise the removal himself or at least delegate the duty to another person whom he knows is careful and competent. Each hand should be enclosed in a bag, secured at the wrist by adhesive tape or string. A similar bag should be placed over the head. The packaging medium may vary, but generally paper bags are recommended.

The body should be placed gently in a 'body-bag', which has a zip closure, or moved on to a large, new plastic sheet, at least 2 metres square. If a sheet is used, the edges should be wrapped over the body and secured with adhesive tape. The object of the exercise is to retain any loose objects, hairs and fibres that may be adhering to the body or the clothing. The sheet or bag is taken by the forensic laboratory after the body is removed in the mortuary so that they may screen it for trace evidence. The transport of the body is the responsibility of the police or other agency such as the coroner or his officer. The body in its plastic wrapping should be placed in a rigid fibreglass 'shell' or ordinary coffin, and taken by hearse, van or police transport to the chosen mortuary.

Physical damage during the removal should be avoided as much as possible, though in difficult or inaccessible sites this is easier said than done. In fires, the body may be seriously damaged before or during recovery, sometimes because its presence is not suspected in the smoke-filled, often waterlogged, debris of a conflagration. Handling brittle, charred, bodies can easily cause the splits at joints that may mimic ante-mortem injuries.

In summary, the function of a forensic medicine expert at any scene of suspicious death is to observe the situation, to conserve any fragile evidence, to supervise the removal of the body and offer an opinion, based on experience, about the nature of death where this can reasonably be done. He is not there to act as a latter-day Sherlock Holmes, voicing unsubstantiated theories on non-medical matters, nor attempting to overinterpret the situation from the flimsiest of facts. The forensic medicine expert is part of a team of specialists, all experts in their own field, and it is as a member of such a cooperative, coordinated group that his best contributions can be made (Saukko & Knight, 2004).

5. Homicide

In the community, the most serious crime is that of the intentional killing of one person by another and it is therefore necessary that each of these events be thoroughly investigated by a team of specialists (Horswell, 2005b).

Death scenes may be indoors or outdoors. The death may have occurred at the scene or the body may have been "dumped." The death scene may be untouched since the crime was committed or it may have been contaminated by the untrained or the unwary. The murderer may have intentionally altered the scene in an effort to mislead investigators or make a statement, usually a defiant one. A crime scene altered in this manner is said to have been staged.

The forensic medicine expert's focus is mainly on the body. What is the position of the body? What clothes are on the body and are they intact, dirty, torn, or rearranged? If there is blood, is it spattered or pooled? Detailed photographs of the body and the surroundings are critical. What is the temperature of the body? What is the ambient temperature? What injuries are visible? What is the state of rigor mortis? Are there any signs of a struggle? Does anyone know the identity, or presumptive identity, of this person? If there are bullet wounds, the forensic medicine expert determines where the entrance wound or wounds are. If there are exit wounds, the forensic medicine expert notes the presence of bullet holes in the walls or other objects to help determine the position of the victim when the shots were fired. Here, the expertise of the ballistics or firearm expert is crucial (Adelman, 2007).

Homicide victims need to be examined front and back to determine the nature and extent of injuries. For example, once the nature of the injuries is confirmed (gunshot wounds with no casings on the scene), the police will be able to focus their efforts on finding a shooter with a revolver, as opposed to searching for an assailant with another type of weapon such as an ice pick. Once the extent of injuries is seen, the forensic medicine expert will know how many radiographs are required. A beating death will alert the team that a struggle may have ensued, and scalp hair and fingernail scrapings/clippings are required, in addition to a blood standard obtained during the autopsy. Whenever sexual assault/battery is a possibility, specimens for a sexual battery kit must be obtained from the deceased victim prior to cleaning the body. Bodies with patterned injuries from an object or weapon still at the scene should be photographed with the object close to, but not touching, the injured part of the body. The patterned injury and the object should be photographed separately with a scale. A weapon may be brought to the autopsy for comparison with the wounds only after the weapon has been processed for trace evidence, DNA, and fingerprints to prevent allegations of contamination at the autopsy (Rogers, 2004; Lew & Matshes, 2005).

It is always advantageous for the forensic medicine expert to visit the death scene of a possible homicide. By visiting the scene and actually seeing the position of the body and the pattern of injuries to the deceased and the arrangement of objects in the surrounding areas, the forensic medicine expert can put the pieces of the puzzle together and attempt to reconstruct the circumstances that led to the event (Fig. 3). The autopsy becomes a major item in the solution of this puzzle (Adelman, 2007).

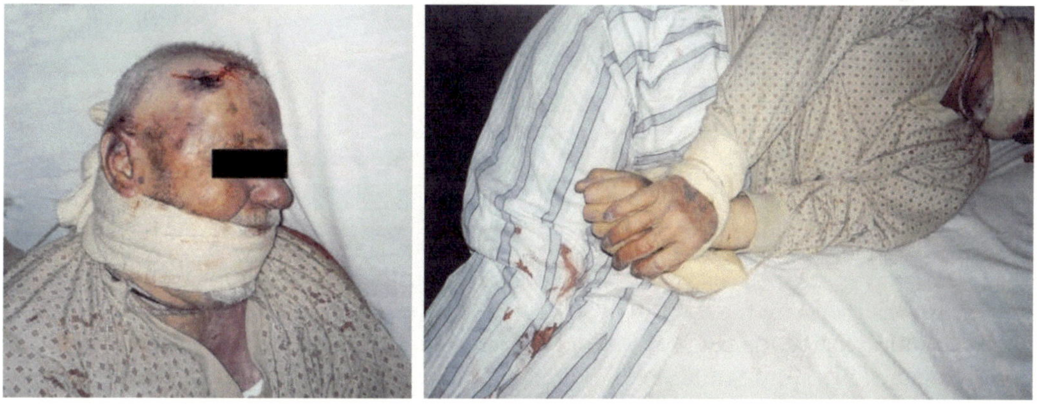

Fig. 3. The murderer sometimes binds the victim's hands and mouth before killing the victim. 65-year-old man was found dead in his bed, his hands and mouth were bound. The cause of death was strangulation and blunt head trauma.

Always be professional—remember that onlookers, including the decedent's family, and news media may be at the perimeter of the scene, so do not say or do anything that would reflect poorly on yourself and the organization you represent. Trash (discarded gloves, etc.) should be placed in bags designated for investigators' refuse, and not in the garbage cans that are part of the scene because in actuality, they are evidence. Never remove items from a scene for souvenirs (Rogers, 2004; Lew & Matshes, 2005).

In any given case of suspected homicide, it is self-evident that the forensic medicine expert who performs the autopsy should visit the death scene because all injuries must be examined within the context of the event. There are still far too many cases where this does not occur, thus making it impossible to carry out an exact reconstruction of the sequence of events in later stages of the criminal investigation. In numerous cases, however, the initial situation is inadvertently changed by police forces or rescue teams that first arrive at the crime scene. As a result, the initial scene is often not sufficiently documented, and changes may lead to misinterpretation in the future analyzing process (Schröer & Püschel, 2006). Don't forget: The victim himself or herself is the most important crime scene (Trestrail, 2007) (Fig. 4) .

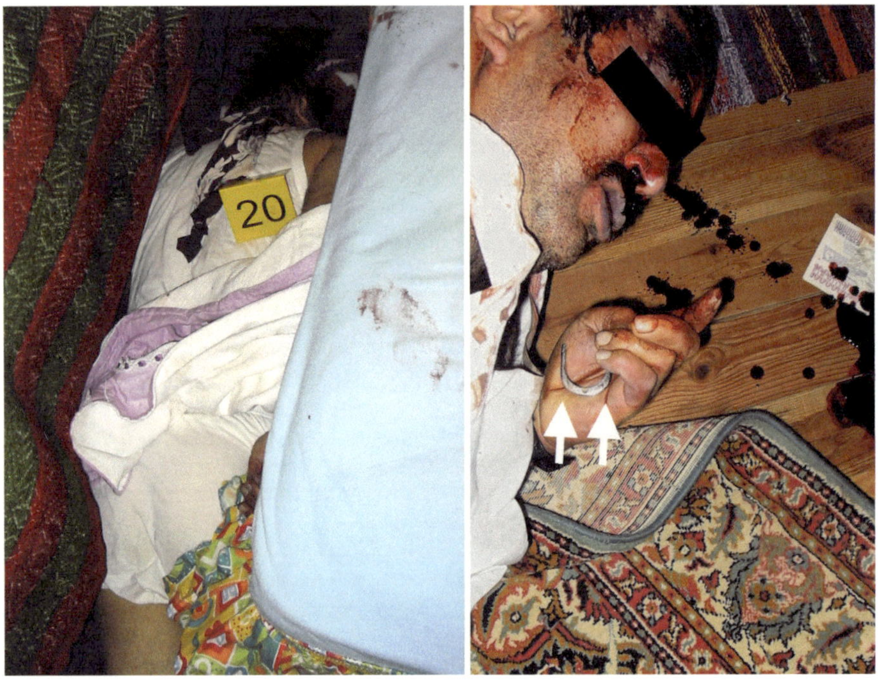

Fig. 4. The murderer killed his 36-year-old brother by strangulation and blunt head trauma. The victim was found on the floor in prone position near his bed. The belt buckle of the killer was found inside the hand of the victim (arrows) and this belt buckle helped in identifying the killer. Strangulations should be presumed to be homicidal unless proved otherwise. In order to determine the origin of ligature strangulation, it is necessary to perform a detailed investigation of death scene and examine the type of ligature on the neck of the victim carefully (McMaster et al., 2001; Verma & Lal, 2006).

In some murders, after killing the victim, the murderer uses a very sharp cutting weapon (a saw, axe, etc.) to sever the limbs and cut the body into small pieces. The operation is generally carried out immediately after the crime, although more rarely a long time may pass between the two events. Dismemberment of the corpse allows the murderer to clear the scene of the crime to delay investigations until the body is found. It also makes it easier to transport the body even for long distances, during times of day when possible witnesses could be about, without raising suspicion (Di Nunno et al., 2006). In a case which authors visited the death scene, a 57-year-old woman's corpse was found between the bed and wardrobe in her house in a prone position. The victim's severed head, right arm and both hands were found in a cardboard box near the bed. After death scene investigation and autopsy the murderer was determined as her 33-year-old schizophrenic daughter (Dogan et al., 2010a) (Fig. 5) .

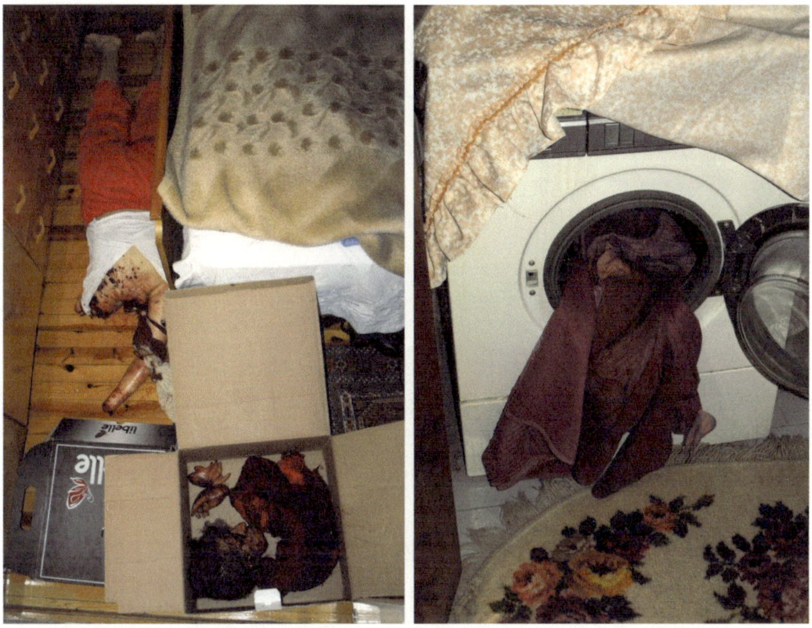

Fig. 5. The 57-year-old woman was found between bed and wardrobe. Her severed head, right arm and both hands were in a cardboard box. On the right, bloody sports suits of the assailant in the washing machine.

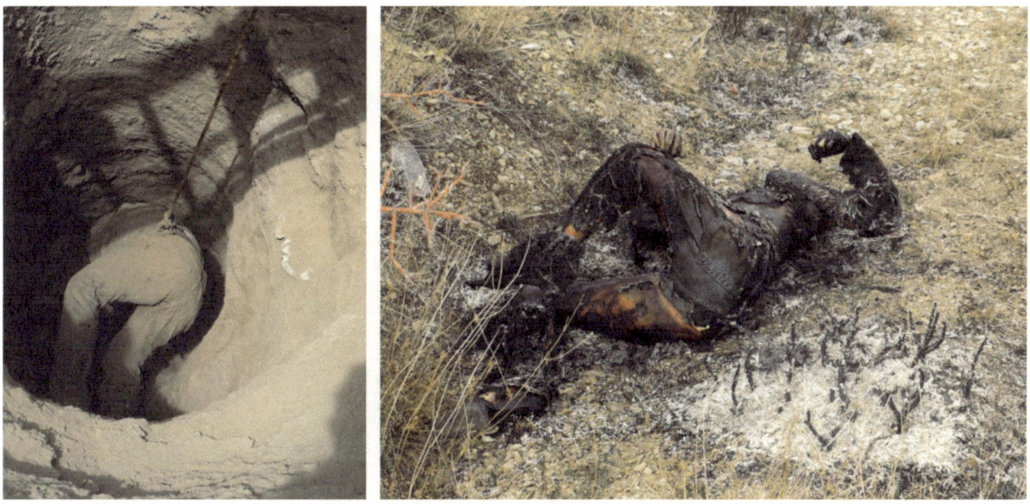

Fig. 6. A homicide victim found in a well (on the left) and a victim who was burned (on the right, note the unburned parts of the clothes which are useful for identification).

Sometimes the assailants, after killing the victims, try to hide their crimes by disposing the corpses by burying, by burning, by throwing them into water or wells, or concealing them in distant places (Figs. 6-8).Corpses found in wells or lime pits must be identified, and the cause and manner of death must be determined. There are several circumstances that may lead to the presence of corpses in wells. People may accidentally fall in wells where safety measures have not been taken. Other people may use wells for the purpose of committing suicide. Also, the victims of a homicide may be thrown into a well for concealment. A murdered victim may be thrown into a well to prevent the body from being found. In the cases of homicide, the wells chosen to dispose of the body are often distant from the victim's district and close to the killer's district. Wells can provide a means for concealing a corpse and that the corpse can sometimes only be found upon a confession by the killer (Dogan et al., 2010c).

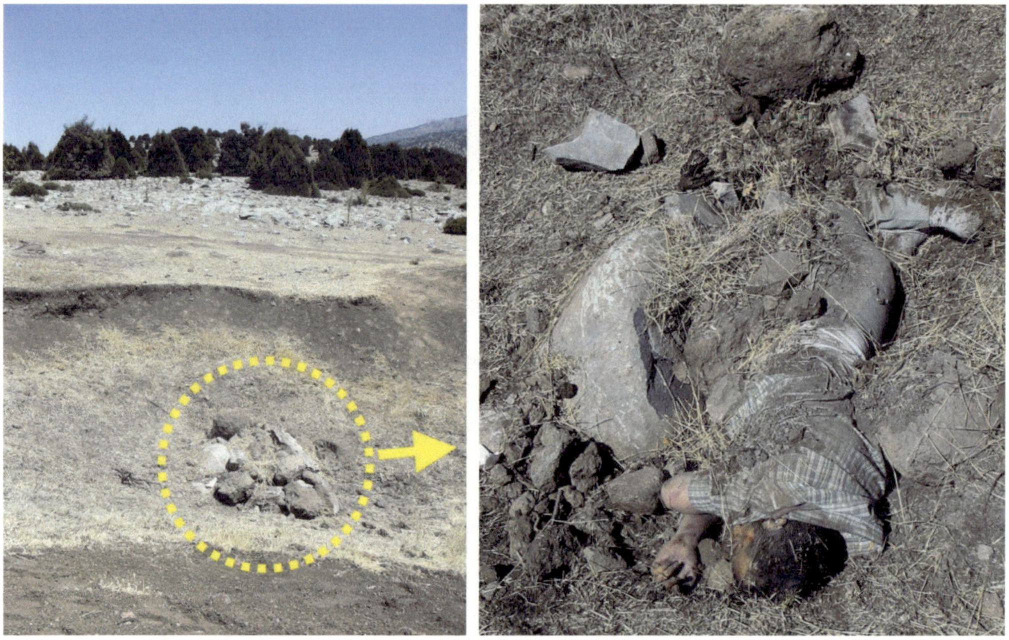

Fig. 7. A buried homicide victim in a desolate land.

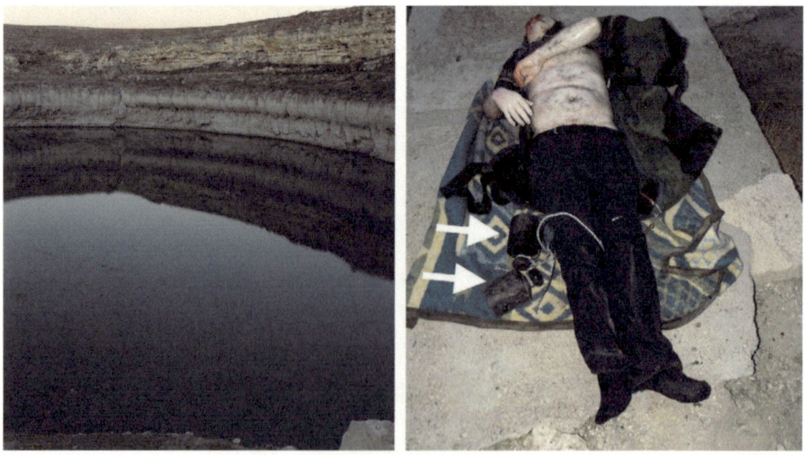

Fig. 8. The victim was killed by blunt head trauma first, then 20 kg iron (arrows) was bound to his legs and thrown into a lake.

Homicide-suicide (HS) events are defined by a perpetrator killing one or more victims before killing him or herself. The term "dyadic death" has also been used for these incidents, because deaths often involve a pair of persons (Milroy et al., 1997). In most of the HS cases, the perpetrator knows the victim (Dogan et al., 2010e) (Fig. 9).

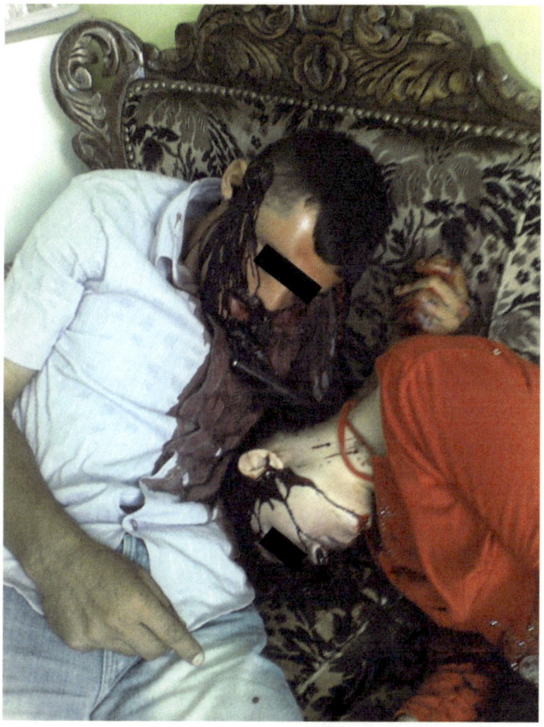

Fig. 9. Death scene of a homicide-suicide. Twenty two-year-old man killed his 16-year-old lover (illegitimate relationship), then killed himself with his handgun. The man was married with another woman. Note the handgun between victims.

5.1 Homicide by poisoning

Our ability to detect poisons has greatly improved over the last 100 years, but our ability to suspect poisoning in the first place has not improved, and may have actually gotten worse.
Some things that might come up in an investigation that should send up a red flag are as follows:

- The death occurred in a normally healthy individual. Certainly a person can die without warning, but when this type of death occurs, a deeper look into the cause is called for, including an autopsy.
- An individual interfered with the victim receiving proper medical attention. This may lead one to wonder if that person does not want educated eyes and minds delving into the possible cause of the condition in question.
- There is no sign of violence to the body. This is always an indication that the death could have been the result of a poisoning misadventure.
- The affliction appeared as a natural disease yet failed to respond to normal treatment methods.

- An illness reoccurred in cycles; that is, the victim became ill at home, went to a medical facility and seemed to recover, then went home and became ill again, and so on. This would indicate that there is something in the home environment that is proving unhealthy for the individual. Could it be the chronic administration of heavy metals (e.g., arsenic) in the person's meals? There certainly have been recorded criminal cases in which this has happened, and the poisoner is often not caught in the initial stages of the homicide attempt.
- There are common mysterious symptoms in a common group of people. This could indicate that there has been a mass tampering, or that the supposed specific target was a off the mark of the poisoner.
- There is an individual who is anxious to dispose of food, drink, or medicine of which the victim partook. In this case, it is clear that the person is attempting to foil the investigation by destroying critical evidence.
- An individual prevented friends or relations from being sent for during the victim's illness. The criminal investigator should question what that person did not want others to witness.
- There is an insistence on no autopsy. The criminal investigator should clearly state that one will take place. Once again, the desire not to have educated minds look at the problem comes to the forefront.
- There is an insistence on a rapid cremation. This could be construed as an attempt to burn the primary evidence of the crime and foil the investigation. The criminal investigator should clearly state that an investigation must take place before cremation can proceed.
- While grieving over the loss of a close family member or friend, a certain individual does not freely begin to offer an explanation for the cause of death. Neither will the person attempt to guide the investigation in any way. If the person does, it could very well be an attempt to divert investigators' attention from his or her crime, and investigators must be aware of this.
- An individual shows a familiarity with poisons and possesses literature about poisons. In this case, not just a red flag should go up, but a whole sky full of mental fireworks (Trestrail, 2007).

It has been stated that poisoning is the least used method of homicide, accounting for only 3-6% of known homicide cases (Adelson, 1974, as cited in Trestrail, 2007). Because of the complexity of poisoning homicide, it is one of the most difficult homicides to prove.

Regarding the death scene, with poisoning multiple locations may have come into play during the planning and execution of the murder. Each location can yield important clues that must be included in the complete case investigation. Some of the locations and the items to look for to yield clues are as follows:

- Where the victim was *found* (vomited material, clothes containing poison residue).
- Where the poison was *administered* (medicine bottles, food/beverage containers).
- Where the poison was *disposed* of (storage areas, trash containers, sink traps, vacuum cleaner bags).
- Where the poison was *prepared* (tools with poison residues, utensils, clothes, containers).
- Where the poison was *procured* (stolen items, receipts of purchase, signature on a poison register, computer files) (Trestrail, 2007).

6. Suicide

The finding of suicide as a manner of death may impact families differently. Suicide carries a stigma on the family name in many cultures. Consequently, objections are often raised by survivors when suicide is documented on the death certificate. Additionally, the finding of suicide can influence the payment of life insurance policies, as most exclude suicide within the first two years after issuance of the policy in order to prevent profit from an individual's death (Moldovan, 2008).

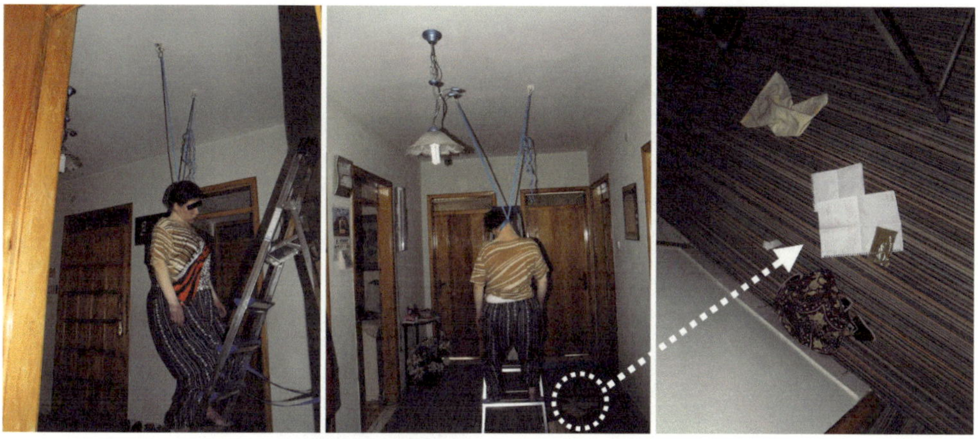

Fig. 10. Thirty seven-year-old woman hanged herself in her house. There was a farewell letter on the floor.

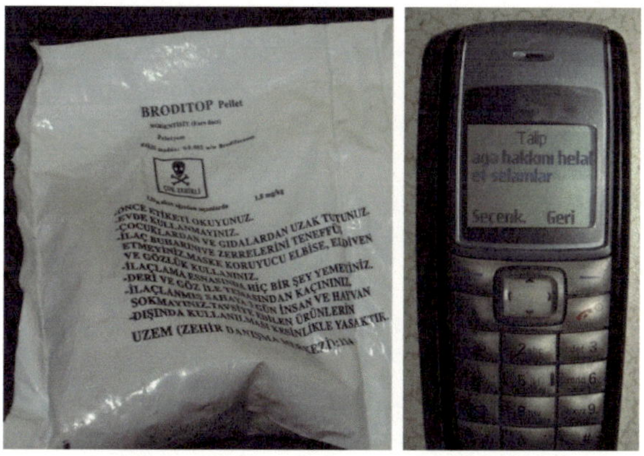

Fig. 11. Two items found at a suicide death scene. The packing of a rodenticide and the last SMS message in the victim's phone which was sent to his friend containing a suicide note.

An experienced death investigator would recognize several ingredients in the scene. A plastic bag, a large rubber band used to hold the bag in place, and drugs or alcohol are often present in suicide scenes. In his book *Final Exit*, Derek Humphry described in detail how a person can take their own life using the equipment and procedure described here (Humphry, 1991, as cited in Moldovan, 2008). Moldovan (2008) had observed this death scene frequently in the many suicide scenes he investigated. He often found the book Final

Exit near the body, indicating that the decedent used it as a reference for the final act of self destruction.

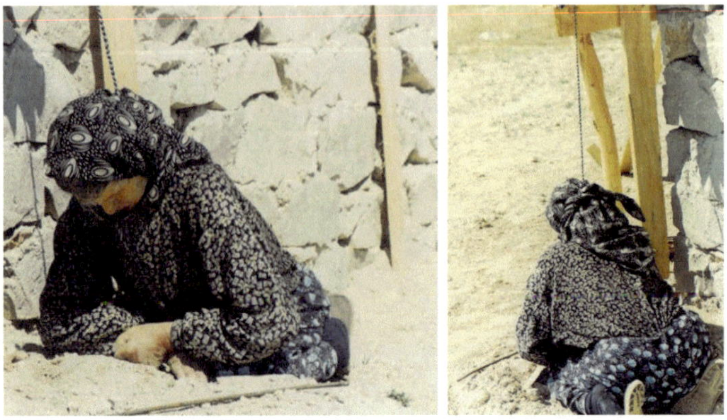

Fig. 12. Seventy eight-year-old woman hanged (partial) herself in the garden of her house.

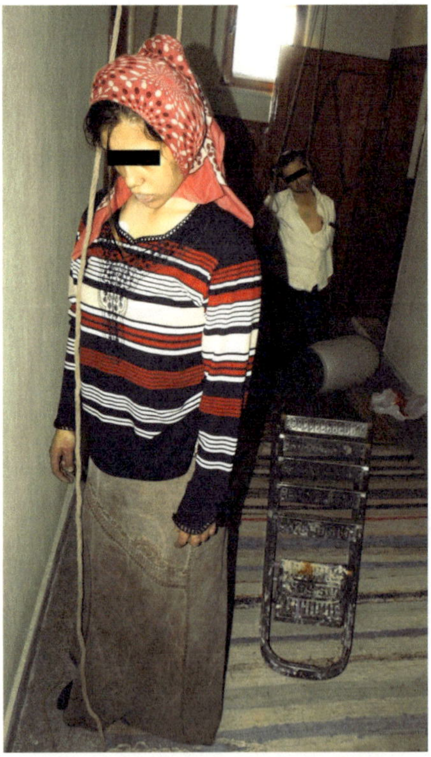

Fig. 13. The father hanged himself to the same place where his daughter hanged herself (as he loved his daughter so much, he couldn't stand up to the pain). There were farewell letters in both of their clothes' pockets.

Hanging is one of the most preferred methods for suicide, but homicidal hangings were also reported (Vieira et al., 1988; Sauvageau, 2009). So it is important to visit a death scene in hanging deaths. To determine the cause of death in hanging cases, while the corpse is still at the death scene and in the suspended position, a detailed investigation should be performed by a team including a forensic medicine expert. Further evidence from the death scene investigation, statements from witnesses, the presence of a suicide note, and autopsy findings can all help to determine whether the victim was responsible for his or her own death (Figs. 10-16).

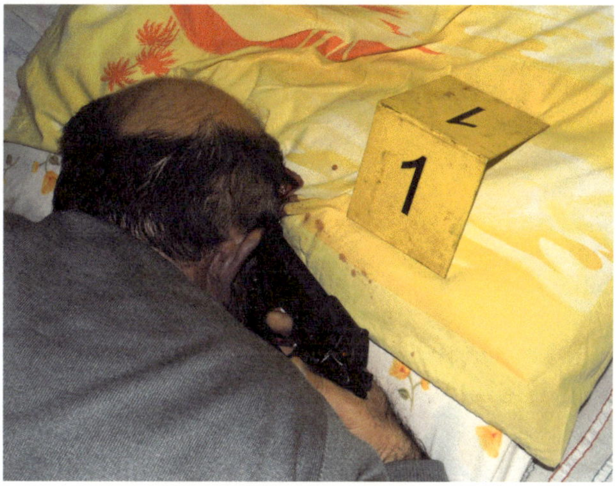

Fig. 14. The hand of the suicide victim is still gripping the handgun (cadaveric spasm).

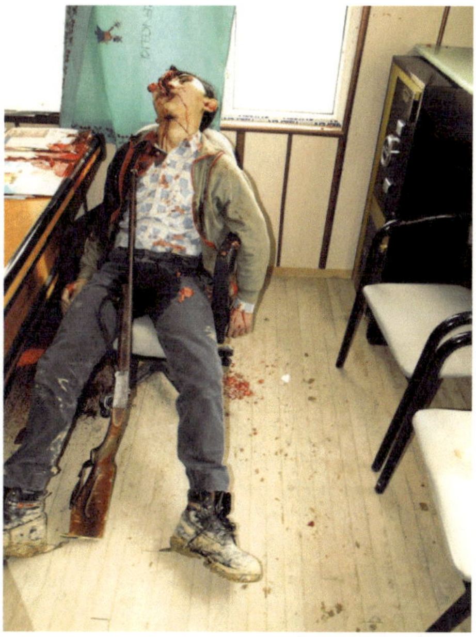

Fig. 15. The death scene of a 13-year-old boy's suicide. The shotgun is in front of the victim, and the entry wound is under the chin. According to the witnesses, after he argued with his father in the garden of his father's office, he had ran into the office of his father and took his father's shotgun and killed himself.

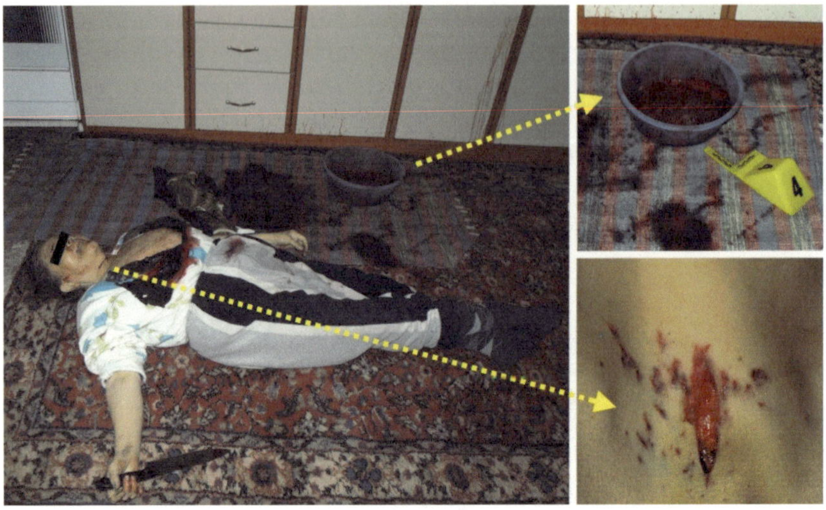

Fig. 16. The death scene of a 75-year-old woman who stabbed herself in the neck. There is a basin which she collected her blood (right top) and there are hesitation wounds on the neck (right bottom). She had psychiatric problems.

The tying together of the wrists in hanging cases is rare, but may not indicate a homicide, so long as the hanging ligature could not have been self-applied. At first glance, a hanging body found with their hands tied together would give the impression of a homicide but some suicidal people try to avoid being rescued by others or themselves. The closing of the mouth with a plastic bag or a scarf was thought to have removed the possibility of calling out for help during the hanging. Both the tying together of the hands and closing of the mouth were regarded as precautions taken by the victims to prevent any change in mind and an indication of their resolve to go through with the suicide (Fig. 17). In addition, placing soft material against the ligature loop was thought to be an attempt to lessen the feeling of pain (Demirci et al., 2009a) (Fig. 18).

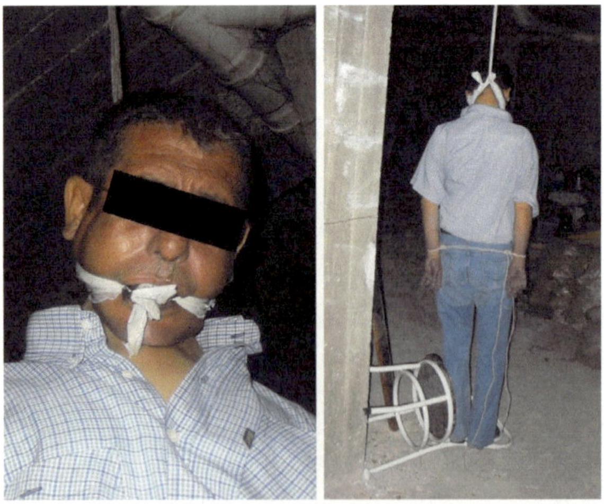

Fig. 17. Fifty two-year-old man who hanged himself. Both hands were tied limply behind his back with clothesline and a plastic bag was tied around the mouth.

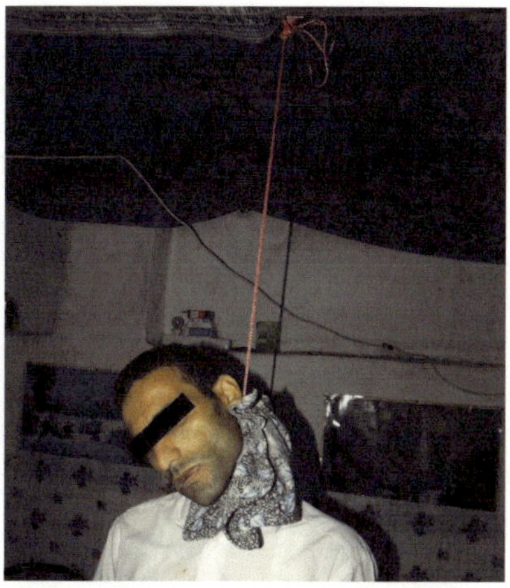

Fig. 18. A soft piece of cloth against the ligature.

In some cultures, religious books and findings indicating praying before suicide may be found at death scene. Demirci et al. (2008a) reported that in investigating medicolegal death cases believed to be of suicidal origin, evidence showing that this action was committed by the victim, the presence of a suicide note at the death scene, and a history of a previous suicidal attempt, the presence of daily axillary and pubic shaving on the external examination of the victim's body, when of the Muslim faith, may also be considered a feature of suicide (Fig. 19).

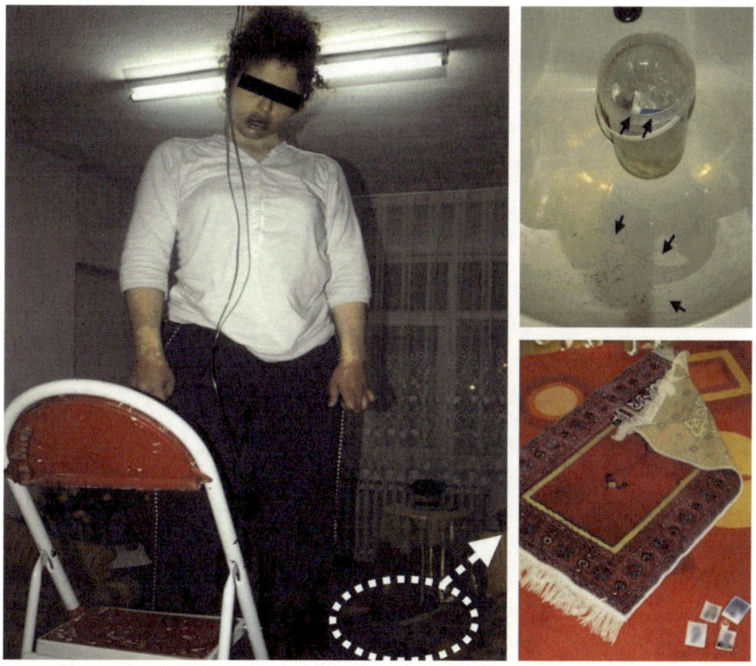

Fig. 19. A death scene of a 42-year-old woman's suicide. There was a razor and cut axillary hair in the sink of the bathroom (arrows on right up). Also a prayer rug, pictures of herself, her husband and two daughters, and her ring were on the carpet of the room (right down).

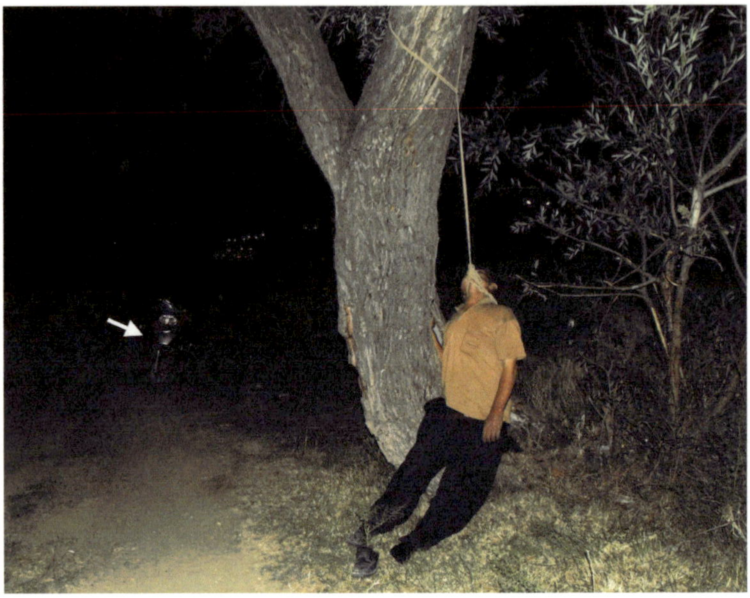

Fig. 20. Forty one-year-old man went to the woodland with his motorcycle (arrow) and hanged himself on a tree. A suicide note about his familial problems was found in his pocket.

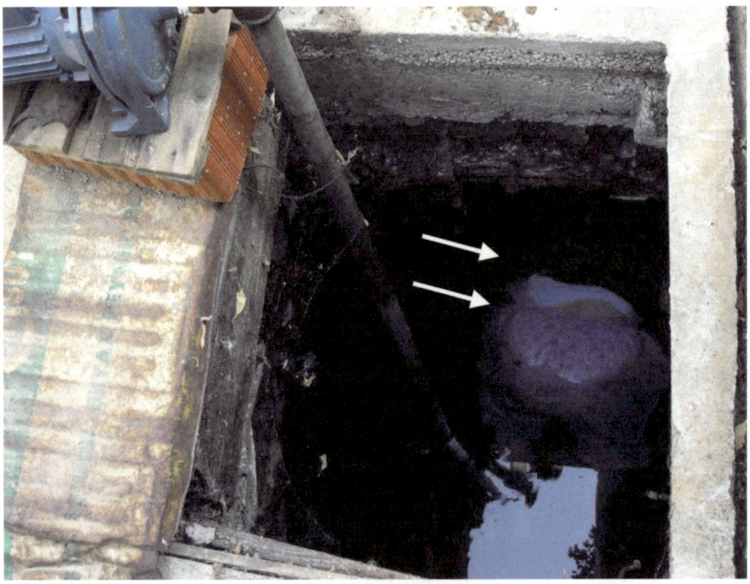

Fig. 21. The corpse of a 70-year-old woman who threw herself into the well in the garden of her house. A farewell letter was found in her house.

Suicidal acts carried out in places open to public can be highly traumatic for witnesses (Owens et al., 2009; Reisch & Michel, 2005; Tranah & Farmer, 1994). Moreover, they are considered more newsworthy than those occurring at home, and media reporting may encourage further suicides (Michel et al., 1995; Pirkis et al., 2007). It was suggested that nearly a third of all suicides occur in public places (Owens et al., 2009). The association of bridges and high buildings with suicide by jumping is well-known, but many other public places offer means or opportunity for suicide. Hanging, car exhaust poisoning and burning involve elaborate preparations and require seclusion. For these deaths, woods and isolated rural car parks provide the perfect opportunity (King & Frost, 2005) (Fig. 20). Wells are a preferred locality for suicides, which is the one reason why individuals may jump into a well, regardless of whether there is water or not. A suicide by drowning, although seen in all age groups, seems to be a preferred method for the elderly individuals (Dogan et al., 2010c) (Fig. 21).

7. Accident

An accidental death scene investigation launches after someone is dead in an automobile or other such accident. The investigation evaluates evidence, usually immediately, as to how the accident occurred. These are some types of accident scenes:
Auto Accident - An auto accident scene investigation may include an accident reconstruction if liability is in dispute. An investigator diagrams and photographs the auto accident scene and evaluates several factors, including points of impact to the vehicles, skid marks, roadway conditions and witness statements.
Fire - The investigator photographs, diagrams and examines the scene. The person who first discovered the fire and the participating fire personnel are interviewed. Physical evidence may be collected for further examination. A report may be drafted about the investigator's conclusions.
Slip and Fall - If a patron slips and falls, the slip and fall accident scene investigation usually begins with one of the employees of the establishment. What kind of fall occurred? Was there a defect in the ground or flooring? Was there a hazardous condition? How long were these conditions exposed? Photographs of the scene may be taken, and available witnesses, including the store employee or manager, are interviewed.

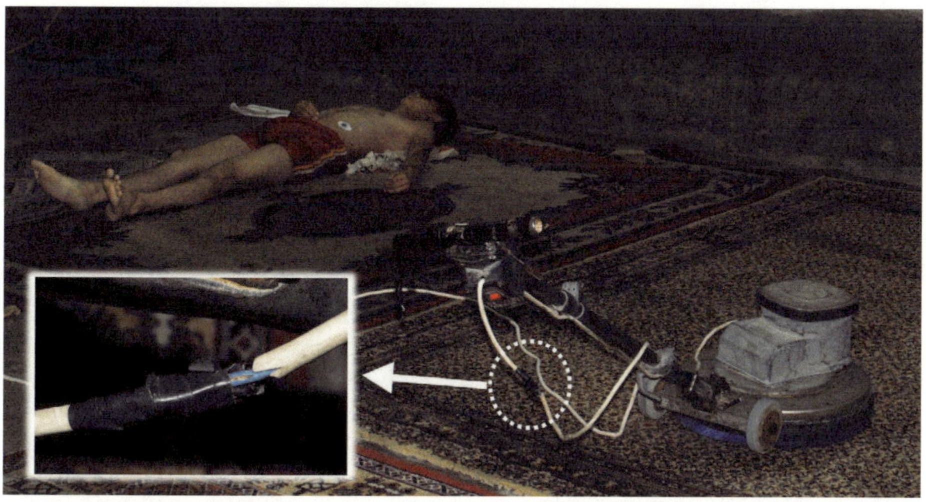

Fig. 22. A 17-year-old worker was dead due to electric shock in his workplace. The scene investigation revealed electrical leakage from the defect of the plastic sheath of the cable of carpet washing machine.

It is sometimes difficult to determine the manner and cause of death, if a detailed death scene investigation is not performed. In a case reported by Demirci et al. (2008b), a 30-year-old man's death was due to throat-cutting. They reported that although the cut in the neck initially suggested homicide, it was found to have occurred as a result of an accident in his workplace after the death scene investigation and autopsy. This case emphasizes the importance of the examination of incident scene and autopsy in determining the origin. Similar cases are deaths due to electric shock. The forensic medicine expert should visit the death scene before the autopsy if it is possible (Fig. 22).
Carbon monoxide (CO) is a colorless and odorless gas, and is lighter than air. It is an incomplete combustion product of hydrocarbons. About 600 accidental deaths due to CO poisoning are reported every year in the United States. CO usually causes accidental deaths, because it is pure and odorless (Thom & Keim, 1989; Cobb & Etzel, 1991; Saukko & Knight, 2004) (Figs. 23,24).

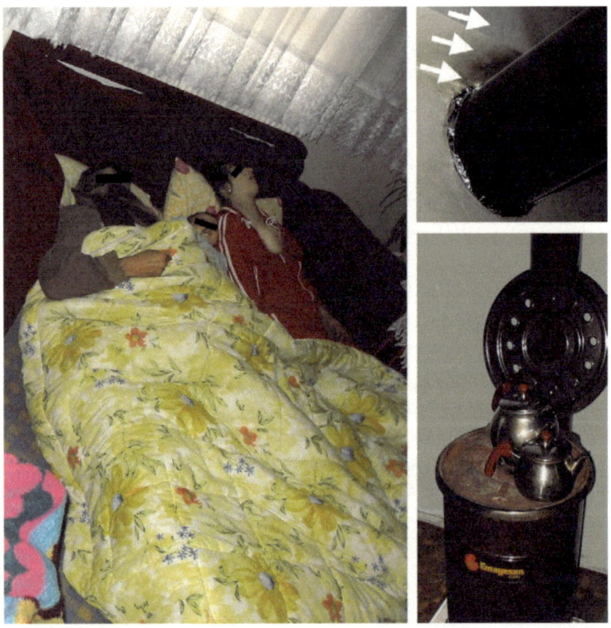

Fig. 23. A family (father, mother and child) was found dead in their bed due to carbon monoxide poisoning. There was a coal stove in the room and soot traces (arrows) were observed at the entry point of the stovepipe on the wall which indicating leakage of smoke of the stove.

Carbon monoxide can affect drivers of a moving vehicle, usually owing to a defective exhaust system that allows gas to percolate through the floor or engine bulkhead into the interior. Rarely, a strong following wind can blow the external exhaust-gas through the open doors of a van or truck. Another cause is a leak in the heat exchanger in vehicles that use a direct air supply from around the exhaust manifold to provide passenger heating (Saukko & Knight, 2004). In motor vehicles in which persons must remain for a long period of time while the vehicle is parked, for example, trucks with sleeping cabs, road service vehicles and mail trucks, a separate heater (working independently of the engine of the vehicle) may be used to heat the vehicle. The engine of the apparatus works with diesel fuel or gasoline. Combustion products burning in the pre-combustion chamber heat the fins of the engine. The air passing through the fins is heated and is transferred into the cabin. Malfunction of such an apparatus may be the cause of CO poisoning or fire. So the supplementary heater in the truck might be the cause of fatal CO poisoning and of the fires in the cabins of the trucks (Demirci et al., 2009c) (Fig. 25).

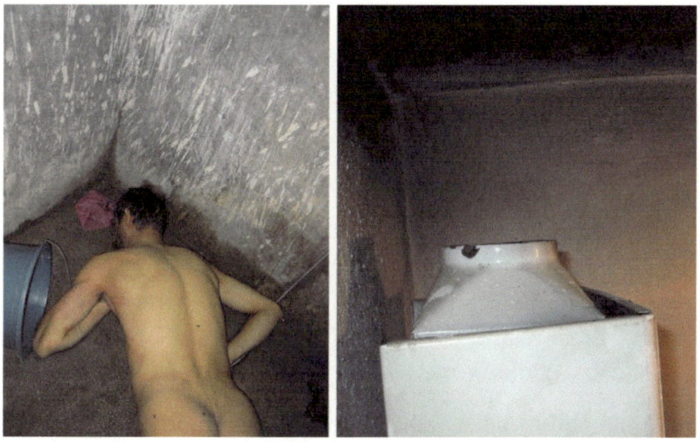

Fig. 24. A 42-year-old man was found dead due to carbon monoxide poisoning in his bathroom. There was an LPG water heater which had not a smoke pipe in the bathroom.

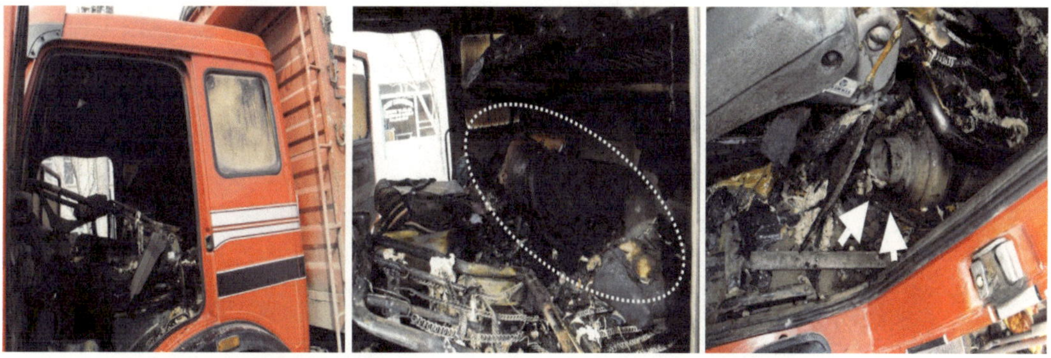

Fig. 25. A 48-year old male truck driver (ellipse) was found dead due to a fire in a truck parked in an open area of the truck garage. Scene investigation revealed that the cause of fire was broken supplementary heater (arrows) in the truck.

Decapitation may be suicidal, homicidal, and accidental. Accidental decapitations can result from traffic accidents, or occupational accidents. Decapitation by industrial trauma can occur at any age, and is often associated with heavy machinery in workshops or farm equipment being towed behind a tractor (Sharma et al., 1995). The helix elevator is an appliance connected to a tractor. It is used for loading grains from a field to any vehicle, such as a trailer, for transportation. In a case Demirci et al. (2009b) reported, the victim was a 41-year-old male farmer. In the stackyard, a helix elevator machine was loading a trailer with barley while the victim was distributing the loaded barley with a shovel in the trailer. He had tied a scarf loosely over his face and neck because he was allergic to the barley dust. When the victim's head and neck were level with the turning helix elevator shaft, the scarf was pulled up and wrapped around the shaft. The scarf then slid around the victim's neck and tightened, causing the head to separate from the body (Fig. 26).

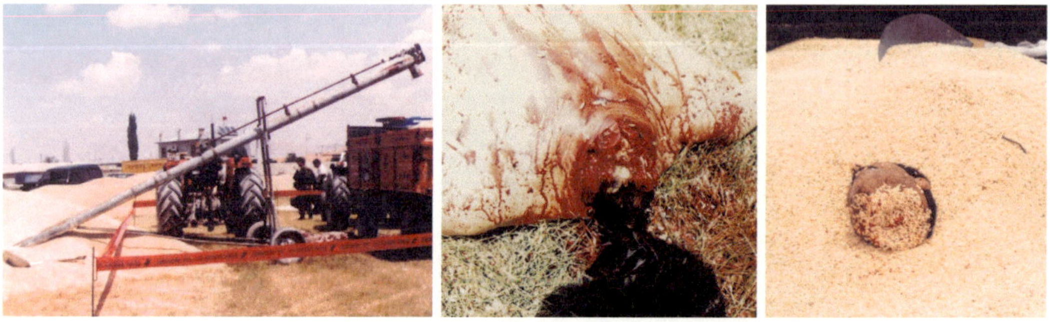

Fig. 26. A 41-year-old male farmer was found decapitated in the stackyard. He was working with a helix elevator machine. He had scarf tied loosely over his face and neck but the scarf was pulled up and wrapped around the shaft of the machine. The scarf then slid around the victim's neck and tightened, causing the head to separate from the body.

Possession of firearms is limited because of the technological requirements in production and strict laws. However, anyone can manufacture a handmade firearm by following some simple instructions and these actions do not a carry any legal liability. A mole gun is an unusual weapon used to kill moles in agricultural areas. Mole guns are primitive weapons produced for the purpose of trapping and are capable of firing a standard shotgun cartridge. Injuries and deaths caused by mole guns are generally a result of an accident while the victim is setting or controlling the gun (Demirci et al., 2008c) (Fig. 27).

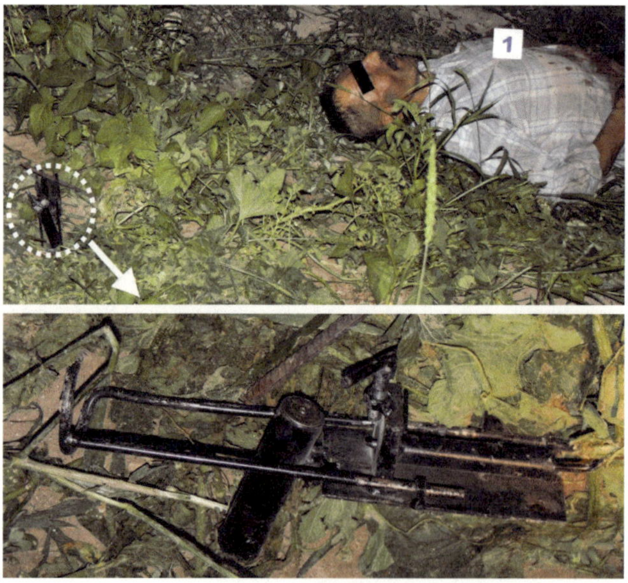

Fig. 27. A 42-year-old man was injured on the right thigh region while he was setting a mole gun to kill moles which were damaging the vegetables in his field, and died shortly after at the incident scene. The mole gun was found at the scene.

In some cases, it is important to distinguish accidental manner from suicidal or homicidal ones. For example, if a ligature mark is present on the neck, this is usually suicide or homicide. But sometimes the death may be accidental origin. In a case reported by Dogan et al. (2010d), a 53-year-old woman who had been working in the laundry of a hospital sat on the counter of the ironing machine to heat her back and leaned her back closer to the machine in a cold winter day. At that point, her coworkers left the room. When they re-entered the room 15 min later, they found her dead and observed that her scarf was caught in the roller cylinder of the ironing machine (Fig. 28).

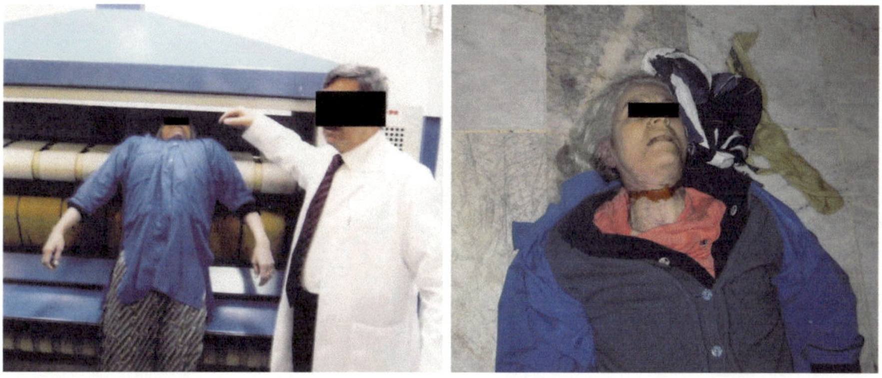

Fig. 28. The chief physician of the hospital showing the victim who was found strangulated with her scarf by the roller cylinder of the ironing machine in the laundry of the hospital. On the right side the ligature mark is seen on the neck.

Children have an increased risk for injury or death from accidents for a variety of reasons compared to adults. Perhaps the greatest reason is their natural curiosity, which leads them to explore their environment and investigate situations where they often do not recognize potential hazards (Byard, 1996). Accidental asphyxia can occur in childhood as a result of a variety situations (Dogan et al., 2010b) (Fig. 29).

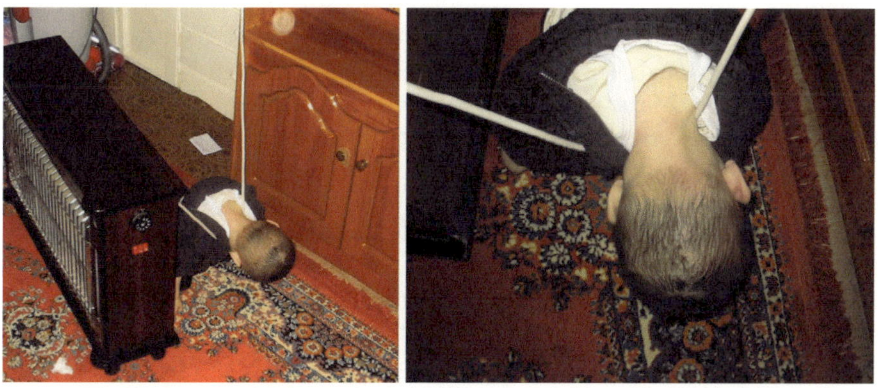

Fig. 29. The one-year-old child's neck was entangled in a tight cable of the electric heater while he was crawling on the floor of the living room.

Farm accidents are a frequent occurrence in many countries; for example, in the United States, farming is rated second only to mining in terms of occupational danger (Rivara,

1985). Unguarded agricultural power take-off (PTO) drivelines and the related components, including secondary drivelines powered by the PTO, have been historically recognized as serious farm-related hazards that can cause severe, permanently disabling injuries and death when entanglement occurs (Beer & Field, 2005). PTOs are rapidly rotating shafts that transfer power from the tractor attached at one end to a piece of farm machinery at the other end. Clothing or body parts can become entangled, resulting in amputation or avulsion of body parts, strangulation, and massive crushing injuries (Karlson & Noren, 1979) (Fig. 30). Dogan et al. (2010f) reported that 5.8% of the farm tractor-related fatalities involved deaths resulting from PTO entanglement. In these cases, there were extensive crush injuries to the chest, abdomen, and extremities. None of the turning shafts in these cases had safety shields.

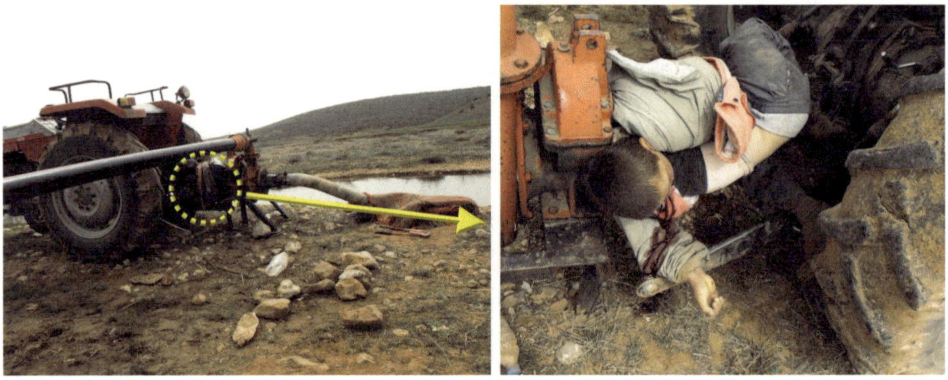

Fig. 30. Fatality involving power take-off (water pump) entanglement.

8. Natural deaths

An important portion of the deaths investigated by forensic medicine experts involve natural diseases, the most common being cardiovascular disease. Natural diseases processes alter the way the body reacts to and repairs from injuries. The older the person, the more likely that natural disease has a role in the death (Figs. 31,32). This concept can work in reverse. One can erroneously assume that because the person is young, natural disease is not a factor in the death. Many people have unknown or undiagnosed natural diseases that manifest in sudden, unexpected death. A common history in these cases is that "he hadn't seen a doctor in years" or "he didn't believe in doctors." The result is that the first doctor he sees is the forensic medicine expert, who diagnoses what was a treatable natural disease such as a cardiovascular disease. "Sudden death" is a term used frequently in death investigation but its meaning can be ambiguous. In some situations, death can literally be *instantaneous*, such as with a massive pulmonary embolus. In others, such as a myocardial infarction, the death can be instantaneous, or take minutes to hours or longer. Sudden cardiac death is a sudden, unexpected death from cardiac causes within one hour of onset of symptoms (Wagner, 2009). Investigating natural deaths might not be very exciting to some but can be interesting and rewarding. For example, Wagner (2009) reported that he found an aortic aneurysm in a 14-year-old girl who died suddenly while running. Knowing this condition to be genetic, a study of 12 family members showed the same abnormality in three, thus saving those individuals the same fate as their relative.

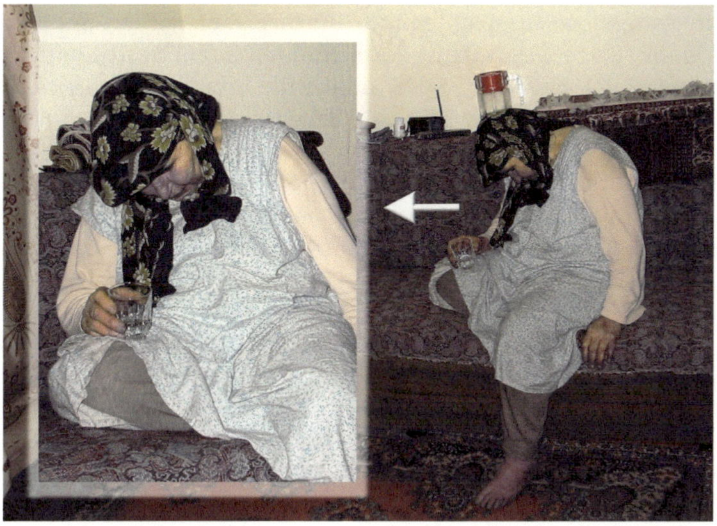

Fig. 31. Seventy six-year-old woman who had been living alone was found dead in her home in sitting position and holding a glass in her hand. Note the livor mortis on face, hands and left foot due to the position of the deceased.

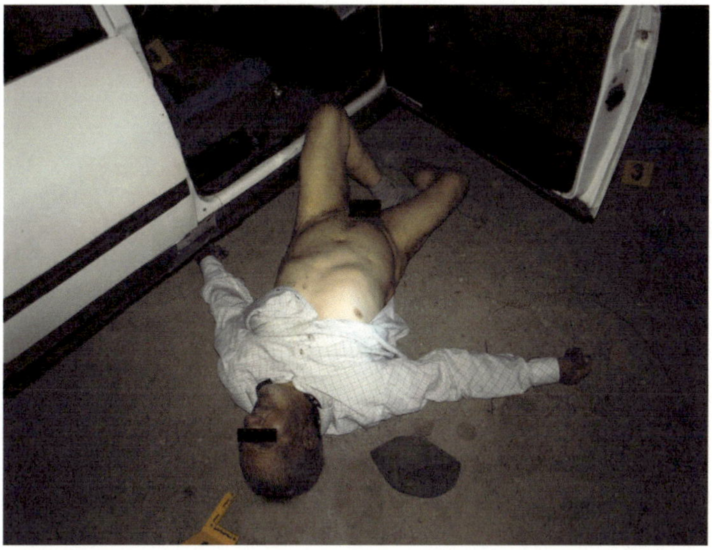

Fig. 32. A 74-year-old man was found dead in half-naked position lying alongside his car. The investigation revealed that when the man and a young woman were having sex, the man suddenly deteriorated and died. The cause of death was determined as myocardial infarction at the autopsy.

9. Sudden and unexplained infant death

Sudden unexplained infant death (SUID) is the sudden and unexpected death of an infant due to natural or unnatural causes. SUID applies to the death of an infant less than 1 year of age, in which investigation, autopsy, medical history review, and appropriate laboratory testing fails to identify a specific cause of death. Sudden infant death syndrome (SIDS) is one of several causes of SUID. However, SIDS, unlike the other SUID causes, is a diagnosis of exclusion. Even with a thorough death scene investigation, review of the clinical history, and autopsy, SIDS is difficult to distinguish from other SUIDs, such as accidental suffocation and asphyxia. In the world of death investigation, infant death investigation is unique. From scene through certification, these investigations require skill and knowledge drawn from disciplines outside those typically considered a part of medicolegal education (Corey et al., 2007; Hanzlick, 2001; Shapiro-Mendoza, 2006). The post mortem examination, ideally should include a history of the gestation, delivery and postnatal development, a death scene investigation, a family psycho-social history, a complete autopsy, and a confidential case conference (Bajanowski et al., 2007).

Having knowledge about the many causes of SUID, in addition to SIDS, is of utmost importance for the death scene investigator. At the scene, the investigator will gather evidence as well as information from the parents or caregivers who were with the infant and who may be in a great deal of distress. All of this information is crucial for distinguishing between a natural death, an accidental death, or a homicide.

The following is a brief overview of known causes of infant death that are oftentimes overlooked during investigation, resulting in the cause of death being listed as SIDS on the death certificate.

Asphyxia or suffocation is caused by the inability to breathe. This condition leads to a lack of oxygen in the body, which can lead to loss of consciousness and death. Asphyxia can be caused by choking, constriction of the chest or abdomen, strangulation, narrowing of airway passages (severe allergic reaction or reactive airway disorders), or the inhalation of toxic gases. Common objects that are involved with asphyxia or suffocation include plastic bags, soft pillows, and soft materials such as bedding or stuffed animals. These objects can occlude the mouth and nostrils, causing suffocation. The most commonly reported cause of asphyxia in infants is accidental suffocation and strangulation in bed.

If the investigator is very observant, knows what to look for, and is particularly careful in talking with the caregiver, he/she may pick up some clues that will help determine the specific cause of asphyxia or suffocation and determine whether the manner of death was accidental or intentionally inflicted. A thorough death scene investigation can help answer questions about environmental factors that may have interfered with breathing (e.g., covering of the nose and mouth) or hazards related to aspiration, choking, electrocution, excessive heat or cold, and other external factors.

There are a number of risk factors associated with asphyxia and suffocation. The following is a list of the typical causes of infant asphyxia and/or suffocation.

- Overlaying or accidental suffocation on a shared sleep surface.
- Accidental strangulation from unsafe surroundings.
- Wedging or entrapment.
- Immersion in water or drowning.
- Choking.
- Neck compression (Shapiro-Mendoza, 2006).

Accidental asphyxia can occur in younger children and infants, who may move into positions in which their airways become occluded, their bodies become wedged so that they are unable to breathe, or they become suspended from their clothing or restraining harnesses (Gilbert-Barness et al., 1991; Nixon et al., 1995; Byard, 1996). Many houses in Turkey (especially those situated in the villages and slums) are built with metal rings mounted in the ceilings, so that the occupants can set up swing-like cradles, which are hammock-like in nature. The cradles are constructed by tying two ropes between the two metal rings and connecting them with cloth. Infants are placed in these cradles on top of cushions, and ligatures (e.g., scarf, rope, or sash) are tied around the cradles to prevent them from falling out. However, the ligature can wrap around the neck and asphyxiate the infant if it leans out of the cradle (Dogan et al., 2010b) (Fig. 33).

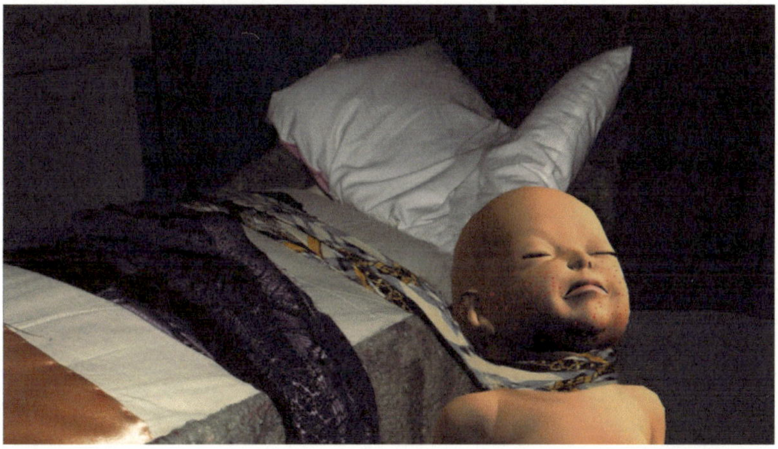

Fig. 33. The position of dead infant in the swing-like cradle. As the victim leaned out of the cradle, the ligature that was tied around the swing-like cradle wrapped around the child's neck, resulting in asphyxia.

There are a number of risk factors associated with the infant's environment that may be connected with the death. The following is a list of causes typically associated with the environment or death scene.

- Poisoning or intoxication.
- Electrocution.
- Hypothermia.
- Hyperthermia.

Inborn errors of metabolism are rare genetic disorders that stop or prevent the body from turning food into energy. These disorders are usually caused by defects in the enzymes that help break down foods in the body. When the body cannot process these foods, a buildup of toxic substances or a deficiency of substances needed for normal body function can occur. This buildup can be fatal if not controlled with diet or medication. Some metabolic diseases are inherited.

Injuries can be fatal or nonfatal, and they can occur unintentionally or intentionally (because of purposeful acts of harm). It is often difficult to determine whether an infant's injury was a result of an unintentional or intentional act. Examples of unintentional injuries include the infant choking on a small toy or rolling over in bed onto the infant.

Shaken baby syndrome (SBS) is one form of abusive head trauma that occurs when an infant or young child is violently shaken or struck against a hard or soft surface. Shaking may cause bleeding over a large portion of the brain. SBS can cause severe brain damage as well as death. In cases where a child receives a head injury from a fall or other impact, there may be external signs of injury, such as bruising or abrasions on the scalp. In SBS, there may be no signs of injury on the infant (Shapiro-Mendoza, 2006).

9.1 SUID scene investigation

The physical environment of the death scene may play an important role in the cause and manner of the infant's death. Some research has indicated that the change of seasons, which requires turning on or off heating or cooling devices (furnace, fireplace, air conditioner, ceiling fan), might precipitate an apneic event. Therefore, it is important to determine, describe, and document the specific environmental conditions of the scene such as room temperature and other factors that may affect the microenvironment of the infant at the time of death (e.g., air current from ceiling fan, humidity levels in a spa, water temperature in a hot tub).

The forensic medicine expert should personally inspect the death scene to gain a thorough understanding of the possible environmental hazards to which the infant might have been exposed. He or she, should observe and document the furnishings in the room/area where the infant was found dead or unresponsive. In addition, the investigator should describe the general state of the room/area; if there is evidence of rodent, insect, or animal activity or a generally unkempt situation, this should be documented as accurately and objectively as possible. The scene should be documented with photographs, diagrams, and descriptions.

Fumes that are noticed at the scene might have contributed to or been the cause of the infant's death and should be noted in the investigative report. A description of the fumes might provide forensic scientists with clues that will assist them in ordering laboratory tests. The investigator should describe the fumes and their intensity and attempt to ascertain the source of the fumes. If necessary, local fire department personnel should be contacted to ensure that the scene's air is clear of harmful substances.

The smell of smoke may indicate a live-fire situation or tobacco use at the scene. Smoke might have contributed to or been the cause of the infant's death. A description of the smoke smell may provide forensic scientists with clues that will assist them in ordering laboratory tests. The investigator should describe the smoke smell, its intensity, and its possible sources.

Mold growth at the scene may have exposed the infant to dangerous airborne pathogens. A description and location of mold growth may provide forensic scientists with clues that will assist them in ordering laboratory tests. The investigator should describe the mold growth and its location in relation to the infant's sleeping/activity area. Photographs of any suspicious material should be taken at this time.

The observance and documentation of peeling paint at the scene may indicate an infant's exposure to dangerous lead-based materials. A description of the room and the location and size of the peeling paint area can provide forensic scientists with clues that will assist them in ordering appropriate laboratory tests. The location and size of the peeling paint and its location in relation to the infant's sleeping/activity area should be described as accurately as possible. The investigator should contact the local health department if the problem presents safety concerns to persons in the vicinity (Ernst et al., 2006).

10. Conclusion

The forensic medicine expert should visit the death scene before the autopsy if it is possible. Although, investigation and legal systems differs from country to country, there is always a crime scene investigation team. If the forensic medicine expert does not have the opportunity to visit the death scene him/herself, he/she would check the documents (notes, sketches, photographs, etc) which crime scene investigation team prepared. Many medicolegal deaths may be resolved by death scene investigation. A forensic medicine expert should never forget: If the death scene investigation is not performed before the autopsy, that autopsy will be an imperfect autopsy.

11. References

Adelman, H.C. (2007). *Forensic Medicine,* Chelsea House Publishing, New York

Avis, S.P. (1993). An unusual suicide. The importance of the scene investigation. Am *J Forensic Med Pathol,* Vol. 14, No. 2, Jun. 1993, pp. 148-150

Bajanowski, T., Vege, A., Byard, R.W. et al., (2007). Sudden infant death syndrome (SIDS)--standardised investigations and classification: recommendations. *Forensic Sci Int,* Vol. 165, No. 2-3, Jan. 2007, pp. 129-143

Beer, S.R. & Field, W.E. (2005). Analysis of factors contributing to 674 agricultural driveline-related injuries and fatalities documented between 1970 to 2003. *J Agromedicine,* Vol. 10, No. 3, Sep. 2005, pp. 3-19

Byard, R.W. (1996). Hazardous infant and early childhood sleeping environments and death scene examination. *J Clin Forensic Med,* Vol. 3, No. 3, Sep. 1996, 115-122

Clark, S.C. (1999). *Death Investigation: A Guide for the Scene Investigator,* US Dept Justice, National Institute of Justice, Washington, DC

Cobb, N. & Etzel, R.A. (1991). Unintentional carbon monoxide-related deaths in the United States, 1979 through 1988. *JAMA,* Vol. 266, No. 5, Aug. 1991, pp. 659-663

Committee for the Workshop on the Medicolegal Death Investigation System. (2003). *Medicolegal Death Investigation System Workshop Summary,* The National Academy Press, Washington, DC, Retrieved from: http://www.nap.edu/catalog/10792.html

Corey, T.S., Hanzlick, R., Howard, J., Nelson, C. & Krous, H. (2007) A functional approach to sudden unexplained infant deaths. *Am J Forensic Med Pathol,* Vol. 28, No. 3, Sep. 2007, pp. 271-277

Demirci, S., Dogan, K.H., Erkol, Z. & Deniz, I. (2008a). Is daily shaving of axillary and pubic hair a feature of suicide in the Muslim community? *Am J Forensic Med Pathol,* Vol. 29, No. 4, Dec. 2008, pp. 330-333

Demirci, S., Dogan, K.H. & Gunaydin, G. (2008b). Throat-cutting of accidental origin. *J Forensic Sci,* Vol. 53, No. 4, Jul. 2008, pp. 965-967

Demirci, S., Gunaydin, G., Dogan, K.H. & Erkol, Z. (2008c). Deaths caused by mole guns: three case reports. *Int J Legal Med,* Vol. 122, No. 4, Jul. 2008, pp. 323-325

Demirci, S., Dogan, K.H., Erkol, Z. & Deniz, I. (2009a). Precautions taken to avoid abandoning the act of hanging and reducing pain in suicidal hanging cases. *Am J Forensic Med Pathol,* Vol. 30, No. 1, Mar. 2009, pp. 32-35

Demirci, S., Dogan, K.H., Erkol, Z. & Gunaydin, G. (2009b). Accidental decapitation: a case report. *Am J Forensic Med Pathol,* Vol. 30, No. 3, Sep. 2009, pp. 270-272

Demirci, S., Dogan, K.H., Erkol, Z. & Gunaydin, G. (2009c). Two death cases originating from supplementary heater in the cabins of parked trucks. *J Forensic Leg Med,* Vol. 16, No. 2, Feb. 2009, pp. 97-100

Di Nunno, N., Costantinides, F., Vacca, M. & Di Nunno, C. (2006). Dismemberment: a review of the literature and description of 3 cases, *Am J Forensic Med Pathol,* Vol. 27, No. 4, Dec. 2006, pp. 307-312

DiMaio, V.J. & DiMaio, D. (2001). *Forensic Pathology* (2nd ed), CRC Press, Boca Raton, FL

Dix, J., Calaluce, R. & Ernst, M.F. (1999). *Guide to Forensic Pathology,* CRC Press, Boca Raton, FL

Dix, J. & Ernst, M.F. (1999). *Handbook for Death Scene Investigators,* CRC Press, Boca Raton, FL

Dogan, K.H., Demirci, S., Deniz, I. & Erkol, Z. (2010a). Decapitation and dismemberment of the corpse: a matricide case. *J Forensic Sci,* Vol. 55, No. 2, Mar. 2010, pp. 542-545

Dogan, K.H., Demirci, S., Erkol, Z. & Gulmen, M.K. (2010b). Accidental hanging deaths in children in Konya, Turkey between 1998 and 2007. *J Forensic Sci,* Vol. 55, No. 3, May. 2010, pp. 637-641

Dogan, K.H., Demirci, S., Erkol, Z., Gulmen, M.K. & Deniz, I. (2010c). Dead bodies found in wells. *Am J Forensic Med Pathol,* Vol. 31, No. 3, Sep. 2010, pp. 208-212

Dogan, K.H., Demirci, S., Gunaydin, G. & Buken, B. (2010d). Accidental ligature strangulation by an ironing machine: an unusual case. *J Forensic Sci,* Vol. 55, No. 1, Jan. 2010, pp. 251-253

Dogan, K.H., Demirci, S., Gunaydin, G. & Buken, B. (2010e). Homicide-suicide in Konya, Turkey between 2000 and 2007. *J Forensic Sci,* Vol. 55, No. 1, Jan. 2010, pp. 110-115

Dogan, K.H., Demirci, S., Sunam, G.S., Deniz, I. & Gunaydin, G. (2010f). Evaluation of farm tractor-related fatalities. *Am J Forensic Med Pathol,* Vol. 31, No. 1, Mar. 2010, pp. 64-68

Ernst, M.F., Jentzen, J., Burbrink, D., Robinson, D., Nunez, S., O'Neal, B.J. & Davis, T. (2006). Conducting scene investigations, In: *Sudden Unexplained Infant Death Investigation Training Material,* pp. 140-168, Centers for Disease Control and Prevention, Atlanta, GA, Retrieved from: http://www.cdc.gov/SIDS/TrainingMaterial.htm

Gilbert-Barness, E., Hegstrand, L., Chandra, S., Emery, J.L., Barness, L.A., Franciosi, R. & Huntington, R. (1991). Hazards of mattresses, beds and bedding in deaths of infants. *Am J Forensic Med Pathol,* Vol. 12, No. 1, Mar. 1991, pp. 27-32

Hanzlick, R. (2001). Death scene investigation, In: *Sudden Infant Death Syndrome: Problems, Progress, and Possibilities,* Byard, R.W. & Krovs, H.F., pp. 58-65, Arnold, London

Horswell, J. (2005a). Major incident scene management, In: *Encyclopedia of Forensic and Legal Medicine, Vol 2,* Payne-James, J., Byard, R., Corey, T. & Henderson. C., pp. 12-20, Academic Press, London

Horswell, J. (2005b). Suspicious deaths, In: *Encyclopedia of Forensic and Legal Medicine, Vol 2,* Payne-James, J., Byard, R., Corey, T. & Henderson, C., pp. 32-36, Academic Press, London

Karlson, T. & Noren, J. (1979). Farm tractor fatalities: the failure of voluntary safety standards. *Am J Public Health,* Vol. 69, No. 2, Feb. 1969, pp. 146-149

King, E. & Frost, N. (2005). The New Forest Suicide Prevention Initiative (NFSPI). *Crisis,* Vol. 26, No. 1, Jan. 2005, pp. 25-33

Lee, H.C., Palmback, T. & Miller, M.T. (2000). *Henry Lee's Crime Scene Handbook,* Academic Press, San Diego, CA

Lew, E. & Matshes, E. (2005). Death scene investigation, In: *Forensic Pathology: Principles and Practice,* Dolinak, D., Matshes, E. & Lew, E., pp. 9-64, Elsevier, San Diego, CA

McMaster, A.R., Ward, E.W., Dykeman, A. & Warman, M.D. (2001). Suicidal ligature strangulation: case report and review of literature. *J Forensic Sci,* Vol. 46, No. 2, Mar. 2001, pp. 386-388

Michel, K., Frey, C., Schlaepfer, T. & Valach, L. (1995). Suicide reporting in the Swiss print media: frequency, form and content of articles. *Eur J Public Health,* Vol. 5, No. 3, Sep. 1995, pp. 199-203

Miller, M.T. (2003). Crime scene investigation, In: *Forensic Science: An Introduction to Scientific and Investigative Techniques,* James, S.H. & Nordby, J.J., pp. 115-135, CRC Press, Boca Raton, FL

Milroy, C.M., Dratsas, M. & Ranson, D.L. (1997). Homicide-suicide in Victoria, Australia. *Am J Forensic Med Pathol,* Vol. 18, No. 4, Dec. 1997, pp. 369-373

Moldovan, E. (2008). The Medicolegal Death Investigator. An Evolution in Crime Scene Investigations Relating to Unexpected Deaths, In: *Discovery Guides,* 18 Feb 2011, Available from: http://www.csa.com/discoveryguides/medicolegal/review.pdf

Nixon, J.W., Kemp, A.M., Levene, S. & Sibert, J.R. (1995). Suffocation, choking, and strangulation in childhood in England and Wales: epidemiology and prevention. *Arch Dis Child,* Vol. 72, No. 1, Jan. 1995, pp. 6-10

Owens, C., Lloyd-Tomlins, S., Emmens, T. & Aitken, P. (2009). Suicides in public places: findings from one English county. *Eur J Public Health,* Vol. 19, No. 6, Dec. 2009, pp. 580-582

Pirkis, J., Burgess, P., Blood, R. & Francis, C. (2007). The newsworthiness of suicide. *Suicide Life Threat Behav,* Vol. 37, No. 3, Jun. 2007, pp. 278-283

Prahlow, J. (2010). *Forensic Pathology for Police, Death Investigators, Attorneys and Forensic Scientists,* Humana Press Inc, Totowa, NJ

Reisch, T. & Michel, K. (2005). Securing a suicide hot spot: effects of a safety net at the Bern Muenster Terrace. *Suicide Life Threat Behav,* Vol. 35, No. 4, Aug. 2005, pp. 460-467

Rivara, F.P. (1985). Fatal and nonfatal farm injuries to children and adolescents in the United States. *Pediatrics,* Vol. 76, No. 4, Oct. 1985, pp. 567-573

Rogers, T.L. (2004). Crime scene ethics: souvenirs, teaching material, and artifacts. *J Forensic Sci,* Vol. 49, No. 2, Mar. 2004, pp. 307-311

Saukko, P. & Knight, B. (2004). *Knight's Forensic Pathology* (3rd ed), Arnold, London

Sauvageau A. (2009). True and simulated homicidal hangings: a six-year retrospective study. *Med Sci Law,* Vol. 49, No. 4, Oct. 2009, pp. 283-290

Schröer, J. & Püschel, K. (2005). Special aspects of crime scene interpretation and behavioral analysis: The phenomenon of "undoing", In: *Forensic Pathology Reviews, Vol 4,* Tsokos M, pp. 193-202, Humana Press Inc, Totowa, NJ

Shapiro-Mendoza, C. (2006). Sudden, unexplained infant deaths, In: *Sudden Unexplained Infant Death Investigation Training Material,* pp. 12-23, Centers for Disease Control and Prevention, Atlanta, GA, Retrieved from: http://www.cdc.gov/SIDS/TrainingMaterial.htm

Sharma, G.K., Sarangi, M.P. & Tyagi, A.K. (1995). Decapitation death. *Med Sci Law,* Vol. 35, No. 1, Jan. 1995, pp. 85-86

Spitz, W.U. (2006). *Medicolegal Investigation of Death: Guidelines for the Application of Pathology to Crime Investigation* (4th ed), Charles C. Thomas, Springfield, IL

Thom, S.R. & Keim, L.W. (1989). Carbon monoxide poisoning: a review epidemiology, pathophysiology, clinical findings, and treatment options including hyperbaric oxygen therapy. *J Toxicol Clin Toxicol,* Vol. 27, No. 3, May. 1989, pp. 141-156

Tranah, T. & Farmer, R. (1994). Psychological reactions of drivers to railway suicide. *Soc Sci Med,* Vol. 38, No. 3, Feb. 1994, pp. 459-469

Trestrail, J.H. 3rd. (2007). Crime Scene Investigation, In: *Criminal Poisoning: Investigational Guide for Law Enforcement, Toxicologists, Forensic Scientists, and Attorneys* (2nd ed), Trestrail, J.H. 3rd, pp. 69-81, Humana Press Inc, Totowa, NJ

Verma, S.K. & Lal, S. (2006). Strangulation deaths during 1993–2002 in East Delhi (India). *Leg Med (Tokyo),* Vol. 8, No. 1, Jan 2006, pp. 1-4

Vieira DN, Pinto AE, Sá FO. (1988). Homicidal hanging. *Am J Forensic Med Pathol,* Vol. 9, No. 4, Dec. 1988, pp. 287-289

Wagner, S.A. (2009). *Death Scene Investigation-A Field Guide,* CRC Press, Boca Raton, FL

3

Diagnostic of Drowning in Forensic Medicine

Audrey Farrugia and Bertrand Ludes
Institute of Legal Medicine,
11 rue Humann 67085,
Strasbourg Cedex
France

1. Introduction

The diagnostic of drowning is described in the literature as one of the most difficult in the field of forensic medicine (Piette & De letter, 2006). In fact, the external examination and the autopsy findings are in most of the cases not specific and the laboratory investigations are controversially appreciated by the scientific community. The main goal in this field is to differentiate a death by submersion from a immersion of a body. Death of a victim found in water should not always be related to drowning (Knight, 1991).

It is important to remind that the death by drowning is defined as a death due to submersion in a liquid and the mechanism in acute drowning is hypoxemia and irreversible cerebral anoxia (D.J. Di Maio & V.J.M. Di Maio 1989).

2. Physiopathology

Considering the pathophysiology of human drowning, the role of mechanical airways obstruction and the washing out of alveoli surfactant as well as the shifts of fluid and electrolytes are still debated. In fact, several phases were described during the drowning process, first a breath-holding phase, followed by involuntary inspiration, gasping for air and loss of consciousness. The death is secondary of the development of cerebral hypoxia leading to irreversible brain damage. The duration of the phases is dependent on various factors, such as age, previous diseases, breath holding tolerance of the victims and the temperature of the water. Consciousness is usually lost within 3 minutes of submersion.

The inhaled water enters the alveolar spaces of the lungs and destroys the surfactant inducing pulmonary edema with the transudation of protein-rich fluid into the alveolar spaces. The surfactant washout decreases the lung compliance and ventilation-perfusion mismatch resulting to an hypoxemia secondary of non oxygenation of blood flowing through underventilated portions of the lung. A non cardiogenic pulmonary edema will result with secondary metabolic acidosis. This is the main pathophysiological mechanism of drowning and the fluid and electrolyte shifts are quite secondary.

It was stated that fresh water is hypotonic and hyponatremic relative to blood inducing, after inhalation, a movementt of water from the alveoli into the blood and movement of sodium from the blood into the alveoli. These changes induce haemodilution, hypervolemia, hypnonatremia, hyperkalemia and haemolysis (Jeanmonod et al., 1992). As the sea water is very hypertonic relative to the blood, the water movement goes from blood into the alveoli and the electrolytes (sodium, chloride, magnesium) from the alveoli into the blood. The consequences of the sea water drowning should be haemoconcentration, hypovolemia and hypernatremia. The biochemical tests that proposed to assess the diagnostic of drowning are based on these fluids and electrolytes shifts. It is during the phases where water is penetrating from the alveoli into the blood circulation that particles like diatom passing through the alveolar-capillary interface before reaching internal organs.

A vagal reflex may be also induced by inhalation of water, it will increase peripheral airway resistance with pulmonary vasoconstriction, decreased lung compliance and reduction of ventilation - perfusion ratios (Ornato, 1986).

An intense stimulation of nerve endings at the skin, the mucosa of the ear drum, the pharynx or the larynx by cold water can lead to a cardiac reflex arrest. It was assumed that 10% of the drowned humans die after laryngospasm or breath-holding without actually aspirating fluid (Ludes & Fornes, 2003). A discussion was also hold about the volumes of inhalated water and the effect on the circulation. In drowning, the inhalated volume of water can range, from relatively small to very large. It has been showed that small amount of water, particularly cold water, may induce vaso vagal reflex or cardiac arrest reflex. When great amounts of water are inhalated and pass through the alveolar-capillary interface and enter the circulation, the phenomenon of destruction of surfactant and of the alveoli architecture leads to asphyxia. During the entering of water into the blood stream, the diatoms present in the drowning fluid may reach the internal organs.

To establish the diagnosis of drowning it is of particular importance to correlate informations about the circumstances preceding the death, the past medical history of the victim if known, the circumstances of the body recovery from the water, the external examination, the autopsy findings and the results of the complementary analyses (histologic, biochemical, toxicological analyses and diatom test).

3. Autopsy findings

The majority of the autopsy findings are related to asphyxia and have no specific link to drowning. The signs of drowning depend on the delay in recovering the body and on the development of the putrefaction phenomenon which alter the positive signs of drowning. One of the signs of drowning would be large amounts of froth present around nostrils and mouth in freshly drowned bodies. This froth is also present in the upper and lower airways. Froth can also be observed in cases of edema of left ventricular failure but in drowning cases the volume of froth is generally much more abundant than in other origins.

It is admitted that lung weights are higher in drowning cases but it was shown that normal weights are possible in the drowning cases after cardiac arrest reflex or vaso vagal reflex. After water inhalation, the lungs may be over inflated, filling the thoracic cavity, generally water logged referred to as "emphysema aquosum". So the surfaces of lungs have a marbled appearance with dark red areas linked with collapsed alveoli, interspersed with more aerated tissues areas. The fluid is trapped in the lower airways and blocks the passive collapse of the bronchi that normally occurs after death. Subpleural bullae of emphysema, sometimes hemorrhagic may be found and are related to the rupture of the alveolar walls (Pounder, 2005). Even if these signs are mostly evocating of drowning, none of them is pathognomonic of water inhalation.

The body having sunk to the bottom of the site of drowning, will show a pattern of post mortem injuries such as post-mortem abrasion over the forehead, the prominent points of the face, the anterior trunk, the backs of the hands and the fronts of the lower legs. Injuries may also inflicted by passing watercraft in navigable waters by stumbling against rocks or by animal activities. Accidental or suicidal injuries due to the way the person falls or enters into the water may also be observed. Post-mortem injuries linked to the way of recovery of the body using ropes and hooks can also be seen. These kinds of post-mortem injuries can mimic ante-mortem wounds and the differentiation between ante and post-mortem injuries is quite difficult because of the lack of the usual criteria of ante-mortem wounds.

It can also be found sand, silt, seashells and weeds in the airways, lungs, stomach and duodenum of drowned victims. If this material is fund in abundance within the alveoli, it can be related to an immersion during life as long as it concerns a freshly drowned body. This material may also enter the upper airways during the post-mortem immersion period and it is possible that small quantities may enter the oesophagus and stomach but it is unlikely that it will reach the alveoli to any significant extent if the post-mortem submersion is short.

One of the sign of immersion is skin maceration becoming visible after various time interval depending on the temperature of the immersion water. The skin becomes wrinkled, pale and sodden like a "washer woman's skin". These changes appear at the finger tips, palms, backs of the hands, and later, the soles. The next step is the detachment of the thick keratin of hands and feet which pull off in "glove and stoking fashion". Nails and hair become loosened after a few days. Other signs of immersion are *cutis anserine* and post-mortem distribution of hypostasis. The presence of mud, silt or sand on the body was described but has no diagnostic value.

4. Complementary investigations

4.1 Histology

The microscopic investigations must be performed on all the organs of non putrefied bodies in the aim to make the difference between a death by drowning and other causes of death. The lung examinations can show over-distension of the alveoli, thinning of the alveolar septa and compression with narrowing of the capillary network (Pounder, 2005).

The modifications in lungs are heterogeneous distributed and multiple sections must be performed to assess the diagnostic. In fact the microscopic appearance may be entirely normal in some part of the lungs.

Several staining techniques must be performed such as the staining for elastic fibers (orcein) and reticulin fibers (Fornes et al., 1988 ; Ludes & Fornes, 2003). The examination of other organs (brain, heart, liver) shows none specific histological changes indicative of hypoxia such as acute congestion and swelling of the capillary endothelia.

4.2 Biological tests

The chemical changes in plasma after drowning were based on the fluid and electrolyte shifts after the penetration of either sea or fresh water in the alveoli and in the blood stream (Modell & Davis, 1969). It was proposed the measurement of the specific gravity of blood, of the concentration of sodium, chloride and potassium. For the electrolytes, the diagnosis of drowning was based on changes of these electrolytes between the blood samples taken from the right versus left ventricle (Bray, 1985; Couteselinis & Boukis 1976; Karkola & Neittaanmaki, 1981). Such electrolyte shifts were described in many other causes of death and do not provide reliable evidence of drowning.

A special mention must be made for the blood strontium analysis. The toxicological analysis are performed to show the presence of medicaments or alcohol, taken before death in suicidal or accidental conditions and to determine the serum level of strontium which is described as a good parameter of drowning in sea water (Piette & Timperman, 1989). In case of fresh water drowing, the water concentration of strontium must be higher than the serum concentration to be a valuable parameter in favour of drowning.

Authors such as Kane et al. (1996, 2000) and Nübel et al. (1997) proposed the detection by molecular biology techniques of the 16S rRNA subunits of ribosomal RNA for plankton detection in tissues samples indicating an active water inhalation and may assess the diagnostic of drowning. According to these authors, the sequence comparison of the variable regions of 16S rRNA could provide sufficient information to allow the discrimination of both close and distant phylogenetic relationships.

Abe et al. (2003) and Suto et al. (2003) proposed the detection of chlorophyll-related genes of *Euglena gracilis* and *Skeletonema costatum* to identify plankton in the victim's tissues. It is important to emphasize that these methods give only qualitative results (He et al., 2008) but the quantitative approach can only be achieved by the diatom test which may also give an indication of the site of drowning.

In fact, diatoms can be considered as particles present in the submersion water which are inhalated during drowning and once in the blood stream which reach the closed organs. Under strict extraction and identification conditions, these particles are good markers of drowning.

Diatoms are unicellular algae belonging to the class of bacillariophycae which includes more than 15 000 species living in fresh, brakish or sea water. The skeleton of these algae is called a frustule which is constituted by two valves fitting together to enclose the cytoplasm (Ludes & Fornes, 2003) and made of hard silice.

Due to this hard silicaceous skeleton, diatoms can be recovered from putrefied or burnt tissues by either enzymatic or acid digestion (Ludes et al., 1994). The identification of these algae is based on the structure of their valves showing different symmetry allowing the distinction of two main groups namely the centric diatoms and the elongated or pennate diatoms.

After a long period of time where the use of the diatom test was very controversial due to false positive results linked to the presence of diatoms in closed organs of non drowned victims (Foged, 1983; Gylseth & Mowe, 1979; Schellmann & Sperl, 1979; Schneider, 1980, 1990; Schneider & Kolb, 1969), it was stated by several authors that under strict defined analytical conditions this test could discriminate between drowning and none drowning cases (Auer & Möttönen, 1988 ; Neidhard & Greedyke, 1967; Peabody, 1977; Pollanen, 1997,1998; Pollanen et al., 1997). Auer & Möttönen (1988) were one of the first authors to propose that 20 diatoms per microscope slide obtained from lung samples should be a sufficient concentration to exclude false positive due to contaminations. We also proposed qualitative and quantitative criteria for a positive drowning diagnostic with the diatom test.

For us, an analysis will be considered as positive when at least 20 diatoms are identified per 100 µl of a pellet sediment extracted from a 2 g lung sample and the identification of more than 5 complete diatoms (with exclusion of fragments) per 100 µl of a pellet sediment extracted from a 2 g tissue samples such as brain, kidney, liver and bone marrow. Bone marrow is described as a sanctuary organ and if diatoms reach this tissue, the diagnostic of drowning could be assessed.

In controlled samples belonging to non drowned victims, we newer find a number of diatoms above the fixed criteria. When diatoms were found in closed organs of drowned victims, the results in lung samples were in each case also above the 20 algae per 100 µl pellet. To assess the diagnostic of drowning, it is of high importance to perform a qualitative analysis of the found diatoms and the comparison of the diatoms present in the closed organs and the microflora of the presumed site of drowning.

In this aim, water samples must be collected at the drowning site (two samples of 100 ml) as well as algae scraped from stones present in the water.

The samples are disposed in clean containers and the extraction and identification protocols on water and tissue samples were described by our group (Ludes et al., 1999). All reagents and glass containers must be checked for the absence of diatoms before use, and contamination from exogenous diatoms must be avoided by using diatom-free water and by protecting the organs during autopsy from the clothes of the victims and from the skin surface.

At each step of the analyses and the identification of diatoms, a potential contamination must be considered. This test cannot be proposed to assess the diagnostic of drowning in bathtub or in water containing very few algae, for example in iced water.

If water samples are not available, it is possible to compare the diatoms found in the organs with data collected in the rivers by a continuous water monitoring which can be set up by, for example, the Agencies in charge of the survey of water quality.

We set up a continuous water monitoring of the main rivers of our area (Ludes et al., 1996). Seasonal variations of the concentration of diatoms and the diatom profile are determined at a given month by the five most frequent species. The relative abundance of each diatom may also vary along the course of the river. So, the site of drowning may be determined by comparison between the water microflora with the diatoms found in the lungs. In fact, diatoms of more than 50 - 60 µm in size rarely pass the alveoli-capillary barrier even after the rupture of the alveoli by the inhalation of water.

The diagnostic of drowning can be achieved when the qualitative analysis shows that the algae found in the organ belongs to the water microflora and the quantitative criteria are fulfilled (Hendey, 1973, 1980 ; Ludes et al., 1999).

5. Conclusion

The diagnostic of drowning may be achieved after having considered all the forensic investigations performed in those cases, i.e: external examination, autopsy findings, histological and toxicological analysis, blood strontium determination, biochemical analysis and diatom test. The diatom test was still considered controversial by the by the literature but we defined qualitative and quantitative criteria which could exclude false positive results. It is of particular interest in case of putrefied bodies where the other investigations have failed.

6. References

Abe S, Suto M, Nakamura H, Gunji H, Hiraiwa K, Suzuki T, Itoh T, Kochi H, Hoshiai G (2003). A novel PCR method for identifying plankton in cases of death by drowning. Med. Sci. Law 43: 23-30.

Auer A, Möttönen M (1988). Diatoms and drowning. Z Rechtsmed 101: 87-98.

Bray M (1985). Chemical estimation of fresh water immersion intervals. Am J Forensic Med Pathol 61: 133-139.

Coutselinis A, Boukis D (1976). The estimation of magnesium concentration in cerebrospinal fluid as a method of ,drowning diagnosis in seawater. Forensic Sci 7: 109-111.

Davis J (1986). Bodies found in the water: an investigative approach. Am. J. Forensic Med Pathol 7: 281-287.

DiMaio DJ, DiMaio VJM (1989) Drowning. In: DiMaio DJ, DiMaio VJM, eds. Forensic pathology. Elsevier, Amsterdam pp. 357-365.

Foged N (1983). Diatoms and drowning. Once more. Forensic Sci Int 21: 153-159.

Fornes P, Pepin G, Heudes D, Lecomte D (1988) Diagnosis of drowning by computer-assisted histomorphometry of lungs with blood strontium determination. J Forensic Sci 43(3): 772-776.

Gylseth B, Mowe G (1979). Diatoms in the lung tissue. Lancet 29: 1375.

He F, Huang D, Liu L, Shu X, Yin H, Li X (2008). A novel PCR - DGGE - based Method for Identification Plankton 165 r DNA for the Diagnosis of Drowning. Forensic Sci Int 176 : 152-156.

Hendey NI (1973). The diagnosis value of diatoms in the cases of drowning. Med Sci Law 13(1): 23-34.

Hendey NI (1980). Letter to the Editor, diatoms and drowning —A review. Med Sci Law 20(4): 289.

Jeanmonod R, Staub Ch, Mermillod B (1992). The reliability of cardiac haemodilution as a diagnostic test of drowning. Forensic Sci Int 52: 171-180.

Kane M, Fukunaga T, Maeda H, Nishi K. (2000). Phylogenetic analysis of picoplankton in Lake Biwa and application to legal medicine. Electrophoresis 21: 351-354.

Kane M, Fukunaga T, Maeda H, Nishi K. (1996). The detection of picoplankton 16S rDNA in case of drowning. Int. J. Leg. Med. 108: 323-326.

Karkola K, Neittaanmaki H (1981). Diagnosis of drowning by investigation of left heart blood. Forensic Sci Int 18: 149-153.

Knight B (1991). Immersion deaths. In: Knight B, ed. Forensic Pathology, E.Arnold, London pp. 360-374.
Ludes B, Fornes P. (2003). Drowning in : Forensic Medicine : Clinical and Pathological Aspects. Payne-James J, Busuttil A, Smock W eds, Greenwich Medical Media, pp 247-257.
Ludes B, Coste M, North N, Doray S, Tracqui A, Kintz P (1999). Diatom analysis in victim's tissues as an indicator of the site of drowning. Int J Legal Med 112: 163-166.
Ludes B, Coste M, Tracqui A, Mangin P (1996) Continuous river monitoring of the diatoms in die diagnosis of drowning. J Forensic Sci 41(3): 425-428.
Ludes B, Quantin S, Coste M, Mangin P (1994). Application of a simple enzymatic digestion method for diatom detection in the diagnosis of drowning in putrefied corpses by diatom analysis. Int J Med 107: 37-41.
Modell JH, Davis JH (1969). Electrolyte changes in human drowning victims. Anesthesiology 30: 414-417.
Neidhart DA, Greedyke RM (1967). The significance of diatom demonstration in the diagnosis of death by drowning. Am J Clin Pathol 48(4): 377-382.
Nübel U, Garcia-Pichel F, Muyzer G (1997). PCR primers to amplify 16S rRNA genes from cyanobacteria. Appl. Environ. Microbiol 63: 3327-3332.
Ornato JP (1986). The resuscitation of near-drowning victims. JAMA 256: 75-77.
Peabody AJ (1977). Diatom in Forensic Science. J Forensic Soc 17: 81-87.
Piette M, Timperman J (1989). Serum strontium estimation as a medico-legal diagnostic indicator of drowning. Med Sci Law 29: 162-171.
Piette M.H.A, De Letter E.A (2006). Drowning : still a difficult autopsy diagnosis. Forensic Sci. Int 163 1-9.
Pollanen MS (1997). The diagnosis value of the diatom test for drowning, II. Validity: analysis of diatoms in bone marrow and drowning medium. J Forensic Sci 42(2): 286-290.
Pollanen MS (1998). Forensic diatomology and drowning. Elsevier (Amsterdam) ed.
Pollanen MS, Cheug C, Chiasson DA (1997). The diagnosis value of the diatom test for drowning, I. Utility: a retrospective analysis of 771 cases of drowning in Ontario, Canada. J Forensic Sci 42(2): 281-285.
Pounder DJ (2005). Drowning in: Encyclopedia of Forensic and Legal Medicine. Payne-James J, Byard RW, Corey TS, Henderson C eds, Elsevier Academic Press pp 227-232.
Schellmann B, Sperl W (1979). Nachweis im Knochenmark (Femur) Nichtertrunkener. Z Rechtsmed 83: 319-324.
Schneider V (1980). Detection of diatoms in the bone marrow of non-drowning victims. Z Rechtsmed 85(4): 315-317.
Schneider V (1990). Zur Diatomeen Assoziations Methode: Alt-bekannte "neu" entdeckt? Z Kriminalistik 44: 461.
Schneider V, Kolb KH (1969). Uber den nachweis von radioaktiv markierten Diatomeen in den Organen in den Organen. Beitr Gerichd Med 25: 158-164.

Suto M, Abe S, Nakamura H, Suzuki T, Itoh T, Kocbi H, Hoshiai G, Hiraiwa K (2003). Phytoplankton gene detection in drowned rabbits. Leg. Med. 5: S142–S144.

4

Forensic Investigation in Anaphylactic Deaths

Nicoletta Trani, Luca Reggiani Bonetti, Giorgio Gualandri[1],
Giuseppe Barbolini and Margherita Trani[2]
[1]*Azienda USL of Reggio Emilia,*
[2]*Nuovo Ospedale di Sassuolo (MO)*
Department of Diagnostic Services, Pathology and Legal Medicine, section of Legal Medicine, University of Modena and Reggio Emilia, Modena
Italy

1. Introduction

Deaths anaphylaxis related have always been very difficult in objectification in autopsies. So they are object of study for pathologists and legal doctors. In this work we want to propose a methodological protocol based on the various available diagnostic tools to use when an anaphylaxis related death is suspected.

2. Pathogenesis

The anaphylaxis is an allergic reaction. An allergic reaction is a spontaneous and exaggerate reaction of the body to a particular substance. These substances, called allergens, cause production of antibodies when enter the body. The exposition with the substance happens by inhalation, ingestion, contact or inoculation of the allergen. Every substance can act as allergen. Among the more frequent substances we remember the heterologous proteins (hormone like insulin, vasopressin, parathormon; enzymes like trypsin, chemotrypsin, penicillinases; pollens, food like eggs, fish, hazel-nuts, cereals, beans, chocolate; antiserums, hymenoptera venom); polysaccharides (iron dextran); drugs (antibiotics like penicillins, cephalosporins, Amphotericin B, nitrofurantoin, local anesthetics like procaine and lidocaine; vitamins like thiamine and folic acid); diagnostic substances (iodated means of contrast, sodium dehydrocoled, sulfobromoftaleine); industrial chemical products (ethylene oxide). (Fauci et al., 2009)

The concept of anaphylaxis comes from the study of the actinotoxins on the dogs' arterial blood pressure (Richet, 1902).

It is well known that the anaphylactic shock is an example of the immediate type of hypersensitivity reaction inducing a diffuse organ hypoperfusion. It has been defined (Delage & Irey, 1972) as the failure of the peripheral circulation induced by an antigen (allergen)-antibody reaction in already sensitized subjects for a foreign substance. Whenever the hypoperfusion is complicated by increased capillary permeability, a rapidly irreversible circulatory fatal damage occurs (anaphylactic death).

Delage and Irey (Delage & Irey, 1972), in their clinico-pathological study of 43 validated cases of drug-induced fatal anaphylactic shock, the predominant role of penicillin, subsequently confirmed (Di Maio & Di Maio 2001; Menchel et al., 1987; Weeden, 1988), is reported. In these as well as in other cases immunoglobulin E (IgE) antibodies have been tested to various allergens, present in contrast media (Di Maio & Di Maio 2001; Lang et al., 1995; Pumphrey & Roberts, 2000; Risgaard et al., 2008), sera (Vance & Strassmann, 1942; Johann-Liang et. Al., 2011), insect venom (Pumphrey, 2000; Riches et al., 2001; Yunginger et al., 1991), and food (Di Maio & Di Maio 2001; Pumphrey, 2000; Pumphrey & Roberts, 2000; Yunginger et al., 1991) are thought to initiate anaphylactic reaction in patients previously sensitized towards that allergen (often unknowingly).

A register including all fatal anaphylactic reactions in the UK is operative since 1992 (Pumphrey, 2008). In France and Belgium since 2001 a university research team has founded the Allergy Vigilance Network, that in addition to reporting cases of severe anaphylaxis, to determine the prevalence of sensitization to risk allergens and screening and long-term monitoring of dangers related to new foods, ingredients and adjuvant sensitizing factors, with the French National Institute for Food Safety (AFSSA) and the Ministry of Consumer Affairs (DGCCRF) and various patient associations, also analyzes dangers related to the allergenicity of natural and modified food proteins (Moneret-Vautrin et al., 2002; Moneret-Vautrin, 2007).

Allergy depends on the individual "predisposition". In certain people the contact between the allergen and the human body causes an abnormal immune reaction that clinically appears with the wide spectrum of manifestations of the allergic reaction (Crane, 2006; Liccardi et al., 2006)

Hypersensitivity reaction can be classified according the four type of immuno-pathological reaction of Gell and Coombs (Fauci, 2009):

- type I: they are the result of an IgE-mediated reaction that leads to an immediate hypersensitivity
- type II: IgG or IgM mediated. These antibodies are directed against cellular surface's antigens altered by the drug that provoke a complement-mediated cytotoxicity.
- type III: immuno-complexes mediated. The immunocomplexes' dimensions determine the site of deposition and the consequent immunological damage.
- type IV: retarded hypersensitivity. They come out by the interaction of the antigen with T lymphocyte and determine a cell-mediated reaction.

Type I reaction is characterized by a rapid activation (in few minutes)of vasoactive and spasmogen substances by antibodies that are on the surface of the mastcells and basophils. It's composed of three phases:

1. sensitization, when the immune system come into contact with the allergen for the first time and stimulates IgE antibodies by B cells (the IgE production is under the control of TH2 CD4+ that increases its production and under the control of TH1 that reduces the production). The IgE bind mastcells' and basophils' receptors making them sensible to a next exposition to the antigen.
2. initial reaction: Immune system has a memory; so at the second exposition to the allergen there's a binding between the antigen and the IgE antibodies localized on the mast-cells and basophils (sensitized). High affinity receptors (IgE) are almost exclusively on the mast-cells and on the basophils while low affinity receptors are also in other cytotypes (eosinophils, macrophages, platelets).

   When the allergen binds to the high affinity receptor there's the activation of the mastcells that leads to the degranulation of the mastcells and release of primary mediators (preformed) such as histamine, adenosine, chemiotactic mediators (e.g. the ones for the eosinophils), enzyme (tryptases, kynases), proteoglicans. There's also the release of secondary mediators of 'de novo' synthesis such as leucothrienes, prostaglandines, platelets' aggregation stimulation factors, cytokines, chemokines. In the first 30-60 minutes after exposition symptoms happen. Histamine is characterized by a very short half-life in the circulation, tryptase and chymase, are stable post-mortem (Edston et al., 2007; Nishio et al., 2005) and respectively used in post-mortem diagnosis of acute anaphylaxis (Edston, 2007; Nishio, 2005; Pumphrey, 2000; Riches et al., 2001; Schwartz, 1987; Yunginger et al., 1991). Tryptase is a serine protease stored mainly in mast cell granules, not found in circulating basophils, eosinophils, platelets or any other cell, represented by two varieties: an active free form (β) and an inactive tetramere (α) (Ansari et al., 1993; Schwartz et al. 1995).

The former is a protein released from mast cell granules during anaphylactic reactions, the latter is a similar protein secreted by resting mast cells and raised in mastocytosis (Pumphrey & Roberts, 2000; Schwartz et al. 1995).

Chymase is a mast cell-derived serine protease, characterized as an angiotensin II-generating enzyme (Nishio, 2005) and used to determine mast cells and thus to assess the timing of wounds after deaths (Bonelli et al., 2003; Urata et al., 1990).

It is quite stable in serum and a significant positive correlation between serum chymase and tryptase levels was found in post-mortem diagnosis of anaphylaxis (Nishio, 2005). Heterogeneity of human mast cells is known (Irani & Schwartz, 1994; Weidner & Austen, 1993) and recently different subsets of mast cells (MC) are distinguished by immunohistochemistry (Perskvist & Edston, 2007), as follows:

MC-TCs (formerly connective tissue mast cells) mainly composed of histamine, heparin, tryptase, chymase, cathepsin G and carboxypeptidase, preformed and stored in granules.

- MC-T (formerly mucosal mast cells) lacking or containing only small amounts of chymase, carboxypeptidase and cathepsin.
- MC-C lacking tryptase and not further characterized

3. Late phase: after 2 hours from the initial response the presence of antigen is not necessary and the tissue infiltration begins by inflammatory cells (neutrophils, eosinophils, basophils, monocytes) with consequent tissue lesions (in particular epithelia and mucosas).

This is the typical allergic reaction that usually brings to vasodilatation, skin rash, edema, itching; but the clinical spectrum is very wide and the allergic disturbs can be poor or get the death for anaphylactic shock.

Anaphylaxis is the most dangerous among the allergic reaction and it is a severe systemic reaction, with an often sudden and important beginning, with an acute response that happens in a variable time from few seconds to few minutes after the antigen exposition.

Anaphylaxis can be elicited for every concentration of the antigen (also minimal, sometimes it happens during skin test for drugs, etc.) (Bernstein et al., 2004; Blanton & Sutphin, 1949; Eleuterio Gonzàlez et al., 1997; Harris & Sure, 1950; Liccardi et al., 2006; Lockey et al., 1987; Riezzo, 2010; Weber-Mani & Pichler, 2008).

The typical anaphylaxis consists of sudden weakness, itching and urticaria, chest oppression, respiratory distress (wheezing) followed by cardio-circulatory collapse. Symptoms maybe very variable and could be involved almost all the functions/apparatus.

Could be involved: cardio-vascular system(tachycardia, hypotension, arrhythmias, ischemia/ myocardial infarction, heart arrest, symptoms from hypoperfusion are constant), nervous system (vertigo, asthenia, syncope, convulsions), eye (conjunctival injection, lachrymation), upper airway (nasal congestion, sneezing, hoarseness, stridor, pharyngeal or laryngeal edema, cough, obstruction, laryngospasm), lower airway (dyspnea, bronchospasm, tachypnea, involvement of the accessory respiratory muscles, cyanosis, respiratory arrest), skin (rash, erythema, itching, urticaria or urticarial reaction, edema, maculo-papular rash), gastrointestinal apparatus (nausea, vomiting, abdominal pain, diarrhea)(Crane et al. 2006; Fauci, 2009; Rovere-Querini, 2010).

Lethal cases are mainly due to: acute respiratory distress derived by the glottis edema or by bronchial obstruction/bronchospasm; cardio-vascular collapse also without an important respiratory distress.

In the lethal cases between the contact with the allergen and the anaphylaxis there's a very short time. The anaphylaxis shows immediately or in few minutes after the exposition; in the most of the cases by 15-20 minutes. Reactions after 60 minutes from the exposition are very rare. As soon the reaction occurs as easier the death is; sometimes death can be immediate and, however by 1-2 hours. More rarely death occurs by 24 hours.

3. Proposal of a methodological protocol

In most of the cases the diagnosis of anaphylactic death represents a challenging deal. So it's very important that the anatomo-pathological and/or medico-legal investigations must be very scrupulous and must analyze:

- medical history of the deceased and eventual investigations on the spot;
- necropsy with:
- lab tests, for which it's better to use peripheral blood sample and not central ones;
- histological tests
- histochemical and immuno-histochemical tests.

3.1 Medical history and investigations on the spot

To make diagnosis of anaphylactic death it's important to make a correlation between the symptoms and an insect bite, the ingestion of food, drugs or other substances.

So we should collect anamnesis by family and general practitioner, especially if related to an history of allergy. Some patients, however, doesn't know to have allergies and anaphylaxis is the first (and last) allergic reaction they have in their life.

Especially in the cases with medical history negative for past allergic reaction it's important, when possible, going on the spot where the death occurred to get the eventual syringes used for injection and/ or to evaluate the presence of nests of wasps. It's important hearing to witnesses that could tell the symptoms of the victim. Sudden weakness, itching and urticaria, chest oppression and respiratory distress (wheezing) followed by cardio-circulatory collapse may occur. Symptoms maybe very variable and could be involved almost all the functions/apparatus as we remembered before.

3.2 Complete necroscopic exam

It's very important beginning with an accurate external exam to verify the presence of signs such as rash, urticaria or angioedema; to verify the skin integrity finding out eventual site of inoculation: it's important to investigate also the sites covered by hair. If there a positive finding it's opportune to proceed, during the successive autopsy, also to get a skin sample after the examination of the route in the case of subcutaneous or intramuscular injection. During the autopsy the pathological findings are often aspecific.

Usually we find multivisceral congestion, aspecific finding in various different types of death. (Barnard, 1967; Da Broi & Moreschi, 2011; Delage & Irey, 1972; Di Maio & Di Maio, 2001; Edston & van Hage-Hamsten, 2005; James & Austen, 1964; Low & Stables, 2006; Lu et al., 2006; Menchel et al, 1987; Pumphrey & Roberts, 2000; Shen et al.,2009; Yilmaz et al., 2009).
You can find:

- glottis edema and/or of the pharyngo-laryngeal districts;
- congestion and/or pulmonary edema;
- hyperinflation of the alveoli with acute emphysema;
- endo-luminal bronchial secretions- this finding is more frequent if there's an asthmatic factor and it's usually related to a almost immediate death;
- hemorrhagic petechiae: it's suggestive of an asphyxial component of the death and it's usually associated with an almost immediate death.

These findings can change according to the allergen type, to the way of administration and to the time passed between the exposition and the death (Edston & van Hage-Hamsten, 2005; Low & Stables, 2006; Pumphrey & Roberts, 2000). If the death is very fast the only macroscopic finding is an important multivisceral congestion associated or not with the petechial hemorrhages (Edston & van Hage-Hamsten, 2005; Low & Stables, 2006; Pumphrey & Roberts, 2000; Roberts & Pumphrey, 2001).
In the table n. 1 there are the results of different studies present in literature (Barnard, 1967; Delage & Irey, 1972; Greenberger et al, 2007; James & Austen, 1964; Low & Stables, 2006; Pumphrey & Roberts, 2000; Shen et al.,2009; Yilmaz et al., 2009).

Autopsy findings	Study		
	Delage & Irey (1972)	James & Austen (1964)	Barnard (1967)
Number of cases	40	6	50
		3 cases penicillin, 1 case guinea-pig haemoglobin; 1 case bee venom; 1 case ragweed extraxt	Insect-Stings
Erythematous skin rash/cutaneous edema			35
Pulmonary congestion and edema	36	5	35
Upper airway edema	15	4	14
Hyperinflation of the lungs and/or mucous plugging of airways	18	5	16
Petechial hemorrahages			10

Autopsy findings	Study						
	Pumphrey & Roberts (2000)			Low & Stables (2006)			
Number of cases	56			18			
	Venom (19)	Food (16)	Drugs (21)	Venom (4)	Food (2)	Drugs (10)	Undetermined (2)
Erythematous skin rash/cutaneous edema	1	2	0	0	0	0	2
Pulmonary congestion and edema	14	9	18	3	0	5	2
Upper airway oedema	6	10	7	3	0	0	1
Hyperinflation of the lungs and/or mucous plugging of airways	7	5	3				
Petechial hemorrahages	4	5	1				

Autopsy findings	Study		
	Greenberger et al. (2007)	Shen et al. (2009)	Yilmaz et al. (2009)
Number of cases	25	28	36
Erythematous skin rash/cutaneous edema	3	4	2
Pulmonary congestion and edema	18	28	29
Upper airway edema	16	15	11
Hyperinflation of the lungs and/or mucous plugging of airways	3	11	5
Petechial hemorrahages	6		3

Table 1. Autopsy findings.

A complete autopsy, with histo-pathological and chemical-toxicological investigations, is mandatory in every case.

3.3 Laboratory tests

A very useful first investigation is the research of the total and specific IgE for specific substances: The Igs are very stable also after death (Hieda et al, 1991).

The finding of total IgE doesn't demonstrate the anaphylaxis but indicates that the subject was sensible for particular substances (e.g. insect venom, antibiotics, etc..). However , in there's a positive history or suspect for allergies for specific substances, every suspected substance must be tested with specific IgE. If there isn't an accurate anamnesis or an history of allergy it's a good idea testing the most common allergens. (Calvani et al., 2007; Hamilton & Adkinson, 2003; Horn et al., 2004).

A second investigation on the cadaverous blood sample is the dosage of beta-tryptase. As we already said, the degranulation of the mast-cells releases powerful chemical mediators (histamine, tryptase, etc..) (Ansari et al., 1993, Carson et al., 2009; Way & Baxendine 2002).

The tryptases, instead, are relatively stable post-mortem (values can remain high for some days in a serum sample kept at room temperature and for some months if freezed) (Joint Task Force on Practice Parameters et al., 1998; Horn, 2004) and their dosage is very useful in the diagnostics of acute anaphylaxis. As already said, in addition to mast cells also the basophiles produce tryptases but fewer than 300-700 times compared to skin and lung mast cells. So the serum concentration of tryptase is considered an index of mast cells activation. In particular we must determine the beta-tryptases that are usually released by mast cell degranulation (while the alfa-tryptase is secreted constitutively by mast cells and represent an index of the mast cells mass and so it is present in the mastocytosis) (Kanthawatana et al, 1999; Schwartz 2004).

For this reason the ratio between total tryptase (alfa + beta) and beta-tryptase is important to distinguish between an episode of anaphylaxis and patients with systemic mastocytosis: a ratio less than 10 is usually indicative of an anaphylactic reaction while a ratio <20 suggests a systemic mastocytosis (Joint Task Force on Practice Parameters et al., 2005; Lieberman et al, 2010; Schwartz et al., 1995, Schwartz & Irani, 2000). Serum levels of tryptase quickly increase and are detectable by 30 minutes (the concentration peak is reached in the first 2-3 hours) and remain high for about 5 hours (Joint Task Force on Practice Parameters et al., 2005; Lieberman et al, 2010). High levels of beta-tryptase point out a degranulation and, so, support the diagnosis of anaphylaxis.

Usually the increase of the serum level of tryptase is bigger as much as the anaphylaxis has been severe. It's important underline that the negativity of this test doesn't exclude an anaphylactic death. In fact Sampson has demonstrated that the rise of this enzyme could be absent in the anaphylaxis by food, maybe because of the involvement of other cells such as basophils or monocytes/macrophages (Sampson et al., 1992).

Therefore tryptase concentrations in femoral blood (not influenced by position at death or resuscitation efforts) (Edston et al., 2007) and serum chymase and tryptase levels (Nishio et al., 2005; Shen et al., 2002) have been suggested in postmortem cases to validate the diagnosis of anaphylactic deaths.

The histamine is another product of mast cell degranulation. This mediator, even if is very valid in vivo (it's an index of mast cell activation even though not specific of the mastcells alone) , isn't an effective indicator after death because has a very short half-life (2 minutes).

So the N-methylhistamine, that is a product of histamine degradation and is stable in the urine, but in the cases of anaphylactic death the time is too short to find it into the urine (Sthephan et al. 1990; Edston et al, 2005, 2007).

Among the other possible tests we remember the serum titration of a mastcell-specific chymase (Nishio et al., 2005; Osawa et al. 2008), that is a serum protein mainly kept into the mastcell granules.

It's important to note that the positivity to total IgE or of the serum tryptase cannot be considered , by the forensic profile, as a sure indication of a death by anaphylaxis because the positivity of one or both the markers has been found also in other pathologies (Randall et al., 1995; Horn et al., 2004) such as traumatic death or the sudden infant death syndrome (Buckley et al., 2001; Edston et al., 1999; D'Errico et al., 2008; Holgate et al, 1994; Nishio & Suzuki, 2004; Schwartz, 2001) but must be integrated with the results of other investigations that must be done in every case of death.

3.4 Histology

Finally the histo-pathological diagnosis is very important and may show eosinophilia (Delage ande Irey, 1972) especially in the upper and lower airway, in the liver and in the spleen (Voigt, 1966); the presence of glottis edema and/or pharyngo-laryngeal edema that, histologically, could be associated with a wide dissociation of collagen fibers and of the glandular elements, eosinophilic infiltration and vascular congestion (Pumphrey and Roberts, 2000).

Sometimes, using hematoxylin-eosin stain, there's lung hyperinflation with emphysema, endo-luminar mucous and peri-bronchial congestion, edema and eosinophilic infiltrate.

Another method is the mast cell count in the various organs and tissues: unfortunately specific stainings for mast-cells are based on the metachromatic properties of the cytoplasmic granules and showed limited:

1. the positivity of the mast cells varies according the technique used to fix and stain (Strobel et all., 1981);
2. the counts in the tissue 'post-mortem' after the anaphylaxis is underestimated because of the mast cells' degranulation during anaphylaxis. The staining can't put in evidence the degranulated mast cells; so, because the number of mast cells varies from each one it's impossible decide how many cells have degranulated.
3. the base -level of mast-cell concentration after death is strongly underestimated.

In literature, however, there is a case (Heard et all., 1989) where the authors compare the pulmonary concentration of mast-cells in the allergic subject pre- (biopsy) and post-mortem showing a diminution in the latter sections.

3.5 Auxiliary techniques: histochemical and immuno-histochemical

Since histology alone cannot give absolute results, it have been studied more complex techniques such as histochemistry and immuno-histochemistry.

In 1960 Glenner and Cohen (Glenner & Cohen, 1960) identified the proteases of mast cell granules using histo-chemical procedures. The main morphologic characteristic to distinguish mast cells is the presence, in cytoplasm, of many roundish granules, homogeneous in man, soluble in water, that stain methacromatically with basic dyes such as Toluidine blue, or with dyes for glycosaminoglycans polymerized such as Alcian blue. The granules are coated with membrane and contain heparin and histamine. In particular, the presence of heparin, an anticoagulant glycosaminoglycan, accounts for the staining of these granules. In the anaphylaxis the massive degranulation could be emphasized with this technique with the highlight of the granules next to mast cells. Furthermore it has been identified antibodies against histamine but they are not useful for post-mortem evaluation since histamine is poorly stable (Johansson et al., 1992)

Pagoda red stain is another histo-chemical procedure successfully employed for the histological demonstration of several substances with fibrillar periodical structure, like amyloids (Battaglia et al., 1985; Yanagihara et al. 1984), cellulose, siloxanes, polysiloxanes and polyethylene polymers and more rarely to put in evidence eosinophilia in various tissues (Kyono et al, 1982). This technique displays a mixing of cytotypes, contemporaneously on the same slide, easily identifiable, since degranulated mast cells and their outside granules appear brilliant red over a pale blue background (Trani et al., 2008).

Cytotypes	EMBP	Chymase	Tryptase	CD117	Pagoda red
Eosinophils	++	-	-	-	+++
Mast cell	-	+++	+++	-	+++

- negative reaction ++ moderate reaction +++ strong reaction

Table 2. Panel of identification of eosinophils and mast cells: a comparative evaluation (Trani et al. 2008).

Pagoda Red stain is a dye originally employed in the industrial field to dye clothes and occasionally carried out in cytopathology in case of nasal (Rivasi & Bergamini, 1988) or ocular (Rivasi et al., 1992) allergic processes possibly related to the presence of airborne, nonhuman elements.

Immuno-histo-chemical investigations although more expensive than histo-chemical ones allow to characterize the immuno-phenotype of the various cells in the inflammatory infiltrate associated with anaphylaxis; especially specific antibodies can bind superficial antigens in these cells such as tryptases and chymases (Akin et al. 2007; Carson & Cook, 2009; Irani et al., 1989; Perskvist & Edston, 2007).

Human mast cell tryptases comprise a family of trypsin-like neutral serine proteases that are predominantly expressed in mast cells. This antibody is useful for the identification of very atypical or immature mast cells (MC) in mast cell leukemia, and for the detection of small, even minute, dense focal MC infiltrates in staging procedures in patients with known cutaneous mastocytosis. Using an avidin-biotin enhanced immunoperoxidase procedure, with monoclonal antibodies (AA1, AA3, and AA5) directed against human mast cell tryptase, it's possible to obtain an intense staining of mast cells in paraffin-embedded tissue. It represents an highly specific and sensitive means for the detection of mast cells in routinely processed tissues.

Chymases belong to a family of serine proteases like intracellular granule and it's involved in regulating extracellular matrix proteolysis and promoting tissue remodelling (Doggrell & Wanstall, 2004). This substance is mainly found in mast cell cytoplasm but also outside the mast cells in the connective tissues surrounding vascular walls and, in less concentration, in basophils. (Hamada et al. 1999). Chymase antibodies is available for formaldehyde-fixed tissue and can be used simultaneously to tryptase by a sandwich technique applying the two antibody (Buckley et al. 1999).

The eosinophilic major basic protein, also known as MBP, PRG2, a proteoglycan 2, BMPG or bone marrow natural killer cell activator, is a constituent of the eosinophilic granules. High levels of the pro-EMBP are present in pregnancy serum and in placenta where it develops a complex with other proteins. It may influence antiparasitic defense mechanisms as cytotoxin and helminthotoxin and immune hypersensitivity reactions (Trocme et al. 1989).

The role of EMBP is to modulate inflammation and lead to tissue destruction resulting in cytotoxic effects (Butterworth & David, 1981). It has been demonstrated to be elicited in mast cell and basophil (Trocme et al. 1989) degranulation.

4. Conclusions

Post-mortem diagnosis of anaphylactic death is very difficult and it's possible only excluding every other cause of death and taking into considerations the results of other exams: accurate medical history, complete necroscopic examination integrated with histological examination, lab tests, and auxiliary techniques of histochemistry and immuno-histo-chemistry. This diagnosis, in particular for the medico-legal aspect, cannot be based on the positivity of one only type of investigation (e.g. bioumoral tests) because that positivity can be found also in other pathologies (Horn, 2004) but must be integrated with the results of more investigations.

5. Acknowledgment

Many thanks to Aldo Ferrucci and Mr Vidic for their kind patience and to everyone that supported the authors in writing this chapter.

6. References

Akin, C.; Scott, L.M.; Kocabas, C.N.; Kushnir-Sukhov, N.; Brittain, E.; Noel, P.; Metcalfe, D.D. (2007) Demonstration of an aberrant mast-cell population with clonal markers in a subset of patients with "idiopathic" anaphylaxis. *Blood,* Vol. 110, No. 7, (October 2007), pp. (2331–2333), ISSN 0006-4971

Ansari, M.Q.; Zamora, J.L.; Lipscomb, M.F.; (1993) Postmortem diagnosis of acute anaphylaxis by serum tryptase analysis: a case report. *American Journal of Clinical Pathology,* Vol. 99, No. 1, (January 1993), pp. (101–103), ISSN 0002-9173

Barnard, J.H. (1967) Allergic and pathologic findings in fifthy insect-sting fatalities. *The Journal of Allergy,* Vol. 40, No. 2, (August 1967), pp. 107-114), ISSN 0021-8707

Battaglia, S.; Barbolini, G.; Botticelli, A.R.; Trentini, G.P. (1985) Apoptotic amyloid: a study on prostatic amyloidosis with particular reference to corpora amylacea. *International Academy of Pathology.* Vol. 3, No. 1-2, pp. (105-114), ISSN 0252-1172

Bernstein, D.I.; Wanner, M.; Borish, L.; Liss, G.M.; The Immunoteraphy Committee of the American Academy of Allergy, Asthma and Immunology. (2004) Twelve-year survey of fatal reactions to allergen injections and skin testing: 1990-2001. *The Journal of Allergy and Clinical Immunology,* Vol. 113, No. 6, (June 2004), pp. (1129-1136), ISSN 0091-6749

Blanton, W.B.; Sutphin, A.K. (1949). Death during skin testing. *The American journal of the medical sciences,* Vol. 217, No. 2, (February 1949), pp. (169-173), ISSN 0002-9629

Bonelli, A.; Bacci, S.; Norelli, G.A. (2003). Affinity cytochemistry analysis of mast cells in skin lesions: a possible tool to assess the timing of lesions after death. *International Journal of Legal Medicine,* Vol. 117, No. 6, (December 2003), pp. (331–334), ISSN 0937-9827

Buckley, M.G.; McEuen, A.R.; Walls, A.F. (1999) The detection of mast cell subpopulations in formalin-fixed human tissues using a new monoclonal antibody specific for chymase. *Jthe Journal of Pathololy,* Vol. 189, No. 1, (September 1999), pp. (138-143), ISSN 0022-3417

Buckley, M.G.; Variend, S.; Walls, A.F. (2001) Elevated serum concentrations of beta-tryptase, but not alpha-tryptase in Sudden Infant Death Syndrome: investigation of anaphylactic mechanisms. *Clinical and experimental allergy,* Vol. 31, No. 11, (November 2001), pp. (1696-1704), ISNN 0954-7894

Butterworth, A.E.; David, J.R. (1981) Eosinophil function. *N Engl J Med,* Vol. 304, No. 3, (January 1981), pp. 154-156, ISSN 0028-4793

Calvani, M.; Cardinale, F.; Martelli. A.; Muraro, M.A.; Pucci. N.; Savino, F. (2007) *Anafilassi in pediatria,* Springer-Verlag Italia, ISBN 978-88-470-0620-1, Milano, Italia

Carson, H.J.; Cook, B.A. (2009) Mast cell tryptase in a case of anaphylaxis due to repeat antibiotic exposure. *Legal medicine (Tokyo),* Vol. 11, No. 5, (September 2009), pp. (234-236), ISNN 1344-6223

Crane, J.; von Mutius, E.; Custovic, A.; (2006) Epidemiology of allergic disease. In: Holgate ST, Church MK, Lichtenstein LM, eds, *Allergy* 3rd ed. Mosby Elsevier, pp. (233-246), Elsevier Ltd., ISBN 0323032273, London, U.K.

Da Broi, U.; Moreschi, C. (2011) Post-mortem diagnosis of anaphylaxis: a difficult task in forensic medicine. *Forensic Science International.* Vol. 204, No. 1-3, (January 2011), pp. (1-5), ISSN 0379-0738

D'Errico, S.; Neri, M.; Riezzo, I.; Rossi, G.; Pomara, C.; Turillazzi, E.; Fineschi, V. (2008) Beta-tryptase and quantitative mast-cell increase in a sudden infant death following hexavalent immunization. *Forensic Science International.* Vol. 179, No. 2-3, (August 2008), pp. (25-29), ISSN 0379-0738

Delage, C.; Irey N.S., (1972) Anaphylactic deaths: a clinicopathologic study of 43 cases, *Journal of Forensic Sciences,* Vol. 17, No. 4, (October 1972), pp. (525–540), ISSN: 0022-1198

Di Maio, V.J.; Di Maio, D. (2001) *Forensic Pathology,* second ed., CRC Press, ISBN 0-8493-0072-X, Boca Raton, USA

Doggrell, S.A.; Wanstall, J.C. (2004) Vascular chymase: pathophysiological role and therapeutic potential of inhibition. *Cardiovascular research,* Vol. 61, No. 4, (March (2004), pp. 653-662, ISSN 0008-6363

Edston, E.; Eriksson, O.; Van Hage, M.; (2007) Mast cell tryptase in postmortem serum-reference values and confounders, *International Journal of Legal Medicine,* Vol. 121, No. 4, (July 2007), pp. (275–280), ISSN 0937-9827

Edston, E.; Gidlund, E.; Wickman, M.; Ribbing, H., van Hage-Hamsten, M. (1999) Increased mast cell tryptase in sudden infant death syndrome--anaphylaxis,hypoxia or artefact? *Clinical and experimental allergy* Vol. 29, No. 12, (December 1999), pp. (1648-1654), ISNN 0954-7894

Edston, E.; Van Hage-Hamsten, M.; (2005) Diagnosis of Anaphylaxis in: *Forensic Pathology Reviews,* Vol. 3, part. 6, Tsokos, M., pp. (267-281), Humana Press, ISBN 978-1-59259-910-3, Totowa, New Jersey

Eleuterio Gonzàlez, J.; Leal de Hernàndez, L.; Gonzàlez Spencer, D. (1997) Anaphylactic reaction caused by the performance of skin tests: report of a case. *Revista Alergia México,* Vol. 44, No. 3, (May-June 1997), pp. (74-76), ISSN 0002-5151

Fauci, A.S.; Barunwald, E.; Kasper, L.; Hauser, S.L.; Longo, D.L.; Jameson, J.L.; Loscalzo, J.; (2009). Anafilassi, In: *Harrison-Principi di medicina interna,* Mc Graw Hill, pp (114-115), ISBN: 9788838624629, Milano, Italy

Glenner, G.G.; Cohen, L.A. (1960) Histochemical demonstration of a species-specific trypsin-like enzyme in mast cells. *Nature,* Vol. 185, (March 1960), pp. (846-847), ISSN 0028-0836

Greenberger, P.A.; Rotskoff B.D.; Lifschultz, B. (2007) Fatal anaphylaxis: postmortem findings and associated comorbid diseases. *Annals of allergy, asthma & immunology,* Vol. 98, No. 3, (March 2007), pp. (252-257), ISSN 1081-1206

Hamada, H.; Terai, M.; Kimura, H.; Hirano, K.; Oana, S.; Nimi, H. (1999) Increased expression of mast cell chymase in the lungs of patients with congenital heart disease associated with early pulmonary vascular disease. *American journal of respiratory and critical care medicine,* Vol. 160, No. 4, (October 1999), pp. 1303-1308, ISSN 1073-449X

Hamilton, R.G.; Adkinson, N.F.jr. (2003) 23. Clinical and laboratory assessment of IGE-dependent hypersensitivity. *The Journal of allergy and clinical immunology,* Vol. 111, No. 2 suppl., (February 2003), pp. 687-701, ISSN 1534-4436

Hard, B.E.; Nunn, A.J.; Kay, A.B. (1989) Mast cells in human lungs *Journal of Pathology,* Vol. 157, No. 1, (January 1989), pp. 59-63, ISSN 0022-3417

Harris, M.C.; Shure, N. (1950) Sudden death due to allergy tests. *The Journal of Allergy,* Vol. 21, No. 3 (May 1950), pp. (208-216), ISSN 0021-8707

Hieda, Y.; Kageura, M.; Hara, K.; Kashimura, S. (1991) Postmortem changes in hapten-specific IgE antibody responses in mice. *International Journal of Legal Medicine,* Vol. 104, No. 3, pp. (133-135), ISSN 0937-9827

Holgate, S.; Waiters, C.; Walls, A.F., Lawrance, S.; Shell, D.J.; Variend, S.; Fleming, P.J.; Berry, P.J.; Gilbert, R.E.; Robinson, C. (1994) The anaphylaxis hypothesis of sudden infant death syndrome (SIDS): mast cell degranulation in cot death revealed by elevated concentrations of tryptase in serum. *Clinical and experimental allergy,* Vol. 24, No. 12, pp. (1115-1122), ISSN 0954-7894.

Horn, K.D.; Halsey, J.F.; Zumwalt, R.E. (2004) Utilization of serum tryptase and immunoglobulin E assay in the postmortem diagnosis of anaphylaxis. *The American journal of forensic medicine and pathology,* Vol. 25, No. 1 (March 2004), pp. 37-43), ISSN 0195-7910

Irani, A.M.; Bradford, T.R.; Kepley, C.L.; Schechter, N.M.; Schwartz, L.B. (1989) Detection of MCT and MCTC types of human mast cells by immunohistochemistry using new monoclonal anti-tryptase and anti-chymase antibodies *The journal of histochemistry and cytochemistry,* Vol. 37, No. 10, (October 1989), pp. (1509-1515), ISSN 0022-1554

Irani, A.M.; Schwartz, L.B. (1994). Human mast cell heterogeneity. *Allergy Proceedings,* Vol. 15, No. 6, (November-December 1994), pp. (303–308), ISSN 1046-9354

James, L.P.; Austen K.F. (1964) Fatal systemic anaphylaxis in man. *The New England Journal of Medicine.* Vol. 270, (March 1964), pp. (597-603), ISSN 0028-4793

Johann-Liang, R.; Josephs, S.; Dreskin, S.C.; (2011). Analysis of anaphylaxis cases after vaccination: 10-year review from the national vaccine injury compensation. *Annals of allergy, asthma, and immunology,* Vol. 106, No. 5, (May 2011), pp. (440-443), ISSN 1534-4436

Johansson, O.; Virtanen, M.; Hilliges, M.; Yang, Q. (1992) Histamine immunohistochemistry: a new and highly sensitive method for studying cutaneous mast cells. *The Histochemical journal.* Vol. 24, No. 5, (May 1992), pp. (283-287), ISSN 0018-2214

Joint Task Force on Practice Parameters, American Academy of Allergy, Asthma and Immunology, American College of Allergy, Asthma and Immunology, and the Joint Council of Allergy, Asthma and Immunology. (1998) The diagnosis and management of anaphylaxis. *The Journal of allergy and clinical immunology,* Vol. 101, (June 1998) pp. (465-528), ISNN 0091-6749

Joint Task Force on Practice Parameters; American Academy of Allergy, Asthma and Immunology; American College of Allergy, Asthma and Immunology; Joint Council of Allergy, Asthma and Immunology. (2005) The diagnosis and management of anaphylaxis: an updated practice parameter. *The Journal of allergy and clinical immunology,* Vol. 115, No. 3 suppl. 2, (March 2005), pp. (483-523), ISNN 0091-6749

Kanthawatana, S.; Carias, K.; Arnaout, R.; Hu, J.; Irani, A.M.; Schwartz, L.B. (1999) The potential clinical utility of serum alpha-protryptase levels. *The Journal of allergy and clinical immunology,* Vol. 103, No. 6, (June 1999), pp. (1092-1099), ISSN 0091-6749

Kiyono, J.; Tada, T.; Wakabayashi, T.; Kishimoto, H.; Nitta, M. (1982) Eosinophile granule staining with Dylon. *Rinsho Byori.* Vol. 30, No. 10, (October 1982), pp. (1137-1141), ISSN 0047-1860

Lang, D.M.; Alpern, M.B.; Visintainer, P.F.; Smith, S.T. (1995) Gender risk for anaphylactoid reaction to radiographic contrast media. *The Journal of Allergy and Clinical Immunology;* Vol. 95, No. 4, (April 1995), pp. (813-817), ISSN 0091-6749

Liccardi, G.; D'Amato, G.; Canonica, G.W.; Salzillo, A.; Piccolo, A.; Passalacqua, G. (2006) Systemic reactions from skin testing: literature review, *Journal of investigational allergology & clinical immunology,* Vol. 16, No. 2, pp. (75-78), ISSN 1018-9068

Lieberman, P.; Nicklas, R.A.; Oppenheimer, J.; Kemp, S.F.; Lang, D.M.; Bernstein, D.I.; Bernstein, J.A.; Burks, A.W.; Feldweg, A.M.; Fink, J.N.; Greenberger, P.A.; Golden, D.B.; James, J.M.; Kemp, S.F.; Ledford, D.K.; Lieberman, P.; Sheffer, A.L.; Bernstein, D.I.; Blessing-Moore, J.; Cox, L.; Khan, D.A.; Lang, D.; Nicklas, R.A.; Oppenheimer, J.; Portnoy, J.M.; Randolph, C.; Schuller, D.E.; Spector, S.L.; Tilles, S.; Wallace, D. (2010) The diagnosis and management of anaphylaxis practice parameter: 2010 update. *The Journal of allergy and clinical immunology.* Vol. 126, No. 3, (September 2010), pp. (477-480), ISSN 0091-6749

Lockey, R.F.; Benedict, L.M.; Turkeltaub, P.C.; Bukantz, S.C. (1987) Fatalities from immunotherapy and skin testing. *The Journal of allergy and clinical immunology.* Vol. 79, No. 4, (April 1987), pp. (660-677), ISSN 0091-6749

Low, I.; Stables, S. (2006) Anaphylactic deaths in Auckland, New Zealand: a review of coronial autopsies from 1985 to 2005. *Pathology,* Vol. 38, No. 4, (August 2006), pp. 328-332), ISSN 0031-3025

Lu, P.; Bao, C.S.; Wang, L.X. (2006) Analysis on 27 autopsy cases died of anaphylactic shock induced by mainline. *Fa Yi Xue Za Zhi,* Vol. 22, No. 4, (August 2006), pp. (305-306), ISSN 1004-5619

Menchel, S.M.; Gorevic, P.D.; Adkinson, N.F. (1987) An immunologic approach to the evaluation of deaths due to penicillin anaphylaxis, *Proceedings of the 39th Annual Meeting of the American Academy of forensic sciences,* San Diego, February 1987

Moneret-Vautrin, D.A. (2007) Allergic risk and role of the Allergy Vigilance Network, *Bulletin de l'Académie nationale de médecine.* Vol. 191, No. 4-5, (April-May 2007), pp. (807-814), ISSN 0001-4079

Moneret-Vautrin, D.A.; Kanny, G.; Parisot, L. (2002) First survey from the "Allergy Vigilance Network": life-threatening food allergies in France. *Allergie et immunologie,* Vol. 34, No. 6, (June 2002), pp. (194-198), ISSN 0397-9148

Nishio, H.; Takai, S.; Miyazaki, M.; Horiuchi, H.; Osawa, M.; Uemura, K.; Yoshida, K.; Mukaida, M.; Ueno, K.; Suzuki, K. (2005) Usefulness of serum mast cell-specific chymase levels for postmortem diagnosis of anaphylaxis. *International Journal of Legal Medicine,* Vol. 119, No. 6, (November 2005), pp. (331–334), ISSN 0937-9827

Nishio, H.; Suzuki, K. (2004) Serum tryptase levels in sudden infant death syndrome in forensic autopsy cases. *Forensic Science International,* Vol.139, No. 1, (January 2004), pp. (57-60), ISSN 0379-0738

Osawa, M.; Satoh, F.; Horiuchi, H.; Tian, W.; Kugota, N.; Hasegawa, I. (2008) Postmortem diagnosis of fatal anaphylaxis during intravenous administration of therapeutic and diagnostic agents: evaluation of clinical laboratory parameters and immunohistochemistry in three cases. *Legal medicine (Tokyo).* Vol. 10, No. 3, (May 2008), pp. (143-147), ISSN 1344-6223

Perskvist, N.; Edston, E. (2007) Differential accumulation of pulmonary and cardiac mast-cell-subsets and eosinophils between fatal anaphylaxis and asthma death. A postmortem comparative study. *Forensic Science International,* Vol. 169, No. 1, (June 2007), pp. (43-49), ISSN 0379-0738

Pumphrey, R.S.H; Roberts, I.S. (2000) Postmortem findings after fatal anaphylactic reactions. *Journal of Clinical Pathology.* Vol. 53, No. 4, (April 2000), pp (273-276), ISSN: 0021-9746

Pumphrey, R.S.H (2000) Lessons for management of anaphylaxis from a study of fatal reactions. *Clinical and Experimental Allergy.* Vol. 30, No. 8, (August 2000), pp. (1144-1150), ISSN 0954-7894

Pumphrey, R. S. H.; (2008) Fatal Anaphylaxis in the UK, 1992–2001, in Anaphylaxis: Novartis Foundation Symposium 257 (eds G. Bock and J. Goode), pp. (116-132), John Wiley & Sons, Ltd, ISBN: 9780470861196, Chichester, UK

Randall, B.; Butts, J.; Halsey, J.F. (1995) Elevated postmortem tryptase in the absence of anaphylaxis. *Journal of Forensic Science.* Vol. 40, No. 2, (March 1995), pp. (208-211), ISSN 0022-1198

Riches, K.J.; Gills, D.; James, R.A. (2002) An autopsy approach to bee sting-related deaths. *Pathology;* Vol. 34, No. 3, (June 2002), pp. (257–262), ISSN: 0031-3025

Richet, C.; (1902) Des effets anaphylactiques de l'actinotoxine sur la pressi on artérielle, *Comptes rendus des séances de la Société de biologie et de ses filiales.* 54, pp. 837-838, Available from: http://www.biodiversitylibrary.org/pdf3/005324000100655.pdf

Riezzo, I.; Bello, S.; Neri, M.; Turillazzi, E.; Fineschi, V. (2010) Ceftriaxone intradermal test-related fatal anaphylactic shock: a medico-legal nightmare. *Allergy,* Vol. 65, No. 1, (January 2010), pp. (130-131), ISSN 0105-4538

Risgaard, O.; Søe, C.K.; Zejden, A. (2008) Lethal reaction after contrast medium administration. *Ugeskr Laeger.* Vol. 170, No. 17, (April 2008), p. (1474), ISSN 0041-5782

Rivasi, F.; Bergamini, G. (1988) Nasal cytology in allergenic processes and other syndromes caused by hyperreactivity. *Diagnostic cytopathology,* Vol. 4, No. 2, pp. (99–105), ISSN 8755-1039

Rivasi, F.; Cavallini, G.M.; Longanesi, L. (1992) Cytology of allergenic conjunctivitis. Presence of airbone, non human elements. *Acta cytologica,* Vol. 36, No. 4, (July-August 1992), pp. (492–498), ISSN 0001-5547

Roberts, I.S.D.; Pumphrey, R.S.H. (2001) The autopsy in fatal anaphylaxis. In *Recent Advances in Histopathology*. Vol. 19, Lowe, D.G.; Underwood J.C.E., pp. (145-162), Churchill Livingstone, ISBN 0443063478, London, U.K.

Rovere-Querini, P. (2010) Anafilassi, In: *Medicina interna sistematica,* C. Rugarli., p. (1632-1633), Elservier, ISBN 8821431096, Milano, Italy

Sampson, H.A.; Mendelson, L.; Rosen, J.P. (1992) Fatal and near-fatal anaphylactic reactions to food in children and adolescents. *The New England Journal of Medicine.* Vol. 327, No. 6, (August 1992), pp. (380-384), ISSN 0028-4793

Schwartz, L.B. (1987) Mediators of human mast cells and human mast cell subsets. *Annals of Allergy*. Vol. 58, No. 4, (April 1987), pp. (226–235), ISSN 0003-4738

Schwartz, L.B. (2000) Effector cells of anaphylaxis: mast cells and basophils. *Novartis Foundation symposium.* Vol. 257, pp. 65-74, pp. (65-74), ISSN 1528-2511

Schwartz, L.B. (2001) Light is recognized best through darkness: mast cells and Sudden Infant Death Syndrome. *Clinical and experimental allergy,* Vol. 31, No. 11, (November 2001), pp. (1657-1659), ISNN 0954-7894

Schwartz, L.B.; Irani A.M. (2000) Serum tryptase and the laboratory diagnosis of systemic mastocytosis. *Hematology/oncology clinics of North America,* Vol. 14, No. 3, (June 2000), pp. 641-657, ISSN 0889-8588

Schwartz, L.B.; Sakai, K.; Bradford, T.R.; Ren, S.; Zwelman, B.; Worobec, A.S.; Metcalfe, D.D. (1995) The alpha form of human tryptase is the predominant type present in blood at base line in normal subjects and is elevated in those with systemic mastocytosis. *The Journal of clinical investigation,* Vol. 96, No. 6, (December 1995), pp. (2702–2710), ISSN 0021-9738

Shen, Y.; Li, L.; Grant, J.; Rubio, A.; Zhao, Z.; Zhang, X.; Zhou, L.; Fowler, D. (2009) Anaphylactic death in maryland (United States) and Shangai (China): a rewiew of forensic autopsy cases from 2004 to 2006. *Forensic Science International,* Vol. 186, No. 1-3, (April 2009), pp. (1-5), ISSN 0379-0738

Shen, Y.W.; Lu, C.; Zhao, Z.Q. (2002) Tryptase and fatal anaphylaxic reaction. *Fa Yi Xue Za Zhi,* Vol. 18, No. 3, (August 2002), pp. 132-134, ISSN 1004-5619

Stephan, V.; Zimmermann, A.; Kühr, J., Urbanek, R. (1990) Determination of N-methylhistamine in urine as an indicator of histamine release in immediate allergic reactions. *The Journal of allergy and clinical immunology.* Vol. 86, No. 6 part 1, (December 1990), pp. 862-868, ISSN 0091-6749

Strobel, S.; Miller, H.R.; Ferguson, A. (1981) Human intestinal mucosal mast cells: evaluation of fixation and staining techniques. *Journal of clinical pathology,* Vol. 34, No. 8, (August 1981), pp. (851-858), ISSN 0021-9746

Trani, N.; Bonetti Reggiani, L.; Gualandri, G.; Barbolini, G. (2008) Immediate anaphylactic death following antibiotics injection: splenic eosinophilia easily revealed by pagoda red stain. *Forensic Science International.* Vol. 181, No. 1-3, (October 2008), pp. (21-25), ISSN 0379-0738

Trocme, S.D.; Kephart, G.M.; Allansmith, M.R.; Bourne, W.M.; Gleich, G.J. (1989) Conjunctival deposition of eosinophil granule major basic protein in vernal conjunctivitis and contact lens-associated giant papillary conjunctivitis. *American journal of ophthalmology,* Vol. 108, No. 1, (July 1989), pp. (57-63), ISSN 0002-9394

Urata, H.; Kinoshita, A.; Misono, K.S.; Bumpus, F.M.; Husain, A. (1990) Identification of a highly specific chymase as the major angiotensin II-forming enzyme in human heart. *The Journal of Biological Chemists,* Vol. 265, No. 36, (December 1990), pp. (22348–22357), ISSN 0021-9258

Vance, B.M.; Strassmann, G.; (1942) Sudden death following injection of foreign protein. *Archives of Pathology*; Vol. 34 , pp (849-865)

Voigt, J. (1966) Eosinophils in the spleen in cases of lethal anaphylactic shock. *Medicine, science, and the law,* Vol. 6, No. 3, (July 1966), pp. (162-163), ISSN 0025-8024

Way, M.G.; Baxendine, C.L. (2002) The significance of post mortem tryptase levels in supporting a diagnosis of anaphylaxis. *Anaesthesia.* Vol. 57, No. 3, (March 2002), pp. (310-311), ISSN 0003-2409

Weber-Mani, U.; Pichler, W.J. (2008) Anaphylactic shock after intradermal testing with betalactam antibiotics. *Allergy,* Vol. 63, No. 6, (June 2008), pp. (785), ISSN 0105-4538

Weedn, W. (1988) Anaphylactic death (Letters to the Editor), *Journal of Forensic Sciences,* Vol. 33, No. 5, (September 1988), pp. (1108–1110), ISSN: 0022-1198

Weidner, N.; Austen, K.F. (1993) Heterogeneity of mast cells at multiple body site. Flurorescent determination of avidin binding and immunofluorescent determination of chymase, tryptase and carboxypeptidase content. *Pathology, Research and Practice,* Vol. 189, No. 2, (March 1993), pp. (156–162), ISSN 0344-0338

Yanagihara, M.; Mehregan, A.H.; Mehregan, D.R. (1984) Staining of amyloid with cotton dyes. *Archives of Dermatology.* Vol. 120, No. 9, (September 1984), pp. (1184-1185), ISSN 0003-987X

Yilmaz, R.; Yuksekbas, O.; Erkol, Z.; Bulut, E.R.; Arslan, M.N. (2009). Postmortem findings after anaphylactic reactions to drugs in Turkey. *The American journal of forensic medicine and pathology* ,Vol. 30, No.4, (December 2009), pp. 346-349, ISSN 0195-7910

Yunginger, J.W.; Nelson, D.R.; Squillace D.L.; Jones, R.T.; Holley, K.E.; Hyma, B.A.; Biedrzycki, L.; Sweeney, K.G.; Sturner, W.Q.; Schwartz, L.B.; (1991) Laboratory investigation of deaths due to anaphylaxis. *Journal of Forensic Sciences,* Vol. 36, No. 3, (May 1991), pp. (857–865), ISSN: 0022-1198

5

Forensic Age Estimation in Unaccompanied Minors and Young Living Adults

Andreas Schmeling[1], Pedro Manuel Garamendi[2], Jose Luis Prieto[3] and María Irene Landa[4]
[1]*Forensic Physician Institute of Legal Medicine of Münster*
[2]*Forensic Physician Council of Forensic Medicine of Istanbul*
[3]*Forensic Physician Complutense University of Madrid*
[4]*Forensic Phsycian Institute of legal Medicine of the Basque Country*
[1]*Germany*
[2]*Turkey*
[3,4]*Spain*

1. Introduction

1.1 FAE a need in nowadays everyday forensic practice

Forensic Age Estimation (FAE) defines an expertise in forensic medicine which aims to define in the most accurate way the chronological age of person of an unknown age involved in judicial or legal proceedings. The term "estimation" defines more precisely than other as "diagnosis" the real limits inherent to this expertise. The state of the art in FAE is such that nowadays there is no medical test or a group of tests that absolutely and accurately let us know the exact chronological age of a human being (Ritz Timme et al., 2000).

Nevertheless, in everyday practice, Justice Courts and other Public Institutions require this type of experts reports to forensic physicians and Legal Medicine Institutes. In this expertise it´s needed a collaborative knowledge of very diverse disciplines like Forensic and Physical Anthropology, Odontology and even some general medical specialities like Radiology of Pediatrics all of them ideally centered in Legal Medicine Institutes.

FAE is not at all a recent field of expertise in Forensic Sciences and Judiciary History. In old Roman Empire, the eruption of second molar indicated the moment in which a young male was considered for military service (Schmeling, 2008). During XIX century age estimation was mainly performed by dentists. In 1837, Edwing Saunders published "The Teeth a Test of Age" and British Parlament decided to teeth eruption as an accurate method to determine the age of kids. At those ages, minimum criminal age was 7 years old in Britain and also in 1883 minimum required age for mining workers was 9 years. Nevertheless, at that time, also some voices expressed their criticism with this practice for an age estimation. In 1846, Dr. Pedro Mata in his text book of Legal Medicine expressed his concern on assuring without any kind of a doubt an age estimation based solely on teeth eruption (Mata, 1846).

In 1895, Röntgen discovered X rays. His discover opens a new dimension for age estimation in living subjects. The applications of his discovery in Legal Medicine were nearly immediate and age estimation in living subjects rapidly changed to include these new tests based on radiographies of the skeleton as a complement to the teeth eruption classical methods. In 1886 in Munchen, Angerer was first to suggest that radiographies from carpus could be indicator of an age in young persons (Brogdon, 1998). In 1887, Behrendsen published the first systematic review of age variations in carpus (Schmeling, 2008).

During the next 40 years, different researches focused in defining the standard radiological maturation of human skeleton with age (Stevenson,1924; Flecker,1933; Galstaun, 1937; Sidhom & Derry, 1931; Pryor, 1908; Borovansky & Hnévkovsky, 1927; Davies & Parsons, 1927; Paterson, 1929; Meenes & Holly, 1932; Adair & Scammon, 1921). The lack of consciousness on the harms inherent to X-rays exposure lead to a massive amount of X-rays expositions only on investigation purposes. Between decades of 50 to 80 of XX century, main definitive methods of age estimation based on radiological analysis of carpus (Greulich & Pyle, 1959; Tanner et al, 1983) and dental maturation (Nolla, 1960; Demirjian, 1975) were defined.

Until recent years, forensic physicians in European Countries weren´t usually required for a FAE in living subjects. Census and Birth Registration in Europe was really accurate and only exceptionally an expert report was needed to assess an age of a European citizen. But in the last two decades European countries have received a flood of immigrants from extracommunitarian countries. In many cases these non European citizens don´t have any documents that ascertain their chronological age or there are doubts on the certainty of chronological age alleged. This situation is specially complex in a case of an immigrant supposedly minor of age. European Legislation and International Traits assure an special treatment of these immigrant minors when they are unaccompanied and they must be consider under the trusteeship of European authorities. This special treatment must also be assured in case of criminal proceedings in which minors have a special protection as victims and also as responsible of criminal activities. In all those cases, Justice Courts and Public Institutions require forensic doctors a FAE expert report (European Migration Network, 2010).

It´s very difficult to ascertain the total number of immigrants supposedly minors unaccompanied with an known chronological age in European Countries. In our legal framework, unaccompanied minors is the term to define this population. There are many different reasons in each European country to determine the uncertainty of a statistics on the total number of unaccompanied minors. In countries like Germany or Spain, the division of the Government in Lander or Autonomous Communities turn difficult to maintain a central register of minors unaccompanied. In most European Countries it was also observed that many minors under trusteeship of authorities suddenly disappear from the asylum institutions. Some studies also stress the fact that there is a group of minors unaccompanied who don´t seek for asylum and they keep as immigrants in many European cities unknown to the authorities (European Migration Network, 2010).

During 2008 in Germany the census of minors unaccompanied was a total of 763 subjects. From these 324 were up to 15 years old and 438 were aged 16 to 17. Most of them were detected at the airports and they came mainly from Iraq and Afghanistan during 2007 and 2008. During 2003 to 2006, the most usual nationalities were Turkish and Chinese, and other nationalities more unusual were Russian, Serbian, Vietnamese and Nigerian (Federal Office for Migration and Refugees, 2009).

In Spain, the census of unaccompanied minors by the end of 2008 was an estimation of 6000 minors under trusteeship of Spanish authorities. Nearly all of them came from Magreb and

Sahel African Subsaharian countries, being most usual nationality Moroccan. Until 2003 most of them arrived at Spain inside trucks and industrial vehicles crossing Mediterranean Sea in Algeciras (Andalucia). Since 2003, this changed and most of the minors detected arrived at Southern Spanish and Canary Islands coast by sea in "pateras" or "cayucos", different light and dangerous boats that illegally cross Atlantic and Mediterranean sea waters (Bravo, 2005; PICUM, 2008).

In both cases, Spain and Germany, nearly all of the unaccompanied minors are male. Only in Somalian nationality girls are more frequent than boys (Bueno & Mestre, 2006; European Migration Network, 2010).

Nowadays, there is still no consensus in European countries on which methods must be applied when an age estimation of a supposedly minor is needed. All Member States attempt to determine this using a variety of techniques. European Statistical data are also uncertain about the methods really applied in every country. Nevertheless, official data from EU indicate that in some countries like United Kingdom authorities usually only apply an interview with the minor by a social worker without a medicine doctor examination. UK Border Agency accepts the "Merton compliant age assessment" carried out bt two specially trained social workers when assessing the individual´s asylum claim, unless there is evidence to the contrary. On the other side, Austria since 2010 applies the so called "multifactorial examination methodology" that consists of three elements: an inspection by a doctor, a dental analysis and X-ray examinations, the latter performed only with the consent of the minor. If the age of the minor cannot be determined exactly, the benefit of the doubt is given to the individual concerned. In France, also a psychological interview is used for age estimations of unaccompanied minors. In six out of all Member States no skeletal development estimation by radiographies was applied and in other eight ones no dental analysis was performed (European Migration Network, 2010).

ACNUR has recently recommended EU authorities to unify methodology applied in age estimation to ensure the protection of children and the defense of immigrants Human Rights in Member States. Different international groups of experts have published guidelines and recommendations on FAE, like American Board of Forensic Odontologists (ABFO), International Organization for Forensic Odonto-Stomatology (IOFOS) or Study Group of Age Estimation of the German Society of Legal Medicine (AGFAD). This chapter aims to spread these recommendations on FAE by these international groups of experts (UNHCR, 2000,2001,2002).

2. Methods

2.1 Selection of the methods

In the infant and juvenile stage the use of morphological methods based on radiological examination of dental and skeletal development is recommended (Ritz Timme et al., 2000).

However, the methodology employed varies, while the criteria followed internationally for official application of these techniques are disparate, with some countries arguing the dubious validity that much scientific research currently accords this type of proof, whose margins of error do not permit the diagnostic reliability required in such cases (UNHCR, 2000, 2001, 2002). For this reason, in certain countries X-ray tests are only used in criminal cases (Solari & Abramovitz, 20202). Despite this, the programs developed by official institutions and NGOs have established protocols of good practice which include the elements corresponding to age assessment (UNHCR, 1997).

In accordance to the guidelines proposed by Ritz-Timme et al for an age assessment method to be considered acceptable, it must fulfill the following requirements:

1. The method must be transparent and provable, presented to the scientific community, as a rule by publication in peer-reviewed journals.
2. Clear information concerning accuracy of age assessment by the method should be available.
3. The method needs to be sufficiently accurate to fulfill the specific demands of the single case to solve the underlying questions.
4. In cases of age assessment in living individuals principles of medical ethics and legal regulations have to be considered, especially if medical intervention is involved.

Reference material used must fulfill certain requirements (Solari & Abramovitch, 2002):

- Adequate simple size. The number of subjects of each sex and age group should be ten times the number of the examined features.
- The age indicated by the subjects should be verified.
- An even distribuition of subjects across all age groups.
- All data have to be collected separately for both sexes.
- The time of the examination should be recorded.
- The examined features should be defined unambiguously.
- The technique used in the examination should be described precisely.
- Information on genetic-geographic origin, socio-economic status and health of the reference population is indispensable.
- The simple size, mean value and statistical parameters of deviation should be provided for every feature examined.
- Information on inter- and intra-observer error is desirable.

Meinl et al stand out in questioning the terms "genetic-geographic origin" "socio-economic status" and "state of health", given the difficulty of establishing a definition of these parameters and the ethical aspects of these terms, which would condition their use in a reliable manner in a study (Meinl et al. 2007).

Many papers have been published concerning age estimation, and numerous different methods developed, although some of them have been considered inaccurate. The choice of a particular method will depend on the specific conditions of each case and mainly on the accuracy required.

In the opinion of the mentioned authors (Ritz-Timme et al. 200), the published data which fulfill the demands listed above in childhood and adolescence, are those based on the examination of dental and/or skeletal development, applied by trained personnel. In childhood (0-14 years) radiological examination of dental development includes all tooth types of teeth. In adolescence (14-21 years), thirds molars are the only teeth undergoing maturation, resulting to a lesser degree in accuracy. In both cases, sex and race influence tooth development, so those factors have to be into account.

The German age study group considers that age diagnosis examination should include (AGFAD, 2001):

- A physical examination which also records anthropometric data, signs of sexual maturation and any age-relevant developmental disorder.
- An X-ray examination of the left hand.
- A dental examination which records dentition status and evaluates an orthopantomogram.

It also recommends that these methods are used in combination for the purpose of increasing accuracy in age assessment and to facilitate the identification of age-relevant developmental disorders (Schmeling et al. 2004).
Each part of the examination is recommended to be performed by a specialist experienced in setting up expert reports and participating in regular ring experiments (see below) for quality assurance, with a coordinating expert giving a comprehensive assessment on the basis of the different parts of the evaluation performed by the respective specialists (Garamendi et al.2011).

3. Physical examination

Physical examination in cases of age determination should include measurements such as body height and weight, body type and body mass index, as well as any visible signs of sexual maturity and the results of a general physical examination, and should describe any signs suggestive of a pathological condition which may interfere with the maturation rate of the child.
There seems to be general agreement among authors that the interpretation of results obtained from anthropometric variables is an imprecise factor for the prediction of chronological age. Some studies have shown that individuals of greater height and weight and those with an athletic body type and an above-average BMI are among those who, in a specific population, may exhibit a more advanced bone age in relation to actual chronological age (Bueno et al. 1996).
Signs of sexual maturation are examined by evaluating the stage of development of the penis and scrotum, pubic hair growth, axillary hair growth, facial hair growth, and laryngeal prominence in male subjects; and breast development, axillary hair growth, and shape of the hip in female subjects.
The most widely used method for the study of secondary sexual characteristics is the staging described by Tanner (Marshall & Tanner, 1969, 1970). The method was devised to estimate the stage of development or physiological age for medical, educational or sports purposes, and to identify delayed or advanced sexual maturation when the chronological age of the subject is known. The method uses a five-stage scale to evaluate the status of pubic hair growth and breast development in girls, and pubic hair growth and development of the penis, scrotum and testes in boys.
Breast development stages (girls) (Marshal & Tanner, 1969):

- Stage 1: Prepubertal, papilla elevation only.
- Stage 2: Breast bud stage, elevation of breast and papilla as a small mound, enlargement of areola diameter.
- Stage 3: General enlargement of breast and areola.
- Stage 4: Projection of areola and papilla as secondary mound.
- Stage 5: Mature stage, adult contour with areola in same contour as breast and only papilla pojecting.

Pubic hair growth stages (girls) (Marshal & Tanner, 1969) :

- Stage 1: Prepubertal, no pubic hair.
- Stage 2: Sparse growth of long, slightly pigmented, downy hair, straight or only slightly curled, chiefly along the labia.
- Stage 3: Considerably darker, coarser and more curled, with an increase in amount. The hair spreads sparsely over the junction of the pubes.

- Stage 4: Hair resembles adult type, but no spread to the medial surface of the thighs.
- Stage 5: Adult in quantity and type, spread to medial thighs.

Genital development stages (boys) (Marshal & Tanner, 1970):

- Stage 1: Prepubertal, no change in size or proportion of testes, scrotum and penis from early childhood.
- Stage 2: Enlargement of scrotum and testes, reddening and change in the texture of the scrotal skin.
- Stage 3: Increase first in length then breadth of penis, further growth of testes and scrotum.
- Stage 4: Enlargement in lenght and breadth of penis and development of glans, further growth of testes and scrotum, darkening of the scrotal skin.
- Stage 5: Genitalia adult in size and shape.

Pubic hair stages (boys) (Marshal & Tanner, 1970):

- Stage 1: Prepubertal, no pubic hair.
- Stage 2: Sparse growth of long, slightly pigmented, downy hair, straight or slightly curled, chiefly at the base of the penis.
- Stage 3: Considerably darker, coarser and more curled, with an increase in amonut. The hair spreads sparsely over the junction of the pubes.
- Stage 4: Hair resembles adult type, but no spread to the medial surface of the thighs.
- Stage 5: Adult in quantity and type, spread to medial thighs.

Axillary hair growth, facial hair growth and laryngeal prominence development may also be assessed using the four-stage classification proposed by Nezy et al (Neizy et al, 1975).

Of the forensic methods recommended for age determination, assessing age on the basis of physical traits is the least precise. Evaluating sexual maturity has the greatest margin of error and should be used for age determination only in conjunction with an evaluation of skeletal maturity and tooth development. Multiple pathological conditions and non-pathological, idiosyncratic conditions cause a large range of variation in the onset of external changes associated with sexual maturation in different subjects. Therefore, age determination cannot be made on the basis of these examination data alone.

Moreover, irrespective of the difficulty in interpreting the results due to interobserver and intraobserver differences, there are few series analysing the progression of these parameters with chronological age in different populations, and the few available are mainly focused on developed countries (Koc et al, 2001; Cameron, 1993).

However, the physical examination is extremely useful for evaluating the potential impact of pathological factors on the maturation status estimated using other methods. The great discrepancy between height, weight and external signs of maturation and the bone and dental age estimated using radiographic methods should guide the examiner on the potential interference of pathological conditions and to a weighted estimation of age.

Most diseases delay development and are thus conducive to underestimation of age. Such underestimation of age would not disadvantage the person concerned in the judicial framework. By contrast, overestimating age due to a disease that accelerates development should be avoided at all costs. Certain diseases which occur very rarely, in particular endocrine disorders, may affect not only the attainment of height and sexual development, but also skeletal development. Endocrine diseases that may accelerate skeletal development include precocious puberty, adrenogenital syndrome, and hyperthyroidism.

Similarly, a general physical examination may show symptoms such as exophthalmos, virilisation of girls, acromegaly and gigantism, which are indicative of pathological disorders and must also redirect the estimation of age. Another indication of a possible endocrine disorder is a discrepancy between skeletal age and dental age, as dental development normally remains unaffected by endocrine disorders (Schmeling et al. 2007).

4. Bone age in carpus

The most studied anatomical region for age diagnosis, in particular before full maturity is reached at the age of 18, is the carpus and the hand (Garamendi & Landa, 2003).

Among the primitive series which analyzed epiphyseal maturation of the carpus as the main object of study or in the context of a general series of long bones are those by Stevenson in 1924, Galstaun G in 1930, Sidhom G and Derry DE in 1931, Borovansky L and Hnevkovsky O in 1929, Davies DA and Parsons FG in 1927, Paterson RS in 1929, Meenes TO and Holly LE in 1932, Adair FL and Scammon RE in 1921, Francis CC and Werle PB in 1939, and Pryor JW in papers published between 1908 and 1933. The latter author was among the first to note that ossification occurs earlier in females than in males, even during the foetal period.

However, it was not until large longitudinal population studies were carried out in the early 20th century under the auspices of private foundations in both Europe and the U.S. that the study of the carpus took a prominent role among the anatomical regions studied for age determination, in particular in adolescence (Bañón, 2004).

In 1937, Todd compiled hand radiographs taken of individuals during a study conducted by the Western Reserve University in Cleveland, Ohio, and together with comparisons made against the examination of a series of skeletons, he published his *Atlas of Skeletal Maturation* (Todd, 1937) based on the selection of a representative radiograph of the hand for each age and sex. The radiograph had to meet two requirements: have the same degree of development for the 28 bones and ossification nuclei which were the subject of the study, and be from an individual with a degree of body development which was within the average for their age and sex.

Todd's Atlas was used as a standard of reference until it was revised by WW Greulich and SI Pyle in 1950, who used it to compile their well known Atlas still widely used today, *Radiographic atlas of skeletal development of the hand and wrist*, published in two editions in 1951 and 1959 (Greulich & Pyle, 1950-1959). The Greulich and Pyle series was based on a total sample of 6,879 healthy middle-upper class North American children. Essentially, the method evaluates a "mean" bone age by matching an X-ray against the bones of a standard atlas, and normality estimates based on a range of results are made using standard deviation values.

During World War II the Oxford Health Survey was started and conducted by John Ryle on 470 children. The measurement data included radiographs of the carpus, which were analysed by Roy Acheson. Acheson looked to improve the Todd system by increasing the accuracy of the assessment. Under his proposal:

- Each bone or ossification nucleus was studied individually.
- Each bone or ossification nucleus was pre-assigned an identifiable stage as it matured, and each stage was given a progressive score.
- A final maturity score was calculated by adding up all of the partial scores obtained for each individual bone.

The skeletal maturity stage then yields a continuous value which can be used for growth measurements, such as height or weight.

Acheson's procedure was later refined by Tanner and Whitehouse into the Tanner-Whitehouse charts (Tanner et al, 1983). With this method, the study of each hand yields a total score which can be used to calculate an overall maturity stage which is then matched to distribution tables by age and sex based on percentile distributions.

Therefore, there are two main types of methods for bone age assessment based on carpal bones: atlas methods, with the Greulich and Pyle atlas being the main international standard of reference, and numerical methods, with the three editions of the Tanner-Whitehouse method being the main reference. There are some other mixed methods, such as the Thieman-Nitz method based on a German population. There are adaptations of these methods to virtually all populations in practically every country.

In principle it would appear that a numerical method such as the Tanner-Whitehouse method should be more reliable, however, in practice it is subject to intra- and interobserver errors similar to the GP method, and is negatively affected by technical problems arising from an incorrect positioning of the hand while the X-ray is taken, which can be better solved by graphical methods. Some authors recommend the application of the GP method instead of the TW3 for clinical purposes, on the basis of economy of means criteria after ascertaining that the TW3 method is far more costly in terms of time and the results are similar to those obtained through the GP method (Garamendi & Landa, 2003).

Several attempts have been made to develop TW2 and TW3 numerical system software for automated evaluation of X-ray plates. In theory, this would allow for a uniform quantification of results without interference from distortion factors derived from the observer. However, the results are not yet comparable to those obtained through the manual method, and collaboration between radiologists and IT experts is still needed to improve hardware and software systems.

The interpretation of bone age results obtained by any of the available methods must be adapted to the characteristics of the population of the subject of the study. The factors which may modify bone age progression in a particular subject are not perfectly defined, although several studies have identified differences associated with pathological, racial or socio-economic factors. The overall impression from the most recent research is that socio-economic factors, which affect the nutrition patterns and hygiene and health conditions of the subjects, are the most significant in terms of their capacity to modify results (Schmeling et al, 2000, 2001). Racial factors are discussed by several authors in different studies, and while they alone do not seem to justify significant differences in bone age, there are no unquestionable data allowing one to categorically affirm or deny the specific impact of this factor. On the contrary, the studies conducted are conclusive that certain pathological conditions may affect the results of bone age assessment, albeit the list of those pathological conditions cannot be considered in any way exhaustive.

There is a large number of studies in the context of ethnic and racial impact, some of them of questionable methodological basis and at times contradictory results, mainly conducted on populations of European Caucasians, North American Caucasians, other North American ethnic groups (including the genetically questionable racial group of Hispanics), different Mongoloid and Caucasian populations from Asia, and some incomplete studies on central and southern African Negroid populations.

The most recent studies in Europe appear to indicate that maturation rates for European Caucasians are close to those described in the GP and TW2 systems or are slightly delayed or advanced in relation to them. In some cases, the differences with the original methods were small yet so statistically significant that the need to create charts and atlases specific to these populations has been proposed.

Classical studies conducted in the seventies and eighties on Mongoloid Asian populations showed that the bone ages of the Chinese and Japanese groups were delayed in relation to chronological age during the prepubertal period; however, accelerated growth in the postpubertal period resulted in maturity being reached at a similar age as for European and American Caucasians. The most current series on modern populations with better socio-economic status show a trend to adjust results even further to the rate of bone age maturation of western populations. Similar findings have been reported in India and Pakistan, where studies have shown advances in bone age in relation to chronological age during the postpubertal period, more obvious in subjects from an upper social class.

In the U.S., studies indicate that Caucasian subjects either closely fit the GP and TW2 standards or often show a certain advance in maturation. By contrast, studies on Negroid subjects show contradictory results in the series. For Gross et al. the black race fits the GP standard better than the white race (Gross et al, 1995). In the series conducted by Ontell et al. and Lodler et al. the black race is advanced in relation to the GP standard (Lodler et al, 1993; Ontel et al, 1996). The series obtained by Marshall WA on black Jamaicans compared to the TW2 UK60 indicates delayed bone age from age 13 irrespective of socio-economic factors (Marshall et al, 1970). Lastly, in a study of black and white subjects in the U.S., Gilsanz V found no significant differences between bone age and chronological age in both races after the socio-economic factors were made equal (Gilsanz et al, 1988).

As far as our knowledge extends, the inhabitants of Muslim countries in the Near East and northern Africa, and populations of these countries who have migrated to developed countries have not been systematically studied and it is not known whether their rate of bone maturation is in keeping with the progression described for other populations (Souguir, 2002). The only studies available are those by Koc et al (Koc et al, 2001), Büken et al (Büken et al, 2007) and Garamendi et al (Garamendi et al., 2005). The study conducted by Koc A et al. on a modern Turkish population showed delayed bone age up until the age of 13, and a discreet advance after that age in relation to the GP atlas. A major objection to this study is that the population sample had a chronological age of only up to 17. This problem was later solved in a recent study reported by Büken et al., who examined carpal radiographs of 409 Turkish boys and girls of Caucasian background aged 11 to 19. Similarly to Koc et al., their study indicated that their population cohort exhibited advanced bone age between ages 13 and 17, and a relative delay in the 18 to 19 age group. In 2005, Garamendi et al. published a study of 114 Moroccan immigrants with a confirmed age of 12 to 25, presenting a joint analysis of the variations from the Greulich and Pyle standard for carpal X-rays as well as of the dental age assessed by orthopantomography.

Some authors consider that the socio-economic characteristics of each population are the most significant factors affecting variation in the rate of bone age maturation. Other studies, on the contrary, fail to confirm this hypothesis. A study on a black Jamaican population reported by Marshall WA found no variations according to the upper or lower social class of the subjects (Marshall et al., 1970). However, modern specific studies of this variable by authors such as Jahari AB et al on an Indonesian population (Jahari, 2000), Fleshman AK on an African population (Fleshman, 2000), and Melsen B et al on a population of adopted foreign minors in Denmark (Melsen et al, 1996) clearly identify socio-economic factors and poverty as causing significant delay in the rate of the bone maturation sequence during the prepubertal period.

Pathological factors clearly identified as altering bone age maturation rate include, among others, nocturnal enuresis (Dundaroz et al., 2001), GH deficit (Vallejo-Bolaños et al., 1999), obesity (Bueno et al, 1996), high-level competitive sport activities (Theintz et al., 1993) or bone malformations, and exposure to physical agents causing injury such as frostbite (Freyshmidt et al., 2001).

5. Dental age

Dental age can be assessed accurately in childhood, because many of the teeth are developing simultaneously.

5.1 Dental eruption

Visual inspection of dental eruption was the first and most usual method for dental age assessment. In a work entitled "The Teeth, a Test of Age", Edwin Saunders in 1837 proposed to the English parliament the use of the degree of dental eruption as a method to determine the age of child workers in factories, where the age limit was nine years (Bang, 1989). For a long time, and even up to the present day in many parts of the world where birth registers do not exist, dental development is used as a child age indicator, adopted as a biological-legal indicator.

However, although this method is fast, cheap and not very influenced by intra- and interobserver error, eruption is not a good age indicator when used alone, due to factors like interindividual or populational variation (Garn et al., 1959; Moorees et al, 1963), systemic or local diseases (Ungar, 1937) or the elapsed time without changes (Teivens & Mörnstad, 2001).

Numerous authors have investigated the chronology and sequence of eruption in different populations (Foti et al., 2003; Fulton & Price, 1954; Giles et al., 1963; Logan & Kronfield, 1933; Olze et al, 2007; Planells et al, 1993; Saunders et al 1993; Tanguay et al. 1984; Van der Linden, 1980). Some of this research examines the correlation between dental eruption and other development parameters; for example Lewis and Garn (Garn & Lewis, 1959) which evaluates parameters such as somatic and sexual growth, personality and state of health, or Green (Green, 1961) which attempts to establish correlations between dental, skeletal and chronological age and weight and height, finding a stronger correlation between dental and chronological age even than that existing between dental and bone development. Hagg and Taranger (Hagg & Taranger, 1980) study the relationship between dental eruption and maximum puberal growth, finding a low correlation between somatic and dental development. Baume and cols (Baume et al., 1954) have shown changes in dental eruption related to hypophyseal hormonal levels.

5.2 Dental maturation

Mineralization of deciduous tooth crowns begins at around 3 or 4 months of intrauterine life, with calcification continuing after birth during the neonatal period (Burdi, 1992). Root formation is generally completed between 18 months and 3 years of age.

Mineralization of adult teeth meanwhile takes around nine years, beginning with the first permanent molar around the moment of birth (Evans & Knight, 1981).

The dental development process correlates with different morphological stages of mineralization that can be observed with radiographic techniques, and undergo much more uniform and gradual changes than eruption; more controlled by genetics and less influenced by external factors than all other measurable criteria of maturity (Frucht et al., 2000). This is the reason why several methods of dental age assessment have been developed.

All the age assessment methods based on dental maturation follow the same procedure. First the stage of development of each of the teeth is evaluated from radiographic records, the method of choice being panoramic radiography or orthopantomography (OPT). Next the stage of development is related to the age of each tooth, derived from study of a sample of known age. This estimation method is based on subjective evaluation of the stages and has many defects. The biological variation in development is also wide for all teeth.

Due to the differences existing between methods and populations of different origin, these elements must be expressed as well as the confidence interval. Numerous studies have provided maturation scales in both deciduous and permanent teeth populations, identifying the successive states of development, though they show differences in the methodology employed (longitudinal versus transversal methods, definition of the development stages, etc)(Demirjian et al., 1973; Moorrees et al., 1963; Nolla, 1960). During the infant period where simultaneous development of several teeth can be observed the majority of these age assessment methods show variations of around 2 years to the average for confidence intervals of 90-95%, indicating rather low accuracy. Studies carried out on samples of known ages (Liversidge, 1994; Saunders et al., 1993), show differences of some 6 months to the real ages.

Nolla classified dental development into 10 calcificación stages from crypt state to closure of the root apex (Nolla, 1960). The Nolla study warned that mineralización development began and ended earlier in females, though there appear to be no differences in the sequence of development finalization. The Nolla method is one of the most widely used clinically as a reliable procedure for dental development estimation in permanent teeth. Diverse studies (Bolaños et al, 2003; Haavikko, 1974; Staaf et al, 1991), applying the Nolla method find an average assessment error of around 2 years for a 95% confidence interval.

One of the systems most universally used to evaluate the degree of permanent dental development is that proposed by Demirjian, Goldstein and Tanner (Demirjian et al., 1973), based on analysis of a sample of French-Canadian children. The original method evaluates the degree of calcification of the seven teeth in the left mandibular hemiarch, excluding the third molar, from radiographic records. 8 maturation stages (A to H) are established for each tooth, from the start of crown calcification to the root apex close, in a similar way to the Nolla method. Each tooth is attributed a formation stage, then converted into a score depending on the sex, following the same mathematical technique used to evaluate skeletal development by the Tanner-Whitehouse method (Tanner et al., 1975). The scores of the seven teeth are added to obtain the so-called dental maturity score on a scale of 0 to 100. This score is transformed through the corresponding tables into dental age. The method has the disadvantage that it does not include a valuation of the third molars, so can only be used for preadolescent ages.

Subsequently the same author has produced updates to the original method, proposing a valuation system for four teeth (both premolars and molars) with different standards (Demirjian, 1976).

In all cases, given that maturation development is different for the two sexes, the sex must be determined beforehand (Levesque et al., 1981).

The widespread use of this method as an infant age assessment procedure has meant that the results of the Demirjian study have been tested in other populations. Numerous studies over recent decades show a slight delay in maturation of the original French-Canadian population, causing overestimation when the original results of the method are applied to other populations (Bolaños et al., 2003; Davis & Hagg, 1994; Eid et al., 2002; Frucht et al.,

2000; Koshy & Tandom, 1998; Liversigde etl., 1999; Loevy & Goldberg, 1999; MacKenna et al., 2002; Nykanen et al., 1998; Nystro et al., 1986; Prabhakar et al., 2002; Staaf et al., 1991; Willems et al., 2001). The aforesaid overestimation varies between some months and several years in age, and it is recommended that standard values based on studies of the same population to which the method is applied are used.

Seeking a more accurate statistical model that explains as well as possible the correlation between the degree of dental development and chronological age, Teivens and Mönstard (Teivens & Mönstard, 2001) have recently produced diverse mathematical functions modifying the original Demirjian method, obtaining the best results when a cubic regression model is used (R2 = 0.95). This model has been tested in a comparative study between Swiss and Korean subjects, showing statistically significant differences, with earlier development in the Swedish sample of 2 months for males and 6 months for females.

5.3 The third molar in age assesment.

Age assessment becomes more complicated once the root apex of the second permanent molar has closed (at around 14 years of age) due to the variablilty of third molar development. The third molar is the tooth showing greatest frequency of agenesia (Garn & Lewis, 1962), the most irregular in its maturation sequence (Kieser, 1990) and, in contrast to the rest of dentition, tends to appear earlier in males than females (Levesque et al., 1981). However, due to the scarcity of alternative indicators maturity evaluation in this tooth is one of the prime tools in age assessment in these cases

Recent years have seen a proliferation of studies focusing on third molar maturation as an age assessment method, with the purpose of contributing data enabling us to better understand the factors influencing the maturation of this tooth and establish more specific reference values providing more reliable diagnosis.

Despite this, the continual increase in immigration of young people from third world to industrialised countries, and the need to have a reliable and sound age assessment procedure in the absence of documents showing the date of birth, have for some years now prompted studies based on third molar development (Harris & Nortjé, 1984; Micci & Buzzanca, 1998; Robetti et al., 1982; Robetti et al., 1993). The third molar is the only tooth undergoing maturation during juvenile years, and is especially attractive as a study subject because the degree of mineralization can be easily ascertained through non-invasive methods such as radiology.

Of the numerous methods for third molar maturation evaluation, there seems to be a broad current consensus that the Demirjian method (Demirjian et al., 1973), is the most suitable, for several reasons:

The Demirjian stages are defined by morphological changes more objectively valued than speculative estimates of length (Olze et al, 2005, 2006). Stages of root formation are more clearly defined and show the highest values for inter-observer and intra-observer agreement and for correlation between the defined stages and true age (Dhanjal et al., 2006).

In comparison with other age diagnosis methods, those used in estimating legal age or minor status should minimise false positives with the aim of avoiding mistaken classification of a minor as of legal age.

Intra-observer and inter-observer agreement are reported to be high (Dhanjal et al., 2006; Orhan et al., 2007; Prieto et al., 2007) with best agreement for mandibular third molar when Demirjian's method is employed (Arany et al., 2004; Dhanjal et al., 2006).

In a study carried out by the Research Committee of the American Board of Forensic Odontology Mincer et al (Mincer et al., 1993) evaluate precision in age assessment from the development state of the lower third molar, valued according to the Demirjian method. According to this study, stages A to D (up to complete crown formation) and stage H (complete apex closure) would show respectively a strong probability that the individual is younger or older than 18. Accuracy, established based on the difference between the real age and that calculated from the degree of dental development, is situated at 4.8 years for the 95% range (two standard deviations). Using the same valuation system in a Swedish population sample Thorson and Hägg (Thorson & Hägg, 1991) observed a weak relation between chronological and dental age (underestimation of chronological age), with a mean difference between the estimated and the chronological age of about ±4.5 years in girls (95% confidence interval) and ±2.8 years in boys, and intra-observer error of ±0.8 years (95% confidence interval) which for the authors rules out this method for age assessment.

Kullman et al (Kullman et al., 1992) obtain similar results using a system based on classifying root development into 7 development stages, with standard deviations of 1 to 2 years to the average age in the different development stages.

In the review carried out by Rirz-Timme et al (Rotz Timme et al., 2000) the third molar gives standard error values (SEE) varying in a range of 1-2.5 years, with correlation ratios (r) between 0.32 and 0.85.

The use of standard error as a measure of accuracy has been criticised by diverse authors (Aykroyd et al., 1997; Giles & Klepinger, 1988) and recent papers propose the use of Bayesian probability as an alternative to regression analysis (Braga et al., 2005), though more studies with respect to these items are desirable.

Perhaps due to the fact that a good part of the third molar formation process occurs once puberty is reached, sexual dimorphism contrary to the rest of the dental maturation processes can be observed, with males reaching the different development stages earlier than females, independently of their ethnic origin. Studies published to date agree in this respect (Arany et al., 2004; Garn et al., 1959; Gunst et al., 2003; Haavikko, 1974; Harris, 2007; Harris & Nortjé, 1984; Köhler et al., 1994; Levesque et al., 1981; Meinl et al, 2007; Orhan et al., 2007; Prieto et al., 2007; Solari & Abramovitch, 2002; Throson & Hägg, 1991; Willerhausen et al., 2001).

Studies evaluating third molar development in the maxillary and mandibular arch appear to agree in the greater advance in maturation of maxillary molars versus mandibular ones (UNHCR, 2002; 6),(14),(37),Meinl et al., 2007; Orhan et al., 2007; Solari & Abramovitch, 2002; Willerhausen et al., 2001). For Mincer (Mincer et al., 1993) this could reflect different control mechanisms in the process of development of the two arches. He also observes that combining the results of the teeth of both arches seems to improve accuracy slightly.

Though impaction of the third molars has been put forward as a cause of delay in root formation (Köhler et al., 1994), a recent work by Friedrich (Friedrich et al., 2005) concludes that the topography of the wisdom teeth did not influence the timing of root development.

All studies coincide in the absence of significant differences depending on the side (left or right) (Meinl et al., 2007; Orhan et al., 2007; Prieto et al., 2007; Willerhausen et al., 2001).

Dental development can be altered by long term conditions, congenital syndromes, nutrition deficiencies or hormonal disorders, among others. Meanwhile, the factors influencing dental formation are difficult to identify.

Meinl et al (Meinl et al., 2007) call attention to the consequences of exclusion of subjects showing certain pathologies or irregular development, so that age assessment methods would be only applicable to individuals with a pretended normal dental state. In their study they decide not to carry out exclusions for such motives and include all the subjects of the original sample, observing that none of the outliers had characteristics associated with altered growth, and also that individuals with severe development alterations did not show precarious findings. In accordance with these results they assume the hypothesis that dental development underlies strong regulation mechanisms which seem difficult to alter, even under pathological conditions.

As in all anthropological analysis, the characteristics of the reference population are a very significant element. The influence of genetic, nutritional, and geographical factors must be taken into account, when standards are developed. The applicability of standards generated to members of ethnic groups that are different from the reference population has been the subject of controversial discussion. Up to now several studies have been undertaken in different populations, with the aim of observing the usefulness of the third molar as a reliable indicator of age(Arany et al., 2004; Blankenship et al., 2007; Bolaños et al., 2003; Garamendi et al., 2005; Gunst et al., 2003; Gunst et al., 2003; Harris, 2007; Harris & Nortjé, 1984; Kullman, 1992; Martín, 2007; Meinl et al., 2007; Micci & Buzzanca, 1998; Mincer et al., 1993; Nambiar, 1996; Olze et al., 2004, 2006, 2007; Prieto et al. 2007; Robetti et al., 1982; Solari & Abramovitch, 2002; illerhausen et al., 2001; Yaacob et al., 1996). These studies have proved that dental development shows slight variations among different populations, making specific studies necessary.

Although certain heterogeneity is observed when comparing the results of studies carried out on different populations, the results of a work (Prieto et al., 2007) performed on a sample of 1050 ortopantomographs of young Spaniards aged 14 to 21 show that the Spanish population undergoes maturation development of the lower third molars faster than the North American, French-Canadian , Austrian and Scandinavian populations, while more similar to the Hispanic population of the United States.

Garamendi et al (Garamendi et al., 2005) studied a sample of 114 illegal Moroccan immigrants, whose real age was subsequently obtained. The examination included radiográphical dental study to estimate third molar maturation following the Demirjian and Goldstein method previously commented. The results show that this constitutes a good age diagnosis method -though the standards used were those obtained from the original French-Canadian population - while efficiency was increased by combining bone maturation valuation methods.

The lack of data on the influence of the ethnic factor in mineralization represents a restriction in the reliability of age assessment and therefore in the value of forensic information essential to legal soundness. This has come about for diverse reasons, such as the use of different assessment methods, small sample sizes, or African population birth data not checked, which prevent data being directly comparable.

In various studies together with South African and Japanese colleagues, Olze et al (Olze et al., 2004, 2006, 2007) evaluate the possible influence of the ethnic factor in third molar mineralization and eruption, observing a slower maturation process in the mongoloid population, which could reach the predominant stages of mineralization 1-2 years older and Africans 1-2 years younger, than Caucasoids and similar behaviour as regards third molar eruption. These authors think that these differences could be owed to the difference in the palate dimensions, smaller in mongoloids, which could cause a delay in eruption and because of this in mineralization.

Blankenship et al (Blankenship et al. 2007) and Harris (Harris, 2007) evaluate the differences between black and white North Americans. The results coincide with those of Olze et al. showing greater maturation speed in the black population.

The scientific studies performed, though representing an important contribution to our knowledge of third molar maturation, do not resolve the problem facing us in determining the age of a young illegal immigrant. In the case of Spain and the majority of European countries, these immigrants come in different proportions from Morocco, the sub-Sahara, Latin America and Eastern Europe.

Martín de las Heras et al (Martín, 2007) evaluates the development of the third molar in in the northern Spanish population and the Spanish and Moroccan population resident in one of the Spanish cities of North Africa (Ceuta). The interest of this work centres on the fact that the Maghreb population is one of the most frequent illegal immigrant groups in Spain and other Mediterranean European countries.

The lack of maturation standards for African countries and the difficulty of carrying out studies in the countries of origin makes it necessary to perform studies enabling us to evaluate dental maturation in these countries to arrive at more reliable data.

The inter-populational differences shown by these studies underline the need for specific work in this area. More research is needed in this field.

The results of the work published agree in stating that once the third molar reaches the H stage of Demirjian, the probability that an individual is of legal age is greater than 90%, independently of ethnic origin, sex or the tooth evaluated (Arany et al., 2004; Meinl et al., 2007; Mincer et al, 1993; Solari & Abramovitch, 2002). For this reason this element can be considered a useful marker to resolve the question of whether an individual of unknown age can be considered an adult for legal effects.

Only in criminal cases is the use of radiography justifiable.

In practice it is not habitual to request the express consent of a minor to carry out the exploration and complementary examinations, including radiological tests. Given that the examination will affect their privacy and that radiological tests mean exposure to radiation with potentially harmful effects, as we understand it it should be obligatory to obtain the consent of the subject, and to suspend examination in the absence of consent. This aspect is included in the guide of good practice of the program for unaccompanied minors in Europe.

It must further be appreciated that using techniques developed for clinical purposes - to seek possible pathologies - in evaluating the degree of maturation for a specific age represents a perversion, as it inverts the application in the search for evidence to deduce the age of an individual from their maturation level when there is no clinical reason justifying such use.

Attempts to standardisation, calibration and evaluation procedures have been scarce up to now, pointing to the need for guidelines on this and all other aspects.

The difficulty involved hence in diagnosis and the potential sources of evaluation makes it necessary to draw up common guidelines for action, based on scientific evidence and unifying the criteria to be followed, such as those of the Study Group on Forensic Age Diagnosis (AGFAD), founded in Berlin in 2000. The group has published guidelines on age diagnosis on living individuals for criminal, civil and asylum proceedings among others (Schmeling et al., 2007).

The International Organization for Forensic Odonto-Stomatology (IOFOS) has published recommended procedures for quality assurance in forensic dental age estimation http://www.odont.uio.no/foreninger/iofos/quality/Age-IOFOS.htm

Regarding these recommendations, Solheim and Vonen(86) highlight the discrepancies of criteria among experts over the steps to follow between those who only wish to apply a statistical method and report on the results and those who prefer to express the expert opinion taking into consideration the life conditions of the individual such as state of health and nutrition, clinical findings and of course the results of the statistical scientific methods. These authors coincide with the German Interdisciplinary Working Group for Age Diagnostic (34) that the conclusions should end with a complete assessment of the most likely chronological age.

Just as Ritz-Timme et al (Ritz-Timme et al., 2000) recommend, efforts should be made to develop external quality control, something perfectly possible in the field of age assessment, with the aim of guaranteeing quality standards enabling an adequate response given the important role played by forensic medicine in the legal and social fields of age assessment.

5.4 Age estimation in the clavicle

To answer the question of whether a person has reached the age of 18 it is particularly helpful to evaluate the ossification status of the medial epiphysis of the clavicle, because all other examined developmental systems may already have completed their growth by that age.

A number of studies have been conducted on the time frame for the ossification of the medial clavicular epiphyseal cartilage in the age group concerned for forensic age diagnostics in living individuals. One group of studies adopted an anatomical perspective, assessing ossification by means of autopsy or direct skeletal inspection (Todd & D'Errico, 1928; McKern & Stewart, 1957; Owings Webb & Myers Suchey, 1985; MacLaughlin, 1990; Ji et al., 1994; Black & Scheuer, 1996; Shirley, 2009; Singh & Chavali, 2011), while the other group took a radiological approach.

Several authors pointed out, that data from dry bone material are not directly comparable with data from radiological studies. Krogman and Isçan (Krogman & Isçan, 1986) as well as Kreitner et al. (Kreitner et al, 1998), for example, argued that commencement of fusion can be detected in radiographs before any union of epiphysis and metaphysis can be visible on dry bone. Therefore reference values from dry bone studies should not be applied to assessments based on radiographs.

Radiological methods to examine the medial clavicular epiphysis in living individuals are conventional radiography (CR) (Flecker, 1933; Galstaun, 1937; Jit & Kullkarni, 1976; Schmeling et al., 2004; Garamendi et al. 2011), computed tomography (CT) (Kreitner et al., 1997, 1998; Schulz et al., 2005; Schulze et al., 2006; Bassed et al., 2010; Kellinghaus et al., 2010a, b), as well as new approaches using magnet resonance imaging (Schmidt et al., 2007; Hillewig et al., 2011) and ultrasoundsonography (Schulz et al., 2008b; Quirmbach et al., 2009; Schulz et al., 2010).

While traditional classification systems differentiate between four stages of clavicle ossification (stage 1: ossification centre not ossified; stage 2: ossification centre ossified, epiphyseal plate not ossified; stage 3: epiphyseal plate partly ossified; stage 4: epiphyseal plate fully ossified), Schmeling et al. (Schmeling et al., 2004) divided the stage of total epiphyseal fusion into two additional stages (stage 4: epiphyseal plate fully ossified, epiphyseal scar visible; stage 5: epiphyseal plate fully ossified, epiphyseal scar no longer visible). Figure 1 shows the stages of clavicular ossification for CR and CT.

There is only one study referring to conventional radiography that meets the requirements of a reference study as stated by the Study Group on Forensic Age Diagnostics (Schmeling et al., 2008). In this study the earliest age at which stage 3 was detected in either sex was 16 years. Stage 4 was first observed in women at 20 years and in men at 21 years. Stage 5 was first achieved by both sexes at age 26 (Schmeling et al., 2004). It was concluded that plain chest radiographs can essentially provide a basis for assessing clavicular ossification. If overlap in posterior-anterior views impedes evaluation additional oblique images (Bontrager & Lampignano, 2009) should be taken to facilitate age estimation.

In 1997 and 1998, Kreitner et al. published the first CT-based studies in which the medial epiphyseal ossification of the clavicle was evaluated applying a four stage scheme. Since these studies did not discriminate results by sex, their forensic value is limited. In a CT study conducted by Schulz et al. in 2005, presenting more cases and results discriminated by sex, the five stage classification by Schmeling et al. (Schmeling et al., 2004) was used. The earliest occurrence of stage 3 in females was noted at age 16 and in males at age 17. Stage 4 was first achieved by both sexes at age 21. Stage 5 was first noted in females at age 21 and in males at age 22, which is 4 or 5 years earlier than is reported in the conventional radiographic studies. Schulz et al. (Schulz et al., 2005) raised the question whether CT scans with a slice thickness of > 1 mm could cause misinterpretation of clavicle ossification status and recommended examining the influence of slice thickness on the age intervals of ossification stages in additional studies.

In a study on the influence of the slice thickness on the ability to assess the stages of clavicular ossification Mühler et al. (Mühler et al., 2006) retrospectively analysed the CTs of 40 individuals which have been examined within the scope of age diagnostics. Scans with slice thicknesses of 1, 3, 5, and 7 mm have been reconstructed from the obtained data. Seven out of 80 clavicular epiphyseal plates showed differences depending on the slice thickness in the particular stages of ossification. In 1 case a slice thickness of 1 mm led to a different diagnosis of the ossification stage than a slice thickness of 3 mm, in 3 cases the diagnoses differed between the slice thicknesses of 3 mm and of 5 mm, and in another 3 cases between 5 and 7 mm. The authors therefore concluded that for age estimation purposes the slice thickness should be 1 mm in order to ensure maximum accuracy and diagnostic reliability. The findings of this study were confirmed by Kaur et al. (Kaur et al., 2010).

Recently, Kellinghaus et al. (Kellinghaus et al., 2010) published data from a thin-slice CT study. In this study stage 3 was first achieved by male individuals at age 17 and in females at age 16. The occurrence of stage 4 was first found in both sexes at the age of 21. In either sex, the earliest observation of stage 5 was at age 26. These findings are consistent with the data from the conventional study of the clavicle (Schmeling et al., 2004).

A further improvement of age diagnostics based on clavicular ossification was the subdivision of stages 2 and 3 by Kellinghaus et al. (Kellinghaus et al., 2010). The sub-classification stages were defined as follows (see figure 2):

Stage 2a: The lengthwise epiphyseal measurement is one third or less compared to the widthwise measurement of the metaphyseal ending

Stage 2b: The lengthwise epiphyseal measurement is over one third until two thirds compared to the widthwise measurement of the metaphyseal ending

Stage 2c: The lengthwise epiphyseal measurement is over two thirds compared to the widthwise measurement of the metaphyseal ending

Stage 3a: The epiphyseal-metaphyseal fusion completes one third or less of the former gap between epiphysis and metaphysis

Stage 3b: The epiphyseal-metaphyseal fusion completes over one third until two thirds of the former gap between epiphysis and metaphysis

Stage 3c: The epiphyseal-metaphyseal fusion completes over two thirds of the former gap between epiphysis and metaphysis

Stage 3c first appeared at age 19 in both sexes. If stage 3c is found, it is therefore possible to substantiate that an individual has already reached the legally important age threshold of 18 years.

For forensic age estimations in living individuals, non-ionising procedures for the presentation of the medial clavicular epiphyseal cartilage would be desirable, as the radiation exposure from the necessary imaging examination could be decreased considerably. Against this background Schmidt et al. (Schmidt et al., 2007) prospectively evaluated magnetic resonance (MR) scans of 54 sternoclavicular joints of bodies aged between 6 and 40 years. All of the examined medial clavicular epiphyseal cartilages permitted an assessment of the degree of ossification. Stage 2 was first observed at the age of 15 years, the earliest age at which stage 3 was observed was 16 years, and stage 4 was first observed at the age of 23 years. Very recently Hillewig et al. (Hillewig et al., 2011) published a four-minute approach for MRI of the medial clavicular epiphysis in living individuals.

In a comparative study using CR, CT and MRI for staging of 15 sternoclavicular joints the ossification stage was in agreement in each of the three imaging methods used in 6 cases (Vieth et al., 2010). In the remaining cases the ossification stage was assessed either one stage higher or lower in one of the applied imaging methods than in the other two techniques. In five cases (compared to CT), respectively seven cases (compared to MR), CR showed a higher ossification stage than CT and MR imaging. In two cases CR resulted in the determination of a lower stage than in CT and MR imaging. Twice the MR scans showed a less advanced ossification stage than CT-based images. The authors concluded that in age estimation practice, modality-specific reference studies are to be applied in order to guarantee an adequate assessment of the ossification stage of the medial clavicular epiphysis.

Another radiation free approach to evaluate the ossification stage of the medial clavicular epiphyses is ultrasound sonography. Schulz et al. (Schulz et al., 2008) prospectively evaluated 84 right clavicles of test subjects 12–30 years of age by means of ultrasound. For the sonographic assessment of the clavicle ossification, the traditional classification had to be modified as follows (see figure 3):

Stage 1: The medial end of the clavicle is configured acute-angled. A bony center of ossification is not representable.

Stage 2: The medial end of the clavicle is separated from the bony center of ossification by a sound gap.

Stage 3: Both an ultrasound gap with a bony center of ossification and a fully ossified epiphyseal plate with a convex curved end of the clavicle are representable.

Stage 4: The medial end of the clavicle is convex curved. A bony center of ossification is not representable.

The earliest ages at which the respective ossification stages were observed were 17 years for stage 2, 16 years for stage 3, and 22 years for stage 4. Another pilot study by means of sonography was performed by Quirmbach et al. (Quirmbach et al., 2009). In this study stage 4 was first observed at 20 years. These results were reviewed in a reference sample of 601 healthy volunteers aged between 10 and 25 years by Schulz et al. (Schulz et al., 2010). The earliest observation of stage 4 in women was at 19 years in both sexes. Based on these findings it can reliably be stated that an individual with stage 4 has already accomplished 18 years of age.

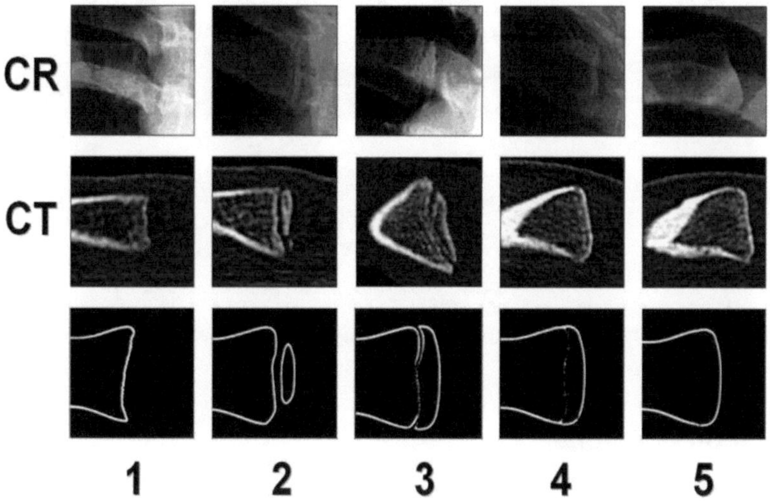

Fig. 1. Schematic drawings and pictures of the stages 1-5 of clavicular ossification as revealed by conventional radiography (CR) and computed tomography (CT)

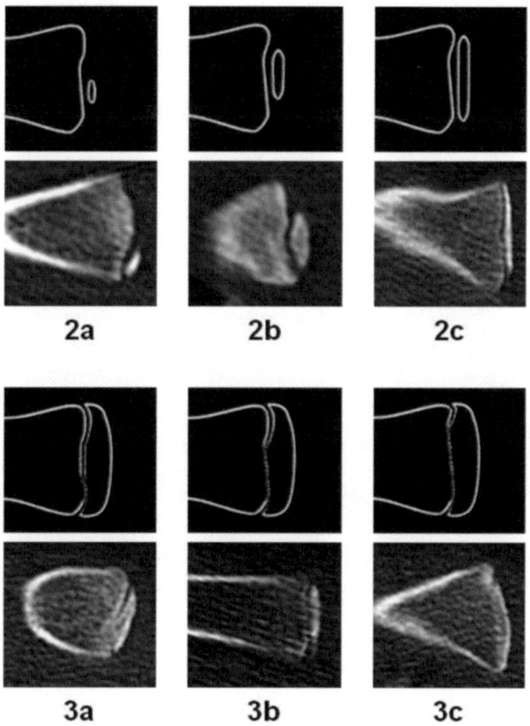

Fig. 2. Schematic drawings and pictures of the stages 2a-3c of clavicular ossification as revealed by means of thin-slice CT

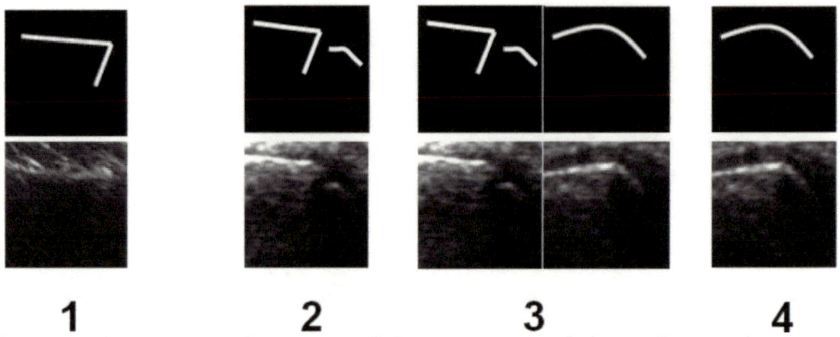

Fig. 3. Schematic drawings and pictures of the stages 1-4 of clavicular ossification as revealed by ultrasound

6. Interpretation of results

6.1 Interpretation of results from combined methods. The clavicle and the twilight zone

AGFAD Guidelines on Age Estimation in Living Subjects recommend that when performing a FAE different methods must applied in the same subject. These recommendations mean that in the same subject different FAE results will be available (AGFAD, 2001).

Previous series (Garamendi et al., 2005) proved that the accuracy of FAE improves when different age estimation methods are simultaneously applied. The under ROC curve area increase when both bone age and dental age methods are applied when assessing if a subject could be older or younger than 18.

In cases of combined analysis of age estimation based on dental age and bone age in carpus, the lowest result of both methods should be used for a final estimation because of ethical reasons and legal accuracy.

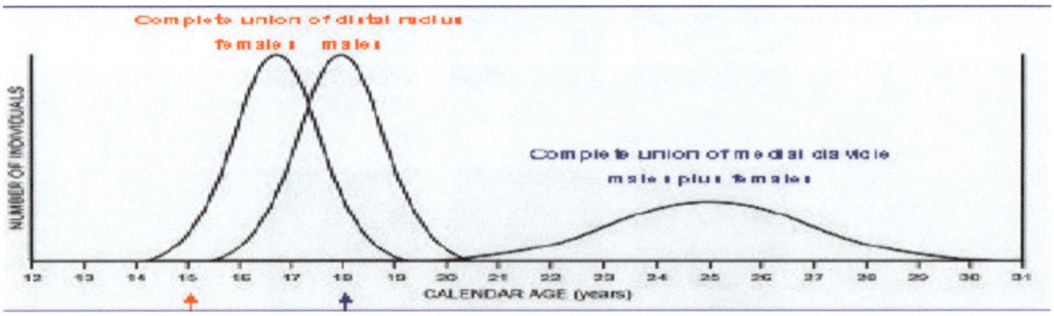

Fig. 4. Simulacra of distribution of results of bone age in carpus and in clavicle in relation with complete fusion of distal radius and complete union of medial clavicle.

More complex is the application of results in case of doubt about an age estimation over or under 18 years or 21 years old based on results of an age estimation in the clavicle. Positive results (clavicle stage 4 of Schmeling´s method) indicate positively that the age of the subject will be most probably older than 21,6 in males and 21,3 in females (Kellinghaus et al., 2010). Nevertheless, stage 3 is observed in subjects up to 26 years old and aritmetical mean of stage 4 is 29,6 +/- 4,2 in males and 8,2+/-4,2 in females. 100% of the sample in stages 4 or 5 of

Schmeling method is observed only in subejcts older than 26 (Kreitner et al., 1997; Schmeling et al., 2004). These statistical results are graphically explained in figure 4 in which it´s clear that a negative result of stage 4 in a subject older than 21 years and younger than 26 is in many cases most probable than a positive result. It turns the range between 18 and 26 years old a twilight zone in which a positive result is definitive but a negative result is the most probable one and suppose the imposibility to assess a FAE of being older than 21 years old in most cases of subjects younger than 26.
Nevertheless, more research is needed in this specific field to define more precisely the best standarized approach to FAE based on simultaneous different methods.

6.2 Ethnical and socioeconomic factors: sexual maturation, ossification, dental development

Since the subjects whose age has to be estimated mostly belong to populations for which no reference studies are available that could be used for forensic purposes, the question arises whether there are significant developmental differences between various ethnic groups which would prohibit the application of relevant age standards to members of ethnic groups other than the reference population. In this respect the term 'ethnicity' shall be used only to identify the affinity of various populations in terms of origin.
Comprehensive studies of the relevant literature revealed that the major ethnic groups of interest to forensic age estimation achieve defined stages of ossification, dentition and sexual maturity in the same natural sequence, so that it is generally possible to apply the relevant reference studies also to other ethnic groups (Schmeling et al., 2001).

6.2.1 Sexual maturation

Data on sexual maturation is relatively scarce. Comparative studies on sexual maturation were conducted by Harlan et al. (Harlan et al., 1979, 1980), Channing-Pearce and Solomon (Channing-Pearce & Solomon, 1987), Wong et al. (Wong et al., 1996) and Huen et al. (Huen et al., 1997). Between 1966 and 1970, Harlan et al. (Harlan et al., 1979) analysed the sexual development of 6,768 male Americans aged between 12 and 17 years. They found no significant differences between blacks and whites. In 1980 Harlan et al. (Harlan et al., 1980) published a representative study examining the sexual maturation of a female American population of the same age group. This study observed relatively faster rates of maturation for blacks compared to whites. Channing-Pearce and Solomon (Channing-Pearce & Solomon, 1987) examined sexual development in a study involving 362 black and 355 white girls in Johannesburg, South Africa. Unlike Harlan et al. (Harlan et al., 1980), they came to the conclusion that black girls on average reached full sexual maturity later than white girls. Wong et al. (Wong et al., 1996) examined sexual maturation in a 1993 study involving 3,872 boys from southern China. They found that the time pattern of sexual maturation was comparable to that of Europeans, with the exception that Asians developed pubic hair later. Huen et al. (Huen et al., 1997) published a similar study including 3,749 girls from southern China. They found that, according to the mean values for the individual stages of maturity, the examined girls were among the earliest to reach sexual maturity worldwide.

6.2.2 Ossification

Numerous studies are available on skeletal maturation of all major ethnic groups (Africans, Australians, Caucasoids and Mongoloids) (Schmeling et al., 2000a). Because there are several potential factors of influence and their simultaneous action makes assessment of population differences a difficult exercise, all the more as the validity of some of those investigations seems to be limited to small sample size, the exclusive consideration of non-relevant age groups, lack of information on health, ethnic identity and socioeconomic status and absence of confirmed data on proband age. Hence, for the problem at hand, greatest relevance may be claimed for studies on various ethnic groups of similar socioeconomic status and living in one and the same region or populations of one and the same socioeconomic status living in different regions. Such studies are available from the USA where research has been conducted on descendants of Caucasoids, Mongoloids and Africans as well as from numerous ethnic groups of the former Soviet Union.

In a comparison with the Greulich-Pyle standards, Sutow (Sutow, 1953) discussed racial differences as one of the causes of retarded skeletal maturation of Japanese children living in Japan. His findings were checked by Greulich (Greulich, 1957) who referred to Japanese individuals living in the USA. He studied hand bone development in 898 children of Japanese descent aged between 5 and 18 years living in the San Francisco Bay area of California. While retarded skeletal maturation, in comparison with the Greulich-Pyle standards was recorded by Sutow for all age groups of Japanese living in their own country, such retardation was detected by Greulich only in boys aged between 5 and 7 years. Boys aged between 13 and 17 and girls between 10 and 17 years even exhibited comparative acceleration. Greulich concluded that the significant retardation, in comparison with the Greulich-Pyle standards, recorded for children living in Japan was attributable to less favourable nutritional and environmental conditions rather than to racial differences. Improved living standards in recent decades resulted in accelerated skeletal maturation even in Japanese living in Japan (Kimura, 1977a, 1977b) which, in the meantime has come to lie within the range of socioeconomically advanced European populations (Beunen et al., 1990; Wenzel et al., 1984).

Whereas some authors (Massé & Hunt, 1963; Garn et al., 1972) reported comparatively accelerated skeletal development in Africans in early childhood, ethnic origin obviously has no significant impact on the bone growth rate in later childhood and adolescence. Platt (Platt, 1956) studied skeletal maturation in 100 black inhabitants of Florida, 143 blacks in Philadelphia and 100 whites in Philadelphia aged between 5 and 14 years. In none of these three groups was skeletal age, as determined by identical X-ray standards, significantly different from chronological age. Platt compared his results with studies on black residents of Africa. Mackay (Mackay, 1952) recorded retardation by 1.5 to 2 years for East Africans, while Weiner and Thambipillai (Weiner & Thambipillai, 1952) recorded an average retardation of 16 months for West Africans. The assumption of an ethnic impact on skeletal maturation would justify expectation of a continuous series of phenomena ranging from severe retardation in blacks in Africa to moderate retardation in black Americans who had mixed with whites to absence of retardation in whites. Such continuous series do not exist, and consequently Platt, postulated that health and nutrition are the major factors influencing skeletal maturation.

Skeletal maturation in 461 black and 380 white Americans in the Lake Erie region was studied by Loder et al. (1993) between 1986 and 1990. Using the atlas method of Greulich and Pyle on the age group of 13-18 years, they recorded comparative acceleration of 0.45 years for white boys, 0.16 years for white girls, 0.38 years for black boys and 0.52 years for black girls. Johnston (Johnston, 1963) studied the same age group of white Americans in

Philadelphia by the same method and found acceleration values of 0.39 years for boys and 0.58 years for girls. Johnston's data for white Americans were almost identical with Loder's findings for black Americans, which seems to clearly underline that in the populations of the age group studied there were no ethnic differences with regard to skeletal maturation. Roche et al. (Roche et al., 1975, 1978) investigated skeletal maturation in the context of race, geographic region, family income and educational standards of parents in a representative cross-section of the US population aged between 6 and 17 years. They found no consistent black-white differences, no significant differences between regions and no urban-rural differences.

Comprehensive studies were conducted on skeletal maturation in different ethnic groups of the former Soviet Union, and 16 studies of 17 ethnic groups in different climatic and geographic zones of the former Soviet Union were evaluated by Pashkova and Burov (Pashkova & Burov, 1980). Included were Russians, Ukrainians, Georgians, Armenians, Azerbaidjanis, Balkarians, Cabardines, Kazakhs, Tadchiks, Uzbeks, Ingushi, Chechenians, Udmurtians, Chukchen, Koryaks, Intelmenians and Evenkians. The range of variation at all stages of skeletal maturation was less than one year in all populations studied. However, the causes of those variations were attributed by the authors to relatively small samples, different methods and techniques used in the studies or undiagnosed clinical conditions of probands but were not attributed to ethnic, regional or climatic differences.

Studies evaluated so far seem to suggest that there is a genetically determined element to skeletal maturation which does not appear to depend on ethnicity and may be exploited under optimum environmental conditions (i.e. high socioeconomic status), whereas a less favourable environment may lead to retardation of skeletal maturation. Applying X-ray standards to individuals of a socioeconomic status lower than that of the reference population, usually leads to underestimating a person's age. In terms of criminal responsibility, this has no adverse effect on the person concerned (Schmeling et al., 2000, 2006).

6.2.3 Dental development

Few comparative studies are available on the subject of third molar mineralization. Gorgani et al. (Gorgani et al., 1990) examined 229 black and 221 white US citizens aged 6-14 years. Among the black subjects crown mineralization of the third molars was completed 1 year earlier. Harris and McKee (Harris & McKee, 1990) studied 655 white and 335 black US citizens aged 3.5-13 years. Whereas the black subjects reached the earlier stages of third molar mineralization about 1 year earlier, the gap appeared to narrow for later stages. This trend is confirmed by the work of Mincer et al. (Mincer et al., 1993). They examined 823 US citizens (80% white, 19% black) aged 14-25 years but did not establish any significant differences in the time frame for third molar mineralization. Daito et al. (Daito et al., 1992) addressed third molar mineralization in 9111 Japanese children aged 7-16 years and compared their data with the values provided by Gravely (Gravely, 1965), Rantanen (Rantanen, 1967) and Haavikko (Haavikko, 1970) for Caucasoid populations. No significant differences were discovered. These studies only lend themselves to limited comparison due to small sample sizes, varying methods and assessment by different observers. A further problem lies in the fact that the age data for subjects of black African origin often was not verified. Moreover, most available studies focus on the earlier stages of mineralization.

A comparative study of third molar mineralization (Olze et al., 2004) was carried out on three population samples: one German, one Japanese and one South African. To this end,

3652 conventional orthopantomograms were evaluated on the basis of Demirjian's stages. Statistically significant differences between the samples investigated were established for the age at which stages D-G of third molar mineralization were achieved. Significant differences between German and Japanese males were noted for stages D-G of mineralization. Significant differences between Japanese and German females were observed for stages D-F. According to these findings, Japanese males and females were approximately 1-2 years older than their German counterparts when they reached stages D-F. Significant age differences between South African and German males applied to stages D-E. Significant age differences between South African and German females were observed for stages E and G. The South African subjects were approximately 1-2 years younger than the German subjects upon achieving these stages of mineralization. Significant age differences between the South African and Japanese samples were ascertained for both sexes at stages D-G. The South African subjects were approx. 1-4 years younger than the Japanese subjects upon reaching these stages.

The population differences observed here may be due to differences in palatal dimensions between the ethnic groups surveyed. The largest palatal dimensions are observed in Africans and the smallest in Mongoloids, with Caucasoids assuming the middle rank (Byers et al., 1997). Inadequate space in the maxillary crest causes delay in third molar eruption, if not retention (Fanning, 1962). In turn, retained third molars mineralize later than teeth whose eruption has not been impeded (Köhler et al., 1994). This would explain why Caucasoid populations occupy the middle position in relative terms when it comes to third molar mineralization, while Mongoloid populations display a comparative delay and African populations a relative acceleration.

With regard to the eruption of third molars, some studies have found significant differences between specific populations (Schmeling et al., 2001). While in Caucasian populations third molars generally do not erupt before age 17 (Müller, 1983), Brown (Brown, 1978), Chagula (Chagula, 1960), Otuyemi et al. (Otuyemi et al., 1997), and Shourie (Shourie, 1946) describe cases of eruption starting in African, Australian and Indian populations already at age 13.

Comparative studies on the relation between age and third molar eruption are available for black and white Americans, Africans, and Asians. Garn et al. (Garn et al., 1972) studied the dentition of all permanent teeth in 953 black and 998 white Americans. In black Americans, the maxillary third molars developed 3.7 years earlier, and the mandibular third molars 5.6 years earlier, than in white Americans. Hassanali (Hassanali, 1985) compared the eruption times of third molars in 1,343 Africans and 1,092 Asians in Kenya. He found that in Africans third molars appeared two to three years earlier. The forensic applicability of these studies is limited, since age data for subjects of African origin are often not verified.

Olze et al. (Olze et al., 2007) analyzed and compared the chronological course of third molar eruption in German, Japanese, and South African populations with proven age of subjects. They found that their German sample had an intermediate rate of dental development as determined by comparing the different ages of third molar eruption. The defined eruption stages occurred at earlier ages in the investigated South African sample, and at later ages in the Japanese sample. Statistically significant population differences were observed in males at stages A and B. The South African males were on average 3.0 to 3.2 years younger than the German males at these stages of development, and the Japanese males were on average 3.1 to 4.2 years older than their South African counterparts for the same developmental stage. The females exhibited statistically significant population differences at stages A, B and C. The South African females reached the target stages on average 1.6 to 1.8 years earlier than the German females, whereas the Japanese females were on average 0.9 to 3.3 years older than their German counterparts. It was concluded that population-specific reference data should be used when evaluating third molar eruption for the purpose of forensic age estimation.

6.3 Pathological factors that produce bone age retardation and acceleration

Pathological conditions alter FAE based on methods of bone and dental age maturation. Albeit being less affected by pathological and ambient conditions than bone age, biomedical literature proves that dental age can be altered by some entities not necessary pathological, like delayed puberty or obesity.

It has been repeatedly demonstrated in the literature that bone age is affected by a wide range of pathological conditions. Main pathological conditions altering bone age maturation are those endocrinological conditions that modify the hypothalamus - hypophysis- gonads axis. Nevertheless other pathological entities affect bone age maturation: some clinical syndromes (as Soto's syndrome or Weaver's syndrome), bone dysplasias (some of them accelerating and other decelerating bone age maturation) and some drugs intake (table 1 and 2) (Taybi & Lachman.1990).

Forensic examiner must be aware of these conditions. The existence of such pathological conditions or drugs intake must must elucidated, as they evidently affect the bone age and dental age maturation. The results of a FAE must include corrections in relation with the existence of such accelerating or decelerating factors.

7. Ethical questions

7.1 Exposition to radiation without clinical indication

When an X-ray examination is carried out exclusively with FAE purposes and without a clinical indication the question arises on the possibility of detrimental effects due to the radiation exposure (European Commision 2004)

The effective dose from an standard X-ray examination of the hands is 0,1 microSievert (μSv), 26 μSv in case of Orthopantomograms, 220 μSv in X-ray examination of the proximal epiphyses of the clavicle and 600 to 800 μSv in case of TC of the sternoclavicular joints. The effective dose in case of a complete thorax TC is 6,6 mSv (Rammstahler et al.2009).

Some authors indicate that an amount of effective annual doses for X-ray examinations of less than 10 μSv are negligible. Other authors have stressed the insignificance of these usual FAE examination doses in comparison with naturally-occurring and civilizing radiation exposure. The effective dose from naturally-occurring radiation exposure has been calculated as an average in Germany at about 1,2 mSv per year and in The Netherlands at about 2,0 mSv. Fly staff of airplanes receive an average of 2000 mSv per year as a result of staying high in air (cosmic radiation). The radiation exposure from intercontinental flight at an altitude of 12000 meters is 0,008 mSv per hour (Schmeling.2008).

It follows that the radiation dose effective in case of an intercontinental flight is equivalent to 2 orthopantomograms and a CT of sternoclavicular joints is equivalent to 3,5 months of naturally occurring radiation exposure. On the basis of these comparisons the health risk as a result of usual X-ray examinations for FAE is negligible (Schmeling.2008)

Nevertheless, radiation exposure produce not only stochastic but non-stochastic damages the physicians must be aware of. Non-stochastic effects appear above 100 mSv and are therefore irrelevant in usual radiological diagnosis. But non-stochastic effects don't have such a threshold and are not dose related, so their eventual appearance in case of X-rays examinations must be cautiously considered. Some authors minimize and other maximize the harm inherent to these non-stochastic effects (Garamendi&Landa.2010)

Bone Age Advanced		Drugs altering bone age
Adrenal Hiperplasia	Gigantism	Amiodarone
Acrodysostosis	Hypertiroidism	Budenoside
Adrenocortical Tumour	Idiopatic isosexual precocious puberty	Buclometasone, Dipropionate
Aldosteronism, primary	Lipodistrophy	Phenitoine
Arthrogryposis	Marshall Smith Syndrome	Metilphenidate
Beckwith-Wiedemann, syndrome	McCune Albright Syndrome	
Cerebral tumour	Neurofibromatosis	
Cockayne syndrome	Obesity	
Congenital Adrenal Hyperplasia	Peripheral dystosis (Brailsford)	
Cushing Syndrome	Sotos syndrome	
Ectopic Gonadotropine Production	Trisomy 8 Syndrome	
Familar Advanced Bone Age	Weaver syndrome	

Table 1. Pathologic factors associated with bine age acceleration and drugs intake that alter bone age process.

Anyway, albeit apparently negligible the possible detrimental effects due to radiation exposure must be considered. A best practice in FAE on the use of X-ray exams without other medical indications should avoid unnecessary repetition of the exams to minimize the radiation dose effective received by probands, should include the practice of the minimum necessary exams to avoid unnecessary exams and should include the elaboration of National Registers of unaccompanied minors to avoid the unnecessary repetition of all tests by different physicians at different dates (Garamendi et al.2011)

7.2 Ethical dimension of the expert report

Forensic physicians involved in FAE case analysis must be conscious of the ethical dimension of the conclusions written on their expert reports. Dr. Mata in 1842 pointed out that expressing an expert opinion in a Justice Court must be cautious (Mata, 1842). This old professor reminds future forensic physicians that writing a report expressing complete reliability in a question without a solid scientific basis could be an error. Some physicians understand that expressing themselves with complete certainty at Justice Court helps judges to decide on questions like FAE more clearly. Oppositely, this is not an advisable attitude as it can give the Court a false impression of certainty in questions not completely certain in the state of the art for the scientific community. This very same principle is the one precluded by Evidence Based Medicine.

Bone Age Retarded			
Addison Disease	Dubowitz syndrome	Juvenil Idiopatic Osteoporosis	Other chronic infections, as Malaria
Amonopterin fetopathy	Elite sports	Juvenil Rhemtaoid Arthritis	Papillon-Lefevre Syndrome
Anemias	Endemic Diarrhea	KBG syndrome	Parasitosis
Aspartylglucosa-minuria	Extreme weight loss	Kocher-Debre-Semelaigne Syndrome	Patterson Syndrome
C Syndrome	Fetal rubella syndrome	Laron Dwarfism	Phenylketonuria
Celiac Disease	Freeman-Seldom syndrome	Larsen Syndrome	Pleonosteosis
Cistis fibrosis	Fucosidosis	Legg, Calvé, Perthes Disease	Prader- Willi Syndrome
Cleiodocraneal dysplasia	GAPO syndrome	Lenz-Manjewski hiperostotic dwarfism	Raquitism
Coffin-Lowry Syndrome	Geophagia-dwarfism hipogonadism syndrome	Lesch-Nyhan syndrome	Renal Failure
Coffin-Siris Syndrome	Glycogenosis tipe I	Malnourishement	Renal tubulra acidosis
Crohn Disease	Hipoadrenalism	Marinesco-Sjögren syndrome	Rickets
Cupper Deficiency	Hipogonadism	Mauriac syndrome	Rubinstein-Taybi syndrome
De Lange Syndrome	Hipoparatiroidism	Melnick-Needles osteodysplasty	Silver-Russel syndrome
De Morsier syndrome	Hipopituitarism	Metartropic dysplasia	Talasemia
De Sanctis-Cacchione syndrome	Hipotiroidism	Meyer dysplasia of femoral head	Thalassemia
Deaf mutism-goiter euthyroidism syndrome	Histiocitosis X	Mucolipidosis II	The 3 M syndrome
Deprivation dwarfism	HIV infection	Mucopolysacharidosis	Trichohesis nodosa syndrome
Deprivation Syndrome	Hypogonadysm	Nephrotic syndrome	Trisomy 21
Diabetes Mellitus	Incontinentia pigmenti	Nervous Anorexia	Weill-Marchesani Syndrome
Diabetes Mellitus	Intrauterine growth retardiation	Noonan syndrome	Wilson disease
Drugs	Johanson-Blizzard syndrome	Osteoporosis idiopatic juvenile	Zellweger Syndrome

Table 2. Pathologic factors associated with bone age process retardation.

Case reports like the one published by Nambiar et al in 1998 warns forensic physicians of the real ethical dangers of not correctly expressing the degree of certainty of the results included in their expert reports (Nambiar et al., 1998).

8. Expert report

According to the recommendations of the Study Group on Forensic Age Diagnostics (Schmeling et al., 2008) the collected findings and the determined stages are to be presented in detail in the expert report. The used stage classifications and reference studies are to be mentioned.

Reference studies used for forensic age estimation should meet the following requirements:

- Adequate sample size
- Proven age of subjects
- Even age distributions of subjects
- Analysis separately for both sexes
- Information on the time of examination
- Clear definition of the examined features
- Detailed description of the methods
- Data on the reference population regarding ethnicity, socioeconomic status, state of health
- Data on the sample size, mean value, and range of scatter for each examined feature

Examples of reference studies are Greulich and Pyle (Greulich & Pyle, 1959), Gunst et al. (Gunst et al., 2003), Kahl and Schwarze (Kahl & Schwarze, 1988), Kellinghaus et al. (Kellinghaus et al., 2010a, b), Mincer et al. (Mincer et al., 1993), Olze et al. (Olze et al., 2003, 2004b, 2006), Ruhstaller (Ruhstaller, 2006), Schmeling et al. (Schmeling etl., 2004), Tanner et al. (Tanner et al., 2001), Thiemann et al. (Thiemann et al., 2006).

For each examined feature, the report must indicate the most likely age and the range of scatter of the reference population. While mean values and medians show the most likely age for a certain age characteristic standard deviations and interquartile differences are common measurement data for the ranges of scatter. Mean values and standard deviations are valid only for normally distributed features. 68% of the test persons of the reference population with a certain feature lie between the mean value plus/ minus one standard deviation and 95% of the test persons lie between the mean value plus/ minus two standard deviations. Medians and percentiles are distribution independent parameters. 50% of the test persons with a special feature lie within the 25th and the 75th percentiles. This difference is also called interquartile difference.

It has to be pointed out that means and medians can not be used for the last stage of the age characteristics because they depend on the upper limit of the examined age group. Instead of mean values the 50% probability value should be used for the last stage of an age characteristic. This value can be calculated by means of logistic regression (Knell et al., 2009).

The results of the individual examinations should be compiled in a final age diagnosis. The individual's most likely age is estimated on the basis of all partial diagnoses and a critical discussion of the individual case. This final age diagnosis should include a discussion of the age-relevant variations resulting from application of the reference studies in an individual case, such as different ethnicity, different socioeconomic status or diseases that may affect the development of the individual examined.

However, for age diagnoses obtained with a combination of methods there is still no satisfactory way to scientifically determine the margin of error. While a number of reference studies collected data on individual features and some studies both on skeletal maturation and tooth mineralization (Grön, 1962; Lacey, 1973; Lamons & Gray, 1958; Pfau & Sciulli,

1994), there is still no reference study available analysing all required features for one single reference population. If independent features are examined as part of an age diagnosis that combines several methods, it may be assumed that the margin of error of the combined age diagnosis would be smaller than that for each individual feature. So far it has not been possible to quantify this difference. Since combining methods also makes it possible to identify statistical outliers, the margin of error of the combined age diagnosis should decrease to a certain extent, which unfortunately is also not quantifiable.

Indirect conclusions about the range of scatter of the summarizing age diagnosis were possible after verifying age estimates carried out at the Institute of Legal Medicine in Berlin. To this effect, the court's case files of the persons originally examined for age estimation purposes at the institute were consulted to see whether the actual age of these persons was established during the court proceedings. In all cases where the age of the person concerned could be verified beyond doubt deviation between estimated and actual age ranged between plus or minus 12 months (Schmeling et al., 2003).

Furthermore the expert report should give the degree of probability that the stated age is the actual age or that the individual's age is above the relevant age limit. To this purpose the following probability ratings can be used:

- "almost certain probability (beyond reasonable doubt)": probability > 99.8% (This probability refers to the threefold standard deviation).
- "very probable" or "high probability": probability > 90%
- "probable": probability > 50%
- "undecided": probability = 50%
- "less probable" or "improbable": probability < 50%
- "very improbable": probability < 10%
- "almost certainly improbable": probability < 0.2%

The following phrasing gives an example for an adequate conclusion:

"Summarizing all test results the following can be established:

- There is a very high probability that the given date of birth is not correct but that an earlier date can be assumed,
- there is a very high probability of an age of above 14 years and a high probability of one above 16,
- there is but very low probability that the 18th year of age has been reached,
- and there is almost certain probability that the 21st year of age has not been reached."

9. Practical cases

Case 1

The accused, of Afghan origin, was under investigation on murder charges. According to his own statement he was 13 years and 5 months old at the time of examination. As the investigative authorities had considerable doubts relative to the age given by the person concerned, a court order was issued for forensic age estimation with inclusion of X-ray examinations.

In the course of physical examination, a body length of 168 cm was measured, body weight was 55 kg. The upper lip and chin were covered with 5 mm-long beard growth, the cheeks manifested an after-shave condition. The larynx was prominent. The armpits displayed 5 mm-long hair stubble. The genital region manifested a dense area of curly hair rising up sparsely to the navel. Genital development was to be placed in the second phase of puberty. The physical stature and the pattern of body hair corresponded to those of an adolescent. No indications of developmental disorders were detected.

Fig. 5 shows the hand radiograph of the person concerned. The X-ray morphology of the carpal bones appeared normal. The former epiphyseal plates of the metacarpals and phalanges were completely ossified and in part still slightly marked. The distal epiphyseal plates of the radius and ulna were for the most part open and presented incipient ossification only in the middle section. On the basis of the morphological findings of the X-rays, a skeletal age of 16-17 years according to Thiemann et al. (Thiemann et al., 2006) emerged. In the reference study by Schmeling et al. (Schmeling et al., 2006), for a skeletal age of 16 years a mean age of 15.3 years with a standard deviation of 0.8 years was reported. For a skeletal age of 17 years, the mean age is 16.8 years, whilst standard deviation amounts to 1.1 years. A reference study which gathered data from a socioeconomically highly developed population was used. For this reason, it may be assumed that the actual age of the person concerned does not lie below the estimated age. As the development of the hand skeleton was not complete, no X-ray examination of the clavicles was performed.

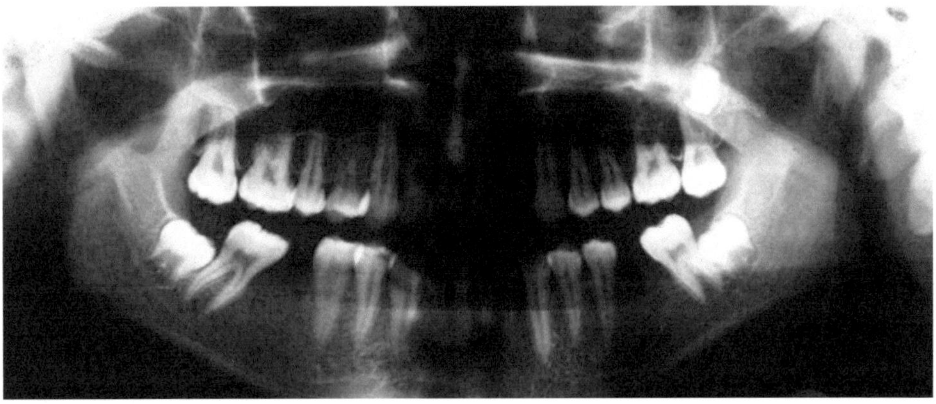

Fig. 5. Case 1: orthopantomogram

In the course of dental examination it was ascertained that the third molars had not erupted into the oral cavity. An evaluation of the orthopantomogram revealed that tooth 18 was congenitally absent and that impacted tooth number 28 presented a mineralisation stage D according to Demirjian whilst teeth 38 and 48 presented a stage E (fig. 6). In the reference study by Olze et al. (Olze et al., 2003), a mean age of 16.3 years was given for mineralisation stage D of tooth number 28 with a standard deviation of 3.2 years. The mean age for stage E of the lower third molars is 16.7 years with standard deviations of 2.1 to 2.3 years. On the basis of the ethnicity of the person concerned, a reference study for Caucasians was used.

In the synopsis of the findings it was determined that the person concerned was most probably 16-17 years old at the time of examination. At the time of examination the 14th year of life had been completed beyond reasonable doubt. The age stated by the person concerned was not consistent with the examination findings. In the course of the court case it came to light that the actual age of the person concerned at the time of examination was 16 years and 4 months.

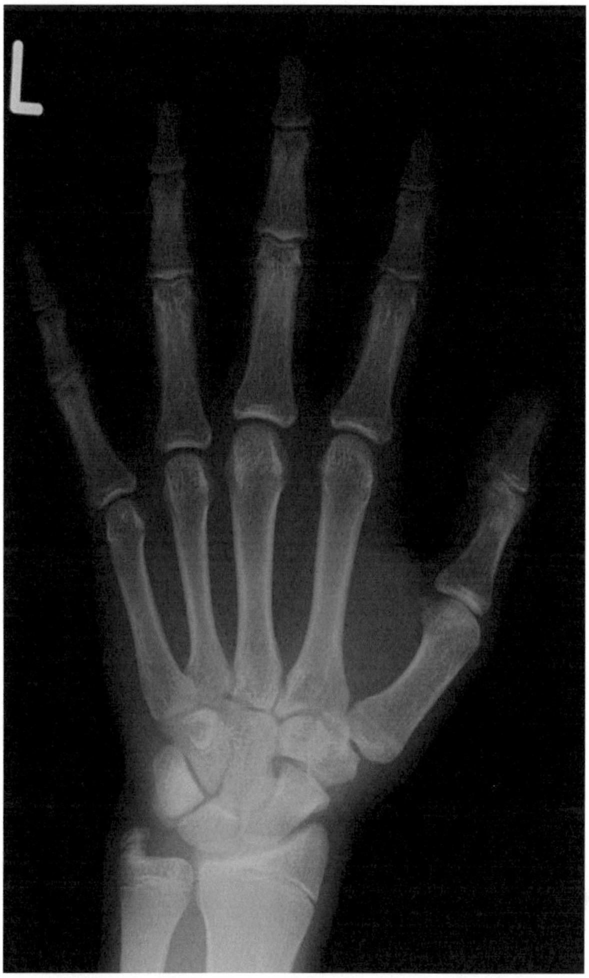

Fig. 6. Case 1: hand radiograph

Case 2

The person to be examined was under investigation for a drug offence. According to his own statement the accused came from Guinea-Bissau and was 17 years and 8 months old at the time of examination. As the investigative authorities had considerable doubts relative to the age given by the person concerned, a court order was issued for forensic age estimation with inclusion of X-ray examinations.

In the course of physical examination, a body length of 178 cm and a body weight of 68 kg were measured. The upper lip, chin and cheeks manifested an after-shave condition. The larynx was prominent. The armpits displayed an area of dense curly hair. The genital region was covered with a horizontally restricted area of dense curly hair. The external genitalia were mature. The physical stature and the pattern of body hair corresponded to those of an adult. No indications of developmental disorders were detected.

Fig. 7 shows the hand radiograph of the person concerned. The X-ray morphology of the carpal bones appeared normal. The former epiphyseal plates of the metacarpals and phalanges were completely ossified and no longer detectable. The former epiphyseal plate of the radius was completely ossified and only very discretely marked in the middle third. The former epiphyseal plate of the ulna was completely ossified and no longer detectable. Ossification of the hand skeleton was thus complete. In line with this, skeletal age according to Thiemann et al. (Thiemann et al., 2006) was 18 years. In the reference study by Schmeling et al. (Schmeling et al., 2006), for a skeletal age of 18 years a mean age of 18.2 years with a standard deviation of 0.7 years was reported. The minimum age was 16.7 years. A reference study which gathered data from a socioeconomically highly developed population was used. For this reason, it may be assumed that the person concerned was not younger than 16.7 years at the time of examination.

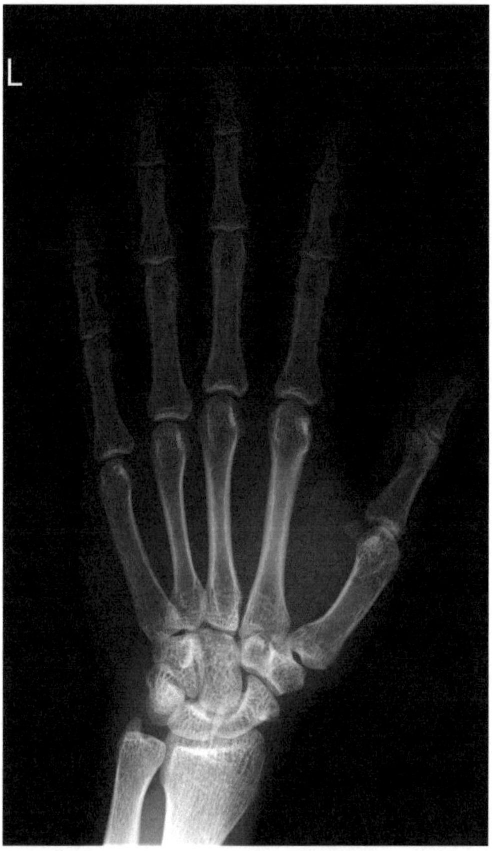

Fig. 7. Case 2: hand radiograph

As development of the hand skeleton was complete, a CT examination of both sternoclavicular joints was performed with a slice thickness of 1 mm. The former medial clavicular epiphyseal plate was completely ossified on both sides. In the region of the former epiphyseal plates, remnants of the epiphyseal scar still remained both on the right and the left (fig. 8 and 9). Thus, a stage 4 was present on both sides according to Schmeling et al. (Schmeling et al., 2004). In the reference study by Kellinghaus et al. (Kellinghaus et al., 2010) the mean age for stage 4 was 29.6 years with a standard deviation of 4.2 years. The minimum age was around 21.6 years.

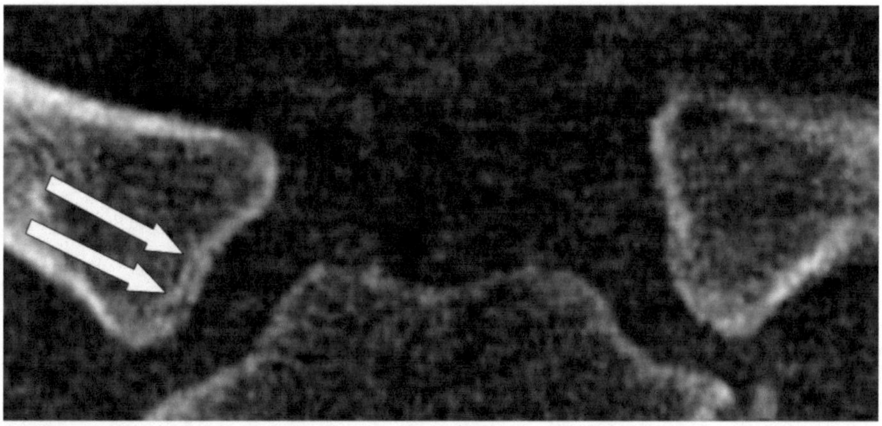

Fig. 8. Case 2: CT scan of the sterno-clavicular joints, the arrows show remnants of the epiphyseal scar of the right clavicle

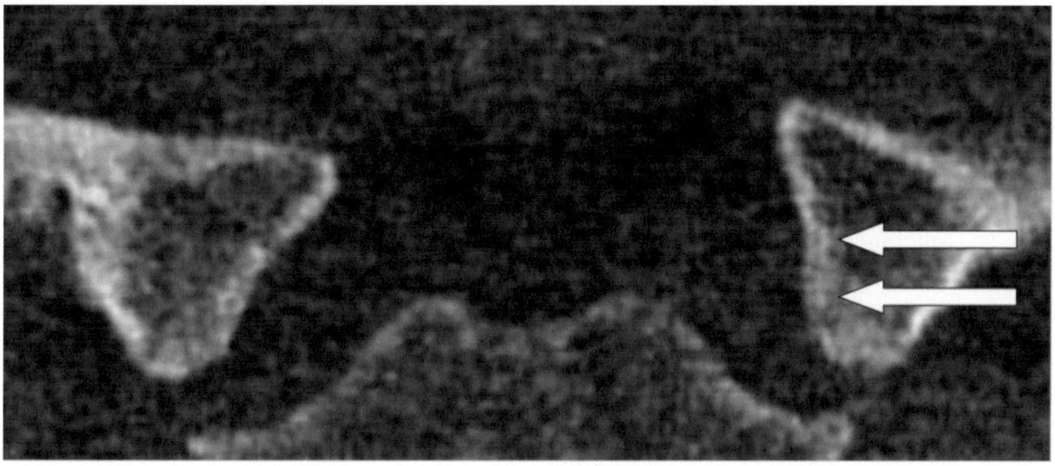

Fig. 9. Case 2: CT scan of the sterno-clavicular joints, the arrows show remnants of the epiphyseal scar of the left clavicle

In the course of dental examination it was ascertained that the person concerned had an incomplete set of teeth. Teeth numbers 11, 12, 21, 22 and 37 were missing. All four third molars had erupted into the oral cavity and had reached the occlusal plane. An evaluation of the orthopantomogram revealed that all the third molars presented a mineralisation stage H according to Demirjian (fig. 6). In the reference study by Olze et al. (Olze et al., 2006) a mean age of between 22.7 and 22.9 years was given for mineralisation stage H of the third molars with standard deviations of between 2.3 and 2.5 years. The minimum age was given as 17 years (Olze et al., 2004). On the basis of the ethnicity of the person concerned a reference study for black Africans was used.

In the synopsis of the findings it was determined that the absolute minimum age of the person concerned was 21.6 years. At the time of examination both the 18th and the 21st year of life had been completed beyond reasonable doubt. The age stated by the person concerned was not consistent with the examination findings.

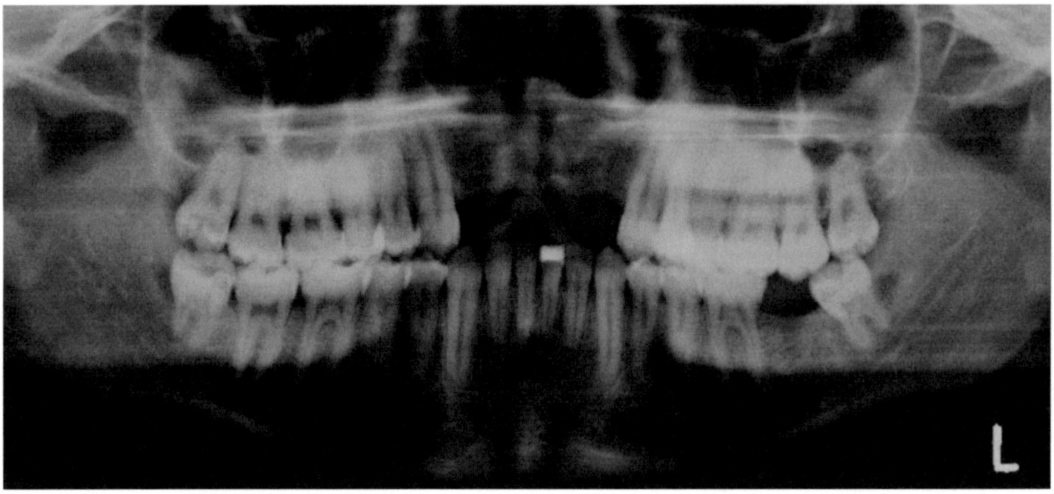

Fig. 10. Case 2: orthopantomogram

10. Reference

Adair FL, Scammon RE. Ossification centers of the wrist, knee and ankle at birth with particular reference to the physical development and maturity of the newborn. Am J Obst Gynec.1921;2:35-60.

Arany S, Iino M, Yoshioka N (2004) Radiographic survey of third molar development in relation to chronological age among Japanese juveniles. J Forensic Sci 49(3):534-8

Aykroyd RG, Lucy D, Pollard AM, Solheim T (1997) Technical note: regression analysis in adult age assessment. Am J Phys Anthopol 104 259-265.

Bang G (1989) Age Changes in teeth: developmental and regressive. In: Iscan MY Age Markers in the Human Skeleton: 213. Charles C Thomas (ed). Springfield. Illinois.

Bañón R. El estudio de la edad ósea en el carpo y en otras regiones anatómicas aplicado a la estimación de minoría de edad. Jornadas sobre Determinación de edad en menores indocumentados. Donostia, marzo de 2004.

Baume LJ, Becks H, Evans HM (1954) Hormonal control of tooth eruption. III. The response of the incisors of hypophysectomized rats to a growth hormone, thyroxin, or the combination of both. J Dent Res 33(1):104-14.

Bassed RB, Drummer OH, Briggs C, Valenzuela A (2010) Age estimation and the medial clavicular epiphysis: analysis of the age of majority in an Australian population using computed tomography. Forensic Sci Med Pathol, doi 10.1007/s12024-010-9200-y

Beunen G, Lefevre J, Ostyn M, Renson R, Simons J, Van Gerven D (1990) Skeletal maturity in Belgian youths assessed by the Tanner-Whitehouse method (TW2). Ann Hum Biol 17:355-376

Black SM, Scheuer JL (1996) Age changes in the clavicle: from the early neonatal period to skeletal maturity. Int J Osteoarcheol 6:425-434

Blankenship JA, Mincer HH, Anderson KM, Woods MA, Burton EL (2007) Third molar development in the estimation of chronologic age in american blacks as compared with whites. J Forensic Sci 52(2):428-33.

Bolaños Bolaños MV, Moussa H, Manrique MC, Bolaños MJ (2003) Radiographic evaluation of third molar development in Spanish children and young people. Forensic Sci Int 133(3):212-9.
Bontrager KL, Lampignano (2009) Bontrager's handbook of radiographic positioning and techniques. Mosby
Borovansky L, Hnévkovský O. Growth of the body and process of ossification in Prague boys from 4 to 19 years. Anthropologie Praha.1929;7:169-208.
Braga J, Heuze Y, Chavadel O, Sonan NK, Geramy A (2005) Non-adult dental age assessment: correspondence analysis and linear regression versus Bayesian predictions. Int J Legal Med 119:260-274.
Bravo RM. La situación de menores no acompañados en España. Conferencia regional sobre las migraciones de los menores no acompañados: actuar de acuerdo con el interés superior del menor. European Council. Strasbourg.2005.
Brogdon BG. Forensic Radiology. CRC Press 1998.
Brown T (1978) Tooth emergence in Australian Aboriginies. Ann Hum Biol 5:41-54
Bueno JR, Mestre FJ. La proteccion de menores migrantes no acompañados: un modelo de intervención social. Revista Alterantivas. Cuadernos de Trabajo Social.2006;14:155-170
Bueno M, Sarria A, Bueno M. Estudio de la maduración ósea en niños obesos aragoneses de ambos sexos. An Esp Pediatr 1996;45:29-32.
Bueno M, Sarría A, Bueno M. Estudio de la maduración ósea en niños obesos aragoneses de ambos sexos. An Esp Pediatr, 1996; 45: 29-32.
Büken B, Safak AA, Yazici B, Büken E, Mayda AS. Is the assessment of bone age by the Greulich-Pyle meted reliable at forensic age estimation for Turkish children? Forensic Sci Int. 2007;DOI:10.1016/j.forsciint.2007.02.023
Burdi A.R. Desarrollo de la dentición y la oclusión.Moyers R.E. Manual de ortodoncia. Buenos Aires: Panamericana; 1992.
Byers SN, Churchill SE, Curran B (1997) Identification of Euro-Americans, Afro-Americans, and Ameridians from palatal dimensions. J Forensic Sci 42:3-9.
Cameron M. Assessment of growth and maturtion during adoelsecence. Horm Res 1993;39(Suppl 3):9-17.
Chagula WK (1960) The age of eruption of third permanent molars in male East Africans. Am J Phys Anthrop 18:77-82
Chaning-Pearce SM, Solomon L (1987) Pubertal development in black and white Johannesburg girls. S Afr Med J 71:22-24
Convention on the Rights of the Child, G.A. res. 44/25, annex, 44 U.N. GAOR Supp. (No. 49) at 167, U.N. Doc. A/44/49 (1989), entered into force Sept. 2, 1990.
Daito M, Tanaka M, Hieda T (1992) Clinical observations on the development of third molars. J Osaka Dent Univ 26:91-104
Davies DA, Parsons FG. Age order of appearance of epiphyses and their fusion with the diaphyses. J Anat.1927;62:58-71.
Davis PJ, Hagg U (1994) The accuracy and precision of the "Demirjian system" when used for age determination in Chinese children. Swed Dent J 18(3):113-6.
Declaration of the Rights of the Child, G.A. res. 1386 (XIV), 14 U.N. GAOR Supp. (No. 16) at 19, U.N. Doc. A/4354 (1959).
Demirjian A, Goldstein H, Tanner JM (1973) A new system of dental age assessment. Human Biology 42:211-27.

Demirjian A. (1976) New systems for dental maturity based on seven and four teeth. Annals for Human Biology 3(5):411-21.

Dhanjal KS, Bhardwaj MK, Liversidge HM (2006) Reproducibility of radiographic stage assessment of third molars. Forensic Sci Int 15;159 Suppl 1:S74-7.

Dundaroz MR, Sarici SU, Denli M et al. Bone age in children with nocturnal eneuresis. Int Urol Nephrol, 2001; 32(3): 389-391.

Eid RM Simi R Friggi MN Fisberg M (2002) Assessment of dental maturity of Brazilian children aged 6 to years using Demirjian's method. Int J Paediatr Dent 12(6):423-8.

European Commission. Radiation protection (2004). Medico-legal exposures, exposures with ionising radiation without medical indication. Proceedings of the International Symposium. Dublin, 4-6 September 2002.

European Migration Network. Policies on reception, return and integration arrangements for Unacompannied minors- an EU comparative study. Eurepaen Comission. Brussels. 2010.

Evans KT, Knight B (1981) Radiology in forensic medicine. Oxford: Blackwell Scientific Publications.

Fanning EA (1962) Third molar emergence in Bostonians. Am J Phys Anthropol 20:339-346.

Federal Office for Migrationa nd Refugees. Uncompanied minors in Germany: reception, return and integration arrangements. European Migration Network. European Comission. Brussels.2008

Flecker H (1933) Roentgenographic observations of the times of appearance of epiphyses and their fusion with the diaphyses. J Anat 67:118-164

Fleshman K. Bone age determination in a pediatric population as an indicator of nutritional status. Trop Doct, 2000; 30(1): 16-18.

Foti B, Lalys L, Adalian P, Giustiniani J, Maczel M, Signoli M et al (2003) New forensic approach to age determination in children based on tooth eruption. Forensic Sci Int 132(1):49-56.

Freyschmidt J, Brossmann J, Wiens J, Sternberg A. Borderlands of normal and early pathological findings in skeletal radiography. 5th English Edition, 2.001. George Thieme Verlag.

Friedrich RE, Ulbricht C, von Maydell LA, Scheuer HA (2005) The impact of wisdom teeth topography on chronology of root formation--forensic consequence for forensic-odontologic age estimation of adolescents and young adults. Radiographic investigations using orthopantomography. Arch Kriminol 216(1-2):15-35.

Frucht S, Schnegelsberg C, Schulte-Monting J, Rose E, Jonas I (2000) Dental age in southwest Germany. A radiographic study. J Orofac Orthop 61(5):318-29.

Fulton JT, Price B (1954) Longitudinal data on eruption and attack of the permanent teeth. J Dent Res 33:65-79.

Galstaun G. A study of ossification as observed in Indian subjects. Indian J Med Res. 1937;25:267-324

Garamendi PM, Landa MI. Estimación forense de la edad en torno a 18 años. Revisión bibliográfica. Cuad Med For. 2003(31):13-24.

Garamendi PM, Landa MI. Estimación forense de la edad en torno a 18 años. Revisión bibliográfica. Cuad Med For. 2003(31):13-24.

Garamendi PM, Landa MI (2010). Determinación de la edad mediante la radiología. Rev Esp Med Legal.36(1):3-13.

Garamendi PM, Landa MI, Ballesteros J, Solano MA (2005) Reliability of the methods applied to assess age minority in living subjects around 18 years old. A survey on a Moroccan origin population. Forensic Sci Int 10;154(1):3-12.

Garamendi PM, Landa MI, Ballesteros J, Solano MA. Reliability of the methods applied to assess age minority in living subjects around 18 years old. A survey on a Moroccan origin population. Forensic Sci Int.2005;154:3–12

Garamendi PM, Landa MI, Botella MC, Alemán I (2011) Forensic age estimation on digital X-ray images: Medial epiphyses of the clavicle and first rib ossification in relation to chronological age. J Foensic Sci 56:S3-S12

Garamendi PM, Bañón R, Pujol A, Aguado F, Landa MI, Prieto JL, Serrulla F. Recomendaciones sobre métodos de estimación forense de la edad de los menores extranjeros no acompañados. Documento de Consenso de Buenas Practicas entre los Institutos de Medicina Legal de España (2011). Rev Esp Med Legal.37(1):22-29.

Garn SM, Lewis AB (1962) Relationship between third molar agenesis and reduction in tooth number. Angle Orthodontist 32(1):14-8.

Garn SM, Lewis AB, Polachek DL (1959) Variability of Tooth Formation. J Dent Res 38:135-48.

Garn SM, Sandusky ST, Nagy JM, McCann MB (1972) Advanced skeletal development in low income Negro children. J Pediatr 80:965-969

Geneva Declaration of the Rights of the Child of 1924, adopted Sept. 26, 1924, League of Nations O.J. Spec. Supp. 21, at 43 (1924).

German interdisciplinary working group for age diagnostics (2001) Recommendations on Age Diagnostics of Living Persons in Criminal Proceedings. Newsletter. German Association Of Forensic Odonto-Stomatology (AKFOS) 8(2).

Giles E, Klepinger LL (1988) Confidence intervals for estimates based on linear regression in forensic anthropology. J. Forensic Sci 33:1218-1222.

Giles NB, Knott VB, Meredith HV (1963) Increase in intraoral height of selected permanent teeth during the quadrennium following gingival emergence. Angle Orthodontist 33:195-206.

Gilsanz V, Skaggs DL, Kovanlikaya A et al. Differential effect of race on the axial appendicular skeletons of children. J Clin Endocrinol Metab, 1988; 83: 1420-1427

Gorgani N, Sullivan RE, DuBois L (1990) A radiographic investigation of third-molar development. J Dent Child 57:106-110

Gravely JF (1965) A radiographic survey of third molar development. Brit Dent J 119:397-401

Green LJ (19619 The interrelationships among height, weight and chronological dental and skeletal ages. Angle Orthod 31:1890-6.

Greulich WW (1957) A comparison of the physical growth and development of American-born and native Japanese children. Am J Phys Anthrop 15:489-515

Greulich WW, Pyle SI. Radiographic atlas of skeletal development of the hand and wrist. ment of the hand and wrist. Standford University Press, 1950- 1959.

Grön A-M (1962) Prediction of tooth emergence. J Dent Res 41:573-585

Gross GW, Boone JM, Bishop DM. Pediatric skeletal age: determination with neural networks. Radiology, 1995;195:686-695.

Gunst K, Mesotten K, Carbonez A, Willems G (2003) Third molar root development in relation to chronological age: a large sample sized retrospective study. Forensic Sci Int 136(1-3):52-7.

Haavikko K (1970) The formation and the alveolar and clinical eruption of the permanent teeth. Suom Hammaslääk Toim 66:103-170

Haavikko K (1974) Tooth formation age stimated on a few selected teeth. A simple method for clinical use. Procc Finn Dent Soc 70:15-9.

Hagg U, Taranger J (1980) Skeletal stages of the hand and wrist as indicators of the puberal growth. Acta Odontol Scand 38:187-200.

Harlan WR, Grillo GP, Cornoni-Huntley J, Leaverton PE (1979) Secondary sex characteristics of boys 12 to 17 years of age - United States Health Examination Survey. J Pediatr 95:293-297

Harlan WR, Harlan EA, Grillo GP (1980) Secondary sex characteristics of girls 12 to 17 years of age - United States Health Examination Survey. J Pediatr 96:1074-1078

Harris EF (2007) Mineralization of the mandibular third molar: a study of American blacks and whites. Am J Phys Anthropol. 2007 Jan;132(1):98-109.

Harris EF, McKee JH (1990) Tooth mineralisation standards for Blacks and Whites from the Middle Southern United States. J Forensic Sci 35:859-872

Harris MJ, Nortjé CJ (1984) The mesial root of the third mandibular molar. A possible indicator of age. J Forensic Odontostomat 2(2):39-43.

Hassanali J (1985) The third permanent molar eruption in Kenyan Africans and Asians. Ann Hum Biol 12:517-523

Hillewig E, De Tobel J, Cuche O, Vandemaele P, Piette M, Verstraete K (2011) Magnetic resonance imaging of the medial extremity of the clavicle in forensic bone age determination: a new four-minute approach. Eur Radiol 21:757-767

Huen KF, Leung SS, Lau JT, Cheung AY, Leung NK, Chiu MC (1997) Secular trend in the sexual maturation of southern Chinese girls. Acta Paediatr 86:1121-1124

Jahari AB, Haas J, Husaini MA, Pollitt E. Effects of an energy and micronutrient supplement on skeletal maturation in undernourished children in Indonesia. Eur J Clin Nutr, 2000; 54 (suppl 2): 74-79

Ji L, Terazawa K, Tsukamoto T, Haga K (1994) Estimation of age from epiphyseal union degrees of the sternal end of the clavicle. Hokkaido Igaku Zasshi 69:104-111

Jit I, Kullkarni M (1976) Times of appearance and fusion of epiphysis at the medial end of the clavicle. Indian J Med Res 64:773-782

Johnston FE (1963) Skeletal age and its prediction in Philadelphia children. Hum Biol 35:192-202

Kahl B, Schwarze CW (1988) Aktualisierung der Dentitionstabelle von I. Schour und M. Massler von 1941. Fortschr Kieferorthop 49:432-443

Kaur G, Khandelwal N, Jasuja OP (2010) Computed tomographic studies on ossification status of medial epiphysis of clavicle: effect of slice thickness and dose distribution. J Indian Acad Forensic Med 32:298-302

Kellinghaus M, Schulz R, Vieth V, Schmidt S, Pfeiffer H, Schmeling A (2010a) Enhanced possibilities to make statements on the ossification status of the medial clavicular epiphysis using an amplified staging scheme in evaluating thin-slice CT scans. Int J Legal Med 124:321-325

Kellinghaus M, Schulz R, Vieth V, Schmidt S, Schmeling A (2010b) Forensic age estimation in living subjects based on the ossification status of the medial clavicular epiphysis as revealed by thin-slice multidetector computed tomography. Int J Legal Med 124:149-154

Kieser JA (1990) Human Adults Odontometrics: The Study of Variation in Adult Tooth Size. New York: Cambridge University Press.

Kimura K (1977a) Skeletal maturity of the hand and wrist in Japanese children by the TW2 method. Ann Hum Biol 4:353-356

Kimura K (1977b) Skeletal maturity of the hand and wrist in Japanese children in Sapporo by the TW2 method. Ann Hum Biol 4:449-454

Knell B, Ruhstaller P, Prieels F, Schmeling A (2009) Dental age diagnostics by means of radiographical evaluation of the growth stages of lower wisdom teeth. Int J Legal Med 123:465-469.

Koc A, Karaoglanoglu M, Erdogan M et al. Assessment of bone ages: is the Greulich-Pyle method sufficient for Turkish boys?. Pediatr Int, 2001; 43(6): 662-665.

Koc A, Karaoglanoglu M, Erdogan M, Kosecik M, Cesur Y. Assessment of bone ages: is the Greulich-Pyle method sufficient for Turkish boys? Pediatr Int 2001;43(6):662-665.

Köhler S, Schmelzle R, Loitz C, Püschel K (1994) Development of wisdom teeth as a criterion of age determination. Ann Anat 176(4):339-45.

Koshy S, Tandon S (1998) Dental age assessment: the applicability of Demirjian's method in south Indian children. Forensic Sci Int 94(1-2):73-85.

Kreitner K-F, Schweden F, Schild HH, Riepert T, Nafe B (1997) Die computertomographisch bestimmte Ausreifung der medialen Klavikulaepiphyse - eine additive Methode zur Altersbestimmung im Adoleszentenalter und in der dritten Lebensdekade? Fortschr Röntgenstr 166:481-486

Kreitner K-F, Schweden FJ, Riepert T, Nafe B, Thelen M (1998) Bone age determination based on the study of the medial extremity of the clavicle. Eur Radiol 8:1116-1122

Krogman WM, Iscan MY (1986) The human skeleton in forensic medicine. 2 ed. Springfield: Charles C Thomas

Kullman L, Johanson G, Åkesson L (1992) Root development of the lower third molar and its relation to chronological age. Swed Dent J 16:161-7.

Lacey KA (1973) Relationship between bone age and dental development. Lancet 302:736-737

Lamons FF, Gray SW (1958) A study of the relationship between tooth eruption age, skeletal development age, and chronological age in sixty-one Atlanta children. Am J Orthod 44:687-691

Levesque GY, Demirjian A, Tanguay R (1981) Sexual dimophism in the development, emergence and agenesis of the mandibular third molar. J Dent Res 60(10):1735-41.

Liversidge HM (1994) Accuracy of age stimation from developing teeth of a population of known age (0 to 5,4 years). Int Journal Osteoarchaeol 4:37-46.

Liversidge HM, Speechly T, Hector MP (1999) Dental maduration in British children: are Demirjian's standars applicable. Int J Pediatr Dent 9:263-9.

Loder RT, Estle DT, Morrison K, Eggleston D, Fish DN, Grennfield ML, Guire KE (1993) Applicability of the Greulich and Pyle skeletal age standards to black and white children of today. Am J Dis Child 147:1329-1333

Lodler R, Estle DT, Morrison K et al. Applicability of the Greulich and Pyle skeletal age standards to black and white children of today. AJDC, 1993; 147: 1329-1333.

Loevy HT, Goldberg AF (1999) Shifts in tooth maturation patterns in non-French Canadian boys. Int J Pediatr Dent 9(2):105-10.

Logan WH, Kronfield R (1933) Development of the human jaws and surrounding structures from birth to the age of fiftten years. J Am Dent Assoc 20:379-427.

Mackay DH (1952) Skeletal maturation in the hand: a study of development in East African children. Trans R Soc Trop Med Hyg 46:135-150

MacLaughlin SM (1990) Epiphyseal fusion at the sternal end of the clavicle in a modern Portugese skeletal sample. Antropol Port 8:59-68

Marshall WA and Tanner JM. Variations in the pattern of pubertal changes in boys. Arch Dis Childh 1970;45:13-23.

Marshall WA and Tanner JM. Variations in the pattern of pubertal changes in girls. Arch Dis Childh 1969;44:291-303.

Marshall WA, Ashcroft MT, Bryan G. Skeletal maturation of the hand and wrist in Jamaican children. Human Biol, 1970; 42: 419-435.

Martin-de Las Heras S, García-Fortea P, Ortega A, Zodocovich S, Valenzuela A (2007) Third molar development according to chronological age in populations from Spanish and Magrebian origin. Forensic Sci Int 23 (ahead of print).

Massé G, Hunt EE (1963) Skeletal maturation of the hand and wrist in West African children. Hum Biol 35:3-25

Mata P. Cirugía y Medicina Legal. 2ª Edición.1846; Vol. 1, p. 314-315 1842.

McKenna CJ, James H, Taylor JA, Townsend GC (2002) Tooth development standards for South Australia. Aust Dent J 47(3):223-7.

McKern TW, Stewart TD (1957) Skeletal age changes in young American males. Analysed from the standpoint of age identification. In: Technical report EP 45. Quartermaster Research and Development Center, Environmental Protection Research Division. Natick, Massachusetts, pp. 89-97

Meinl A, Tangl S, Huber C, Maurer B, Watzek G (2007) The chronology of third molar mineralization in the Austrian population--a contribution to forensic age assessment. Forensic Sci Int 169(2-3):161-7.

Melsen B, Wenzel A, Miletic T et al. Dental and skeletal maturity in adoptive children: assessment at arrival and after one year in the admitting country. Ann Human Biol, 1986; 13(2): 153-159

Micci M, Buzzanca R(1998) Age and mineralization of third molars in a group from Enna and Caltonissetta provinces. Stomatol Mediterr 8(2):123-5.

Mincer HH, Harris EF, Berryman HE (1993) The A.B.F.O. study of third molar development and its use as an estimator of chronological age. J For Sci 38(2):379-90.

Moorrees CFA, Fanning EA, Hunt EE (1963) Formation and resorption of three deciduous teeth in children. Am J Phys Anthropol 21:99-108.

Morrees CFA, Fanning EA, Hunt EE (1963) Age variation of formation stages for ten permanent teeth. J Dent Res 42(6):149-502.

Mühler M, Schulz R, Schmidt S, Schmeling A, Reisinger W (2006) The influence of slice thickness on assessment of clavicle ossification in forensic age diagnostics. Int J Legal Med 120:15-17

Müller HR (1983) Eine Studie über die Inkonstanz des dritten Molaren (Fehlen, Anlage, Durchbruch). Ddissertation. Dresden: Univ. of Dresden

Nambiar P (1996) Third molars in the stablisment of adult status. A case report. J Forensic Odontostomatol 14(2):30-3.

Neizy O, Alp A, Yalcindag A, Yakacikli S, Orphon A. Sexual maturation in Turkish boys. Ann Hum Biol 1975;2(3):251-259.

Nolla CM (1960) The development of the permanent teeth. J Dent Child 27:254-66.

Nykanen R, Espeland L, Kvaal SI, Krogstad O (1998) Validity of Demirjian method for dental age assessment when applied to Norwegian children. Acta Odontol Scand 56(4):238-44.

Nystrom M, Haataja J, Kataja M, Evalahti M, Peck L, Kleemola-Kujala E (1986) Dental maturity in finnish children, estimated from the development of seven permanent mandibular teeth. Acta Odontol Scand 44(4):193-8.

Olze A, Schmeling A, Rieger K, Kalb G, Geserick G (2003) Untersuchungen zum zeitlichen Verlauf der Weisheitszahnmineralisation bei einer deutschen Population. Rechtsmed 13:5-10

Olze A, Bilang D, Schmidt S, Wernecke KD, Geserick G, Schmeling A (2005) Validation of common classification systems for assessing the mineralization of third molars. Int J Legal Med 119(1):22-6.

Olze A, Reisinger W, Geserick G, Schmeling A (2006) Age estimation of unaccompanied minors. Part II. Dental aspects. Forensic Sci Int 159 Suppl 1:S65-7.

Olze A, Schmeling A, Taniguchi M, Maeda H, van Niekerk P, Wernecke KD, Geserick G (2004a) Forensic age estimation in living subjects: the ethnic factor in wisdom tooth mineralization. Int J Legal Med 118(3):170-3.

Olze A, Taniguchi M, Schmeling A, Zhu B-L, Yamada Y, Maeda H, Geserick G (2004b) Studies on the chronology of third molar mineralization in a Japanese population. Legal Med 6:73-79

Olze A, van Niekerk P, Ishikawa T, Zhu BL, Schulz R, Maeda H, Schmeling A (2007) Comparative study on the effect of ethnicity on wisdom tooth eruption. Int J Legal Med 121:445-448

Olze A, van Niekerk P, Schmidt S, Wernecke KD, Rosing FW, Geserick G, Schmeling A (2006) Studies on the progress of third-molar mineralisation in a Black African population. Homo 57(3):209-17.

Ontell FK, Ivanovic M, Ablin DS, Barlow TW. Bone age in chil- dren of diverse ethnicity. AJR, 1996; 167: 1395-1398.

Orhan K, Ozer L, Orhan AI, Dogan S, Paksoy CS (2007) Radiographic evaluation of third molar development in relation to chronological age among Turkish children and youth. Forensic Sci Int 165(1):46-51.

Otuyemi OD, Ugboko VI, Ndukwe KC, Adekoya-Sofowora CA (1997) Eruption times of third molars in young rural Nigerians. Int Dent J 47:266-270

Owings Webb PA, Myers Suchey J (1985) Epiphyseal union of the anterior iliac crest and medial clavicle in a modern multiracial sample of American males and females. Am J Phys Anthropol 68:457-466

Pashkova VI, Burov SA (1980) Possibility of using standard indices of skeletal ossification for the forensic medical expertise of determining the age of children and adolescents living throughout the whole territory of the USSR (in Russian). Sud Med Ekspert 23 (3):22-25

Paterson RS. Radiographic investigation of the epiphyses of the long bones. J Anat. 1929; 64:28-46.

Pfau RO, Sciulli PW (1994) A method for establishing the age of subadults. J Forensic Sci 39:165-176

PICUM (Platform for International Cooperation n Undocumented Migrants). Los niños indocumentados en España: víctimas invisibles de las restricciones a la inmigración. PICUM. Brussels. 2008.

Planells P, De Nova J, Barbería E (1993) Cronología de la erupción dentaria II. Comparación entre arcadas. Rev Iberoamer de Ortod 12(1):41-9.

Platt RA (1956) The skeletal maturation of Negro school children. M. A. Thesis, Philadelphia

Prabhakar AR, Panda AK, Raju OS (2002) Applicability of Demirjian's method of age assessment in children of Davangere. J Indian Soc Pedod Prev Dent 20(2):54-62.

Prieto JL, Barbería E, Ortega R, Magaña C (2007) Evaluation of chronological age based on third molar development in the Spanish population. Int J Legal Med 119(6):349-54.

Pryor JW. Chronology and order of ossification of the bones of the human carpus: x-ray method. Bull State Coll Kentucky.1908; 1(1)

Quirmbach F, Ramsthaler F, Verhoff MA (2009) Evaluation of the ossification of the medial clavicular epiphysis with a digital ultrasonic system to determine the age threshold of 21 years. Int J Legal Med 123:241–245

Ramsthaler F, Proschek P, Betz W (2009). How reliable are the risks estimates for X-ray examinations in forensic age estimations? A safety update. Int J Leg Med 123:199-204.

Rantanen AV (1967) The age of eruption of the third molar teeth. Acta Odontol Scand 25 (Suppl):1-86

Ritz-Timme S, Cattaneo C, Collins MJ, Waite ER, Schutz HW, Kaatsch HJ, Borrman HI (2000) Age estimation: the state of the art in relation to the specific demands of forensic practise. Int J Legal Med 113(3):129-36.

Robetti I, Iorio M, Guglielmetti Mugion T (1982) Age of third molar mineralization. A bibliographic review and synoptic table. Minerva Stomatol 31(6):837-9.

Robetti I. Iorio M, Dalle Molle M (1993) Orthopantomography and the determination of majority age. Panminerva Med 35:3.

Roche AF, Roberts J, Hamill PVV (1975) Skeletal maturity of children 6-11 years: racial, geographic area and socioeconomic differentials, United States. (Vital and health statistics-series 11. no. 149). U.S. Government Printing Office, Washington, D.C.

Roche AF, Roberts J, Hamill PVV (1978) Skeletal maturity of youth 12-17 years, racial, geographic area and socioeconomic differentials, United States, 1966-1970. (Vital and health statistics-series 11. no. 167). U.S. Government Printing Office, Washington, D.C.

Ruhstaller P (2006) Zahnärztliche Altersdiagnostik durch röntgenologische Evaluation der Entwicklungsstadien des unteren Weisheitszahnes: Auswertung von 1260 Orthopantomogrammen von Jugendlichen und jungen Erwachsenen. Med Diss, Zürich

Saunders S. De Vito C. Herrig A. Southern R. Hoppa R (1993) Accuracy tests of tooth formation age estimations for human skeletal remains. Am J Phys Anthropol 92:173-88.

Schmeling A, Schulz R, Reisinger W, Mühler M, Wernecke K-D, Geserick G (2004) Studies on the time frame for ossification of medial clavicular epiphyseal cartilage in conventional radiography. Int J Legal Med 118:5-8

Schmeling A, Geserick G, Reisinger W, Olze A (2007) Age estimation. Forensic Sci Int 165(2-3):178-81.

Schmeling A, Olze A, Reisinger W et al. Age estimation of living people undergoing criminal proceedings. The Lancet, 2001; 358(9276): 89-90.

Schmeling A, Olze A, Reisinger W, Geserick G (2001) Der Einfluß der Ethnie auf die bei strafrechtlichen Altersschätzungen untersuchten Merkmale. Rechtsmedizin 11:78-81

Schmeling A, Olze A, Reisinger W, König M, Geserick G (2003) Statistical analysis and verification of forensic age estimation of living persons in the Institute of Legal Medicine of the University Hospital Charité. Legal Med 5:S367-S371

Schmeling A, Olze A, Reisinger W, Geserick G (2004) Forensic age diagnostics of living people undergoing criminal proceedings. Forensic Sci Int 144(2-3):243-5.

Schmeling A, Reisinger W, Geserick G, Olze A. Age estimation of unaccompanied minors. Part 1. General considerations. Forensic Sci Int 2006:S61-S64.

Schmeling A, Reisinger W, Loreck D et al. Effects of ethnicity on skeletal maturation: consequences for forensic age estimation. Int J Legal Med, 2000; 113(5): 253-258

Schmeling A, Schulz R, Danner B, Rösing F (2006) The impact of economic progress and modernization in medicine on the ossification of hand and wrist. International Journal of Legal Medicine 120:121-126.

Schmeling A, Grundmann C, Fuhrmann A, Kaatsch H-J, Knell B, Ramsthaler F, Reisinger W, Riepert T, Ritz-Timme S, Rösing FW, Rötzscher K, Geserick G (2008) Criteria for age estimation in living individuals. Int J Legal Med 122:457-460

Schmeling A, Reisinger W, Geserick G, Olze A (2008). Forensic Age estimation of live adolescents and Young Adults. En: Forensic Pathology reviews. Vol 5. Editor: Michael Tsokos. Forensic Pathology Reviews, vol 5. Humana Press. 2008.

Schmidt S, Mühler M, Schmeling A, Reisinger W, Schulz R (2007) Magnetic resonance imaging of the clavicular ossification. Int J Legal Med 121:321-324

Schulz R, Mühler M, Mutze S, Schmidt S, Reisinger W, Schmeling A (2005) Studies on the time frame for ossification of the medial epiphysis of the clavicle as revealed by CT scans. Int J Legal Med 119:142-145

Schulze D, Rother U, Fuhrmann A, Richel S, Faulmann G, Heiland M (2006) Correlation of age and ossification of the medial clavicular epiphysis using computed tomography. Forensic Sci Int 158:184-189

Schulz R, Mühler M, Reisinger W, Schmidt S, Schmeling A (2008a) Radiographic staging of ossification of the medial clavicular epiphysis. Int J Legal Med 122:55-58

Schulz R, Zwiesigk P, Schiborr M, Schmidt S, Schmeling A (2008b) Ultrasound studies on the time course of clavicular ossification. Int J Legal Med 122:163-167

Schulz R, Schmidt S, Schiborr M, Pfeiffer H, Schmeling A (2010) Referenzstudie zur sonographischen Beurteilung der Ossifikation der medialen Schlüssel beinepiphysenfuge. Rechtsmed 20:327

Shirley NR (2009) Age and sex estimation from the human clavicle: an investigation of traditional and novel methods. Dissertation. Knoxville: University of Tennessee

Shourie KL (1946) Eruption age of teeth in India. Ind J Med Res 34:105-118

Sidhom G, Derry DE. Dates of union of some epiphyses in Egyptians from xray photographs. J Anat.1931;65:196-211.

Singh J, Chavali KH (2011) Age estimation from clavicular epiphyseal union sequencing in a Northwest Indian population of the Chandigarh region. J Forensic Legal Med 18:82-87

Solari AC, Abramovitch K (2002) The Accuracy and Precision of Third MOlar Development as an Indicator of Chronological Age in Hispanics. J Forensic Sci 47(3):531-5.

Solheim T, Vonen A (2006) Dental age estimation, quality assurance and age estimation of asylum seekers in Norway. Forensic Sci Int 159 Suppl 1:S56-60.

Souguir MK, Ben Dhiab M, Masmoudi T, Zemni M. La détermi- nation de l'âge chez le jeune tunisien. À propos de 200 cas. Journal de Médicine Légale Droit Médical, 2002; 45(2-3):89-91.

Staaf V, Mönstard H, Welander U (1991) Age stimation based on tooth development: a test of reliability and validity. Scand J Dent Res 99:281-6.

Stevenson PH. Age order of epiphyseal union in man. Am J Phys Anthropol.1924;7:53-93

Sutow WW (1953) Skeletal maturation in healthy Japanese children, 6 to 19 years of age. Comparison with skeletal maturation in American children. Hiroshima J Med Sci 2:181-193

Taybi H, Lachman RS (1990). Radiology of syndromes, metabolic disorders and skeletal dysplasias. Year Book Medical Publishers, Chicago. 3rd ed.

Tanguay R, Demirjian A, Thilbaut HW (1984) Sexual dimorphism in the emergence of deciduous teeth. J Dent Res 63(1):65-8.

Tanner JM, Whitehouse RH, Cameron N, Marshall WA, Healy M, Goldstein H (1983). Assessment of skeletal maturity and prediction of adult height (TW2). London Academy Press, 2nd edition.

Tanner JM, Whitehouse RM, Marshall WA, Healy MJR, Goldstein H (1975) Assessment of skeletal maturity and prediction of adult height TW2 method. Academic Press. London.

Tanner JM, Healy MJR, Goldstein H, Cameron N (2001) Assessment of skeletal maturity and prediction of adult height (TW3 method). Saunders, London

Teivens A, Mörnstad H (2001) A modification of the Demirjian method for age stimation in children. J Forensic Odontostomatol 19(2):26-30.

Theintz GE, Howald H, Weiss U et al. Evidence of reduction of growth potential in adolescent female gymnasts. J Pediatr, 1993; 122: 306-313.

Thiemann H-H, Nitz I, Schmeling A (2006) Röntgenatlas der normalen Hand im Kindesalter. Thieme, Stuttgart, New York

Thorson J, Hagg U (1991) The accuracy and precision of the third mandibular molar as an indicator of chronological age. Swed Dent J 15(1):15-22.

Todd TW. Atlas of skeletal maturation (Hand). CV Mosby Co. St. Louis, 1937.

Todd TW, D'Errico J (1928) The clavicular epiphyses. Am J Anat 41:25-50

Ungar AL (1937) Incidence and effect of premature loss of deciduous teeth. Int J Orthod 24:613-25.

UNHCR NEWSLETTER. Separated Children in Europe Programme. 2000 Dec-2001 Jan;(2).

UNHCR NEWSLETTER. Separated Children in Europe Programme. 2001 Feb-2001 Mar;(3).

UNHCR NEWSLETTER. Separated Children in Europe Programme. 2001 Oct-2001 Nov;(9).

UNHCR NEWSLETTER. Separated Children in Europe Programme. 2002 Jun-2002 Jul;(11).

UNHCR, Guidelines on Policies and Procedures in dealing with Unaccompanied Children Seeking Asylum, Geneva 1997

Vallejo-Bolaños E, España-López AJ, Muñoz-Hoyos A, Fernández-García JM. The relationship between bone age, chrono- logical age and dental age in children with isolated growth hormo- ne deficiency. In J Pediatr Dent, 1999; 9(3): 201-206.

Van Der Linden F (1980) La transición de la dentición humana. Rev Esp Ort 10:1-96.

Vieth V, Kellinghaus M, Schulz R, Pfeiffer H, Schmeling A (2010) Beurteilung des Ossifikationsstadiums der medialen Klavikulaepiphysenfuge. Vergleich von Projektionsradiographie, Computertomographie und Magnetreso nanztomographie. Rechtsmed 20:483-488

Weiner JS, Thambipillai V (1952) Skeletal maturation of West-African negroes. Am J Phys Anthrop 10:407-418

Wenzel A, Droschl H, Melsen B (1984) Skeletal maturity in Austrian children assessed by the GP and the TW-2 methods. Ann Hum Biol 11:173-177

Willems G, Van Olmen A, Spiessens B, Carels C (2001) Dental age assessment in Belgian children: Demmirjian's technique revisited. J Forensic Sci 46(4):893-5.

Willershausen B, Loffler N, Schulze R (2001) Analysis of 1202 orthopantomograms to evaluate the potential of forensic age determination based on third molar development stages. Eur J Med Res 28(6):377-84.

Wong GW, Leung SS, Law WY, Yeung VT, Lau JT, Yeung WK (1996) Secular trend in the sexual maturation of southern Chinese boys. Acta Paediatr 85: 620-621

Yaacob H, Nambiar P, Naidu MD (1996) Racial characteristics of human teeth with special emphasis on the Mongoloid dentition. Malays J Pathol 18(1):1-7.

6

Epidemiology and Diagnostic Problems of Electrical Injury in Forensic Medicine

William Dokov and Klara Dokova
Medical University of Varna,
Bulgaria

1. Introduction

The first fatal electrical injury reported in scientific literature was in France in 1879 (Jex-Blake, 1913). A stage carpenter was killed at Lyon by the alternating current of a Siemens dynamo giving a voltage of about 250 volts at the time. The first electrocution death in UK was in 1880, close to Birmingham (Jex-Blake, 1913). Samuel W. Smith was the first person in the United States to die after electrocution by a generator in Buffalo, New York, in 1881 (Daley, 2010). Since those first cases the annual number of electrical injuries and deaths from electric shock have steadily increased as a result of the widespread use of electricity and the application of electrically powered machinery.

Although electricity is a relatively recent invention, humans have always been exposed to the devastating electrical power of lightning and understandably attributed it to supernatural powers (Koumbourlis, 2002). Beginning around 700BC the ancient Greeks depicted lightning as a tool of warning of their god of thunder Zeus (O'Keefe Gatewood, 2004). In Roman mythology Jupiter used thunderbolts as a tool of vengeance and condemnation, thus those stuck by lighting were denied burial rituals. For the Vikings, lightning was produced by the hammer of Thor the Thunderer as he rode through the heavens. In the East, early statues of Buddha show him carrying a thunderbolt with arrows at each end. In Chinese mythology the goddess of lightning, Tien Mu, used mirrors to direct bolts of lightning. African tribes, the Native American Navajo culture and many others also have specific beliefs about lightning.

Benjamin Franklin is generally regarded as the father of electrical science, the person who proved that lightning is an electric phenomenon and that thunderclouds are electrically charged with his famous kite experiment (O'Keefe Gatewood, 2004). He constructed a kite and flew it during a storm. When the string became wet enough to conduct, Franklin, who stood under a shed and held the string by a dry silk cord, put his hand near a metal key attached to the string, causing a spark to jump.

Today it is known that lightning is a phenomenon not restricted to the Earth planet only. It is observed in the atmosphere of Jupiter (Little, 1999), and in this sense lightning presents danger to flying craft and their crew as well (Uman, 2003).

1.1 Definitions and terms

Electrical injury, electrical shock, electrocution are often used as synonyms when trauma caused by electric current is being discussed. In this text "electrical injury" is used as the term with the broadest meaning. The existing various definitions of "electrical injury" are principally similar. The Russian Bolshaya medicinskaya encyclopedia defines electrical injury as an injury caused by electric current or a result from contact with lightning. K. Duff and McCaffrey distinguish between electrical injury and lightening injury (Duff, 2001). The former they define as the sequelae due to accidental contact with man-made or generated electrical power and the later as a sequelae of naturally occurring lightening strike. According to the Merck manual electrical injury is a damage caused by generated electrical current passing through the body (Cooper, 2009).

1.1.1 Terms

Information for the following terms is presented as a basic explanation of electricity and the effects of electrical energy (CDC, 1998).

- *electricity* (electric current) - is the directed flow of an atom's electrons (the negatively charged outer particles of an atom) through a conductor such as wire. Its main characteristics which determine the hazard effect of electricity on the human body are:
- *voltage* - the force or pressure that causes electricity to flow through a conductor, measured in volts (V). Usually household current is 110 to 220V. Anything over 500V is considered high voltage. Life threatening levels of voltage are above 50-60V. Death occurs in 25% of cases in contact with electricity of 127-380V; in 50% of contacts with 1000V; and in 100% if the voltage is 3000V. A more important characteristic is the difference of the voltage at the entrance and exit of the electric chain. A difference up to 24 V is considered acceptable according to international safety norms;
- *power/strength* –is the flow of electrons from a source of voltage through a conductor and is measured in amperes (Amps). The contact with a current with more than 60 mA per 1 sec is life threatening , and above 100 mA is usually lethal. Current up to 50 mA is accepted as less dangerous for direct current and up to 10 mA for alternating current.
- *type of current* - electrical current is categorized as direct current (DC) or alternating current (AC). Direct is the current which flows in one direction only (as in a car battery). Sources of direct current are batteries, solar cells, dynamo, etc. Alternating current (AC) is the current which flows back and forth (a cycle) through a conductor. It is more dangerous than the direct current.
- *rate* - the rate of the cycles (back and forth) of the alternating current per second is measured in Hertz. The normal rate in Europe is 50 cycles per second or 50 Hertz. In the United States it is 60 cycles per second [or 60 Hertz (Hz)]. Most dangerous is electricity with a rate of 40-60 Hertz; electricity with a rate of approximately 500 kilohertz is not dangerous.
- *resistance* - is the ability to impede the flow of electricity. Most of the body's resistance is concentrated in the skin. The thicker the skin is, the greater its resistance. A thick, callused palm or sole, for example, is much more resistant to electrical current than an area of thin skin, such as an inner arm. The skin's resistance decreases when broken (for example, punctured or scraped) or when wet. If skin resistance is high, more of the damage is local, often causing only skin burns. If skin resistance is low, more of the damage affects the internal organs. Thus, the damage is mostly internal if people who are wet come in contact with electrical current, for example, when a hair dryer falls into a bathtub or people step in a puddle that is in contact with a downed electrical line

- *duration of exposure* - the longer the person is exposed to the current, the worse the injury
- *pathway of current* - the path that the electricity takes through the body tends to determine which tissues are affected. Because alternating current continually reverses direction, the commonly used terms "entry" and "exit" are inappropriate. The terms "source" and "ground" are more precise. The most common source point for electricity is the hand, and the second most common is the head. The most common ground point is the foot. A current that travels from arm to arm or from arm to leg may go through the heart and is much more dangerous than a current that travels between a leg and the ground. A current that travels through the head may affect the brain
- *electric arc* – continuous, high-density electric current between two separated conductors in a gas or vapour with a relatively low potential difference, or voltage, across the conductors. According to the power the current can jump from centimetres up to a meter. Electric arcs across specially designed electrodes can produce very high heats and bright light.
- *lightning* – an abrupt, discontinuous natural electric discharge in the atmosphere, characterised with a high strength in the range of 100 000 amps and voltage of several millions volts for a very short period – less than 0,0001 sec. A lightening has thermal, light, acoustic and mechanic damaging influence.
- *electric sign / burn mark* – a specific skin damage at the point of contact of the current with the skin. It is a coagulating necrosis. Their typical macroscopic characteristics are relatively small size - diameter up to 1cm or less, craterlike, round or with a groove form, grey-whity colour, thick bottom and shaft-like edges. Their existence is a morphological proof for the influence of electrical current. Most often they appear at the point of entrance of the current in the human body, so the mechanism of connection between the body and the chain can be clarified.
- *metallization* – a process of coating metal on the surface of non-metallic objects; in the case electrical injury the metal from the current conducing object is coated on the point of contact with the skin. The colour of the metal depends on the type of the metal contained in the conducting object. This is a morphological sign for the influence of electric current. It determines the point of contact between the body and the current; it can provide information for the conducting object.
- *electroshock weapons* – a group of incapacitating weapons used for subduing a person by administering electric shock aimed at disrupting superficial muscle functions. They achieve continuous, direct, or alternating high-voltage discharge 20 000V-80 000V, causing pain, shock, muscle spasms. Duration of the electroshock for more than sec can cause loss of orientation, coordination , and sometimes sleeplessness (insomnia).
- „lightning figures" – paralytic dilatation of subcutaneous blood vessels with specific form: tree or fern - like, occurring on the path of the current along the body in the cases of a person affected by atmospheric electricity.

2. Classification of electrical injuries

Electrical injuries can be classified in different ways:

2.1 According to the sources of electricity

2.1.1 Injuries from natural sources of electricity

- Injuries from atmospheric electricity – lightning and globe lightning
- Injuries from biological electricity – mostly fish
- Static electricity

2.1.2 Injuries from technical sources of electricity

- domestic electricity – 110 -250 V
- technical electricity – up to tens of thousands volts
- weapons using electricity – electro-shockers, electro-guns

2.2 According to the severity of the damages electrical injuries are principally

2.2.1 Fatal injuries – also called electrocution

2.2.2 Non-fatal subdivided as (CDC, 1998)

- electric shock
- electrical burn
- electrical falls

2.3 According to the circumstances at which electrical injuries occur

2.3.1 Forensic cases

- homicides with electricity
- suicides with electricity

2.3.1 Accidents

- domestic accidents
- occupational accidents
- leisure accidents

3. Epidemiology of electrical injuries

Despite significant improvements in product safety, electrical injuries are still the cause of considerable morbidity and mortality.
The frequency of non-fatal electrical injuries is usually presented based on routinely collected, easily accessible hospital or other medical records. Data from a Survey of Occupational Illnesses and Injuries (SOII) for the period 1992-2002 suggest that rates for electrical shock in USA for the 10 year period remained steady at 2 per 100 000 workers. The electrical burn rate remained steady at 1 per 100 000 workers (Cawley J, 2006). Data of this kind depends largely on the severity of trauma and on the accessibility of health services. Adequate analysis of incidence of nonfatal - electrical injuries would require prospective population studies.
Epidemiology of fatal electrical injuries can be more adequately studied based on vital statistics and national death registers. Electrical injuries fall in the class "External causes of death". In the 10th revision of ICD this is class XX with codes W85, W86 and W87. In the older 9th version of ICD, electrical injuries are included in class 18 under code 925 – accidents caused by electric current. Data from the detailed mortality database of WHO reveals that mortality from electrical injuries in the European region varies more than **hundred times** (figure 1.) (WHO, 2010).

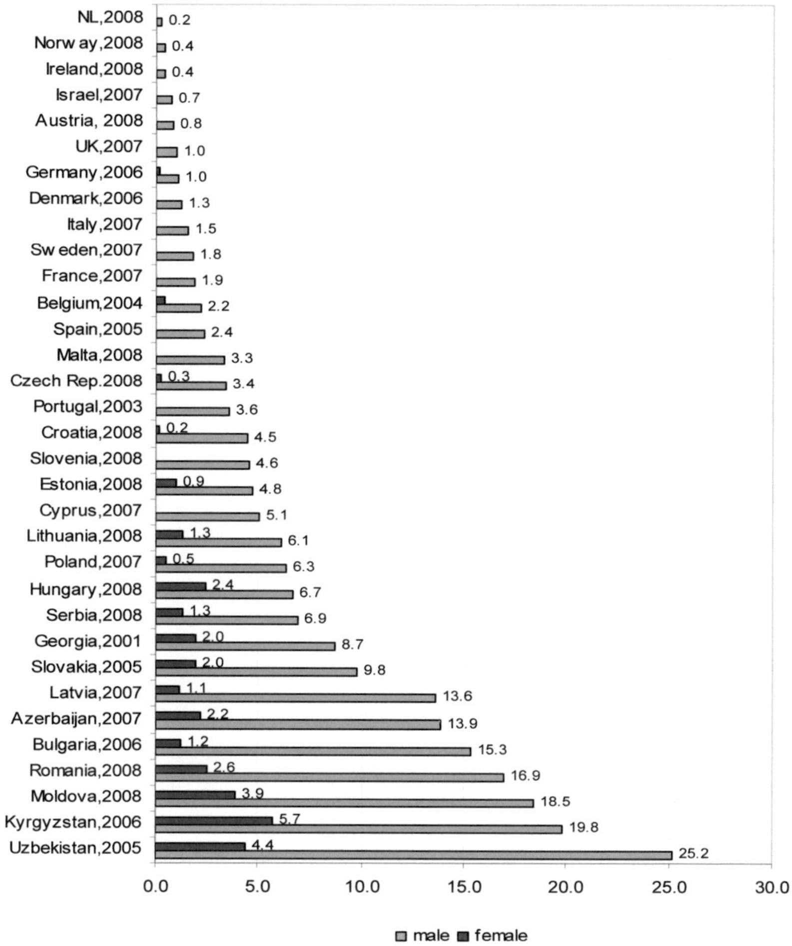

Fig. 1. Age-adjusted mortality rates from electrical injuries per 1 million population, European region

There is a clear East - West gap in relation to fatal electrical injuries mortality in Europe. Rates are much higher in Eastern European countries like Moldova, Romania, Bulgaria, Uzbekistan. This fact clearly needs attention and explanation. While the discrepancy affects both genders men living in Eastern countries are the most affected group.

Because severe electrical injuries tend to occur primarily in the workplace, they usually involve adults between 40 - 50 years of age (figure 2). In Western European countries, where mortality rates are lower, children up to the age of ten years are almost not affected. In eastern European countries with higher mortality rates all age groups are affected including youngest children.

Electrical injuries (excluding lightning) are responsible for approximately 500 deaths per year or 0.63 per million people in the United States (CDC, 1998). For Australia and New Zealand mortality from electrocution for 2007-2008 is also less then 1 per million population (ERAC, 2008). Generally, trends of mortality rates from electrical injuries are decreasing in most of the countries and especially in the developed parts of the world. (WHO, 2010)

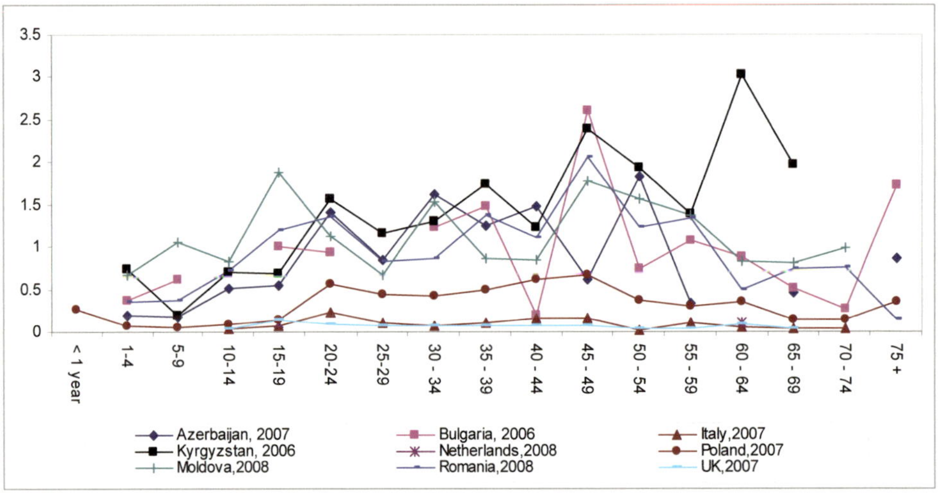

Fig. 2. Age-specific mortality rates from electrical injuries for the European region, per 1 million population, European region (WHO EDMDB)

A substantial number of papers add to the information from routine mortality statistics by reporting numbers of electrical injuries for different geographic areas (table 1).

First author, year	Source of data	Type of el. injury	Area	Period	Cases	Details
Akcan, 2007	Retrospective review of autopsy report	cases of electrocution among children	Adana, Turkey	1999–2004	37 cases; mean age 11.35; age range 18 months - 18 years;	31 (83.8%) cases male; all deaths - accidental
Dokov, 2008	Retrospective review of autopsy reports	electrocution	Central and Northeastern Bulgaria	1980–2006	485 cases, 413 cases in men; mean age 37.3 years, rate of fatalities 1,29 per 100 000 per year	24% occupational injuries; increase in summer
Lindstrom, 2006	Retrospective review of National Cause-of-Death Register;	cases coded with ICD-codes E925 and W85–87; suicides and deaths by lightning excluded	Sweden	1975 - 2000	285 cases; 269 men; mean age 38 years, age range 10 months- 92 years	151 of fatalities in leisure time; 132 in an occupational situation;
Lucas, 2009	retrospective review of autopsy reports at the Northern	electrocution	Northern Ireland	1982 - 2003	59 cases; age range 17 months - 80 years; rate of electrical fatalities	50 cases accidental, 9 suicides; increase in summer

	Ireland State Pathologist's Department				, 1,4 per 1 000 000 per year	
Nguyen, 2004	Retrospective review of 10 provincial and 2 territorial coroners' offices across Canada (no data for Nova Scotia)	fatalities in children 0–19 years from electrocution, including lightning	Canada	1991–1996	21 cases median age 13.2 years; 5 of these were cases of lightning strikes	
Pointer, 2007	Retrospective review of death certificates from Austarlian Bureau of Statistics	Cases coded with T75.4, T75.0, W85, W86, W87, or X33, in underlying cause or additional cause of death,	Australia	1 Jan. 2001 - 31Dec. 2004	162 cases; 2 per 1 mln population for 4 years; 7 cases of deaths from lightning- all males from 16-57 years	42% domestic accidents
Rautji, 2003	Review of autopsy reports and hospital records	electrocution	South Delhi	1996-2001	153 cases	3 cases without burn marks, 1 suicide
Sheikhazadi, 2010	Retrospective review of autopsy report	electrocution	Tehran, Iran	2002 - 2006	295 cases, age range, 11 months - 75 years with a mean age of 28.99; 279 male cases	285 accidents (188 occupational) 10 suicides; no burn marks in 16 cases; increase in summer
Taylor, 2002	Bureau of Labor Statistics Census of Fatal Occupational Injuries	fatal occupational electrocutions	USA	1992 - 1999	2525 cases, 98.6%in males	most among 20–34 yrs, whites and indians; increase in summer,
Tirasci, 2006	Retrospective review of autopsy reports	electrocution; lightning excluded	Diyarbekir, Turkey	1996-2002	123 accidental cases, mean age 20,7, range 2-63 years of age; 86 male	31% of cases b/w 0-10 yrs. of age; lack of burn marks in 11,4%; 56 cases domestic; increase in summer;.
Turkmen, 2008	Retrospective review of autopsy reports	electrocution	Bursa city, Turkey	1996-2003	63 cases (59 males); mean age 32.5; age range 5 to 62 years	Most in 30-39 yrs of age; 63,5% occupational accidents; usually in summer
Wick, 2006	Retrospective review of autopsy reports	electrocution	Adelaide, Australia	1973-2002	96 cases in total, of whom 87 males	

Table 1. Studies of fatal electrical injuries based on forensic records for the period 2000-2010

The diversity of these studies not only in terms of time periods but also age groups, types of electrical injuries covered makes their direct comparison impossible. Generally these studies confirm that electrical injuries are much more common among men. Almost everywhere in the world electrical injuries are more common in the summer season. The reasons for this repeated observations are that during the wormer months of the year people dress lightly and loose the protective effect of clothes, the skin is wet and the threshold for electrical stimulus of the heart is much lower. (Ajibaev, 1978)
Approximately half of the total number of electrocutions are occupational accidents, and constitute the fourth leading cause of work-related traumatic death (5–6% of all workers' deaths). The other half of electrical fatalities are domestic or leisure accidents, mostly associated with malfunctioning or misuse of consumer products.

3.1 Suicide by electrocution

While most deaths due to electrocution are accidental in nature, the forensic specialist should be familiar with electrocution as a method of suicide. Such cases are rare and usually described as casuistical. We have conducted one of the largest studies covering a period of 41 years (1956-2006) and eight regions (from 28 in total) in Bulgaria, a country with a high rate of fatal electrical injuries in Europe (Dokov, 2009).
From 63 825 reviewed autopsy reports 945 were cases of electrocution deaths and 59 of the later were suicides by electrocution. This accounts for 0,09% of all reviewed autopsies and 6,2% of all electrical fatalities. Males prevail definitely (54 of the victims) over females. The mean age of the victims was 45 ± 6 years (ranging from 14 to 75years). The methods used for suicide were quite diverse (figure 3) with high and low voltage electricity used with a similar frequency. This finding contrasts with the reports from Nothern Ireland (Lucas, 2009) where all nine victims identified for a 21 year period had used the domestic electricity supply, usually by removing the insulating sleeving of electrical flex so as to expose the wires.

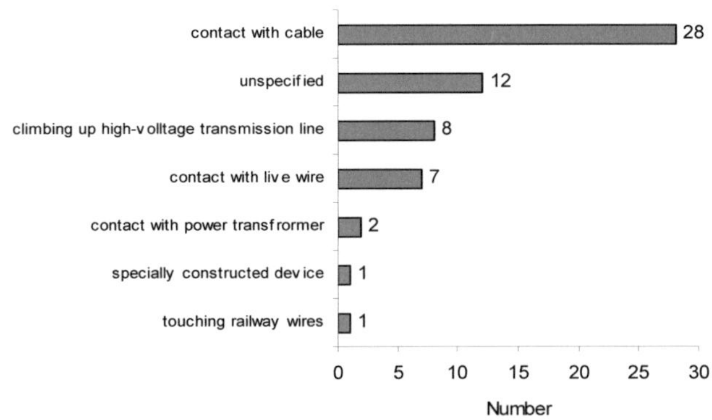

Fig. 3. Methods of suicide by electrocution

In addition we have identified a somewhat cyclical pattern of suicides by electrocution with peaks in the middle of the weak and in September, with summer the typical season.

3.2 Epidemiology of lightning strikes

Lightning strikes cause serious injuries in 1000-1500 individuals each year (Adukauskakeine, 2007). European countries with higher mortality from electrocutions have also a higher rate of lightning fatalities. Romania, Moldova, Bulgaria, have more than 1 fatal lightning strike per million population per year (figure 2).

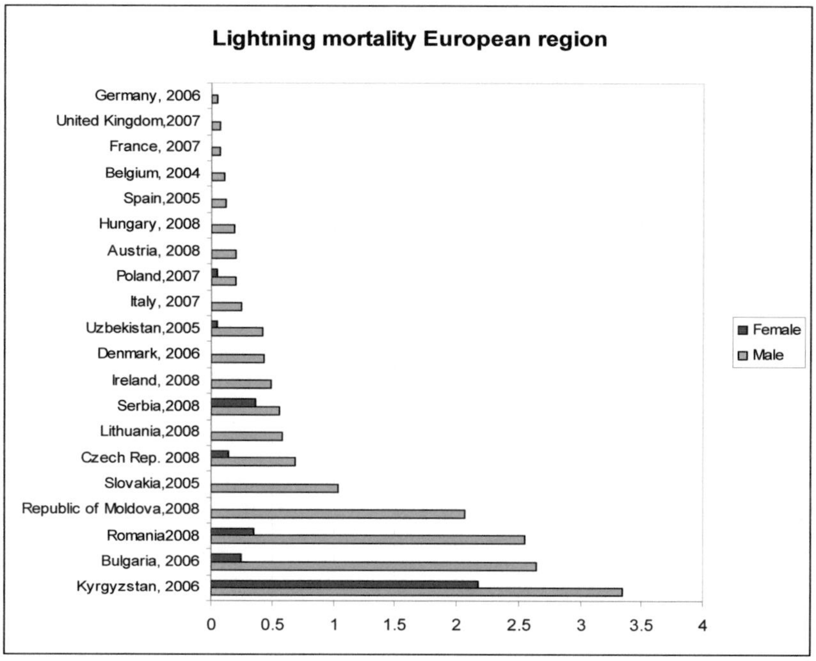

Fig. 2. Lightning mortality in the European regions, by gender, per 1 million population

In a review of lightning strike deaths for the USA, based on data from both the National Centers for Health Statistics (NCHS), the Census of Fatal Occupational Injuries (CFOI), the authors find a total of 374 struck-by-lightning deaths occurring during the period 1995-2000 (**an average annualized rate of 0.23 deaths per million persons**) (Adekoya, 2005). The numbers of lightning deaths are highest in Florida and Texas.

Between 75% and 85% of all lightning deaths are to men in the age group 25-45 years. Thirty per cent of all deaths involve people who work out of doors and 25% involved people participating in outdoor recreations.

Investigations of lightning strikes around the world demonstrate that the predominance of strikes is in summer months in mid-afternoon in moist atmospheric tropical and mountainous environments (Uman, 1971).

Data from WHO data- base regarding the European countries (for a fifteen year period) indicates that lightning fatalities trends are stable. At the same time one of the studies covering the longest - 41 year period (1965-2006) from Bulgaria indicates that lightning fatalities might exhibit a cyclic trend (Dokov, 2009). For Bulgaria it is suggested to be around 30years.

While lightning fatalities can be successfully analyzed based on available mortality data, it is much more difficult to obtain figures on lightning injury. The ratio of deaths to injuries is likely to be between 2 and 10. Those who are fortunate enough to recover from lightning strike frequently suffer severe and prolnged psychological damage, characterized -by withdrawal, depression, fatigue, sleep disturbance, difficulty with fine mental and motor functions, paraesthesias, headaches and storm phobias (Andirews, 1992).

4. The process of forensic medical diagnosis in case of electrical injury

4.1 Examination at the scene of death

In a case of electrical injury the examination at the scene of death has to be carried out from a team of a policeman, forensic medical specialist and a technical expert (power engineer). The tasks of the engineer are to provide evidence for the sources and reasons of electrical flow and to assure all necessary precautionary and safety measures during the inspection.

The forensic medical expert needs to pay special attention to the following problems during the inspection:

In cases of an accident with technical electricity: The forensic expert needs to determine is there a contact with source of electricity – wires, devices etc., and the position of the victim in relation to them. The specialist has to look for circumstances facilitating the accident, such as increased dampness, wet clothes, lack of protective clothing, gloves, shoes, etc. On the clothes can be found signs of electrical influence (burns, other electrical sings); on the shoes there might be breaks at the points of entrance or exit of the electric chain; burns; melted nails; magnetized metal objects. Electrical burn-marks should be looked for carefully on the body, but in up to 20% of cases they might be missing. The outer inspection of the body can provide evidence of mechanic injuries - a result of falling from electrical pylon or a roof, or other not typical burns. In the case of a suicide, uncovered wires can be wrapped or fixed in some way to the body, and a letter might be left.

Information for the beginning and the course of the accident should be collected from witnesses during the process of inspection, together with information on the clinical picture before the time of death of the victim.

In cases caused by high voltage technical electricity or electric arc – deep local burns or even carbonization at the point of contact can be found, metallization, stings or burns of hairs, external traumatic injuries due to throwing back of the body. Such cases do not cause diagnostic difficulties.

In cases of an accident from electric weapons can be found changes identical with electrocution from low voltage electricity – round, point like burns or hyperemia 5-7 mm in a diameter.

In cases of an injury with atmospheric electricity there is a specific surrounding situation. The victim is most often in the open, after a lightning storm, under a tree. Signs of atmospheric electrical influence in the surrounding environment can be found – burns or tree splitting, melted or magnetized metal objects or parts of constructions. Very often the clothes of the victim are severely torn and the body might be denuded. Hairs on the head might be singed, hairs on the chest or genitals might be intertwined, and the typical for electrical influence sequelae as burns of different stages can be observed including carbonization of parts of the body.

4.1.1 Practical tasks of the forensic medical expert during the examination at the scene of death

- To check that all necessary safety measures are in place before the begging of the inspection;
- To prove the fact of death;
- To make a detailed description of the position of the body in relation to the sources of electricity (outlet, wires, devices);
- To describe the status of the clothes (wet/dry), presence of protective gloves, shoes, condition of instruments with which the victim had worked;

- To look for evidence for electrical influence (electric burn signs, non-specific burns, metallization);
- To look for traumatic injuries, their character and relation to the death;
- To estimate the time of death;
- To describe all observations and facts; to inform the leader of the inspection about the observations and assure their existence in the inspection protocol.

4.2 Post-mortem examination in the autopsy room

4.2.1 Outer inspection of the body

The first task of the forensic expert is to look for evidences for the influence of electricity such as the presence of electrical burn, electrical burn-marks, metallization on the skin etc.
In the case of contact with high voltage electricity - wide burn areas on the skin and deeper tissues can be caused and observed reaching to carbonization (Pictures 1-2).

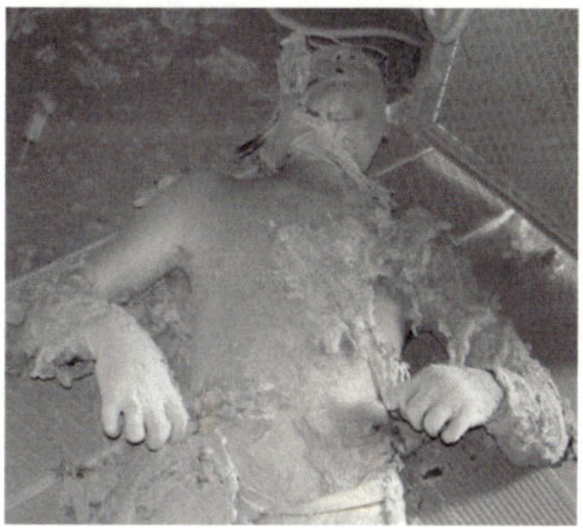

a)

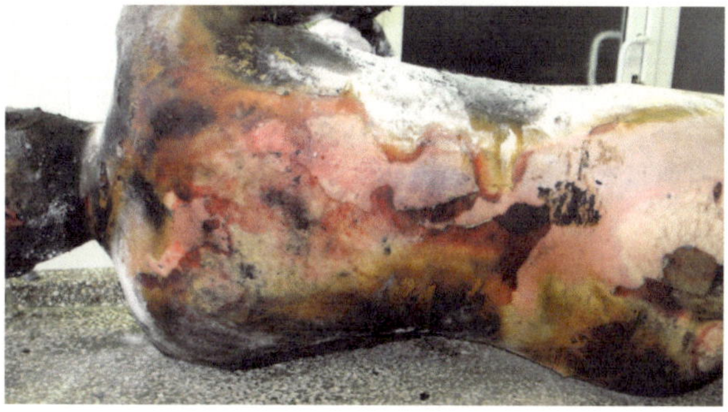

b)

Picture 1. High voltage/20KV/ injuries

High voltage electricity can cause damages from distance - so called electrical arc. It also causes burns. Diagnostics in such cases is not a problem.

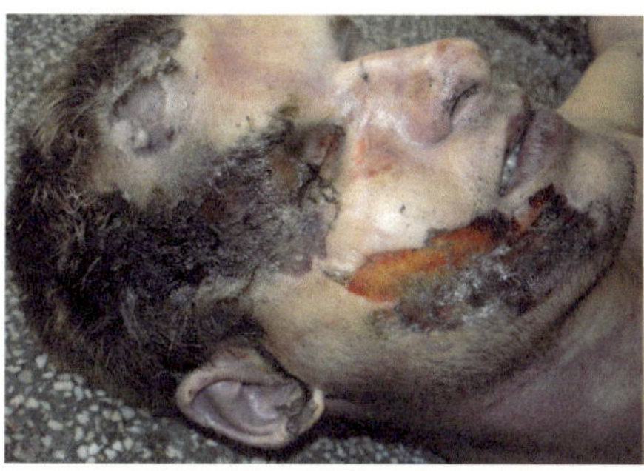

a)

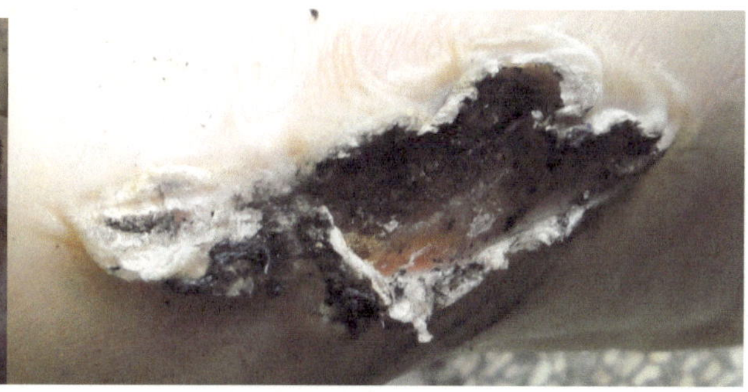

b)

Picture 2. High voltage injuries

In the case of influence of electricity with low voltage, electrical burn marks appear. Their usual macroscopic view is with round-like or oval shape, sometimes they are an imprint of the form of the electro-conductive object (Pictures 3-4).

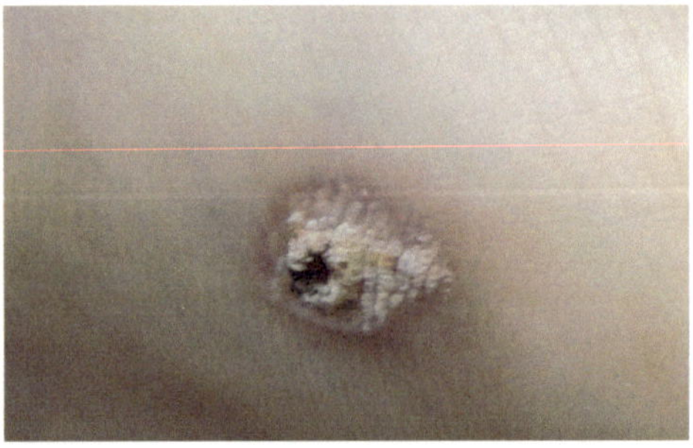

a)

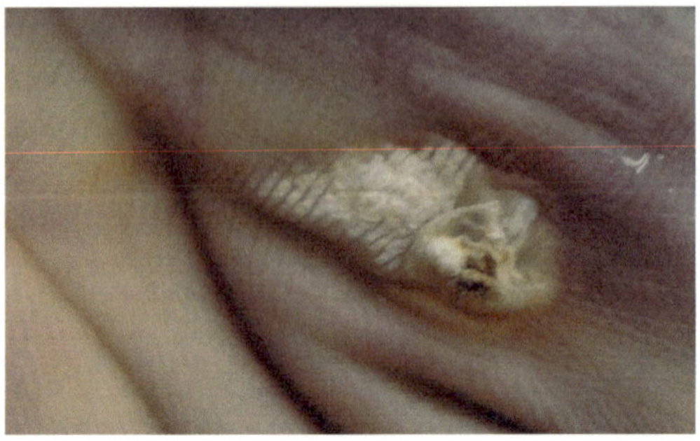

b)

Picture 3. Low voltage injuries on feet

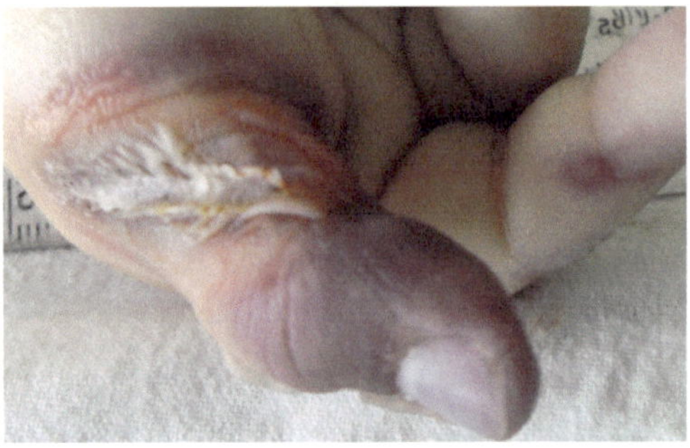

a)

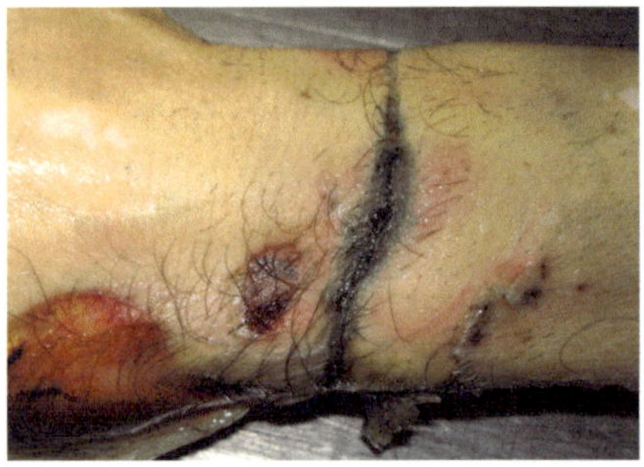

b)

Picture 4. Low voltage injuries on palm (a) and metalization of skin of the leg (b)

The central area of the damage is hollow and the edges are above the level of the surrounding skin. The skin in the damaged area is dry, thick grey-yellowish in color. In areas without horn layer of the skin they look like chafes.

Microscopic view: multiple cavities in the horn layer with various shape can be observed. Often fissures are formed on the borderline with the epidermis, reaching sometimes to complete tearing off of the horn layer. After colouring with haematoxylin eosin some focuses with basophilic colour can be found. Deposition of metal particles from wires can often be observed in such focuses. In the cell layers of the epidermis, cells and their nuclei are with elongated form. Vortex, chains and similar figures are formed at some spots. Blood vessels in the derma reveal various changes - spasm, paresis of some vessel, others are empty, without blood or with haemolysed blood. Such a complex of morphological changes in skin in the zone of contact with electro-conductive surface can be viewed as specific for the influence of technical electricity.

Important:

- The presence of electrical burn marks does not necessarily mean that the cause of death is electrical injury. Electrical burn marks often can be observed for a period of months in people who have survived electrical injury.
- Electrical burn marks can appear after the moment of death.
- A contact with electroconductive object with low voltage can cause death without burn marks which happens in as much as 20% of the cases.

4.2.2 Changes in the internal organs as a result of electricity

In cases of death from domestic or technical electricity a picture of sudden death is usually observed. Broken bones, formation of bone purls and other traumatic injuries of internal organs are possible in cases of high voltage injuries. A specific feature which appears in some cases of death from atmospheric electricity is perforation of the tympanum.

Microscopic changes in internal organs (Naumenko, 1980, Nazarov, 1992):

In the brain - oedema around vessels and cells, focal hemorrhages around vessels, vacuolization and karyolysis in the pyramidal cells. No specific changes have been described in neurons.

In myocardium - dilation of blood vessels, cyanosis to stasis, focal haemorrhages, interstitial oedema, fragmentation of muscle fibres. Often the cross striation of fibres is missing. There are small but multiple focal necrosis in myocardiocytes.

In lungs – spasm of the bronchi with epithelial swelling, interstitial oedema, focal haemorrhages, circulatory disturbances.

Walls of blood vessels – areas with destruction of the intima might be observed, together with necrotic changes of the smooth muscle fibers from medium layer, tendency for thrombosis. (Xuewei, 1992)

Kidneys – oedema of the renal pelvis mucosa, swelling of the epithelium of the kidney channels, homogenization and descvamation, circulatory changes similar to those observed in all other internal organs.

Liver – focal necrotic changes in hepatocytes. Cyanosis in blood vessels with focal haemorrhages around vessels.

Death from electrocution is a result of several different mechanisms – heart ventricle fibrillations, paralysis of respiratory muscles, paralysis of the respiratory center, shock and late sequels (as a result of burns or injury ion the cases of longer survival). In the cases of electrocution the so called delayed death is possible to occur – as a result of fatal arrhythmia, thrombosis or myocardial infarction after two-three hours, sometimes several days after the accident.

4.3 Practical tasks of the forensic medical expert during the post mortem examination

- Repeated examination of the clothes and the body of the victim.
- Description of all external injuries and fixing those through schemes and/or pictures. Finding specific features for the influence of electricity and adequate description of the electrical burn marks in terms of localization, distance from main body lines and points, distance from the feet basis, shape, size, color (gray, black, shades in the case of metallization of the skin), relief of the surface (craterlike, uneven etc.), edges (exfoliated, raised, uneven, thick, friable, burned) is of greatest importance most .
- Performing a full autopsy and exclusion of other causes for death.
- Taking materials for laboratory tests /histological, chemico-spectroscopic etc/

During the autopsy the expert should try to answer the following questions:

- Has death occurred as a result of electricity ?
- What was the position of the victim at the point of the electrical injury?
- Which part of the body was in contact with the source of electricity?
- Which were the entrance and exit points of the electrical current?
- Is there evidence for metallization providing information on the characteristics of the conductor with which there was a contact?

- Are there circumstances facilitating the electrical injury (condition of clothes and surrounding environment, changes as a result of diseases.)?
- Is there evidence for self inflicted electrical injury

5. Conclusion and future research directions in the area

Until the present moment almost all scientific enquiries related to electrical injuries were focused on the changes at the point of contact of the skin with the electric current.
Future work should redirect its attention towards the search for specific changes in target organs as a result of the influence of electric current - such as heart, brain and blood vessels. These are the organs whose damage is directly related to the process of death. It is our deep conviction that such specific changes occur and should be possible to be proved with histological, histochemical, electro-microscopic or other methods.
At present the diagnosis "death from electrical injury" quite often is based on indirect criteria. Strict, definitive unambiguous diagnosis is still awaiting its discoverers.

6. References

Adekoya, N. & Nolte, B. (2005) Struck-by-lightning deaths in the United States. *Journal of Environmental Health.* Vol.67, No.9, pp.45-50, 58.

Adukauskiene, D., Vizgirdaite, V. & Mazeikiene, S. (2007). Electrical injuries, *Medicina (Kaunas),* Vol.43, pp.259-266

Ajibaev K. (1978). *Physiological and pathophysiological mechanisms of electr ical damage,*
Frunze, Ilim, 1978 p.207

Akcan, R., Hilal, A., Gulmen, M., Cekin, N. (2007) Childhood deaths due to electrocution in Adana, Turkey, *Acta Pædiatrica* Vol.96, pp. 443–445

Andirews, C., Cooper M., Darveniza, M. & Mackerras, D. (1992) Lightning injuries: electrical medical and legal aspects. CRC Press, ISBN 0-8493-5458-7, pp. 59-60.

Cawley J. & Homce G. (2006) Trends in Electrical Injury, 1992-2002 Paper No. PCIC- PH-083, available from http://www.docstoc.com/docs/70704806/Trends-in-Electrical-Injury--1992-2002

Centers for Disease Control. (1998). Worker Deaths by Electrocution. *A Summary of NIOSH Surveillance and Investigative Findings,* DHHS (NIOSH) Publication No. 98-131

Cooper, M. (2009). Electrical Injuries, *The Merck manual for healthcare proffesionals,* available from http://www.merckmanuals.com/professional/sec21/ch316/ch316b.html

Daley, B., Aycinena, J. & Mallat, A. (2008) Electrical Injuries, *eMedicine Specialties, Trauma, Multiorgan Trauma Management,* Available from http://emedicine.medscape.com/article/433682-overview

Dokov, W. (2008). Characteristics of Lethal Electrical Injuries in Central and Northeastern Bulgaria for a 27-Year Period (1980–2006), *Eplasty.*Vol.15;8:e11.

Dokov W. (2009). Forensic Characteristics of Suicide by electrocution in Bulgaria. *Journal of Forensic Sciences,* Vol.54, No.3, pp.669-671

Dokov, W. (2009). Lightning fatalities - a review of 98 cases. *Indian Journal of Forensic Medicine,* Vol.3, No.1, pp.1-4

Duff, K. & McCaffrey, R. (2001). Electrical Injury and Lightning Injury: A Review of Their Mechanisms and Neuropsychological, Psychiatric, and Neurological Sequelae.

Electrical Regulatory Authorities Council. (2008). Electrical incident data, Australia and New Zealand 2007-08, Available from http://www.erac.gov.au/downloads/Erac%202007-2008.pdf

Jex-Blake, H. (1913). The Goulstonian Lectures on Death by Electric Currents and by lightning: Delivered before the Royal College of Physicians of London. *British Medical Journal* Vol.1, No2722, pp.425-30

Koumbourlis, A. (2002). Electrical injuries, *Critical Care Med* Vol. 30, Suppl.11, pp. S424 -S430

Lindstrom, R., Bylund, P., & Eriksson, A. (2006). Accidental Deaths Caused by Electricity in Sweden, 1975–2000. *Journal of Forensic Science.* Vol.51, No. 6, pp.1383-1388.

Little, B., Anger, C., Ingersoll,A., Vasavada, Senskec, D., Brenemanc, H., Boruckid, W. &
the Galileo SSI Team (1999). Galileo Images of Lightning on Jupiter *Icarus,* Vol.142, No.2, pp 306-323

Lucas, J. (2009). Electrical Fatalities in Northern Ireland, *Ulster Medical Journal* Vol.78, No.1 pp.37-42

Naumenko, V. & Mitjaeva, N. (1980) Hystological and cytological methods of examination in forensic medicine, Moscow, p.302.

Nazarov, G. & Nikolenko, L. (1992) Fornesic medical examination of electrical injuries, Moscow *Neuropsychology Review* Vol.11, No.2, pp.101-116,

Nguyen, B., MacKay, M., Bailey, B. & Klassen, T. (2004) Epidemiology of electrical and lightning related deaths and injuries among Canadian children and youth, *Injury Prevention* Vol.10, pp.122–124

O'Keefe Gatewood, M. & Zane, D. (2004). Lightning injuries. *Emergency Medicine Clinics of North Americais. Vol.*22 No.2 pp.369–403

Pointer, S. & Harrison, J. (2007). Electrical injury and death, *AIHW National Injury Surveillance Unit,* Number 9, April 2007. Available from http://www.nisu.flinders.edu.au/pubs/reports/2007/injcat99.pdf

Rautji, R., Rudra, A., Behera, C. & Dogra, D. (2003). Electrocution in South Delhi: a retrospective study. *Medicine, Science & the Law.* Vol.43, No.4 pp.350-2.

Sheikhazadi, A., Kiani, M. & Ghadyani, H. (2010). Electrocution-related mortality: a survey of 295 deaths in Tehran, Iran between 2002 and 2006, *The American Journal of Forensic Medicine & Pathology.* Vol.31, No.1, pp.42-45.

Taylor, A., McGwin G., Valent, F. & Rue III L. (2002). Fatal occupational electrocutions in the United States, *Injury Prevention* Vol.8, pp.306–312

Tirasci, Y., Goren, S., Subasi, M. & Gurkan, F. (2006). Electrocution - Related Mortality: A Review of 123 Deaths in Diyarbakir, Turkey between 1996 and 2002. *The Tohoku Journal of Experimental Medicine,* Vol.208, No.2, pp.141-145

Turkmen, N., Eren, B., Fedakar, R. & Durak, D. (2008). Deaths from electrical current injuries in Bursa city of Turkey, *Turkish Journal of Trauma & Emergency Surgery,* Vol.14, No.1 pp.65-69 (in Turkish)

Uman, M. (1971). *Understanding lightning,* Carnegie (PA): Bek Technical Publications;

Uman, M & Rakov, V. (2003). The interaction of lightning with airborne vehicles. *Progress in Aerospace Sciences,* Vol. 39, pp.61-81

Wick, R., Gilbert, D., Simpson, E. & Byard, R. (2006). Fatal electrocution in adults--a 30-year study. *Medicine, Science & the Law.* Vol.46, No.2, pp.166-72

World Health Organization, Regional Office for Europe, (2010). European Detailed Mortality Database, Available from http://data.euro.who.int/dmdb/

Xuewei, W. & Wanrhongb Z. (1983) Vascular injuries in electrical burns —the pathologic basis for mechanism of injury , *Burns,* Vol.9, No.5, pp.335-338

7

Child Deaths

Gurol Canturk, M. Sunay Yavuz and Nergis Canturk
Ankara University, Department of Forensic Medicine,
Celal Bayar University, Department of Forensic Medicine,
Ankara University, Institute of Forensic Sciences
Turkey

1. Introduction

Childhood is the development process which starts with birth and continues till adolescence. According to Convention on the Rights of the Child, every individual is a child till the age of 18. A major proportion of childhood mortality is associated with trauma. Natural mortality during childhood is also high. Accidents have an important place with regards to manner of death; however, child homicide is also standing out with its causes and outcomes.

There is a consensus that children less than 10 has lower tendency to commit suicide. The incidence of child suicides increases during adolescence and young adulthood. Deaths during each and every term of childhood possess some unique differences and features. The aim of this section is to assess deaths due to medico-legal reasons during childhood. Childhood mortality may be analyzed under diverse titles according to age groups and manners of death.

2. Fetal and perinatal deaths

Fetal death is defined as death before 22 completed weeks of gestation when the conceptus exhibits no sign of life after complete separation from the mother. Perinatal infant deaths include deaths over 28th gestational week (late fetal period) and the deaths during postpartum first week. Neonatal deaths occur within 28 days after the delivery; the first week includes early neonatal deaths and the following 2-4 weeks include late neonatal deaths. Neonatal deaths comprise 67% of deaths occurring during the first 1 year of life. The most common causes of death are congenital abnormalities, infections, perinatal asphyxia and metabolic disorders. Perinatal period is of great importance in the perinatal medicine due to higher rate of infant mortality. Natural mortalities, accidents and homicides might occur during this period. Medico-legal investigations are initiated for some perinatal deaths and the cause of death is determined during post-mortem examination. Perinatal deaths include still births, abandoned infants and suspected infanticide (Keeling, 2009a, Pakis & Koc, 2010b, Ozkara et al., 2009).

Childhood mortality globally decreases thanks to socioeconomic development and interventions that keep the child alive. Despite this fact, every year 8.8 million children less than 5 die throughout the world. Infectious diseases (pneumonia 18%, diarrhea 15%, and malaria 8%) comprise 68% of these deaths. 41% (3.6 million) of these die during the first 4 weeks of life (neonatal deaths). Preterm birth complications, birth asphyxia, sepsis and pneumonia are the most important reasons of neonatal deaths. 49% of deaths among children less than 5 occurred in five countries: India, Nigeria, Democratic Republic of the Congo, Pakistan and China. Birth asphyxia, sepsis, preterm birth complications, and congenital abnormalities are to blame as global totals for neonatal causes of death in these five countries. Most of (83%) neonatal deaths occurred in the African region and in the Southeast Asian region (Black et al. 2010, Lawn et al., 2010).

All relevant information with regards to the event before post-mortem examination should be acquired. There are actions to be taken in cases of concealed pregnancy, unattended delivery and abandonment. Fetal maturity, time of death, was the baby born alive, cause of death and evidence of trauma should be scrutinized. Concealed pregnancy and unattended delivery have higher neonatal mortality risk when compared to in-hospital deliveries. Some findings might be helpful in order to learn whether the baby was born alive or not. Maceration of the baby is a sign of stillbirth. Cutaneous maceration occurs six hours after the death. Deep-red discolouration of the umbilical cord at its fetal insertion is a finding which reveals that fetal death occurred at least six hours before the delivery. Inflammatory change on the umbilical cord is a significant finding. Air in stomach and middle ear, food in the stomach, macroscopic and microscopic findings in the inspection of lungs are assessed in terms of live birth. These questions will be difficult to answer if the body decays. Most of the babies defecate a few minutes after the delivery. Meconium within the colons is also a positive sign indicating full time birth (Keeling, 2009a, Pakis & Koc, 2010b).

Lowest gestational ages and birth weights, congenital malformations and SIDS are the factors playing a role in mortality rates. Moreover, socioeconomic status, ethnicity/race, pregnancy at extreme advanced maternal age (≥45 years), obese women, multiple pregnancy, prematurity, diabetic pregnancy, delivering an infant outside the normal working week are reported as risk factors for prenatal, perinatal and neonatal mortality rate (Mathews & MacDorman, 2007, Alexander et al., 2003, Dudenhausen & Maier, 2010, Yogev et al., 2010, Teramo, 2010, Pasupathy et al., 2010, Flick et al., 2010).

Antenatal and perinatal deaths, premature and intrauterine growth retardation should be taken into consideration as risk factors. Placenta insufficiency is the most important cause of intrauterine growth retardation. Some of the studies report that placenta and umbilical cord pathologies, congenital abnormalities, infections, hyaline membrane disease and trauma at a lower degree are the causes of antenatal and perinatal mortality. Detailed anamneses and post mortem examination are crucial especially for cases in which there is a claim of medical malpractice. Cases with undetermined cause of death are more common among intrauterine and neonatal mortalities when compared to adulthood mortality. This rate reaches up to 50% in some of the studies (Pakis & Koc, 2010b).

A study from Istanbul which includes 184 cases reported that; based on the examinations of lesions and the findings from autopsies, there was no sign to indicate that the neonates were battered with a tool in 96.2% of the cases (Ozkara et al., 2009). Although traumatic cases are rare, it should be remembered that fetal and perinatal mortality might be associated with trauma.

3. Sudden infant death syndrome

Sudden infant death syndrome (SIDS) is defined by Beckwith in 1970 as follows: "The sudden death of any infant or young child, which is unexpected by history, and in which a thorough post-mortem examination fails to demonstrate an adequate cause for death" (Beckwith, 2003). Infant is a term used to describe babies under 1 year of age. All infants who died sudden, unexplained, or unexpectedly (SUDI) are not SIDS. According to a research report, only 39% of SUDI's are SIDS cases (Mitchell et al., 2000). SIDS is one of the major causes of infant deaths between 1 month and 1 year old (Moon et al., 2007). SIDS is a status of not being able to determine the cause of death situation in sudden, unexpected death cases of an infant aged between 1 month and 1 year, although crime scene investigation, family history, microbiological, toxicological and histological studies are made. SIDS is very hard to be diagnosed when it is not possible to reach a diagnosis despite the fact that all the investigations are made in sudden and unexpected infant deaths and in cases of exclusion of other possible diagnoses. Such deaths are natural deaths, the causes of which cannot be determined (Keeling, 2009b).

In sudden, unexpected infant deaths, a detailed history, especially the detailed history of death and crime scene investigation, is the most important part of the research (Willinger et al., 1991). Diagnosis cannot be accessed only by external examination. Bajanowski et al reported unnatural death in 17 of 339 sudden and unexpected death cases which have no evidence at external examination (Bajanowski et al., 2005). In the Istanbul study carried out in all children mortality cases under the age of 18, deaths between the ages of 1 month and 1 year were reported as 21.9% (Canturk et al., 2007).

Although pathogenesis is not clear, the number of SIDS reduced in recent years (Van Norstrand & Ackerman, 2010). Possible mechanism is re-breathing carbon dioxide by infants who are thought to have been stayed in a small unventilated area (Patel et al., 2003). (Figure 1). Epidemiological studies trying to identify genes and genetic factors are associated with SIDS. Central nervous system pathways, cardiac channalopathies, immune dysfunction, differences in response to nicotine metabolism and energy pathways are investigated (Van Norstrand & Ackerman, 2010).

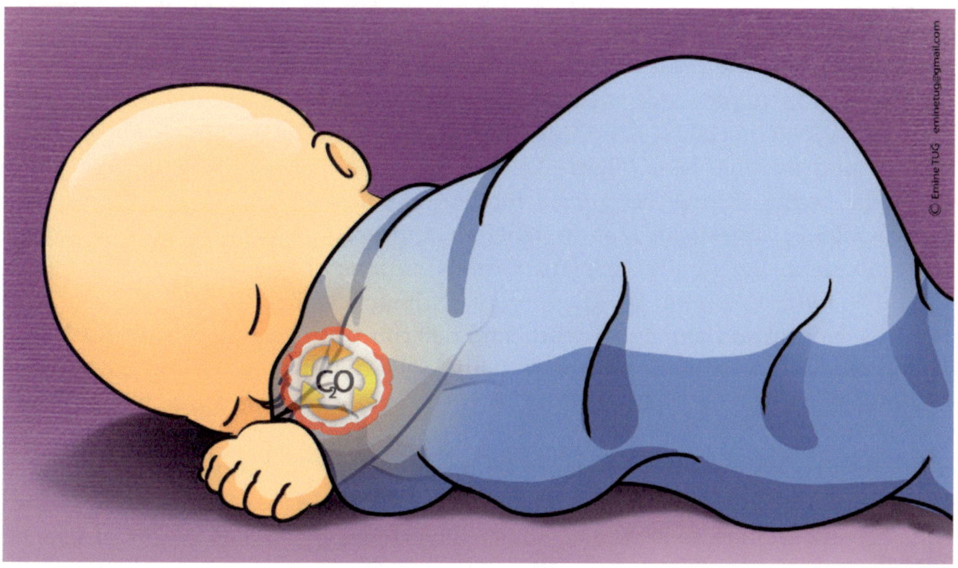

Fig. 1. Infant is re-breathing carbon dioxide.

Prone and side sleeping position, soft bed and sleeping pad, beret, and bonnet use during sleep, bed sharing and too hot sleep environment are risk factors (Kinney & Thacch, 2009). Similarly, being male infant, preterm delivery, high risk pregnancy, twin pregnancy, being multi-parity mother's baby, living within large family are other risk factors. Single and young mothers, mothers who smoked during pregnancy, and who give birth to children with low birth weight are risky. Low socio-economic level is known to be risky (Daltveit et al., 1997, Blair et al., 2006). And it is reported that low socio-economic level also causes other risk factors (Fleming et al., 2003). In a study it is reported that SIDS babies are sharing beds in 70% cases (Brixney et al., 2011). In SIDS cases, most infants die while sleeping in their bedrooms. Death usually occurs in the morning while asleep. (Fleming et al., 2003). Babies are usually 2-4 months old, and usually not followed-up in the prenatal period. Low parental education level, short time drug usage of mothers during pregnancy and winter months are also risky (Byard & Krous, 2003). Bottle feeding and avoiding breast feeding are risk factors, too (Blackwell et al., 2005). Inflammatory changes are often in SIDS cases and infection is a moderate risk factor (Highet, 2008). Staphylococcus aureus, Streptococci and Escherichia coli have been reported to be related pathogens (Blackwell et al., 2005). Also, smoking at home is a risk factor and is associated with the number of cigarettes (Blair et al., 1996). An apparent life-threatening event (ALTE) is a state of emergency, characterized by central or obstructive apnea, skin color change (pallor or cyanosis), decreased muscle tone (hypotonia) and a combination of choking or gagging (National Institutes of Health Consensus Developmental Conference on Infantile Apnea and home monitoring, 1987). ALTE identified in the siblings is thought to be caused by obstruction of the upper airway (Southall et al., 1997). Even if a single episode of unexplained ALTE exists in the anamnesis, SIDS should be suspected (Romanelli et al., 2010, Rosen et al., 1986). Alcohol consumption within family and sleeping together has been reported to be risky in previous studies (Phillips et al., 2011).

History is very important in cases of SIDS. Most of the time before the scene investigation, there may have been an intervention in the scene. The previous death of a baby, who belongs to the same family, the history of pregnancy and the baby's medical history up until death are important. The presence of a dead sibling may cause the investigator to suspect about the possibility of hereditary disease and death as a result of abuse (Meadow, 1999).

In unexpected infant mortality, sleeping environment should be examined carefully in terms of asphyxia and extreme heat (Figure 2). The exact position of the baby, the proximity degree of the bodies during sleep with mother and father, blankets, pillows, quilts and blankets should be investigated as to whether appropriate for use or not. Alcohol and substance abuse in the family, level of parents' fatigue should be questioned (Keeling, 2009b). SIDS, which cannot be diagnosed without detailed main aims in autopsy, differentiates natural and unnatural death, and determines the cause of death (Ozkara et al., 2009). Radiological, microbiological and pathological studies including toxicology and neuropathology contribute to the autopsy. For toxicological examination, blood, urine, and intraocular fluid, if the eyes cannot be examined pathologically, should be sampled (Keeling, 2009b). Genetic analysis should be done in the SIDS cases. (Klaver et al., 2011). When diagnosed ones are subtracted from the SUDI cases, cases with specific criteria for SIDS should be classified as SIDS and others should be classified as deaths of unspecified cause. (Cologlu & Cakalir, 1999). Multidisciplinary, detailed and meticulous research is very important in sudden unexpected child deaths (Inanici et al., 2001).

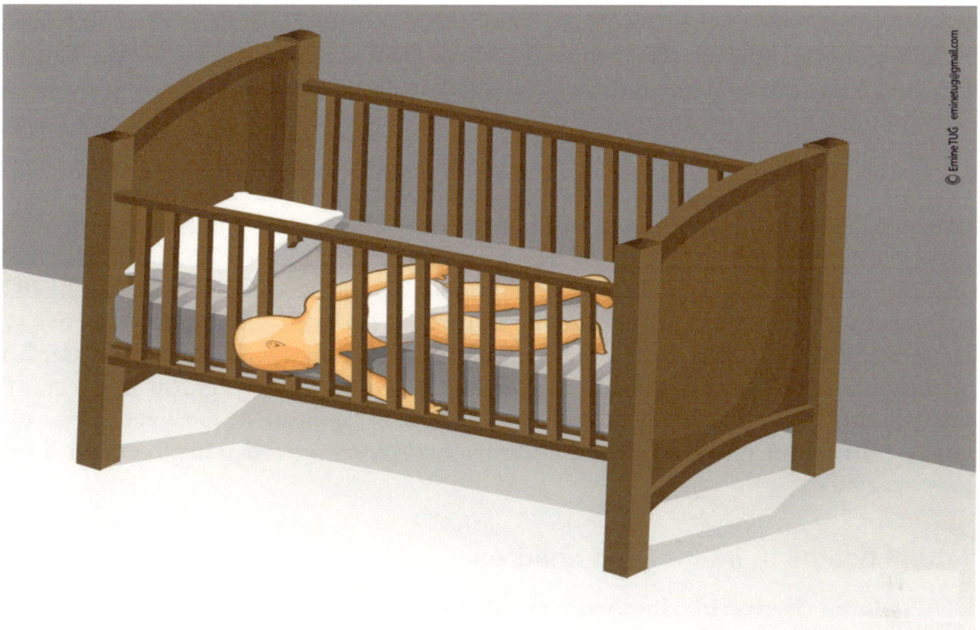

Fig. 2. Broken bed should not be used.

In evaluation of outward appearance, well-groomed infant child can have minor malformations or dysmorphic features. Frothy secretions in nose holes are common. Occurrence of dead marks on the front of the face and chest indicates the prone position of the baby. Hyperemia of internal organs and non-specific changes are seen in asphyxia (Cologlu & Cakalir, 1999). Thymus should be examined carefully. Generally, size of the thymus is found in normal range. A large number of thymic petechiae which is the most important and most common manifestation of SIDS is found especially in the thoracic region and mostly seen on the posterior face (Keeling, 2009b). Small and numerous petechiae also can be found on subpleura (Goldwater, 2008). On epicard and pleural face of diaphragma, petechiae can exist (Cologlu & Cakalir, 1999). Petechiae attend to more than 80% of Becwith's cases (Beckwith, 1988). 61% of SIDS cases in Kleemann's study had petechiae (Kleemann et al., 1995). At this age, mesenteric lymph nodes are often expanded as a reflex to the level of environmental antigenic stimulation (Keeling, 2009b).

The origin of sudden infant death can be natural illness or trauma. This can also be valid for adults (Pakis & Koc, 2010a). Infection is one of the major causes of death in this age group and should be considered in the differential diagnosis (Canturk & Canturk, 2001). In this case, microorganisms can be detected by molecular methods (Baasner et al., 2003). Cardiovascular system-based deaths are common. Cardiomegaly should be warning for researchers about cardiovascular origin. Cardiac malformations, ventricular septal defect (Cohle et al., 1999), coronary artery anomalies should be investigated (Rowley & Shulman, 2010, Lipsett et al., 1994). Although rare, myocardial infarction in the neonatal period is defined (Canturk et al., 2006), severe cardiomyopathy can also be seen (Dettmeyer & Kandolf, 2010). It is important to diagnose these cases, because many of them are familial (Pakis & Koc, 2010a). Dysrhythmias are varied, but complete bundle branch block is common. This diagnosis is important in terms of pregnancies of infant's mothers and close relatives. Postmortem genetic analysis shows that cardiac ion channel mutations like Brugada syndrome, long QT syndrome and short QT syndrome are associated with SIDS (Goldwater, 2008). Other possibilities are genetic-metabolic diseases, and the beta-oxidation defects are considered in this group. Presence of hypoglycemia and hyperammonemia which are common in these diseases can trigger infections (Keeling, 2009b). Sudden unexpected death in epileptic children can be seen (Sillanpää & Shinnar, 2010).

Definitive histological evaluation is important in SUDI cases. Pulmonary edema and congestion are common findings in SUDI cases. Round-cell infiltration is often located on alveolar wall and there are peribronchial lymphoid aggregates (Keeling, 2009b). In 60% of SIDS, focal acute inflammation exists in the upper and lower respiratory tract (Krous et al., 2003). In many SIDS cases, arcuate nucleus hypoplasia, periventricular leukomalacia and brain nucleus subtle gliosis can be found (Keeling, 2009b). Relatively, gliosis in the brain is a common finding (Kinney, 2005). Also continuing hematopoiesis in the liver is one of the findings of SIDS and found to be significantly higher, compared with the control group (Töro et al., 2007).

4. Natural deaths in infants and children

Sudden natural deaths in childhood constitute about 5% of all deaths (Aleszewicz-Baranowska, 2002). Causes of natural death in infants and children relevant with all systems, especially related to the cardiovascular system (Variend, 2009). The most common and mortal cause of childhood cardiovascular system diseases are myocarditis, hypertrophic cardiomyopathy, long QT syndrome and Preexitation syndromes with aortic stenosis, tetralogy of Fallot, transposition of great arteries, Ebstein's syndrome, congenital heart defects, such as coronary artery anomalies (Aleszewicz-Baranowska, 2002, Vetter, 1985). The adolescent period, cardiomyopathies are reported as the most common cause of sudden cardiac death (Thiene et al., 1988).

Causes of natural death in children and infants vary from country to country and due to living in urban or rural areas and age. While in developed countries, congenital anomalies, premature birth, birth trauma, malignancies are the causes of death, in developing countries, preventable causes like infectious diseases, nutritional disorders, etc. are seen primarily. Diseases-related deaths are seen more often in urban than rural areas. While, children between the ages 1-4 infections are main cause, cardiovascular causes, epilepsy, intracranial hemorrhage, and asthma are prevalent in children elder than 14 (Neuspiel & Kuller 1985). In developing countries, sepsis and other infections are among the leading causes of deaths under the age of five. Neonatal tetanus, malaria, measles in Nigeria, congenital syphilis, measles, AIDS in Papua New Guinea and tetanus in India has an important role among the causes of death (Bamgboye & Familusi, 1990, Aikhionbare et al., 1989, Duke et al., 2002, Choudhury et al., 1991). In Tokdemir et al's study; under the age of 18, 178 case of whom autopsies evaluated in Elazıg between 2001-2007, in 7.8% of them death cause were resulted as natural , 92.8% of cases were determined in the 0-5 age group, and the cardiovascular system took the second place, after the respiratory system diseases (Tokdemir et al., 2009).

Mortality rates under 5 years old also vary from country to country. According to 2009, World development indicators of the World Bank, Mortality rates under 5 years old is 7,8 in USA, , 4.2 in Germany, 3.20 in Turkey and 198.6 (for 1000 new-born baby) in Afghanistan (World Bank, World Development Indicators).

5. Asphyxial deaths

Death from asphyxia is common among childhood deaths. Except drowning, entrapment asphyxia, foreign body inhalation, plastic bag asphyxia overlaying and wedging, strangulation, hanging by a ligature, imposed airways obstruction, abuse of inhalants, chemical asphyxia can be considered among the causes of deaths from asphyxia (Byard, 2000, Busuttil, 2009b).

According to ICD asphyxia is defined as follows:

- - Accidental drowning and near drowning
- - Obstruction of the airways due to inhalation or any foodstuff or suffocation
- - Obstruction of the airways due to inhalation or any foreign body or suffocation
- - Accidental mechanical suffocation.

Petechiae is still accepted as the pathognomonic finding of asphyxia. It is not rare to see such haemorrhage in a single zone or only in the eyes. It can be seen on the anterior chest wall and on the body as well in early neonatal deaths and stillbirths due to retroplasental haemorrhage (Busuttil, 2009b).

5.1 Entrapment asphyxia

The curiosity of children related to various objects and spaces can result in difficult situations and they cannot escape from such difficulties and might die. Box type freezers, refrigerators, old cabinets, large chests, suitcases that are left idle within children's reach may lead to problems. To be locked in the trunk of a car can have a similar effect.

There is an accidental asphyxia case reported in the literature, in which the person's head got entrapped in the car window (Byard & James, 2001). In the USA between the years 1987-1998 11 pediatric cases were reported. The children reported were at the age of 6 or younger and kept locked in the trunk of automobiles and died due to hyperthermia and asphyxia (Centers for Disease Control and Prevention,1998). A study conducted in Australia indicated that 13 (31%) out of 47 non-intentional asphyxiation cases were due to head and neck entrapment (Altmann & Nolan 1995). It was also reported that a 19 month old girl died due to the neck compression since her neck got entrapped in the shopping cart (Jensen et al., 2008).

When a child is kept closed in the car in a hot day, heat stroke may develop due to the asphyxial changes together with the heat effect. If the ambient temperature is more than 29.5° C, such deaths may happen. If the ambient temperature is more than 29.5° C, the temperature in the vehicle will be more than 55 ° C (Busuttil, 2009b).

5.2 Plastic bag asphyxia

As plastic bags are common in our daily life, children play games with plastic bags. They put plastic bags over their heads and may die accidentally while they are playing with plastic bags. Such deaths are not rare. Moreover such deaths are common among the children who are solvent abusers (Saint-Martin et al., 2009).

In many countries it is legally obligatory to make holes on plastic bags that will enable air flow (Busuttil, 2009b).

5.3 Hanging by a ligature

Hanging by a ligature is not common among the children under the age of 14. The studies in the literature are mainly case reports and epidemiological studies are missing. It is more common among boys. Cervical spine, hyoid, or thyroid fractures are not frequently seen.

In the USA hanging/suffocation rate among the individuals between the ages 10 and 24 was increased significantly from 1992 to 2006 (Jones et al., 2000). In Australia there is also an increase in hanging by both males and females between the years 1998 and 2007, when compared with the previous decade (Bridge et al., 2010).
In the background there is misery or depression. Post-mortem psychological evaluation shows failure at school and pretension behaviors among the peers. These children might try to hurt themselves before. Autoerotic accidental deaths are reported among children at the age of 9 and above (Busuttil, 2009b,Large & Nielssen 2010).

5.4 Traumatic asphyxia

Traumatic asphyxia is rare in children. It is generally associated with crush injuries. The pathophysiology is different from adults (Large & Nielssen 2010). In the literature there some case reports concerning crush under car or jeep tires, or under some objects or garage door (Wyatt et al., 1998, Nishiyama & Hanaoka 2000). When thorax is stable, but there is no respiratory movement, traumatic asphyxia can occur. Central cyanosis and petechial heamorrhage are classical with congestion findings end up at the level of clavicles at the superior part of the obstruction. In children such findings are observed at the superior part of the obstruction, in case the children are crushed in the crowd or under the walls or any other object due to explosion, conflicts, or natural disasters such as earthquakes and oil explosions.
Another type of accidental asphyxia is related to traffic accidents, in which the child is crushed under the vehicle. Mostly internal organ damage and diffuse soft tissue injuries are seen in children. The abrasions frequently seen on the body of the child show the direction of the car passing over the child in line with the dragging direction. The majority of these children are under the age of 3 and they are male (Busuttil, 2009b).

5.5 Foreign body inhalation

Aspiration of foreign bodies can be fatal particularly in the first year of life. Anatomical and physiological characteristics and behavioral factors cause higher risk in terms of foreign body aspiration among the children under the age of 3 (Hurtado & Della-Giustina 2003).
Frequently toys or foodstuff cause foreign body aspiration in children. Although the majority of these cases show immediate symptoms while the child is eating, there are also some cases that result in the death of the child in the sleep without showing any immediate symptom. Foreign body caused for the death can be identified in the airways during the autopsy.
Aspirated solid or semi-solid foreign body may setin the main bronchi, trachea or larynx of the child. If the foreign body is large enough to close the air way totally, then there will be an immediate asphyxia due to lack of air through the lungs (Busuttil, 2009b).
There is more risk in laryngeal spasm and death due to laryngeal foreign body, when compared to foreign bodies in the trachea and bronchi (Hurtado & Della-Giustina 2003).
It is reported that the foreign bodies mostly go to the right bronchus due to the anatomical position (Hurtado & Della-Giustina 2003).
The inhaled vegetable particles might swell up in the forthcoming hours and even days and cause cough, stridor, wheeziness, short of breath and cyanosis. Peanut and other organic foreign bodies aggravate asphyxia through tissue edema due to acute inflammatory response. The American children between the ages 1 and 3 are under a higher risk. It results in 0.7 deaths per 100.000 annually. Death from foreign body inhalation is due to the

tendency of children to put everything into their mouths. Such young children do not have molar teeth. They tend to chew foodstuff with their incisors. When any foodstuff is sent back they are inclined to inhale due to a reflex reaction (Busuttil, 2009b).
Toddlers possess higher risk in terms of foreign body aspiration. If there is any mastication problem or disphagia in older children, food aspiration might be seen. The fatality risk is more in mentally retarded children or in children suffering from neurological disorders such as cerebral palsy. On the labels of the packaged foodstuff the appropriate consumer group should be stated for the safe consumption of the foodstuff (Byard, 2000).

5.6 Overlaying and wedging

The baby is overlaid by an adult during the deep sleep phase or the baby is accidentally suffocated due to sleep induced extraneous intoxication. The risk of overlaying is the highest in the babies under the age of 5-months. However overlaying can be seen in children until the age of 2. An adult or an older child who is overlaid the child, cause him/her to be kept under the bed or pillow. The child cannot cry due to the pressure in his/her chest and cannot take attention. In some of these babies expected clinical findings and even petechia cannot be seen. In some cases, unusual lividity indicating the pressure zone can be observed besides contusions and abrasions (Busuttil, 2009b).
For many years accidental suffocation cases of infants are considered as the cause of SIDS when infants sleep with their parents. Recently it is being debated that overlaying is a cause of SIDS. The reason for the debate is that the autopsy findings, crime scene investigation, family history and epidemiological findings are not different in SIDS and overlaying (Byard, 2000).
Kirchner reported 515 mortality cases under the age of 2 in a period of 7 years. 121 out of 515 cases died due to overlaying by their parents, siblings or other adults. Kirchner also reported that 77% of these cases were under the age 3-months. 394 out of 515 deaths happened due to entrapment in the bed. 296 of them died in the beds of their parents. According to Kirchner's report 79 cases died in the waterbeds. 2 cases died due to alcohol and substance use. 10 cases died in the adult sunbeds and finally 9 cases died in adult beds with rails (Busuttil, 2009b).

5.7 Strangulation

Although strangulation is a homicide and suicide-related cause of death in adults, it is an accident-related cause of death due to asphyxia in children. It is the 4th most common cause of unintentional injuries for infants under the age of 1 after traffic accidents, drowning and burns (Chinski et al., 2010).
Unintentional or accidental self-strangulation is quite commonly reported in young children mostly by use of a loose wire, rope and other potential ties typically around the house and frequently close to the bed. Tangled death cases account for 14,3% of all childhood mortality in the US. (Busuttil, 2009b).

5.8 Airway obstruction

One way of child abuse is to cover infant's mouth by soft materials such as pillows and to press the infant against the chest by parents or other care givers. The infant may not seem to have tried hard but there might be signs of convulsions due to cerebral hypoxia following hypoxia and cyanosis without the presence of significant traumatic findings; respiratory and cardiac arrest may follow. This situation may be caused by a mother previously diagnosed with Munchausen by Proxy willing to draw attention due to her psychosocial problems. External examination may not indicate any finding, but presence of haemosiderin deposition in lungs both in alveolar cells and interalveolar septa is a quite critical finding. (Busuttil, 2009b).

5.9 Solvent abuse

Inhalable hydrocarbons generally create an impairing effect on mental functions similar to alcohol or substance abuse. They contain petroleum and petroleum products that are present in the composition of many household products such as cleaning and decorating materials, paints, polishers, lacquers, adhesives, room sprays, hair straighteners, dry cleaning solvents, shoe polishes, labels or stain removers. Death may happen in various ways. Reports indicate use of such substances by older children for arousal during autoerotic activity.

Autopsy may reveal limited information in such suspected abuse cases. The body may present rashes and vesicles around the mouth orifice due to the effect caused by the solvent on the skin. Solvent may be olfactive during post-mortem examination. One of the lungs should be taken inside a plastic bag for analysis. Blood, liver and kidneys may also be examined toxicologically (Busuttil, 2009b).

5.10 Reverse suspension

This rare condition presents a situation, where the organs of a child changes position in the upward direction during a game activity resulting in shifting of the diaphragm and air depletion ultimately causing death. Death happens slowly when respiratory efforts are consumed (Busuttil, 2009b, Kurtzman et al., 2001).

5.11 Chemical asphyxia

This is a term used in the presence of non-inhalable gases around the child. For instance, kerosene and paraffin as a fuel, carbon monoxide liberated from fires or from exhaust smoke or barbecue coal in closed spaces or chlorine effusing from swimming pools, hydrogen sulphide and methane emitting from outdated mines and gases dispersing from catch basins may cause mortality. These conditions generally affect elderly individuals, mobile kids and mostly boys in environmental accidents. (Busuttil, 2009b, Meyer et al., 2007).

6. Drowning

Drowning happens due to aspiration of water into upper and lower airways by the reflex at the end of the apnea time (Yorulmaz & Cakalir, 1999). Drowning is the second most common cause of traumatic death for children between the ages of 1-14 (Gilchrist et al., 2004, Bener et al., 2011). In most of the drowning cases, death happens due to hypoxemia and subsequent cerebral hypoxia following inhalation of water down to alveoli (Gok, 1983a). 40% of all drowning cases involve children (Canturk et al., 2009). A study conducted in Istanbul on child mortality reports drowning as the cause of death in 79 out of 736 children (10.73%) (Canturk et al., 2007). Drowning may happen in the bathroom, toilet, buckets and jerry cans, swimming pools, ponds, decorative pools, building sewerage systems, farming reservoirs and tanks, canals, lakes, streams, creeks and sea (Pearn, 2009). The origin of childhood drowning is generally accidental (Brüning et al. 2010). Children between the ages of 1-4 represent the high-risk age group (Iqbal et al., 2007). Summer months are quite risky for drowning events since the weather tends to be warmer than the rest of the year (Canturk et al., 2009). Male gender, African race and adolescent age are the other risk factors (Bener et al., 2011, Hyder et al., 2008). Drowning cases are mostly reported in weekends and between 14.00-19.00 hours (Tyebally & Ang, 2010).

All dead bodies taken out of water should not necessarily be considered to have died of drowning and the person might have died because of

1. A natural disease before he/she has fallen into the water,
2. A natural disease when he/she was in the water,
3. Trauma before having been thrown into the water,
4. Traumatic reasons when in water,
5. Hypothermia and sympathetic inhibition, parasympathetic stimulation in cold water,
6. Drowning (Yorulmaz & Cakalir, 1999,Knight, 1996d).

Every drowning is a forensic case. One should always remember that child abuse or non-accidental injury, homicide, euthanasia and negligence may go along with the anatomical - pathologic characteristics of drowning. A detailed crime scene investigation and witness statement taking process should continue with a thorough anamnesis taking and post-mortem examination, if necessary to be complemented with radiography, chemical examination, diatomeae analysis and photograph taking (Canturk et al., 2009). Drowning does not have any specific laboratory finding to help with the diagnosis and therefore it is one of the most challenging diagnostic works of forensic pathology (Arslan et al., 2005). Since there is no specific histopathological finding to diagnose drowning, other possible causes of death should be ruled out by way of autopsy, histopathological examination, chemical and toxicologic examination. Lung alterations are not specific in drowning cases (Yorulmaz & Cakalir, 1999, Knight, 1991). Diagnosis is even harder in pediatric cases. Since the time of staying in water is only minutes in 99% of pediatric cases, the amount of ingested water may be very small, which challenges the diagnosis (Pearn, 2009).

Mortality due to cardiac arrest that develops by laryngospasm or vasovagal mechanism in absence of fluid in airways is defined as dry drowning (Yorulmaz & Cakalir, 1999). The macroscopic appearance of lungs may differ depending on fresh or salty nature of the drowning water. Since the salty water coming into the alveoli is hypertonic, the water in the vascular bed passes onto the alveoli causing hemoconcentration in blood, hypovolemia and severe pulmonary edema presenting with bloody-fluidy wet appearance in lung cross sections. Drowning in fresh water, on the other hand, presents with hypotonic water coming in the alveoli passing the water from vascular system to the blood and consequently causing hemodilution, hypervolemia and hemolysis creating a drier look in the cross sections of the lung than in drownings in salty water (Demirci & Dogan, 2010). There are age-related risk factors for drowning of children. The most common drowning spot for children is the swimming pools. Buckets, washbowls and Jacuzzis also constitute risky zones for children aged 4 and under. (Tyebally & Ang, 2010). Toddlers may drown when left unattended in the bathtub or when left alone with full buckets, whereas adolescents mostly drown outdoors, in which case possible alcohol intake may be the case (Byard, 2000).

Drowning zones mostly depend on communities and geographical position of their water resources (Byard, 2008, Wang et al., 2010). Nevertheless, the most common drowning zone for childhood events is the swimming pools. (Tyebally & Ang, 2010). In as much as

swimming is the fun and healthy way of refreshing in summer months, it brings along the risk of drowning (Schwebel et al., 2007). Most of the drowning cases in swimming pools and sea involve victims in the age group of 5-15. Boys tend to drown more than girls in swimming pools and sea (Tyebally & Ang, 2010, Pelletier & Gilchrist 2011).
80-90% of child drownings in bathtub are accidental. Particularly, infants under 12 months are under risk (Somers et al., 2006). Drowning cases have been reported by use of bathtub seats and rings when bathing infants in bathtubs (Rauchschwalbe et al., 1997). Inefficient adult attendance and bathing of more than one infant constitute risk factors (Somers et al., 2006). As a classical story, the tired mom starts bathing her children during which the telephone rings or the door knocks causing a sudden and unexpected interruption of the family routine. The mom lets her children stay in the bathtub, when older children get out of the bathtub leaving the younger child alone. The victim is generally the youngest or the second youngest child of the family (Pearn, 2009). Although drownings in buckets or washbowls are generally accidental, the possibility of homicide should not be overlooked in these cases (Pearn, 1992). Most of the victims are younger than 12 months with an age interval of 7-15 months. (Mann et al., 1992)
Children may also drown in rivers, lakes, creeks, sewerage systems and trenches. 90% of cases are boys mostly in the age group of 8-12. They generally drown when playing or swimming in prohibited areas, in which case their friends can't help or more than one child may die (Pearn, 2009).
Presence of fungal foam in external examination would be the strongest finding to indicate drowning in water. Localization of post-mortem stains is consistent with the body position. Goose skin look, wet skin, launderer's hand and foot are the findings that can manifest themselves only in long time stay in water. In drowning cases that present with both non-specific asphyxia symptoms during internal examination (hyperemia, Tardieu's spots, edema and hyperemia in internal organs) and fluid aspiration, lungs are hyperemic, bright and swollen. Furthermore, materials belonging to the drowning site such as algae or sand may be present in the respiratory system. Post-mortem radiologic examination should also be performed to rule out the possibility of child abuse. Besides, alcohol and drug analysis should also be performed as a part of toxicologic workup. Toxicologic workup may reveal content of the drowning fluid from the lung tissue. Although false positive or negative results should be reassessed, diatom analysis from bone marrow is especially important for drowning in the sea. (Yorulmaz & Cakalir, 1999,Canturk et al., 2009, Pearn, 2009, Knight, 1996d,Demirci & Dogan, 2010, Geserick et al. 2010).

7. Poisoning

In parallel with technological developments, there has been an increase in the risk of poisoning due to the increase in the number of chemical substances and drugs. Poisonings are important causes of pediatric emergency service applications and of morbidity and mortality in children and adolescents (Andiran & Sarikayalar 2004, Cheraghali & Taymori 2006).
Reasons for intoxication show variability in a wide range. Among these; drugs, various chemicals, pesticides, solvents, toxic gases or smokes, a variety of metals and minerals, animal bites or stings, and some poisonous plants and foods can be counted (Gurpinar & Asirdizer 2006). Epidemiological features of childhood poisonings differ from country to

country and vary depending on socio-economic and cultural conditions of communities (Senanayeke & Karalliedde 1998, Paritsis et al. 1994).

Based on data from United States of America Poison Control Center, it is indicated that approximately two and a half million poisonings occurred in 2008, 38,7 percent of which were under 3 years of age and more than half of which were under six years of age (Bronstein et al., 2008).

The pattern and risks of intoxication vary depending on age (Marchi et al., 1991, Soyucen et al., 2006). Poisonings in children under one year old include therapeutic errors such as false drug dose adjustment of doctors or families, or prescribing mistakes, while in children between the ages of 1-5 accidental poisonings and over the age of 10, suicidal poisonings are common (Andiran & Sarikayalar 2004).

Food poisoning, which occurs as accidental ingestion of toxic substances, is one of the most important causes of poisoning in children and is most frequently seen among boys between the ages of 1-5 (Marcdante, 2006, Mert & Bilgin 2006, Dart et al., 2007,Busuttil, 2009a, Hoffman & Osterhoudt 2002). Since children can be curious and tend to bring everything in their mouths without noticing that they can be harmful, food poisonings are common in these ages (Roidgers & Matyunas 2002). Intentional (voluntary) poisoning is another cause of poisoning seen in children and is more common among adolescent girls (Soyucen et al., 2006, Marcdante, 2006, Dart et al., 2007, Busuttil, 2009a, Bana, 1997). Compared to adolescents, children are more sensitive to environmental stresses and their emotional reactions are higher due to hormonal changes, and suicide attempts are seen more commonly.

Substances causing intoxication differ from country to country. It is reported that poisonings mostly occur as a result of oral intake of substances and drugs are the most common causing agents of acute toxicity (Andiran & Sarikayalar 2004, Marchi et al., 1991, Soyucen et al., 2006, Dart et al., 2007, Yavuz & Ozguner 2003, Ucar et al., 1993). In Western Europe and North America, domestic products, drugs, carbon monoxide and volatile substances take the first place, while in developing countries, causes such as pesticides, household products, medicines, animal or insect bites are in the forefront (Ellenhorn, 1997, Cardozo & Mugerwa 1972, Jamil, 1990).

The majority of childhood poisonings occur at home and approximately 45% of home accidents are acute poisonings (Asirdizer et al., 2005). It is notified that, in Andiran et al's study performed in Ankara, 93.3% third of poisoning cases occurred at home (Andiran & Sarikayalar 2004); in Petridou et al's study realized in Athens, 88.7% of scene was home and living room, bedroom or kitchen (Paritsis et al. 1994); in Soyucen et al's study performed in Sakarya, 92.7% of poisonings occurred in the house (Marchi et al., 1991). According to the World Health Organization, toxicity-related death rates in children between the ages of 1-14 are 0.05 in Denmark, the 0.12 in USA and Canada, 0.75 in Korea (Busuttil, 2009a).

8. Road traffic accidents

Death due to road traffic accidents is one of the major reasons of childhood mortality (Durkin et al., 1999). The global economic cost of motorized vehicle accidents and injuries of pedestrians is around USD 500 billion.

WHO reports that injuries due to road traffic accidents is still an important public health problem. 1.2 million people die and 50 million people are injured due to traffic accidents in the world annually (Chakravarty et al., 2007). In 27 Member States of the EU around 50000 people, 8500 of whom are pedestrians, die due to traffic accidents (Arrequi-Dalmases et al., 2010).

Road traffic accident issue is a major public health problem for particularly low and medium income countries. Contrary to the low and medium income countries, pedestrians constitute the largest group in the traffic accident related injuries and mortalities in the high income countries (Mabunda et al., 2008). It is reported that low socio-economic status is an increasing risk factor for child pedestrian deaths, and that the children with low socio-economic status has 4-5 folds more mortality risk when compared the children with the highest socio-economic status (Desapriya et al., 2011, Busuttil, 2009d).

In accordance with the National Highway Traffic Safety Administration (NHTSA) report 4641 pedestrians died in 2004 in USA. This number corresponds to 11% of the traffic accident related deaths. Pedestrians generally make fatal mistakes in the afternoon or evening time when crossing a street. Pedestrians at the age of 12 and below are found faulty in the accidents in 90% (Ulfarsson et al., 2010).

The number of in-vehicle deaths in traffic accidents particularly in the developed countries has a decreasing trend in recent years. The ratio of mortality between the ages 0 and 14 due to traffic accidents in Europe is 48 %. The ratio of pedestrians between the ages of 15 and 17 died in traffic accidents is 21 %. Although the pedestrian mortality is high in the less developed countries, this problem is not rare in the developed countries. For instance the number of pedestrian deaths in the USA was 4675 in 2004 and increased up to 4881 in 2005. Recently around 5000 pedestrians die and 600000 pedestrians are injured in the USA annually (Chakravarty et al., 2007, Arrequi-Dalmases et al., 2010). The ratio of pedestrian deaths to the traffic accident related deaths in Hong Kong is more than 50%. This ratio is higher than the ratio in the USA, Japan and many western countries. Children possess high injury and mortality risk in traffic accidents. The risk is highly correlated with driver characteristics, socio-economic environment and demographic characteristics of victims (Sze & Wong 2007). The following factors have a serious impact on the injuries in road traffic accidents: type of the vehicle, speed of the vehicle, size of the vehicle, impact angle of the vehicle, center of gravity of the pedestrian when the vehicle comes into contact with the body of the pedestrian, driver characteristics and alcohol intake (Chakravarty et al., 2007).

The researchers focus on the socio-economic characteristics of children, particularly the pedestrians, undergone traffic accidents. Types of injury depend on the age, gender and socio-economic status of the individual. The risk of death for child pedestrians is found associated with the socio-economic status, economic conditions of the family and ethnicity (Chakravarty et al., 2007, Mabunda et al., 2008, Busuttil, 2009d, Graham et al., 2005, Newbury et al., 2008, Presley et al., 2007).

Pedestrian injuries and deaths have an increasing trend in the world. Children constitute the most sensitive group among the pedestrians in traffic accident related injuries and deaths. Pedestrian injuries are the second most common cause of death among the involuntary injuries between the ages of 5 and 14. Children below the age of 15 have a ratio of 8% in overall pedestrian deaths due to road traffic accidents in the USA. On the other hand this age group comprises 30% of the overall pedestrian injuries (Chakravarty et al., 2007). In-vehicle injuries due to road traffic accidents are mostly seen at the age group of 10-19. Injuries related to bicycle accidents are mostly seen at the age group of 10-14, and the injuries related to motorbike accidents are commonly seen at the age group of 15-19 (Agran et al., 2001). In Africa the traffic accident related pedestrian deaths constitute the most significant group. In four provinces of South Africa 7433 pedestrian deaths were reported between the years 2001 and 2004. 18.8% of the deaths in question were children and adolescents under the age of 20 (Mabunda et al., 2008).

It is reported that children in adverse circumstances are inclined to traffic accidents. It is thought that environmental characteristics play a role in traffic accidents (Durkin et al., 1999). It is stated that around 85% of the deaths due to traffic accidents happen in medium and low income countries (Hyder et al., 2006).

The majority of the injuries due to road traffic accidents happen generally in the afternoon or evening time or on weekends. According to some studies deaths mostly happen in summer. The majority of deaths are seen between 6 p.m and 12.00 p.m. as per the American national data. When it gets dark, the sight distance of drivers may be shortened. Together with alcohol intake and pedestrian traffic, it might affect the occurrence of traffic accidents. It is reported that mostly boys get injured and die due to traffic accidents (Durkin et al., 1999, Chakravarty et al., 2007, Mabunda et al., 2008, Desapriya et al., 2011, Newbury et al., 2008).

Different studies are concluded with different results concerning the scene of traffic accidents - whether in the city center, suburban or rural areas - that resulted in injury or death of children. Some studies indicate that road traffic accidents mostly happen in the city center, whereas some others state that road traffic accidents are mainly seen in rural areas (Chakravarty et al., 2007, Mabunda et al., 2008, Desapriya et al., 2011). However it is generally asserted that accidents happen at the vicinity of the child's home (Busuttil, 2009d).

Alcohol plays an evident role in motorized vehicle accidents likewise in pedestrian injuries. Alcohol intake is common among the drivers and the pedestrians. In 2005 the number of the pedestrians died in alcohol related traffic accidents in USA was 2180. This number comprises around 45% of the overall pedestrian deaths. The pedestrian or the driver might take alcohol (Chakravarty et al., 2007). In accordance with the study conducted on road traffic accidents in four provinces of South Africa, alcohol intake was confirmed in 58% (2326) of the cases tested for alcohol (Mabunda et al., 2008).

The children's body parts injured due to traffic accidents were studied in various studies. Head trauma is the most common injury. The ratio of head trauma differs on the basis of the fact whether the child is a pedestrian, or in the vehicle, or riding bicycle (45.4% among pedestrians, 40.2% among riders, 38.9% in vehicle). Besides head trauma, spinal, thorax and abdominopelvic traumas also result in severe injuries and deaths (Durkin et al., 1999, Arrequi-Dalmases et al., 2010).

According to a study conducted in Manhattan, USA, the number of injuries among the school age children per 100.000 persons is 127.2 for pedestrians, 37.4 per riders and 25.5 for children in the vehicle. The number of the children having accident - whether pedestrian (6-10 ages) or rider (9-15 ages) - peaks in summer and in the afternoon time. The number of the children having accident in vehicle (12-16 ages) shows little variation on the basis of seasons and tends to increase in the evening and night hours. Traffic accidents peak at the age of 15. 22.1% of the severe injuries of the school children between the ages 5 and 16 are related to traffic. Around 2/3 of the individuals severely injured and ¾ of the individuals died in the road traffic accidents are the pedestrians (Durkin et al., 1999).

Riding bicycle is a popular childhood activity. The injuries and deaths among the bicycle riders peak between the ages 9 and 15. Boys are exposed to accidents more than girls. The mortality rate due to bicycle accidents are subjected to the extension of bicycle use on the roads and to the conditions of the roads. The conditions of motorbike accidents are similar to bicycle accidents. The risk factors for the bicycle riders are listed as follows: not to use helmet, crash with motorized vehicles, to ride bicycle at an unsafe environment, male gender and alcohol and substance use. It is asserted that nonuse of helmet would lead to more severe injuries. The most common injury mechanism is reported as fall from the bicycle. The body parts most frequently injured are the upper extremities. They are followed by the head and neck region. And finally comes the lower extremities. Among severe injuries contusion of brain or intracerebral haematoma due to head trauma, blunt abdominal trauma with laceration or rupture of internal organs are reported. It is indicated that the number of chest and abdominal injuries is increasing recently. Similar to road traffic accidents, bicycle accidents also happen in the afternoon time most frequently (Busuttil, 2009d, Agran et al., 2001, Hyder et al. 2006, Kiss et al., 2010, Acton et al., 1995, Linn et al., 1998, Puranik et al., 1998, Klin et al., 2009, Rivara et al., 1997).

The time spent until the injured reach to the trauma center is critical. The percentage of the nonfatal injuries is striking. Millions of people get hurt in the traffic accidents every year in the world. The data suggest that this number increases dramatically until 2020 in the countries particularly, where the number of vehicles increases rapidly (Chakravarty et al., 2007).

During the investigation of fatal road traffic accidents, the evaluation of factors such as the scene of the collision, witness statements, clothes of the dead, vehicles involved in the accident and the laboratory analysis of the autopsies will be helpful to clarify the accidents (Busuttil, 2009d).

Death due to trauma has a significant place among the childhood mortality. Traffic accident is the most common cause among the mortality due to trauma. Children are exposed to road traffic accidents mostly as pedestrians. Mostly the boys generally in summer are seen as the victims of the traffic accidents due to head trauma. In such traffic accidents socio-economic and ethnic factors play an important role (Newbury et al., 2008, Hyder et al. 2006, Mazurek, 1994). Infant seats, toddler seats and safety seats are found helpful in minimizing the injuries and deaths in the vehicle. It is hard to estimate the next move or behavior of the children when they are on foot (Busuttil, 2009d). The children should not be allowed to play on the roads or among the vehicles. The children should wear helmet, while they are riding bicycle or motorbike. Children should fasten seat belts, while seated in vehicles, or they should use infant seats, toddler seats or safety seats. We can only save our children from traffic accidents by taking such precautions. Furthermore the children and drivers should be more careful in the afternoon time when children are off the school, since traffic accidents happen more frequently in the afternoon time. It is also important to train the children both in the school and at home on traffic.

9. Home accidents

Home accidents, occur at home or around the house (Gailerd & Herve 1991). Although home injuries are seen in all age groups, due to being preventable and often, leading up to mortality and morbidity, they are important cause of death for children in both developed and developing countries (Scholer et al., 1997, Harris & Kotch 1992). Among children and adolescents, home accidents are the second most common cause of death after traffic accidents (Jacobsson & Schelp, 1987, Laffoy, 1997).

Home accidents seen in children under 18 years old, are classified as deaths due to poisoning with solid/liquid and gas compounds, falls and blunt trauma, burn, scald or electric shock, drowning and asphyxia, fire arm wounds and stabbing on the basis of "Home

Accident Prevention Inventory" proposed by Tertinger (Tertinger et al., 1984), and has been modified by Asirdizer et al (Asirdizer et al. 2005). Home accidents, are seen in all age groups, especially in children between the ages of 0 and 6 (Asirdizer et al. 2005).
0-6 age group of children, because they spend more time at home, usually in the kitchen, the living room and the bathroom, may face numerous injuries (Bourget & McArtur 1989, Gallagher & Hunter 1995, Kilic et al., 2006). Among children under one year old, drowning and foreign body aspiration and between the ages of 1-4 falling, multiplication, water scalds, flame burns and poisonings are more common. At ages of 2-4, when cleaning agents and drugs are left around; after 5 years old poisonings with drugs stored in the fridge and high places are increasing (Yildirim, 2008).
Home accident types vary according to geographical regions. The most common type of accident is falls and this type of accident is the major cause of childhood injuries and deaths in many regions of the world (Peden et al., 2002, Pomerantz et al., 2001).

9.1 Other accidents

Sports injuries, bicycle accidents and some game accidents are among other childhood accidents. Studies indicate that bicycle accidents usually occur in boys and school-age children (Thompson et al., 1990, Cushman et al., 1990).
If accidents and emergency department visits were examined, bicycle accidents are seen as the frequent cause of multiple system injury and also head and brain injuries are the most common cause of death in children accidents (Ji et al., 2006, Guzel et al., 2006, Clarke & Sibert 1986). In order to prevent head trauma, in many countries of the world's and especially in developed countries, helmet use is made compulsory by law for motorcycle and bicycle drivers, but still helmet use of bicycle drivers in developing countries is at a very low level and the rate has been reported to be around 8% (Brown et al., 2002). Mortality rates of bicycle accidents are indicated between 1.2-4.6% (Ji et al., 2006, Heng et al., 2006).
Sports and game injuries in childhood rarely result with sudden death. Evaluation of these cases necessitates the identification of activities prior to death, medical history and detailed autopsy of the deceased (Byard et al. 2002).

10. Fall from height

Falls from height are important causes of morbidity and mortality in childhood traumas. According to the reports of the World Health Organization, falls from height rank second among the causes of death in children (Sala et al., 2000, Taviloglu et al., 2001, Peden, 2009). The important factors that affect mortality are patient age, drop shape, floor structure, position of the fall, fall height, the injured tissue and the pathology developing in these organs (Sala et al., 2000, Mathis et al., 2003, O'Neill, 2000, Lallier et al., 1999, Chalmers et al., 1996).
In the United States, each year, more than three million children visit emergency departments because of falling (Committee on Injury and Poison Prevention, 2001). In childhood, falls from height hold an important place in home accidents and occur in the form of falling from staircases, balconies, windows or roof (Yagmur et al., 2004, Lallier et al., 1999, Istre et al., 2003).
Etiology of falls from height may vary due to structural and seasonal characteristics of the countries, regions or cities (Yagmur et al., 2004, Lallier et al., 1999). In the United States, in a study investigating the epidemiology of deaths due to trauma in rural areas, deaths due to

falls from height have been determined as such a large percentage of %20 (Campbell, 1988). In the South Eastern Anatolia region of Turkey, falling from the roof of houses is quite common. In this region, in a related study about falling from the roof, %49,4 of the patients were noted as under 10 years of age and mortality rate was noted as %5,8 (Yagmur et al., 2004).
The risk of accidental fall from height is most common among preschool boys and younger children because their neural control mechanisms, sensory systems and cognitive abilities associated with hazard awareness and avoidance skills are insufficient (Chang & Tsai 2007).
According to some studies, the head region is the mainly affected region in the body system (Cassidy et al., 2003, Champion et al., 1989, Potoka et al., 2001, Osmond et al., 2002, Hall et al., 1989). Deaths mostly develop in the early period due to multiple trauma or fatal head trauma (Mosenthal et al., 1995, Buckman & Buckman 1991, Velmahos et al., 1997). In the necropsy studies of Hall et al, head trauma is reported as the most common reason of death in children falls (%70,5) (Hall et al., 1989); because children have a higher head/body ratio than adults (Champion et al., 1989, Buckman & Buckman 1991).
According to the studies about falls from height in childhood, mortality rates are noted between %1,3 and %5,9 (Velmahos et al., 1997, Murray et al., 2000).

11. Deaths due to neglect, starvation and physical agents (heat, cold, electricity)

11.1 Neglect- starvation

Is the situation where fundamental needs of a child like nutrition, health, shelter, clothing, protection and supervision are not properly met by his/her parents (Can et al. 2010). Neglect should be repetitive and should impair the health and development status of the child (Nathanson, 2000).
Accidents rank the first in most cases of child mortality due to neglect. Street accidents (traffic accidents, bicycle accidents, fall from a height), domestic accidents (entrapment in anaerobic places, burns, poisoning, drowning in water), in-car traffic accidents (failure to use child restraints or to put on safety belts, neglecting car maintenance) are the most common ones (Cologlu & Cakalir 1999). It is hardly possible to distinguish between accidental and non-accidental injuries. Post-mortem examination should be performed with relevant post-mortem radiological examination (Nathanson, 2000, Cologlu & Cakalir 1999).
The second most common type of neglect is starvation or forced starvation. Starvation can be due to insufficient delivery or non-delivery of food, delivery of improper food, severe loss of appetite or social hunger (Cologlu & Cakalir 1999) Starvation is the condition where there is severe loss of vitamins, minerals, nutrients and energy (Altun & Altun 2010). During the early days of starvation, the glycogen stored in the liver and muscles are used as energy source but glycogen may be understored in children (Altun et al., 2004). As carbohydrates deplete, proteins and fats become the main source of energy. Abundance of fatty acids are formed and transformed into ketone bodies (Altun & Altun 2010, Milroy & Parai 2011). Body mass index drops down. The child gets slim or cachectic. Shortness in height, dehydration, growth and development retardation are noticeable. The skin is dry, atrophic, cracked and hyperkeratotic in appearance. Post-portem examination indicates subcutaneous and internal adipose tissue depletion and atrophy in organs other than the brain. Gastrointestinal organs shrink. Digestive tract is empty; dilatation may be observed in

the gall bladder; hepatic adiposity may be observed (Cologlu & Cakalir 1999, Altun et al., 2004). Diabetes mellitus findings are absent in mortality due to starvation but ketoacidosis may be present in blood (Milroy & Parai 2011). Most of the neglected death cases are under the age of 1 and measurements such as height-weight, head circumference, femur length and sitting height should be done properly and meticulously (Knight, 1996e).

11.2 Hypothermia

Hypothermia is the condition when the internal body temperature drops under 35°C. Due to limited thermoregulation in children, tissue oxygenation is reduced in prolonged hypothermia resulting in cardiac arrhythmia (Cologlu & Cakalir 1999, Turk, 2010). Hypothermia mostly occurs in infants during delivery at home. This is also called sklerema neonatorum. In the case of premature infants or infection or congenital heart disease, the infant gets more prone to hypothermia. Since infants have a smaller body mass with higher surface area/mass proportion, they suffer from a rapid temperature loss. Subcutaneous adipose tissue is smaller in infants with underdeveloped vasomotor reflexes. Adolescents, on the other hand, may suffer from failure to feel the cold following sports activities and alcohol intake or may be subject to hypothermia in case of fatigue (Cologlu & Cakalir 1999, Eke & Soysal 1999). Hypothermia and hypoglycemia are mostly the cause of death for infants left out in mosque or church gardens or rich neighborhoods. Post-mortem stains are light pink in autopsy with erosion and hemorrhage in the digestive tract mucosa accompanying hemorrhagic pancreatitis and multi-infarct zones in organs (Cologlu & Cakalir 1999).

11.3 Hyperthermia

Hyperthermia is the condition when the body temperature is above 40°C. Hyperthermia may be due to either external reasons (such as heat stroke) or internal reasons (such as infections) (Eke & Soysal 1999). In closed spaces with a high humidity ratio and lack of air flow (such as entrapment in the car in hot weathers) there is a high risk of hyperthermia. Children have a limited thermoregulation capacity when compared to adults. Post-mortem examination indicates non-specific alterations, hyperthermia in internal organs as well as edema in the brain and lungs accompanied with petechial hemorrhages. It is important that both ambient temperature and body temperature are measured during crime scene investigation (Cologlu & Cakalir 1999).

11.4 Burns

Mammalian tissues can preserve viability in a relatively narrow window of temperature between 20- 44°C (Eke & Soysal 1999). Child's skin is softer than adults and is more sensitive to heat (Busuttil, 2009c).

Width and depth of the burnt skin surface as well as its proportion to entire body surface affect morbidity and mortality. Burn surface area is determined according to the classical Rule of Nines. Each arm 9, each leg 18, anterior chest 18, posterior chest 18, head 9 and genitalia 1.

1st degree: is the burn that affects the epidermis. Presents with erythema and mild pain. Sun burns are a good example.

2nd degree: is the burn that affects the epidermis and dermis in varying degrees. Superficial 2nd degree burns only invade upper 1/3 of the dermis, and are characterized with blister formation. Deep 2nd degree burns, on the other hand, penetrate into lower 1/3 of the dermis. 3rd degree burns: are the ones covering the entire epidermis and dermis. (Busuttil, 2009c, Knight, 1996a).

Burns may occur as a result of contact with dry - hot or wet - hot substances or chemicals. The heat damage caused by hot fluids is mostly referred to as scalding. (Busuttil, 2009c, Duke et al., 2011). Burns in children are mostly accidental typically occurring as scalding, but suicide and homicide possibilities should never be overlooked (Hilal et al., 2008). Scalds are severe injuries. Victims generally get to be scalded at home by exposure to hot fluids (Figure 3). There are reports of scalding with boiled milk when making cheese (Cekin et al., 2010). Approximately 10% of abused children have burns and scalds with about 25% of scald injuries resulting from non-accidental reasons (Chester et al., 2006, Jacobi et al., 2010). Abuse-related burns should be differentiated from accidental burns (Figure 4). Arms, face, anterior trunk and neck are risky spots for accidental burns. These are generally asymmetric burns with irregular limits and irregular depth. Abuse-related burns mostly manifest with burns on the thigh and legs, genitalia, hands and feet as glove or sock type burns. These are burns with regular and symmetric limits and depth (Maguire et al., 2008, Maguire, 2010). (Figure 5). Post-mortem examination of a burn case should seek to identify the dead body, indicate cause of death and should try to answer whether the person was trapped alive in fire or not.

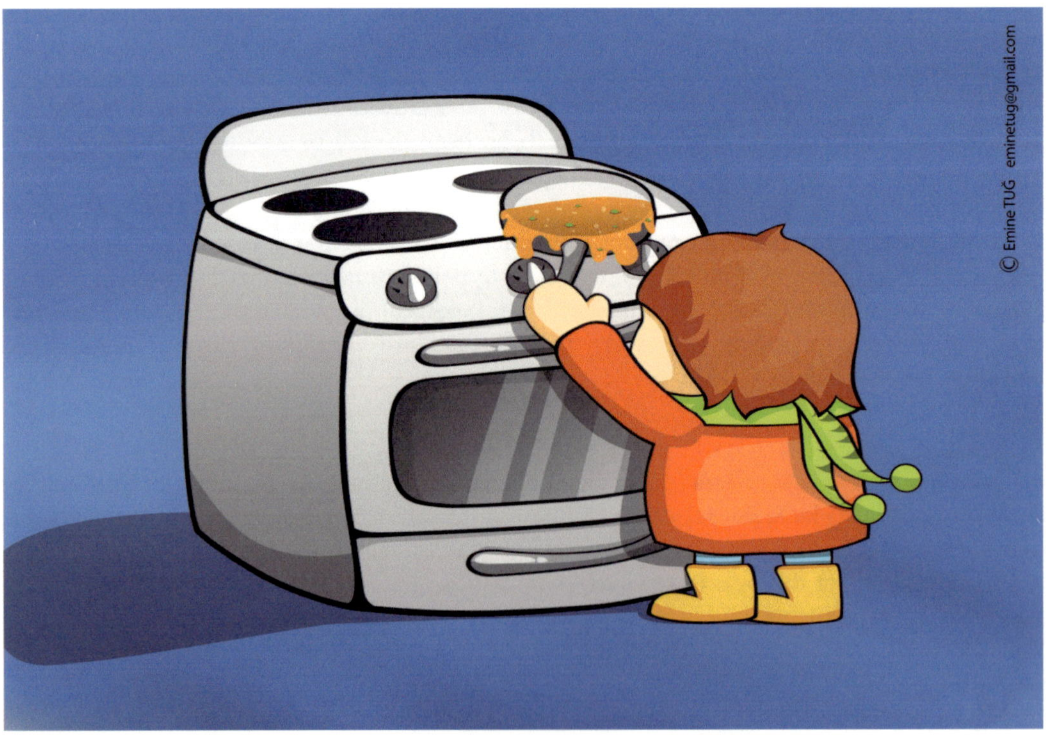

Fig. 3. Children are usually scalding accidentally.

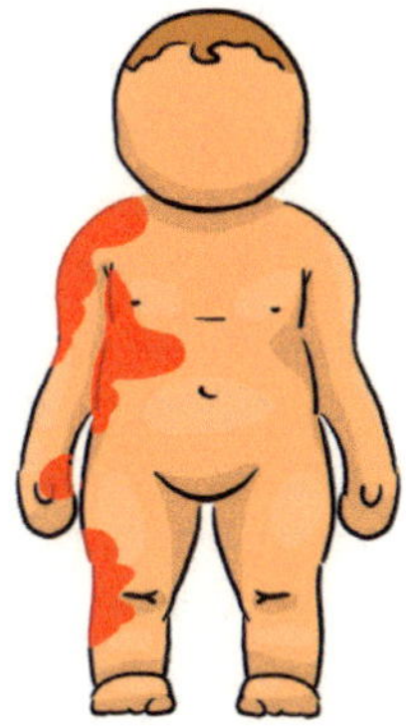

Fig. 4. Accidental burns.

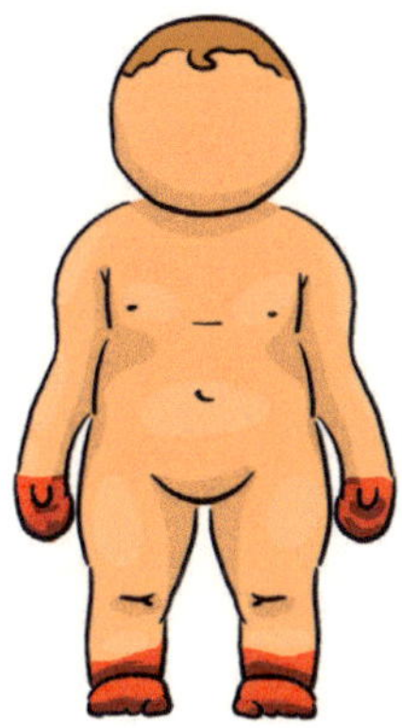

Fig. 5. Abusive burns.

External examination may indicate Pugilistic attitude due to contraction of flexor muscles in upper and lower extremities as a result of denaturation of muscle proteins in exposure to extreme heat. Tissues are dried and toughened due to loss of fluid. There may be bone fractures. Identification of the body may be difficult due to blackened and disintegrated facial features, skin contraction and tightness, scorching of hair and other heat-related changes. Internal examination reveals scalded organs, but the skull may present with extradural hematoma-like, soft, fragmented clots in light chocolate color referred to as heat hematoma (Eke & Soysal 1999, Busuttil, 2009c, Knight, 1996a).

11.5 Electric shock

It is the condition when the electric current (electrons) travels over the child's body as they move from one point to another or in other words, when the body becomes a part of the electricity circuit. The biggest obstacle against the electric current is the skin, which has a stronger resistance than the internal tissues of the body (Eke & Soysal 1999). As dry skin has a resistance of 40.000-100.000 ohms, wet skin manifests a resistance of approximately 1000 ohms and callous skin of 2.000.000 ohms (Busuttil, 2009c). Since the child has a thinner skin, it would have a weaker resistance. It generally develops as a result of accidental contact with an electricity-connected cable. Entry point is generally the hand or the foot, while the exit point is the other hand or the other foot that contacts the ground (Eke & Soysal 1999, Gupta et al., 2009). The most dangerous flow path is the one that goes between the left arm and the right leg. Electricity current may of course run into the body from any spot on the body (Gupta et al., 2009). When it enters the body from the hand, the most important impact that it creates would be the spasm on flexor muscle groups causing a "hold on" effect. As a result, grasping the conductor during electric shock becomes inevitable prolonging the time of electricity to pass the body and worsening the severity of injury (Knight, 1996b). Muscle contractions and spasms may throw away the victim causing extra injuries (Eke & Soysal 1999, Fodor et al., 2011). The origin of the event is mostly accidental in electric shocks that frequently develop as a domestic or occupational accident, and yet the possibility of child abuse or homicide should never be overlooked. It is important to keep the possibility of suicide in mind in adolescent cases (Canturk et al., 2008, Shetty et al., 2010). Death due to electric shock usually develops as a result of ventricular fibrillation or respiratory failure. If the electric current travels through the chest and the abdomen, spasm in intercostal muscles and the diaphragm would cause respiratory paralysis. If it travels through the heart, the result would be arrhythmias, ventricular fibrillation and cardiac arrest. But when it travels through the head and the neck, death would develop as a result of paralysis in the respiratory and circulatory center in the brain stem (Eke & Soysal 1999). There are cases reported with death due to air embolism resulting from electrical injury of neck veins (Kitulwatte & Pollanen 2009). External examination may not indicate any finding in death cases due to electric shock but may as well present with a carbonated body. Electric entry and exit wounds may not always be easily detectable. Entry wound may be in the palms, between the digits, in the oral cavity or in the internal wall of the lips and should be looked for meticulously. Electric burns may present with a grey-white colored parchment look with a typical crater appearance with folded edges. Internal examination indicates non-specific alterations (Eke & Soysal 1999, Polat, 2006).

11.6 Lightening strike

Lightening is the discharge of the electrical potential of the atmosphere between clouds and the earth (Gok, 1983b). With lightening, a DC of 2000- 2 billion Volts gets discharged on earth in an extremely short period of time (in 0,1-1ms) (Busuttil, 2009c). Although rare, it may cause an injury as big as crush injuries (Rash, 2008). Lightening strikes generally occur out in the meadows or forests during spring and summer times (Gok, 1983b). Farmers in small settlements and their children as well as swimmers are under risk (Demirel et al., 2007, Kilbas et al., 2008). Death occurs due to burns, respiratory and circulatory arrest. There may be wide burns on the clothing and on the individual. Metallic parts of clothes have gained a magnetization feature. Clothes may be torn apart or shredded (Eke & Soysal 1999). External examination indicates erythema and fumigation and scorching on burn wounds as well as in the hair. Lichtenberg figures may be present on the skin resembling tree branches originating from dilatation and tearing of small blood vessels. (Eke & Soysal 1999, Polat, 2006, Domart & Garet, 2000, Whitcomb et al., 2002). The most common cause of death is cardiopulmonary arrest (Kilbas et al., 2008). Pulmonary edema, contusion, hemorrhage and ARDS may be seen in the respiratory system. Prolonged Q-T, myocardial infarction and Takotsubo's cardiomyopathy may develop in the heart. Intracranial hemorrhage may be present in the central nervous system (Whitcomb et al., 2002, McIntyre et al., 2010).

12. Wounds

All kinds of damage caused on the body by physical or chemical substances are defined as wounds. The features of the damage on the tissue depend on the energy transferred on the tissue, transfer period to the tissue, width of the transfer area, structure of the substance causing injury, impact angle and the status during the impact, the structure of the body part affected and its status during impact. Wounds caused by substances and tools with diverse features display different characteristics. These wounds can be grouped into five. 1- Blunt traumatic wounds, 2- incised wounds (sharp object wounds), 3- Penetration wounds, 4- penetrating stab wounds, 5- incised & crush wounds (Cetin, 1999, Knight, 1996f).

All the physicians involved with forensic medicine should be familiar with the characterization and images of the wounds. Fatal childhood wounds alone will be assessed here. Blunt traumatic wounds: might be observed as abrasions, ecchymosis, hematoma, laceration and bone fractures (Cetin, 1999). This group of wounds is commonly observed and coexist in deaths due to general body trauma related wounds such as traffic accidents and falling down from height. Internal body, major vessel and medulla spinalis wounds might be fatal (Cetin, 1999, Bilgen et al., 2009). These might be caused by an accident or occur as a result of homicide and neglect. Ecchymosis is the most common abuse wound (Maguire, 2010). Existence of many abrasions, bruises and hematomas can not be assessed as an abuse finding alone. Toddlers and active school age children might have plenty of ecchymosis especially on knees, pretibial area and forehead (Nathanson, 2000). Abrasions with a particular shape and ecchymosis might be helpful in terms of understanding the cause of the wound (Gok, 1983b).

Bite marks, ecchymosis and laceration or combination of three might be observed. Marks should be measured and teeth structure should be defined via the remaining teeth marks in order to assess the possibility that marks may be caused by the bites of another child or an animal (help of the forensic dentist is of value) (Nathanson, 2000).

Existence of many fractured bones is a strong evidence of abuse. Medium shaft fractures, spiral or oblique fractures of long bones, metaphyseal and epiphyseal fractures and smashes, periosteal thickening, numerous rib fractures, linear fractures on skull especially on parietal bone and compression fractures are associated with abuse (Maguire, 2010, Nathanson, 2000, Knight, 1996c).

Incised wounds, penetration wounds, penetrating stab wounds, sharp incised & crush wounds associated mortality might be caused by an accident or a homicide. Suicide is also a possibility for the adolescent groups. Localization and number of the wounds and wound age are important in understanding the cause of the wound. Crime scene investigation, social and medical history of the child and post mortem examination findings should be interpreted together (Ekizoglu & Arican 2010).

13. Firearm fatalities

Injuries are leading causes of mortality throughout the world both for childhood and other age groups (Fraga et al., 2010, Meel, 2007). Firearm fatalities are the most common causes of traumatic death together with deaths from motor vehicle crashes in countries like USA. In 1992, 5367 children and adolescents aged 1 to 19 years were killed by firearms. 63% were the victims of homicides, 27% of suicides and 9% of unintentional injuries. In contrast, during that same year in Britain, firearms were involved in a total of 46 deaths (Mazurek, 1994).

There is a steady nationwide increase in the death toll from firearms and the USA still lacks effective gun control legislation (Mazurek, 1994, Powell et al., 1996). For example, firearms are easily available in the USA and Scandinavian countries (Canturk et al., 2010). Firearm fatalities are common in countries like Columbia, South Africa and Brazil while it is quite low in Japan. Firearm fatalities are more common in countries which legally ensure easy access to firearms and have low-to-mid income level (Meel, 2005). Firearm fatalities are higher among men and the age group 15-44. Minority youth are disproportionately affected by firearm homicides. Availability of firearms at home is reported to increase the risk of firearm fatalities for children and adolescents. Firearm fatalities among children are rarer under the age of 10. The incidence is progressively higher for the age groups 10-14 and 15-19 (Fraga et al., 2010, Meel, 2007, Mazurek, 1994, Powell et al., 1996, Canturk et al., 2010, Meel, 2005, Presley et al., 2007, Grossman et al., 2005, Canturk et al., 2007, Agran et al., 2001).

Fatalities might occur due to negligent behavior with firearms, children playing with firearms and during hunting or firearm cleaning process. Children might shoot themselves or might be shot by a family member or a friend. Pistols are the most common causes of death among other firearms. Shotgun and rifle follow the pistols as a fatality cause (Heninger & Hanzlick 2008, Barber et al., 2002, Bhattacharya et al., 1998). Firearms are mostly to blame for homicides and suicides among children (Mazurek, 1994, Canturk et al., 2007).

Firearm fatalities manner of death is mostly homicide for children. (Meel, 2005, Heninger & Hanzlick 2008, Byard et al., 2009, Sorenson & Berk 1999, Eber et al., 2004). A study which compares the pediatric firearm fatalities in Australia and USA reports that the ratios vary; however, fatalities are more frequently seen among men, the cases are more common respectively as manner of death, homicide, suicide and accidental deaths; the most frequently injured body part was reported to be the head (Byard et al., 2009).

Easy legal access to firearms in some developed countries increases the risk of suicide committed with firearms especially for the adolescents (Canturk et al., 2010, Meel, 2005, Portzky et al., 2005, Grossman et al., 1999). The pediatric suicide risk increases together with the increase in age. The fatal and violent forms of suicide are preferred by boys (Canturk et al., 2010). Hanging is reported to be the most common manner of pediatric suicide. Suicides committed via firearms increase during adolescence and young adulthood (Canturk et al., 2010, Madge, 1999).

Unintentional firearm fatalities are experienced less among children when compared to homicides and suicides. These are sometimes taken as suicides. Children might accidentally die as a result of a bullet fired out of the firearm by family members or aggressors. Access to firearms at home increases the pediatric risk of injury or death. Children or adolescents may lead to an accident while trying to impress others or children might die during the firearm cleaning process or hunting (Grossman et al., 2005, Barber et al., 2002, Karger et al., 2002, Hemenway et al., 2010).

In a study from Istanbul, most of the cases (n=36, 53.4%) were aged 16-20 years (Asirdizer et al., 2010). Firearms other than handgun, rifle, shotgun may cause childhood mortality. Nonpowder firearms are not toys. These may cause serious injuries or fatalities among children and adolescents. 32 of 39 nonpowder gun-related (ball-bearing guns, pellet guns, air rifles, paintball guns) deaths reported in USA between the years 1990 and 2000 were among children less than 15. It is estimated that 3.2 million nonpowder guns are sold every year in USA (Laraque, 2004, O'Neill et al., 2009). A study reports that 16 of 59 simply modified blank cartridge gun related deaths within 4 years occurred among the ages of 11-

20 (Uzun et al., 2009). Nonpowder firearms and blank cartridge guns related child deaths most frequently occur among men as it is the case for other firearm deaths; head injuries are the most common type while most of the cases are suicide cases(Laraque, 2004, O'Neill et al., 2009, Uzun et al., 2009). Celebratory gun shooting injuries are mostly seen among men in metropolitans and crowded places during celebrations or festivals and holidays. However, there are rare cases of women or child injuries or deaths (Ozdemir & Unlu 2009).

14. Acknowledgment

The authors wish to thank Miss Emine Tug for her drawings our figures.

15. References

Acton, CH.; Thomas, S.; Nixon, JW.; Clark, R.; Pitt, WR. & Battistutta, D. (1995). Children and bicycles: what is really happening? Studies of fatal and non-fatal bicycle injury, *Injury prevention*, Vol. 1, No. 2, pp. 86-91, ISSN 1353-8047

Agran, PF.; Winn, D.; Anderson, C.; Trent, R. & Walton-Haynes, L. (2001). Rates of pediatric and adolescent injuries by year of age, *Pediatrics*, Vol. 108, No. 3, pp. (E45), ISSN 1098-4275

Agritmis, H.; Yayci, N.; Colak, B. & Aksoy, E. (2004). Suicidal deaths in childhood and adolescent, *Forensic Science International*, Vol. 142, No. 1, pp. (25-31), ISSN 0379-0738

Aikhionbare, HA.; Yakubu, AM. & Naida, AM. (1989). Mortality pattern in the emergency pediatric unit of Ahmadu Bello University Teaching Hospital, Zaire, Nigeria, *The Central African journal of medicine*, Vol. 35, No. 5, pp. 393-396, ISSN 0008-9176

Aleszewicz-Baranowska, J.; Ulewicz-Filipowicz, J.; Owczuk, R.; Bautembach-Minkowska, J. & Erecinski, J. (2002). Sudden cardiac death in children, *Przegląd lekarski*, Vol. 59, No. 10, pp. (840-843), ISSN 0033-2240 (In Polish)

Alexander, GR.; Kogan, M.; Bader, D.; Carlo, W.; Allen, M. & Mor, J. (2003). US birth weight/gestational age-specific neonatal mortality:1995-1997 rates for Whites, Hispanics, and Blacks, *Pediatrics*, Vol. 111, No. 1, pp. e61-e66, ISSN 1098-4275

Altmann, A. & Nolan, T. (1995). Non-intentional asphyxiation deaths due to upper airway interference in children 0 to 14 years, *Injury prevention*, Vol. 1, No. 2, pp. 76-80, ISSN 1353-8047

Altun, G.; Aansu, B.; Altun, BU.; Azmak, D. & Yilmaz, A. (2004). Deaths due to hunger strike: post-mortem findings, *Forensic Science International*, Vol. 146, No. 1, (Nov 2004), pp. 35-38, ISSN 0379-0738

Altun, G. & Altun, BU. (2010). Evaluation of Starvation and Hunger strikes from Clinical, Ethical and legal perspective, In: *Forensic Medicine in first Step*, Koc, S.; Can, M., pp. 269-277, Istanbul Medical Chamber, ISBN 978-605-5867-33-1, İstanbul, (In Turkish)

Andiran, N. & Sarikayalar, F. (2004). Pattern of Acute Poisonings in Children in Ankara: What has Changed in Twenty Years?, *The Turkish journal of pediatrics*, Vol. 46, No. 2, pp. 147-152, ISSN 0041-4301

Arrequi-Dalmases, C.; Lopez-Valdes, FJ. & Sequi-Gomez, M. (2010). Pedestrian injuries in eight European countries: an analysis of hospital discharge data, *Accident; analysis and prevention*, Vol. 42, No. 4, pp. 1164-1171, ISSN 0001-4575

Arslan, M.; Kar, H.; Akcan, R. & Cekin, N. (2005). Evaluation of diagnostic methods used in drowning, *The Bulletin of Legal Medicine*, Vol. 10, No. 1, pp. (29-34), 1304-5040

Asirdizer, M.; Canturk, G.; Canturk, N.; Yavuz, MS. & Sari, H. (2010). Analyses of Suicidal Deaths with Shotguns in Istanbul, 1998-2007, *Turkish journal of trauma & emergency surgery*, Vol. 16, No. 1, pp. 47-53, ISSN 1306-696X

Asirdizer, M.; Yavuz, MS.; Albek, E. & Canturk G. (2005). Infant and Adolescent Deaths in Istanbul Due to Home Accidents, *Turkish Journal of Pediatrics*, Vol. 47, pp. 141-149, ISSN 0041-4301

Baasner, A.; Dettmeyer, R.; Graebe, M.; Rissland, J. & Madea, B. (2003). PCR-based diagnosis of enterovirus and parvovirus B19 in paraffin-embedded heart tissue of children with suspected sudden infant death syndrome, *Laboratory investigation; a journal of technical methods and pathology*, Vol. 83, No. 10, (Oct 2003), pp. 1451-1455, ISSN 0023-6837

Bajanowski, T.; Vennemann, M.; Bohnert, M.; Rauch, E.; Brinkmann, B. & Mitchell, EA. (2005). Unnatural causes of sudden unexpected deaths initially thought to be sudden infant death syndrome. *International Journal of Legal Medicine*, Vol. 119, No. 4, (Jul 2005), pp. 213-216, ISSN 0937-9827

Bamgboye, EA. & Familusi, JB. (1990). Mortality pattern at a children's emergency ward, University College Hospital, Ibadan, Nigeria, *African journal of medicine and medical sciences*, Vol. 19, No. 2, pp. 127-132, ISSN 0309-3913

Bana, V. (1997). Salicylates, In: *Paediatric Toxicology Handbook of Poisoning in Children*, Bates, N.; Edwards, N.; Roper, J. & Volans, G., pp. 316-320, Macmillan Reference Ltd, ISBN 0333 60951 4 ,New York

Barber, C.; Hemenway, D.; Hochstadt, J. & Azrael, D. (2002). Underestimates of unintentional firearm fatalities: comparing Supplementary Homicide Report data with the National Vital Statistics System, *Injury Prevention*, Vol. 8, No. 3, pp. 252–256, ISSN 1353-8047

Beckwith, JB. (1988). Intrathoracic petechial hemorrhages: a clue to the mechanism of death in sudden infant death syndrome?, *Annals of the New York Academy of Sciences*, Vol. 533, pp. (37-47), 0077-8923

Beckwith, JB.; (2003). Defining the sudden infant death syndrome. *Archives of Pediatrics & Adolescent Medicine*, Vol. 157, No. 3, (Mar 2003), pp. 286-290, ISSN 1072-4710

Bener, A.; Hussain, SJ.; Ghaffar, A.; Abou-Taleb, H. & El-Sayed. (2011). Trends in childhood trauma mortality in the fast economically developing State of Qatar, *World journal of pediatrics*, Vol. 7, No. 1, (Feb 2011), pp. 41-44, ISSN 1708-8569

Bilgen, S.; Turkmen, N.; Eren, B. & Fedar, R.; (2009). Peripheral vascular injury-related deaths, *Turkish journal of trauma & emergency surgery*, Vol. 15, No. 4, (Jul 2009), pp. 357-361, ISSN 1306-696X

Bhattacharya, N.; Bethel, CA.; Caniano, DA.; Pillai, SB.; Deppe, S. & Cooney, DR. (1998). The childhood air gun. Serious injuries and surgical interventions, *Pediatric emergency care*, Vol. 14, No. 3, pp. 188-190, ISSN 0749-5161

Black, RE.; Cousens, S.; Johnson, HL.; Lawn, JE.; Rudan, I.; Bassani, DG.; Jha, P.; Campbell, H.; Walker, CF.; Cibulskis, R.; Eisele, T.; Liu, L. & Mathers, C. (2010). Global, regional, and national causes of child mortality in 2008: a systematic analysis, *Lancet*, Vol. 375, No. 9330, pp. 1969-1987, ISSN 0140-6736

Blackwell, CC.; Moscovis, SM.; Gordon, AE.; Al Madani, OM.; Hall, ST.; Gleeson, M.; Scott, RJ.; Roberts-Thomson, J.; Weir, DM. & Busuttil, A. (2005). Cytokine responses and sudden infant death syndrome: genetic, developmental, and environmental risk factors, *Journal of leukocyte biology,* Vol. 78, No. 6, (Dec 2005), pp. 1242-1254, ISSN 0741-5400

Blair, PS.; Fleming, PJ.; Bensley, D.; Smith, I.; Bacon, J.; Taylor, E.; Berry, J.; Golding, J.; M. & Tripp, J. (1996). Smoking and the sudden infant death syndrome: results from 1993-5 case-control study for confidential inquiry into stillbirths and deaths in infancy. Confidential Enquiry into Stillbirths and Deaths Regional Coordinators and Researchers, *British medical journal,* Vol. 313, No. 7051, (Jul 1996), pp. 195-198, ISSN 0959-8138

Blair, PS.; Sidebotham, P.; Berry, PJ.; Evans, M. & Fleming, PJ.; (2006). Major epidemiological changes in sudden infant death syndrome: a 20-year population-based study in the UK, *Lancet,* Vol. 28, No. 367(9507), (Jan 2006), pp. 314-319, ISSN 0099-5355

Bourget, CC. & McArtur, ER. (1989). Unintentional injuries: Risk factors in preschool children, *American journal of diseases of children,* Vol. 143, No. 5, pp. 556-559, ISSN 0002-922X

Brixey, SN.; Kopp, BC.; Schlotthauer, AE.; Collier, A. & Corden, E.(2011). Use of child death review to inform sudden unexplained infant deaths occurring in a large urban setting, *Injury prevention,* Vol. 17, Suppl 1, (Feb 2011), pp. 23-27, ISSN 1353-8047

Bridge, JA.; Greenhouse, JB.; Sheftall, AH.; Fabio, A.; Campo, JV. & Kelleher, KJ. (2010). Changes in suicide rates by hanging and/or suffocation and firearms among young persons aged 10-24 years in the United States: 1992-2006, *The Journal of adolescent health,* Vol. 46, No. 5, pp. 503-505, ISSN 1054-139X

Bronstein, AC.; Spyker, DA.; Cantilena, LR.; Green, JL.; Rumack, BH. & Giffin, SL. (2008). Annual Report of the American Association of Poison Control Centers' National Poison Data System (NPDS): 26th Annual Report. *Clinical Toxicology,* Vol. 47, pp. 911–1084, ISSN 1556-3650

Brown, RL.; Koepplinger, ME.; Mehlman, CT.; Gittelman, M. & Garcia, VF. (2002). All-terrain vehicle and bicycle crashes in children: epidemiology and comparison of injury severity, *Journal of Pediatric Surgery,* Vol. 37, pp. 375-380, ISSN: 0022-3468

Brüning, C.; Siekmeyer, W.; Siekmeyer, M.; Merkenschlager, A. & Kiess, W. (2010). Retrospective analysis of 44 childhood drowning accidents, *Wiener klinische Wochenschrif,* Vol. 122, No. (13-14), (Jul 2010), pp. 405-412, ISSN 0043-5325 (Article in German)

Buckman, RF. & Buckman, PD. (1991). Vertical deceleration trauma. Principles of management, *The Surgical clinics of North America,* Vol. 71, No. 2, pp. 331-344, ISSN 0039-6109

Busuttil, A. (2009). a) Accidental injuries in children, In: *Paediatric Forenic Medicine&Pahology,* Busuttil, A.; Keeling, JW. pp. (336-344), Edward Arnold Publishers Ltd, 0 340 731 575, London

Busuttil, A. (2009). b) Asphyxial Deaths In Children, In: *Paediatric Forenic Medicine&Pathology,* Busuttil, A.; Keeling, JW. pp. (329-335), Edward Arnold Publishers Ltd, ISBN 0 340 731 575, London

Busuttil, A. (2009). c) Heat-Induced Injury or Death, In: *Paediatric Forenic Medicine & Pathology,* Busuttil, A.; Keeling, JW. pp. 318-328, Edward Arnold Publishers Ltd, ISBN 0 340 731 575, London

Busuttil, A. (2009). d) Road traffic accidents in children, In: *Paediatric Forenic Medicine & Pathology,* Busuttil, A.; Keeling, JW. pp. (385-394), Edward Arnold Publishers Ltd, 1 st ed. ISBN 0 340 731 575, London

Byard, RW. (2000). Accidental childhood death and the role of the pathologist, *Pediatric and developmental pathology,* Vol. 3, No. 5, (Sep-Oct 2000), pp. 405-418, ISSN 1093-5266

Byard, RW. & James, RA. (2001). Car window entrapment and accidental childhood asphyxia, *Journal of paediatrics and child health,* Vol. 37, No. 2, (Apr 2001), pp. 201–202, ISSN 1034-4810

Byard, RW.; James, RA. & Gilbert, JD. (2002). Childhood sporting deaths, *The American Journal of Forensic Medicine and Pathology,* Vol. 23, No. 4, pp. 364-367, ISSN 0195-7910

Byard, RW. & Krous, HF. (2003). Sudden infant death syndrome: overview and update. *Pediatric and developmental pathology,* Vol. 6, No. 2, (Mar-Apr 2003), pp. 112-127, ISSN 1093-5266

Byard, RW. (2008). Rainwater tank drowning. *Journal of forensic and legal medicine,* Vol. 15, No. 8, (Nov 2008), pp. 533-534, ISSN 1752-928X

Byard, RW.; Haas, E.; Marshall, DT.; Gilbert, JD. & Krous, HF. (2009). Characteristic features of pediatric firearm fatalities-comparisons between Australia and the United States, *Journal of forensic sciences,* Vol. 54, No. 5, pp. 1093-1096, ISSN 0022-1198

Campbell-Hewson, G.; Egleston, CV. & Cope, AR. (1997). Traumatic asphyxia in children, *Journal of accident & emergency medicine,* Vol. 14, No. 1, pp. (47-49), 1351-0622

Campbell, JE. (1988). Basic Trauma Life Score, In: *Basic Prehospital Trauma Care,* pp. 23-42, Prentice-Hall Inc.,ISBN 0893031224

Can, M.; Tirtil, L. & Dokgoz, H. (2010). Medical Responsibilities in child abuse cases, In: *Forensic Medicine in first Step,* Koc, S.; Can, M. pp. 181-191, İstanbul Medical Chamber, ISBN 978-605-5867-33-1, Istanbul (In Turkish)

Canturk, G.; Canturk, N.; Teke, HY.; Erkol, Z. & Yavuz, MS. (2010). Suicidal Deaths Among Children and Adolescents in Ankara Between 2001 and 2006, *Journal of Medical Sciences,* Vol. 30, No. 2, pp. 474-481, ISSN 1300-0292

Canturk, N. & Canturk, G. (2001). Waterhouse- Friderichsen Syndrome: a case report, *Journal of Children's Forum,* Vol. 4, No. 3-4, pp. 33-35, ISSN 1301-9872 (In Turkish)

Canturk, N.; Samdanci, E.; Canturk, G. & Yurtman, T. (2006). Acute Myocardial İnfarctus in Newborn: a case report. *13th National Forensic Medicine Days Panels and Poster Presentations Book,* pp. 233-235, Institute of Forensic Medicine, Ministry of Justice Publishs No:17, Istanbul (In Turkish)

Canturk, N.;, Eşiyok, B.; Ozkara, E.; Canturk, G.; Ozata, AB. & Yavuz, MF. (2007). Medico-legal Child Deaths in Istanbul: Data from the Morgue Department, *Pediatrics International,* Vol. 49, pp. 88-93, ISSN 1328-8067

Canturk, N.; Alkan, HA. & Canturk, G. (2008). Evaluation of autopsy cases whom deaths from electricity in Ankara between the years 2002-2006, *Turkish Journal of Forensic Medicine,* Vol. 22, No. 2, pp. 1-7, ISSN 1018-5 (In Turkish)

Canturk, N.; Canturk, G.; Karbeyaz, K.; Ozdes, T.; Dagalp, R. & Celik, S. (2009). Evaluation of the drowning cases in Ankara between the years of 2003-2006, *Journal of Medical Sciences,* Vol. 29, No. 5, pp. 198-205, ISSN 1300-0292 (In Turkish)

Cardozo, LJ. & Mugerwa, RD. (1972). The Pattern of Acute Poisoning in Uganda, *East African medical journal,* Vol. 42, pp. 983-988, ISSN: 0012 835x

Cassidy, LD.; Potoka, DA.; Adelson, PD. & Ford, HR. (2003). Development of a novel method to predict disability after head trauma in children, *Journal of pediatric surgery*, Vol. 38, pp. 482–485, ISSN 0022-3468

Cekin, N.; Akcan, R.; Arslan, MM.; Hilal, A. & Eren, A. (2010). An unusual cause of death at preschool age: scalding by hot milk, *The American journal of forensic medicine and pathology*, Vol. 31, No. 1, (Mar 2010), pp. 69-71, ISSN 0195-7910

Cetin, G. (1999). Wounds. In: *Forensic Medicine vol 1*, Soysal, Z.; Çakalir, C., pp. (475-523), Istanbul University Cerrahpasa Medical Faculty Press, Presidency No: 4165, Faculty No: 224, İstanbul University Press and Film Center, 975-404-540-2, Istanbul, (In Turkish)

Centers for Disease Control and Prevention. (1998). Fatal Car Trunk Entrapment Involving Children—United States, 1987-1998, *Morbidity and mortality weekly report,* Vol. 47, No. 47, pp. 1019-1022, ISSN 0149-2195

Chakravarty, B.; Vaca, FE.; Lotfipour, S. & Bradley, D. (2007). Pediatric pedestrian injuries: emergency care considerations, *Journal of emergencies, trauma and shock* , Vol. 23, No. 10, pp. 738-744, ISSN 0974-2700

Chalmers, DJ.; Marshall, SW.; Langley, JD.; Evans, MJ.; Brunton, CR.; Kelly, AM. & Pickering, AF. (1996). Height and surfacing as risk factors for injury in falls from playground equipment: a case control study, *Injury Prevention*, Vol. 2, No. 2, pp. 98-104, ISSN1353-8047

Champion, HR.; Sacco, WJ.; Copes, WS.; Gann, DS.; Gennarelli, TA. & Flanagan, ME. (1989). *The Journal of Trauma,* Vol. 29, No. 5, pp. 623-629, ISSN 0022-5282

Chang, LT. & Tsai, MC. (2007). Craniofacial injuries from slip, trip, and fall accidents of children, The Journal of trauma, Vol. 63, pp. 70–74 ISSN 0022-5282

Cheraghali, F. & Taymori, M. (2006). Epidemiological Study of Drug Poisoning in Children, *Acta Medica Iranica,* Vol. 44, pp. 37-40, ISSN 0044-6025

Chester, DL.; Jose, RM.; Aldlyami, E. & King, Moiemen, NS. (2006). Non-accidental burns in children--are we neglecting neglect?, *Burns,* Vol. 32, No. 2, (Mar 2006), pp. 222-228, ISSN 0305-4179

Chinski, A.; Foltran, F.; Gregori, D.; Passali, D. & Bellussi, L. (2010). Foreign bodies causing asphyxiation in children: the experience of the Buenos Aires paediatric ORL clinic, *The Journal of international medical research,* Vol. 38, No. 2, pp. 655–660, ISSN 0300-0605

Choudhury, P.; Kumar, P.; Puri, RK.; Prajapati, NC. & Gupta, S.(1991). Childhood morbidity and mortality in a large hospital over last four decades, *Indian pediatrics,* Vol. 28, No. 3, pp. 249-254, ISSN 0019-6061

Clarke, AJ. & Sibert, JR. (1986). Why child cyclists should wear helmets, *Practitioner,* Vol. 230, No. 5, pp. 13-14, ISSN 0032-6518

Cohle, SD.; Balraj, E. & Bell, M. (1999). Sudden death due to ventricular septal defect, *Pediatric and developmental pathology,* Vol. 2, No. 4, (Jul-Aug 1999), pp. 327-332, ISSN 1093-5266

Cologlu, S. & Cakalir, C. (1999). Child deaths, In: *Forensic Medicine Vol 1,* Soysal, Z.; Çakalir, C., pp. 377-404, Istanbul University Cerrahpasa Medical Faculty Press, Presidency No: 4165, Faculty No: 224, İstanbul University Press and Film Center, ISBN 975-404-540-2, Istanbul, (In Turkish)

Committee on Injury and Poison Prevention. (2001). American Academy of Pediatrics: Falls from Heights: Windows, roofs, and balconies, Pediatrics, Vol. 107, No. 5, pp. 1188 - 1191, ISSN 0031-4005

Cushman, R.; Down, J.; MacMillan, N. & Waclawik, H. (1990). Bicycle-related injuries: a survey in a pediatric emergency department, *Canadian Medical Association journal*, Vol. 143, pp. 108-112, ISSN: 0820-3946

Daltveit, AK.; Oyen, N.; Skjaerven, R. & Irgens, LM. (1997). The epidemic of SIDS in Norway 1967-93: changing effects of risk factors, *Archives of disease in childhood*, Vol. 77, No. 1, (Jul 1997), pp. 23-27, ISSN 1743-0585

Dart, RC.; Rumack, BH.; Hay, WW.; Levin, MJ.; Sondheimer, JM. & Deterding RR. (2007). Current pediatric diagnosis and treatment, In: *Poisoning*. 18th ed. NY:Mc Graw-Hill 2007; 335-360.

Demirci, S. & Dogan, KH. (2010). Asphyxia types and dead examination at asphyxial cases, In: *Forensic Medicine in first Step*, Koc, S.; Can, M. pp. 38-56, Istanbul Medical Chamber, ISBN 978-605-5867-33-1, Istanbul, (In Turkish)

Demirel, B.; Yagan, M.; Balseven, A.; Canturk, N. & Dinc, AH. (2007). Death from lightning strike: a case report, *Gazi Medical Journal*, Vol. 18, No. 2, pp. 92-94, ISSN 1300-056X (In Turkish)

Desapriya, E.; Sones, M.; Ramanzin, T.; Weinstein, S.; Scime, G. & Pike, I. (2011). Injury prevention in child death review: child pedestrian fatalities, *Injury prevention*, Vol. 17, No. 1, pp. i4-i9, ISSN 1353-8047

Dettmeyer, RB. & Kandolf, R. (2010). Cardiomyopathies--misdiagnosed as Sudden Infant Death Syndrome (SIDS), *Forensic Science International*, Vol. 194, No. 1-3, (Jan 2010), pp. 21-24, ISSN 1872-6283

Domart, Y. & Garet, E. (2000). Images in clinical medicine. Lichtenberg figures due to a lightning strike, *The New England journal of medicine*, Vol. 343, No. 21, (Nov 2000), pp. 1536, ISSN 0028-4793

Dudenhausen, JW. & Maier, RF. (2010). Perinatal problems in multiple births, *Deutsches Ärzteblatt international*, Vol. 107, No. 38, pp. 663–668, ISSN 1866-0452 (In Germany)

Duke, J.; Wood, F.; Semmens, J.; Edgar, DW.; Spilsbury, K.; Hendrie, D. & Rea,S. (2011). A Study of Burn Hospitalizations for Children Younger Than 5 Years of Age: 1983-2008, *Pediatrics*,Vol. 127, No. 4, (Mar 2011), pp. e971-977, ISSN 1098-4275

Duke, T.; Michael, A.; Mgone, J.; Frank, D.; Wal, T. & Sehuko, R. (2002). Etiology of child mortality in Goroka, Papua New Guinea: a prospective two-year study, *Bulletin of the World Health Organization*, Vol. 80, No. 1, pp. 16-25, ISSN 0042-9686

Durkin, MS.; Laraque, D.; Lubman, I. & Barlow, B. (1999). Epidemiology and prevention of traffic injuries to urban children and adolescents, *Pediatrics*, Vol. 103, No. 6, pp. (e74), ISSN 1098-4275

Eber, GB.; Annest, JL.; Mercy, JA. & Ryan, GW. (2004). Nonfatal and fatal firearm injuries among children aged 14 years and younger: United States, 1993-2000, *Pediatrics*, Vol. 113, No. 6, pp. 1686-1692, ISSN 0031-4005

Eke, M. & Soysal, Z. (1999). Damages Composed Physical Agents In: *Forensic Medicine vol.2*, Soysal, Z.; Çakalir, C., pp. (607-765), Istanbul University Cerrahpasa Medical Faculty Press, Presidency No: 4165, Faculty No: 224, İstanbul University Press and Film Center, ISBN 975-404-540-2, İstanbul (In Turkish)

Ekizoglu, O. & Arican, N. (2010). Wounds, In: *Forensic Medicine in first Step*, Koc, S.; Can, M. pp. (57-73), Istanbul Medical Chamber, 978-605-5867-33-1 Istanbul, (In Turkish)

Ellenhorn, MJ. (1997). Ellenhorn's Medical Toxicology, Williams&Wilkins, ISBN 9780683300314, Baltimore pp.

Fleming, PJ.; Blair, PS.; Ward Platt, M.; Tripp, J. & Smith, IJ. (2003). Sudden infant death syndrome and social deprivation: assessing epidemiological factors after post-matching for deprivation, *Paediatric and perinatal epidemiology*, Vol. 17, No. 3, (Jul 2003), pp. 272-280, ISSN 0269-5022

Flick, AA.; Brookfield, K.; de la Torre, L.; Tudela, CM.; Duthely, L. & lez-Quintero, VHG. (2010). Excessive weight gain among obese women and pregnancy outcomes, *American journal of perinatology*, Vol. 27, No. 4, pp. 333–338, ISSN 0735-1631.

Fodor, L.; Bota, IO.; Abbas, Y.; Fodor M. & Ciuce, C. (2011). Electricity and fishing - a dangerous mix, *Burns*, Vol. 37, No. 3, (May 2011), pp. 495-498, ISSN 0305-4179

Fraga, AM.; Fraga, GP.; Stanley, C.; Costantini, TW. & Coimbra, R. (2010). Children at danger: injury fatalities among children in San Diego County, *European journal of epidemiology*, Vol. 25, No. 3, pp. 211-217, ISSN 0393-2990

Gallagher, SS. & Hunter, PA. (1995). A home injury prevention program for children, Pediatric clinics of North America, Vol. 32, No. 1, pp. 95-113, ISSN 0031-3955

Gailerd, M. & Herve C. (1991). Emergency medical care and severe home accident in children study of 630 cases over 5 years,their significance in traumatic accident, *Annales de pédiatrie*, Vol. 38, No. 5, pp. 311, ISSN 0066-2097

Geserick, G.; Krocker, K. & Wirth, I. (2010). Tardieu's spots and asphyxia--a literature study, *Archiv für Kriminologie*, Vol. 226, No. (5-6), (Nov-Dec 2010), pp. 145-160, ISSN 0003-9225 (Article in German)

Gilchrist, J.; Gotsch, K. & Ryan, G. (2004). Nonfatal and fatal drownings in recreational water settings--United States, 2001-2002, *MMWR. Morbidity and mortality weekly report*, Vol. 53, No. 21, (Jun 2004), pp. 447-452, ISSN 0149-2195

Gok, S. (1983) a) Asphyxias, In: *Forensic Medicine*, Gok, S., pp. 135-149, Filiz Bookstore, ISBN 975-368-022-8, Istanbul (In Turkish)

Gok S. (1983). b) Wounds, In: *Forensic Medicine*, Gok, S., pp. 157-260, Filiz Bookstore, ISBN 975-368-022-8, İstanbul (In Turkish)

Goldwater, PN. (2008). Intrathoracic petechial hemorrhages in sudden infant death syndrome and other infant deaths: time for re-examination, *Pediatric and developmental pathology*, Vol. 11, No. 6, (Nov-Dec 2008), pp. 450-455, ISSN 1093-5266

Graham, D.; Glaister, S. & Anderson, R. (2005). The effects of area deprivation on the incidence of child and adult pedestrian casualties in England, *Accident; analysis and prevention*, Vol. 37, No. 1, pp. 125-135, ISSN 0001-4575

Grossman, DC.; Mueller, BA.; Riedy, C.; Dowd, MD.; Villaveces, A.; Prodzinski, J.; Nakagawara, J.; Howard, J.; Thiersch, N. & Harruff, R. (2005). Gun storage practices and risk of youth suicide and unintentional firearm injuries, *JAMA*, Vol. 293, No. 6, pp. 707-714, ISSN 0098-7484

Grossman, DC.; Reay, DT. & Baker, SA. (1999). Self-inflicted and unintentional firearm injuries among children and adolescents: the source of the firearm, *Archives of pediatrics & adolescent medicine*, Vol. 153, No. 8, pp. 875-878, ISSN 1072-4710

Gupta, BD.; Sing, OG. & Mehta, RA. (2009). Death comes through eye: a rare case of electrocution, *The American journal of forensic medicine and pathology,* Vol. 30, No. 3, (Sep 2009), pp. (301-302), 0195-7910

Gurpinar, T. & Asirdizer, M. (2006). The Responsibility of Physician in Intoxications, *Journal of Medical Sciences,* Vol. 2, No. 50, pp. 56-62, ISSN 1305-3876

Guzel, A.; Ersoy, B.; Dogrusoy, Y.; Kucukugurluoglu, Y.; Altinel, T. & Karasalihoglu, S. (2006). The evaluation of bicycle accidents that were admitted to a pediatric emergency department, *Turkish journal of trauma & emergency vccsurgery,* Vol. 12, pp. 299-304, ISSN 1306-696X

Hall, JR.; Reyes, HM.; Horvat, M.; Meller, JL. & Stein, R. (1989). The mortality of childhood falls. *The Journal of Trauma;* Vol. 29, pp. 1273–1275, ISSN 0022-5282

Harris, J.M. & Kotch, JB. (1992). Unintentional infant injuries sociodemographic and psychological factors, *Public Health Nursing,* Vol. 11, No. 2, pp. 90–97, ISSN: 0737-1209

Hemenway, D.; Barber, C. & Miller, M. (2010). Unintentional firearm deaths: A comparison of other-inflicted and self inflicted shootings, *Accident; analysis and prevention,* Vol. 42, No. 4, pp. 1184–1188, ISSN 0001-4575

Heng, KW.; Lee, AH.; Zhu, S.; Tham, KY. & Seow, E. (2006). Helmetuse and bicycle-related trauma in patients presenting to an acute hospital in Singapore, *Singapore Medical Journal,* Vol. 47, pp. 367-372, ISSN 0037-5675

Heninger, M. & Hanzlick, R. (2008). Nonnatural deaths of adolescents and teenagers: Fulton County, Georgia, 1985-2004, *The American journal of forensic medicine and pathology,* Vol. 29, No. 3, pp. 208-213, ISSN 0195-7910

Highet, AR. (2008). An infectious aetiology of sudden infant death syndrome, *Journal of applied microbiology,* Vol. 105, No. 3, (Sep 2008), pp. 625-635, ISSN 1364-5072

Hilal, A.; Cekin, N.; Arslan, M. & Gulmen, MK. (2008). Deaths due to burns in Adana, Turkey, *Burns,* Vol.34, No.7, (Nov 2008), pp. 982-985, ISSN 0305-4179

Hoffman, RJ. & Osterhoudt, KC. (2002). Evaluation and management of pediatric poisoning. *Pediatrics,* Vol. 2., pp. 51-63, ISSN 0031-4005.

Hurtado, TR. & Della-Giustina, DA. (2003). Traumatic asphyxia in a 6-year-old boy, *Pediatric emergency care,* Vol. 19, No. 3, pp. 167-168, ISSN 0749-5161

Hyder, AA.; Amach, OH.; Garg, N. & Labinjo, MT. (2006). Estimating the burden of road traffic injuries among children and adolescents in urban South Asia, Health policy, Vol. 77, No. 2, pp. 129-139, ISSN 0168-8510

Hyder, AA.; Borse, NN.; Blum, L.; Khan, R.; El Arifen, S. & Baqui, AH.; (2008). Childhood drowning in low- and middle-income countries: Urgent need for intervention trials, *Journal of paediatrics and child health,* Vol. 44, No. 4, (Apr 2008), pp. 221-227, ISSN 1034-4810

Inanici, MA.; Yorulmaz, C. & Canturk, N. (2001). Sudden Infant Death Syndrome: a case report, *The Bulletin of Forensic Medicine,* Vol. 6, No. 3, pp. 130-133, ISSN 1304-5040 (In Turkish)

Iqbal, A.; Shirin, T.; Ahmed, T.; Ahmed, S.; Islam, N.; Sobhan, A. & Siddique, AK. (2007). Childhood mortality due to drowning in rural Matlab of Bangladesh: magnitude of the problem and proposed solutions, *Journal of health, population, and nutrition,* Vol. 25, No. 3, (Sep 2007), pp. 370-376, ISSN 1606-0997

Istre, GR.; McCoy, MA.; Stowe, M.; Davies, K.; Zane, D.; Anderson, RJ. & Wiebe, R. (2003). Childhood injuries due to falls from apartment balconies and windows, *Injury Prevention*, Vol. 9, pp. 349-352, ISSN 1353-8047

Jacobi, G.; Dettmeyer, R.; Banachak, S.; Brosig, B. & Herrmann, B. (2010). Child abuse and neglect: diagnosis and management, *Deutsches Ärzteblatt international*, Vol. 107, No. 13, (Apr 2010), pp. 231-239, ISSN 1866-0452 (In Germany)

Jacobsson, B. & Schelp, L. (1987). Home accidents among children and teenagers in a Swedish rural municipality, *Scandinavian journal of social medicine,* Vol. 15, pp. 31-35, ISSN 0300-8037

Jamil, H. (1990). Acute Poisoning. A review of 1900 cases, *Journal of the Pakistan Medical Association*, Vol. 40, pp. 131-133, ISSN 0030-9982

Jensen, L.; Charlwood, C. & Byard, RW. (2008). Shopping cart injuries, entrapment, and childhood fatality, *Journal of forensic sciences*, Vol. 53, No. 5, pp. 1178-1180, ISSN 0022-1198

Ji, M.; Gilchick, RA. & Bender, SJ. (2006). Trends in helmet use and head injuries in San Diego County: the effect of bicycle helmet legislation, *Accident; analysis and prevention*, Vol. 38, pp. 128-134, ISSN 0001-4575

Jones, LS.; Wyatt, JP. & Busuttil, A. (2000). Plastic bag asphyxia in Southeast Scotland, *The American journal of forensic medicine and pathology*, Vol. 21, No. 4, pp. 401-405, ISSN 0195-7910

Karger, B.; Billeb, E. & Koops, E. (2002). Accidental firearm fatalities. Forensic and preventive implications, *International journal of legal medicine*, Vol. 116, No. 6, pp. (350-353), 0937-9827

Keeling, JW. (2009). a) Fetal And Perinatal Death, In: *Paediatric Forenic Medicine&Pahology*, Busuttil, A.; Keeling, JW. pp. 180-197, Edward Arnold Publishers Ltd, ISBN 0 340 731 575, London

Keeling, JW. (2009). b) Sudden Unexpected Death in infancy: Sudden Infant Death Syndrome or something else?, In: *Paediatric Forensic Medicine&Pahology*, Busuttil, A.; Keeling, JW. pp. 198-221, Edward Arnold Publishers Ltd, ISBN 0340731575, London

Kilbas, Z.; Akin, M.; Gorgulu, S.; Mentes, O.; Ozturk, E.; Kozak, O. & Tufan, T. (2008). Lightning strike: an unusual etiology of gastric perforation, *The American journal of emergency medicine*, Vol. 26, No. 8, (Oct 2008), pp. e5-7, ISSN 1532-8171

Kilic, B.; Meseri, R.; Sonmez, Y.; Kaynak, C.; Demiral, Y. & Ergor, A. (2006). Home accident and the affecting factors, *Syndrome,* Vol. 18, No. 12, pp. 68-74, ISSN 1016-5134 (In Turkish)

Kinney, HC. (2005). Contributions of Larry E. Becker to neuropathologic research in the sıds: a tribute, *Pediatric and developmental pathology*, Vol. 8, pp. 258-267, ISSN 1093-5266

Kinney, HC. & Thacch, BT. (2009). The sudden infant death syndrome. *The New England Journal of Medicine,* Vol. 361, pp. 795-805, ISSN 0028-4793

Kiss, K.; Poto, Z.; Pinter, A. & Sarkozy, S. (2010). Bicyle injuries in children: an analysis based on demographic density, *Accident; analysis and prevention,* Vol. 42, No. 6, pp. 1566-1569, ISSN 0001-4575

Kitulwatte, I. & Pollanen, MS. (2009). Electrical injury of the neck and cardiac air embolism: a novel mechanism of death, *Forensic science, medicine, and pathology*, Vol. 5, No. 1, pp. 32-35, ISSN 1547-769X

Klaver, EC.; Versluijs, GM. & Wilders, R. (2011). Cardiac ion channel mutations in the sudden infant death syndrome, *International journal of cardiology,* (Jan 2011), doi:10.1016/j.ijcard.2010.12.051, 1874-1754

Kleemann, WJ.; Wiechern, V.; Schuck, M. & Tröger, HD. (1995). Intrathoracic and subconjunctival petechiae in sudden infant death syndrome (SIDS), *Forensic Science International,* Vol. 72, No. 1, (Mar 1995), pp. 49-54, ISSN 0379-0738

Klin, B.; Rosenfeld-Yehoshua, N.; Abu-Kishk, I.; Efrati, Y.; Kozer, E.; Jeroukhimov, I.; Eshel, G. & Lotan, G. (2009). Bicycle-related injuries in children: disturbing profile of a growing problem, *Injury,* Vol. 40, No. 9, pp. 1011-1013, ISSN 0020-1383

Knight, B. (1991). Immersion and drowning, In: *Simpson's Forensic Medicine,* Knight, B., pp. 153-159, 10th ed. Edward Arnold, ISBN 0-340-53648-9, London

Knight, B. (1996). a) Burns and scalds, In: *Forensic Pathology,* Knight, B., pp. 305-317, Arnold Publishers, ISBN 0 340 58897 7, London

Knight, B. (1996). b) Electrical fatalities. In: *Forensic Pathology,* Knight, B., pp. 318-331, Arnold Publishers, ISBN 0 340 58897 7, London

Knight, B. (1996). c) Fatal Child Abuse, In: *Forensic Pathology,* Knight, B. pp. 457-473, Arnold Publishers, ISBN 0 340 764 228, London

Knight, B. (1996). d) Immersion death, In: *Forensic Pathology,* Knight, B., pp. 391-406, Arnold Publishers, ISSN 0 340 58897 7, London

Knight, B. (1996). e) Neglect, starvation and hypotermia. In: *Forensic Pathology,* Knight, B., pp. 407-416, Arnold Publishers, ISBN 0 340 58897 7, London

Knight, B. (1996). f) The pathology of wounds. In: *Forensic Pathology,* Knight, B., pp. 133-169, Arnold Publishers, ISBN 0 340 764 228, London

Krous, HF.; Nadeau, JM.; Silva, PD. & Blackbourne, BD. (2003). A comparison of respiratory symptoms and inflammation in sudden infant death syndrome and in accidental or inflicted infant death, *The American journal of forensic medicine and pathology,* Vol. 24, No. 1, (Mar 2003), pp. 1-8, ISSN 0195-7910

Kurtzman, TL.; Otsuka, KN. & Wahl, RA. (2001). Inhalant abuse by adolescents. *Journal of Adolescent Health.* Vol. 28, No. 3, pp. 170-180, ISSN 1054-139X

Laffoy, M. (1997). Childhood accidents at home, *Irish medical journal,* Vol.90, pp. 26-27, ISSN 332-3102

Lallier, M.; Bouchard, S.; St-Vil, D.; Dupont, J. & Tucci, M. (1999). Falls from heights among children: A retrospective review, Journal of Pediatric Surgery, Vol. 34, pp. 1060-1063, ISSN 0022-3468

Laraque, D. (2004). Injury risk of nonpowder gun, *Pediatrics,* Vol. 114, No. 5, pp. 1357-1361, ISSN 0031-4005

Large, MM. & Nielssen, OB. (2010). Suicide in Australia: meta-analysis of rates and methods of suicide between 1988 and 2007, *The Medical journal of Australia,* Vol. 192, No. 8, pp. 432-437, ISSN 0025-729X

Lawn, JE.; Kerber, K.; Enweronu-Laryea, C. & Cousens, S. (2010). 3.6 Million neonatal deaths-what is progreeing and what is not?, *Seminars in perinatology,* Vol. 34, No. 6, pp. 371-386, ISSN 0146-0005

Linn, S.; Smith, D. & Sheps, S. (1998). Epidemiology of bicycle injury, head injury, and helmet use among children İn British Columbia: a five year descriptive study. Canadian Hospitals Injury, Reporting and Prevention Program (CHIRPP), *Injury prevention,* Vol. 4, No. 2, pp. 122-125, ISSN 1353-8047

Lipsett, J.; Cohle, SD.; Berry, PJ.; Russell, G. & Byard, RW. (1994). Anomalous coronary arteries: a multicenter pediatric autopsy study, *Pediatric pathology,* Vol. 14, No. 2, (Mar-Apr 1994), pp. 287-300, ISSN 0277-0938

Mabunda, MM.; Swart, LA. & Sedat, M. (2008). Magnitude and categories of pedestrian fatalities in South Africa, *Accident; analysis and prevention,* Vol. 40, No. 2, pp. 586-593, ISSN 0001-4575

Madge, N. (1999). Youth suicide in an international context, *European child & adolescent psychiatry*, Vol. 8, No. 4, pp. 283-291, ISSN 1018-8827

Maguire, S.; Moynihan, S.; Mann, M.; Potokar, T. & Kemp, AM. (2008). A systematic review of the features that indicate intentional scalds in children. *Burns,* Vol. 34, No. 8, (Dec 2008), pp. 1072-1081, ISSN 0305-4179

Maguire, S. (2010). Which injuries may indicate child abuse?, *Archives of disease in childhood. Education and practice edition*, Vol. 95, No. 6, (Dec 2010), pp. 170-177, ISSN 1743-0585

Mann, NC.; Weller, SC. & Rauchschwalbe, R. (1992). Bucket-related drownings in the United States, 1984 through 1990, *Pediatrics,* Vol. 89, No. (6 Pt 1), (Jun 1992), pp. 1068-1071, ISSN 1098-4275

Marcdante, KJ. (2006). Poisoning, In: *Nelson Essentials of Pediatrics,* Kliegmen RM, Marcdante KJ, Jenson HB. pp. (204-212), Elservier Saunders 2006; 204-212, ISBN 1-4160-0159, Philadelphia

Marchi, AG.; Messi, G. & Loschi, L. (1991). Evaluation of changing patterns in children poisonings and prevention, *Veterinary and human toxicology,* Vol. 33, pp. 244-246, ISSN: 01456296

Mathews, TJ. & MacDorman, MF. (2007). Infant mortality statistics from the 2004 period linked birth/infant death data set, *National vital statistics reports,* Vol. 55, No. 14, pp. 1-32, ISSN 1551-8922

Mathis, RD.; Levine, SH. & Phifer, S. (1993). An analysis of accidental free falls from a height: the 'spring break' syndrome, *The Journal of trauma,* Vol. 34, No. 1, pp. 123-126, ISSN 0022-5282

Mazurek, AJ. (1994). Epidemiology of paediatric injury, *Journal of accident & emergency medicine,* Vol. 11, No. 1, pp. 9-16, ISSN 1351-0622

McIntyre, WF.; Simpson, CS.; Redfearn, DP.; Abdollah, H. & Baranchuk, A. (2010). The lightning heart: a case report and brief review of the cardiovascular complications of lightning injury, *Indian pacing and electrophysiology journal,* Vol. 10, No. 9, (Sep 2010), pp. 429-434, ISSN 0972-6292

Meadow, R. (1999). Unnatural sudden infant death. *Archives of disease in childhood,* Vol. 80, pp. 7-14, ISSN 0003-9888

Meel, B. (2005). Firearm fatalities in the Transkei region of South Africa,1993-2004, *South African medical journal*, Vol. 95, No. 12, pp. 963-967, ISSN 0256-9574

Meel, B. (2007). Trends in firearm-related deaths in the Transkei region of South Africa, *The American journal of forensic medicine and pathology,* Vol. 28, No. 1, pp. 86-90, ISSN 0195-7910

Meller, JL. & Shermeta, DW. (1987). Falls in urban children. A problem revisited, *American journal of diseases of children*, Vol. 141, pp.1271–1275, ISSN 0002-922X

Mert, E. & Bilgin, NG. (2006). Demographical, etiological and clinical characteristics of poisoning in Mersin, Turkey. *Human & experimental toxicology,* Vol. 25, No. 4, pp. 217-213, ISSN 0960-3271

Meyer, S.; Eddleston, M.; Bailey, B.; Desel, H.; Gottschling, S. & Gortner, L. (2007). Unintentional household poisoning in children. *Klinische Pädiatrie,* Vol. 219, No.5, (Sep-Oct 2007), pp. 254-270. ISSN 0300-8630 (Print) - -Milroy, CM. & Parai, JL. (2011). Armanni-Ebstein lesion, ketoacidosis and starvation in a child, *Forensic science, medicine, and pathology,* (Jan 2011), DOI: 10.1007/s12024-010-9213-6, 1556-2891

Mitchell, E.; Krous, HF.; Donald, T. & Byard, RW.; (2000). Changing trends in the diagnosis of sudden infant death. *The Amerian Journal Of Forensic Medicine and Pathology,* Vol.21, No. 4, (Dec 2000), pp. 311-314, ISSN 0195-7910

Moon, R.; Horne, RSC. & Hauk, FR. (2007). Sudden Infant Death Syndrome. *The Lancet,* Vol.370, pp. 1578-1587, ISSN 0099-5355

Mosenthal, AC.; Livingston, DH.; Elcavage, J.; Merritt, S. & Stucker, S. (1995). Falls: epidemiology and strategies for prevention, *The Journal of trauma,* Vol. 38, No. 5, pp. 753-756, ISSN 0022-5282

Murray JA, Chen D, Velmahos GC, Alo, K.; Belzberg, H.; Asensio JA.; Demetriades, D. & Berne, TV. (2000). Pediatric falls: Is height a predictorof injury and outcome?, *The American Surgeon,* Vol. 66, pp. 863–865, ISSN 0003-1348

Nathanson, M. (2000). The physically and emotionally abused child, In: *The Pathology of Trauma,* Mason, JK.; Purdue, BN., pp. 155-175, Edward Arnold, ISBN 0340 691891,London

National Institutes of Health Consensus Developmental Conference on Infantile Apnea and home monitoring, Sep 29 to Oct 1, 1986, *Pediatrics,* Vol. 79, pp. 292-299, ISSN 0031-4005

Neuspiel, DR. & Kuller, LH. (1985). Sudden and unexpected natural death in childhood and adolescence, *JAMA,* Vol. 254, No. 10, pp. 1321-1325, ISSN 0098-7484

Newbury, C.; Hsiao, K.; Dansey, R. & Hamil, J. (2008). Paediatric pedestrian trauma: the danger after school, *Journal of paediatrics and child health,* Vol. 44, No. 9, pp. 488-491, ISSN 1034-4810

Nishiyama, T. & Hanaoka, K. (2000). A Traumatic asphxia in a child, *Canadian journal of anaesthesia,* Vol. 47, No. 11, pp. 1099–1102, ISSN 0832-610X

O'Neill, JA. (2000). Advances in the management of pediatric trauma, *American journal of surgery,* Vol. 180, pp. 365–369. ISSN 0002-9610

O'Neill, PJ.; Lumpkin, MF.; Clapp, B.; Kopelman, TR.; Matthews, MR.; Cox, JC.; Caruso, DM. & Feiz-Erhan, I. (2009). Significant pediatric morbidity and mortality from intracranial ballistic injuries caused by nonpowder gunshot wounds. A case series, Pediatric neurosurgery, Vol. 45, No. 3, pp. 205-209, ISSN 1016-2291

Osmond, MH.; Brennan-Barnes, M. & Shephard, AL. A 4-year review of severe pediatric trauma in eastern Ontario: a descriptive analysis, *The Journal of trauma,* Vol. 52, pp. 8–12, ISSN 0022-5282

Ozdemir, M. & Unlu, A. (2009). Gunshot injuries due to celebratory gun shootings, *Turkish Neurosurgery,* Vol. 19, No. 1, pp. 73-76, ISSN 1019-5149

Ozkara, E.; Canturk, G.; Canturk, N.; Ozata, AB. & Yavuz, MF. (2009). Evaluation of Forensic Perinatal and Neonatal Autopsies in Istanbul, *Indian journal of pediatrics,* Vol. 76, No. 2, pp. 167-170, ISSN 0019-5456

Pakis, I. & Koc, S. (2010) a) Forensic Medicine Approach in sudden unexpected child death, In: *Forensic Medicine in first Step*, Koc, S.; Can, M., pp. (127-139), Istanbul Medical Chamber, ISBN 978-605-5867-33-1, Istanbul (In Turkish)

Pakis, I. & Koc, S. (2010) b) Perinatal and Neonatal Deaths, In: *Forensic Medicine in first Step*, Koc, S.; Can, M. pp. (117-126), Istanbul Medical Chamber, ISBN 978-605-5867-33-1, Istanbul (In Turkish)

Paritsis, N.; Pallis, D.; Deligeorgis, D.; Doxiadis, S.; Phylactou, C. & Vlachonicolis, I. (1994). An epidemiological study of the factors influencing poisoning in children aged 0-5 years. *Paediatric and perinatal epidemiology*, Vol. 8 pp. 79-89, ISSN 0269-5022

Pasupathy, D.; Wood, AM.; Pell, JP.; Fleming, P. & Smith, GCS. (2010). Time of birth and risk of neonatal death term: retrospective cohort study, *British medical journal* , Vol. 341, No.c3498, pp. (1-5), doi: 10.1136/bmj.c3498, 1468-5833

Patel, AL.; Paluszynska, D.; Haris, KA. & Thach, BT. (2003). Occurrence and mechanisms of sudden oxygen desaturation in infants who sleep face down, *Pediatrics*, Vol. 111, pp. 328-332, ISSN 0191-9601

Pearn, J. (1992). Medical aspects of drowning in children, Annals of the Academy of Medicine, Singapore, Vol. 21, No. 3, (May 1992), pp. 433-435, ISSN 0304-4602

Pearn, J. (2009). Drowning and near drowning, In: *Paediatric Forensic Medicine&Pahology*, Busuttil, A.; Keeling, JW., pp. (345-361), Edward Arnold Publishers Ltd, ISBN 0340731575, London

Peden, M.; McGee, K. & Sharma, G. (2002). The Injury Chart Book: a Graphical Overview of the Global Burden of Injuries. Geneva: World Health Organization, pp. 2-6

Peden, M. (2009). World report on child injury prevention calls for evidence-based interventions, *International journal of injury control and safety promotion*, Vol. 16, No. 1, pp. 57-58, ISSN 1745-7300

Pelletier, AR. & Gilchrist, J. (2011). Fatalities in swimming pools with lifeguards: USA, 2000-2008, *Injury Prevention*, (Jan 2011), doi:10.1136/ip.2010.029751, 1475-5785

Phillips, DP.; Brewer, KM. & Wadensweiler, P. (2011). Alcohol as a risk factor for sudden infant death syndrome (SIDS), *Addiction*, Vol. 106, No. 3, (Mar 2011), pp. (526-527), 0965-2140

Polat, O. (2006). Accidents, In: *Clinical Forensic Medicine*, Polat, O. pp. (347-374), Seckin Publishers, ISBN 975 02 0233 3, Ankara (In Turkish)

Pomerantz, WJ.; Dowd, MD. & Buncher, CR. (2001). Relationship between socioeconomic factors and severe childhood ınjuries, *Journal of urban health*, Vol. 78, No. 1, pp. 141-151, ISSN 1099-3460

Portzky, G.; Audenaert, K. & van Heeringen, K. (2005). Suicide among adolescent. A psychological autopsy study of psychiatric, psychosocial and personality-related risk factors, *Social psychiatry and psychiatric epidemiology*, Vol. 40, No. 11, pp. 922-930, ISSN 0933-7954

Potoka, DA.; Schall, LC. & Ford, HR. (2001). Improved functional outcome for severely injured children treated at pediatric trauma centers, *The Journal of trauma*, Vol. 51, pp. 824–834, ISSN 0022-5282

Powell, EC.; Sheehan, KM. & Christoffel, KK. (1996). Firearm violence among youth: public health strategies for prevention, *Annals of emergency medicine*, Vol. 28, No. 2, pp. 204-212, ISSN 0196-0644

Presley, JC.; Barlow, B.; Kendig, T. & Paneth-Pollak, R. (2007). Twenty-year trends in fatal injuries to very young children: the persistence of racial disparities, *Pediatrics*, Vol. 119, No. 4, pp. e875-884, ISSN 1098-4275

Puranik, S.; Long, J. & Coffman, S. (1998). Profile of pediatric bicycle injuries, *Southern medical journal*, Vol. 91, No. 11, pp. 1033-1037, ISSN 0038-4348

Rash, W. (2008). Cardiac injury and death by lightning strike, *Journal of emergency nursing*, Vol. 34, No. 5, (Oct 2008), pp. 470-471, ISSN 0099-1767

Rauchschwalbe, R.; Brenner, RA. & Smith GS. (1997). The role of bathtub seats and rings in infant drowning deaths, *Pediatrics*, Vol. 100, No. 4, pp.(E1), ISSN 1098-4275

Rivara, FP.; Thompson, DC. & Thompson, RS. (1997). Epidemiology of bicycle injuries and risk factors for serious injury, *Injury prevention*. Vol. 3, No. 2, pp. 110-114, ISSN 1353-8047

Roidgers, GC. & Matyunas, NJ. (2002). Poisonings: drugs, chemicals and plants, In: *Nelson Textbook of Pediatrics*, Behram, RE.; Kliegman, RM.; Jenson, HB. pp. (2160-2170), WB Saunders, ISBN 1-4160-0159, Philadelphia

Romaneli, MT.; Fraga, AM.; Morcillo, AM.; Tresoldi, AT. & Baracat, EC. (2010). Factors associated with infant death after apparent life-threatening event (ALTE), *Jornal de pediatria*, Vol. 86, No. 6, (Nov-Dec 2010), pp. 515-519, ISSN 0021-7557

Rosen, CL.; Frost, JD. & Glaze, DG. (1986). Child abuse and recurrent infant apnea, *The Journal of pediatrics*, Vol. 109, pp. 1065-1067, ISSN 0022-3476

Rowley, AH. & Shulman, ST. (2010). Pathogenesis and management of Kawasaki disease, *Expert review of anti-infective therapy*, Vol. 8, No. 2, (Feb 2010), pp. 197-203, ISSN 1478-7210

Saha, A.; Batra, P. & Bansal, A. (2010). Strangulation injury from indigenous rocking cradle, *Journal of emergencies, trauma and shock*, Vol. 3, No. 3, (Jul–Sep 2010), pp. 298, ISSN 0974-2700

Sala, D.; Fernández, E.; Morant, A.; Gasco, J. & Barrios, C. (2000). Epidemiologic aspects of pediatric multiple trauma in a Spanish urban population, Journal of Pediatric Surgery, Vol. 35, pp. 1478-1481, ISSN 0022-3468

Saint-Martin, P.; Prat, S.; Bouyssy, M. & O'Byrne, P. (2009). Plastic bag asphyxia-a case report, *Journal of forensic and legal medicine*, Vol. 16, No. 1, pp. 40-43, ISSN 1752-928X

Scholer, SJ.; Mitchel, EF. & Ray, AW. (1997). Predictors of injury mortality in early childhood, *Pediatrics*, Vol. 100, pp. 342-347, ISSN 0031-4005

Schwebel, DC.; Simpson, J. & Lindsay, S. (2007). Ecology of drowning risk at a public swimming pool, *Journal of safety research*, Vol. 38, No. 3, pp. 367-372, ISSN 0022-4375

Senanayake, N. & Karalliedde, L. (1998). Pattern of Acute Poisoning in Medical Unit in Central Sri Lanka, *Forensic Science International*, Vol. 36, No. (1-2), pp. 101-104, ISSN 0379-0738

Shetty, BS.; Kanchan, T.; Shetty, M.; Naik, R.; Menezes, G.; Sameer, KS. & Hasan, F. (2010). Fatal electrocution by a support metal wire, *Journal of forensic sciences*, Vol. 55, No. 3, (May 2010), pp. 830-831, ISSN 0022-1198

Sillanpää, M. & Shinnr, S. (2010). Long-term mortality in childhood-onset epilepsy. *The New England journal of medicine*, Vol. 363, No. 26, (Dec 2010), pp. 2522-2529, ISSN 0028-4793

Somers, GR.; Chiasson, DA. & Smith, CR. (2006). Pediatric drowning: a 20-year review of autopsied cases: III. Bathtub drownings, *The American journal of forensic medicine and pathology*, Vol 27, No. 2, (Jun 2006), pp. 113-116, ISSN 0195-7910

Sorenson, SB. & Berk, RA. (1999). Young guns: an empirical study of persons who use a firearm in a suicide or a homicide, *Injury prevention*, Vol. 5, No. 4, pp. 280-283, ISSN 1353-8047

Southall, DP.; Plunkett, MC.; Banks, MW.; Falkov, AF. & Samuels, MP. (1997). Covert video recordings of life-threatening child abuse: lessons for child protection, *Pediatrics*, Vol. 100, No. 5, (1997 Nov), pp. 735-760, ISSN 0031-4005

Soyucen, E.; Aktan, Y.; Saral, A.; Akgün, N. & Numanoğlu, AU. (2006). Retrospective analysis of childhood poisoning in Sakarya region. *Journal of Child Health and Diseases*, Vol.49, pp. 301-306. ISSN 0010-0161

Sze, NN. & Wong, SC. (2007). Diagnosis analysis of the logistic model for pedestrian injury severity in traffic crashes, *Accident; analysis and prevention*, Vol. 39, No. 6, pp. 1267-1768, ISSN 0001-4575

Taviloglu, K.; Aydin, A.; Cuhali, BD.; Demiralp, T.; Guloglu, R. & Ertekin, C. (2001). Evaluation of our cases compliance with the criteria of first degree for referral trauma center, *Turkish journal of trauma & emergency surgery*, Vol. 7, No. 3, pp. 146-150, ISSN 1306-696X

Teramo, KA. (2010). Obstetric problems in diabetic pregnancy-The role of fetal hypoxia, *Best practice and research. Clinical endocrinology and metabolism*, Vol. 24, No. 4, pp. 663–671, ISSN 1521-690X

Tertinger, DA.; Grene, BF. & Lutzker, JR. (1984). Home safety: development and validation of one component of an ecobehavioral treatment program for abused and neglected children, *Journal of applied behavior analysis*, Vol. 17, pp. 159-174, ISSN 0021-8855

Thiene, G.; Nava, A.; Corrado, D.; Rossi, L. & Pennelli, N. (1988). Right ventricular cardiomyopathy and sudden death in young people, *The New England journal of medicine*, Vol. 318, No. 3, pp. 129–133, ISSN 0028-4793

Thompson, DC.; Thompson, RS. & Rivara, FP. (1990). Incidence of bicycle-related injuries in a defined population, *American Journal of Public Health*, Vol. 80, pp.1388-1390, ISSN 0090-0036

Tokdemir, M.; Kafadar, H. & Duzer, S. (2009). Evaluation of autopsy cases which aged 0-18 years in Elazig between the years of 2001-2007, *Firat Medical Journal*, Vol. 14, No. 2, pp. 111-114, ISSN 1300-9818 (In Turkish)

Töro, K.; Hubay, M. & Keller, E. (2007). Extramedullary haematopoiesis in liver of sudden infant death cases, *Forensic Science International*, Vol. 170, No. 1, (Jul 2007), pp. 15-19, ISSN 0379-0738

Turk, EE. (2010). Hypothermia, *Forensic science, medicine, and pathology*, Vol. 6, No. 2, (Jun 2010), pp. 106-115, ISSN 1547-769X

Tyebally, A.; Ang, SY. (2010). Kids can't float: epidemiology of paediatric drowning and near-drowning in Singapore, *Singapore medical journal*, Vol. 51, No. 5, (May 2010), pp. 429-433, ISSN 0037-5675

Ucar, B.; Okten, A.; & Mocan, H. (1993). A Retrospective Evaluation of Child Intoxication cases in Blacksee Region, *Journal of Child Health and diseases*, Vol. 36, pp. 363-371, ISSN 0010-0161

Ulfarsson, GF.; Kim, S. & Booth, KM. (2010). Analyzing fault in pedestrian-motor vehicle crashes in North Carolina, *Accident; analysis and prevention*, Vol. 42, No. 6, pp. 1805-1813, ISSN 0001-4575

Uzun, I.; Buyuk, Y.; Erkol, Z.; Agritmis, H. & Kir, Z. (2009). Fatalities Caused by Spherical Bullets Fired from Blank Cartridge Guns in Istanbul, Turkey, *Journal of forensic sciences*, Vol. 54, No. 5, pp. 1127-1130, ISSN 0022-1198

Van Norstrand, DW. & Ackerman, MJ. (2010). Genomic risk factors in sudden infant death syndrome. *Genome medicine*, Vol. 30, No. 11, (Nov 2010), pp. 86, ISSN 1756-994X

Variend, D. (2009). Sudden Natural Death In Infants And Children, In: *Paediatric Forenic Medicine&Pathology*, Busuttil, A.; Keeling, JW., pp. (225-255), Edward Arnold Publishers Ltd, London

Velmahos, GC.; Demetriades, D.; Theodorou, D.; Cornwell, EE., Belzberg, H.; Asensio, J.; Murray, J. & Berne, TV. (1997). Patterns of injury in victims of urban free-falls, *World journal of surgery*, Vol. 21, No. 8, pp. 816-820, ISSN 0364-2313

Vetter, VL. (1985). Sudden death in infants, children, and adolescents, *Cardiovascular clinics*, Vol. 15, No. 3, pp. 301-313, ISSN 0069-0384

Wang, H.; Smith, GA.; Stallonnes, L. & Xiang, H. (2010). Injury-related childhood mortality in migrant households in a southern city of China, *Injury prevention*, Vol. 16, No. 3, (Jun 2010), pp. 161-165, ISSN 1353-8047

Whitcomb, D.; Martinez JA. & Daberkow, D. (2002). Lightning injuries, *Southern medical journal*, Vol. 95, No. 11, (Nov 2002), pp. 1331-1334, ISSN 0038-4348

Willinger, M.; James, LS. & Catz, C. (1991). Defining the sudden infant death syndrome (SIDS): deliberations of an expert panel convened by the National Institute of Child Health and Human Development. *Pediatric Pathology*, Vol.11, pp. 677-684, ISSN 0277-0938

World Bank, World Development Indicators. http://www.google.com/publicdata?ds=wb-wdi&ctype=l&strail=false&nselm=h&met_y=sh_dyn_mort&scale_y=lin&ind_y=false&rdim=country&idim=country:TUR:VIR:AFG:DEU:USA:ASM:ARG&tstart=-315619200000&tunit=Y&tlen=49&hl=tr&dl=tr

Wyatt, JP.; Wyatt, PW.; Squires, TJ. & Busuttil A. (1998). Hanging deaths in children, *The American journal of forensic medicine and pathology*, Vol. 19, No. 4, pp. 343-346, ISSN 0195-7910

Yagmur, Y.; Guloglu, C.; Aldemir, M. & Orak, M. (2004). Falls from flatroofed houses: a surgical experience of 1643 patients, *Injury*, Vol. 35, pp. 425-428, ISSN 0020-1383

Yavuz, MS. & Ozguner, IF. (2003). Evaluation of Preschool Period Toxicity Cases. *Journal of Forensic Medicine*, Vol. 17, No. 2, pp. 22-27, ISSN 1304-5040

Yildirim S. (2008). Socio-demographic Characteristics of Patients Presenting to the Hospital Due to Household Accidents and Evaluation of Miscellaneous Risk Factors Facilitating Accident Exposure. Thesis, 2008. Istanbul.

Yogev, Y.; Melamed, N.; Bardin, R.; Tenenbaum-Gavish, K.; Ben-Shitrit, G. & Ben-Haroush, A. (2010). Pregnancy outcome at extremely advanced maternal age, *American journal of obstetrics and gynecology*, Vol. 203, No. 6, pp. e1-7, ISSN 1097-6868

Yorulmaz, C. & Cakalir, C. (1999). Drowning, In: *Forensic Medicine Vol.1*, Soysal, Z.; Çakalir, C., pp. (459-474), Istanbul University Cerrahpasa Medical Faculty Pres, Presidency No: 4165, Faculty No: 224, İstanbul University Pres and Film Center, ISBN 975-404-540-2, Istanbul, (In Turkish)

8

Child Abuse and the External Cause of Death in Estonia

Marika Väli[1,2], Jana Tuusov[2], Katrin Lang[3] and Kersti Pärna[3]
[1]*Institute of Pathological Anatomy and Forensic Medicine, University of Tartu*
[2]*Estonian Forensic Science Institute*
[3]*Department of Public Health, University of Tartu*
Estonia

1. Introduction

Violence against children cuts across boundaries of geography, race, class, religion and culture. Injury and violence are serious threats to the health and well-being of children worldwide. Children are at high risk from injuries that can lead to death or disability.

A small proportion of violence against children leads to death, but most often the violence does not even leave visible marks. Violence can have severe implications for children's development and in the most severe cases, it can lead to death or injury. However, it can also affect children's health, their ability to learn or even their willingness to go to school at all.

The World Health Organization (WHO) estimates that 40 million children below the age of 15 suffer from abuse and neglect, and require health and social care. In 1998, a UNICEF report quantified the large East-West gap in European child mortality from external causes (injuries and violence). In the past decade, much has changed in central and Eastern Europe, economically, politically and socially. Some positive changes are seen in child injury rates in this region, and hopefully the East-West gap in European child mortality will diminish.

Violence against children is defined as any form of violence, whether physical, mental and sexual, abandonment or negligence, ill-treatment or exploitation that puts their lives in danger or negatively impacts their lives, physical or psychological health dignity, or development.

In this chapter we present recent trends and current situation of child injury mortality in Estonia. We also describe the forensic medical system, examination of the child and the expert report, and give an overview of cases physical and sexual child abuse in Estonia.

In Estonia forensic medical doctors are a medical experts in physical and sexual abuse assisting Law Enforcement, but they are also involved in investigating all child deaths due to external factors.

In all cases including child abuse, an examination by a forensic medical doctor is done only when requested by a police officer, prosecutor or court. In cases where the child is less than 16 years of age, a parent, police officer, teacher, social worker or careworker must be present during the examination. The examination of a child is carried out at the forensic department or at the hospital if the child is admitted for inpatient treatment.

2. The examination of the child and the expert report

In suspected child abuse cases an examination is performed. The aim of the examination is to find out the primary injury, but also to carry out physical examination of the child and record.

During the examination the forensic medical doctor describes the signs and symptoms that could point primarily to the presence of injuries or the complication of injuries. Often the expertise is not timely as the child requires medical attention. In these cases the doctors must document and describe the injuries and sometimes the full examination is performed at the hospital.

As in other countries, the medical doctor may lack knowledge to detect and record injuries, so the forensic examination is needed. From incorrectly completed medical documents the forensic doctor can not decide what kind of injuries the victim has, nor the timeline or the cause of injuries.

The task of the forensic medical doctor is to find the injuries, timing and causes of injuries and answer all questions that may rise during the proceedings. In all cases involving child abuse, an examination by a forensic medical doctor is done only when requested by a police officer, prosecutor or court. In case the child is less than 16 years of age, a parent, police officer, teacher, social worker or careworker must be present during the examination. The examination of a child is carried out at the forensic department or at a hospital if the child is there.

The forensic medical experts report details the existence or the absence of injury to health; the nature of the injury (diagnosis); the way the injury was incurred; assessment to the link between the person's previous state of health and injury to health (if applicable); the injury's threat to life; the duration of the injury; other conclusions related to the assignment. A forensic doctor can use also the opinion of other medical specialists and this will be also mentioned in the examination. In physical abuse cases involving children often a paediatrician is involved in the examination.

In recent years, special rooms have been created for questioning and examining children at the police stations throughout Estonia. Police officers with special training, prosecutors and other specialists use these rooms when dealing with children.

3. Child abuse

Child abuse is a worldwide problem affecting children from birth to 18 years of age. Each year, hundreds of thousands of children suffer abuse or neglect. Many studies have shown a consistent pattern regarding the abuse and neglect inflicted on children of both genders. Approximately 75% of sexual abuse is inflicted upon girls. Girls also are more likely to suffer from emotional abuse and neglect. Boys, on the other hand, are more likely to experience physical trauma (other than sexual abuse). When focusing solely on cause of death, studies indicate fathers are more likely to kill their child via physical abuse, while mothers kill by neglect (for example, starvation).

In most cases, the abuser is someone known to the child – a parent, family member, teacher, or regular careworker. The issue of abused children is an important public health problem since intra-family violence, including child abuse, is a so-called inside-family problem that is usually not discussed in public. The risk of child abuse is higher in families where there are often conflicts between family members, low parental involvement in the family and cold or hostile relationships between children and their parents. Those parents who had been abused during their own childhood were more likely than others to abuse their own children. We found that family sociopathy (alcohol problems) and some family members disability or handicap problems might predict child maltreatment; low family income and poor parental warmth are associated with risk for child neglect. Therefore the number of cases concerning child abuse is relatively low in comparison with other countries.

In Estonia the issue of abused children has been under discussion since 1990. Child abuse in Estonia is probably far more prevalent than generally thought. As elsewhere, national statistics are not available, as the nature of the problem makes it hidden in the society and difficult to detect and record. The pupils from different types of schools who have participated in such studies confess that they have encountered emotional, physical, and sexual abuse as well as negligence. The most common types of abuse according to these inquiries were verbal sexual abuse, negligence of education, emotional abuse, mental sexual abuse, and negligence of health. Physical abuse, physical sexual abuse and physical negligence were less common. Most abused children suffer greater emotional than physical damage. An abused child may become depressed. He or she may withdraw, think of suicide or become violent. An older child may use drugs or alcohol, try to run away or abuse others. However, when comparing the findings of studies performed in pupils from ordinary Estonian schools with those for children with special needs, the incidence of negligence and sexual abuse are far more common in the latter ones. It can be also said that the problem of abused children has gained more attention in the recent years. For example, this is reflected in the discussions about whether to hit children is acceptable or not. The attitude towards hitting a child has changed in recent years. Still, these discussions have not reached the point as to where to draw the line between an accident and child abuse. This to a large extent is a matter of definition. When a two-year-old child drowns in the pond - is it an accident or negligence? In Estonia such cases are usually considered accidents.

3.1 Physical abuse

Physical abuse is physical aggression directed at a child by an adult, but this is very often neglected and without adequate attention. The reason for this is that the specialists of different fields do not cooperate. It is of paramount importance that the specialists of different fields think in the same way in the event of child abuse, and also understand the ways of acquiring injuries in the same way.

The physical signs of child abuse is sometimes called battered child syndrome. Physical abuse tends to occur at moments of great stress. Physical child abuse or non-accidental child trauma refers to fractures and other signs of injury that occur when a child is hit in anger.

According to the data by the Estonian Forensic Institute about 50 children less than 14 years of age annually need physical examination. Most of the cases are related to violence at school or at home, but children are also injured in traffic accidents. During recent years the number of detailed examinations of physically abused children has decreased by 50%. The number of children injured in traffic accidents has also decreased (with only a handful of cases each year). From 2001 to 2009 most of the children examined were between 7 and 14 years old, boys incurred injuries three times more often than girls, and only 10 children under one year old did so.

According to the literature data, the injuries acquired in association with child abuse comprise 7–27% of the total number of injuries to children (Overpeck et al., 1999), and children are most frequently assaulted at the age of less than five years (Laursen & Nielsen,

2008). Among the prevailing injuries are bruises, abrasions and other mild injuries; head, face and extremities are the most frequently affected regions.
Who causes the injuries? Fathers, mothers, adoptive parents, other members of the family. Why are children abused? Often the reason is discord in the family, single mothers, underaged pregnancies, low educational level of the parents and poor living conditions (Lang et al., 2010). Many people who commit physical abuse were abused themselves as children. As a result, they often do not realize that abuse is not appropriate discipline. Often people who commit physical abuse also have poor impulse control. This prevents them from thinking about what happens as a result of their actions.
The causes of hospitalisation have been studied in the case of traumas to children in Estonia, and it appears that the main cause of hospitalisation for children of this age are contusions, bone fractures and wounds associated with a fall. Apart from the falls the others cases of suspected abuse include burns, the occurrence of different objects in throat, and unclear cases.
According to the questionnaire study carried out in Estonian schools during 2001–2009, 45% of children suffer from school violence but most of them do not inform their parents or the police about it. One fifth (20%) of children get hurt at school, one fourth (25%) of children are injured by their schoolmates and 1/10 (10%) of children suffer from domestic violence. One of the causes of physical abuse in small children is definitely the shaking of babies, i.e. Shaken Baby Syndrome (SBS). In Estonia Shaken Baby Syndrome was first diagnosed in 1999.
Shaken Baby Syndrome is most common in children below one year of age, and it is known to occur as a result of child abuse - it is caused by vigorous shaking and/or swinging of the infant. In most cases, an angry parent or caregiver shakes the baby to punish or quiet the child. Such shaking usually takes place when the infant is crying inconsolably and the frustrated caregiver loses control. Many times the caregiver did not intend to harm the baby. When an infant or toddler is shaken, the brain bounces back and forth against the skull. This can cause bruising of the brain (cerebral contusion), swelling, pressure, and bleeding in the brain. The large veins along the outside of the brain may tear, leading to further bleeding, swelling, and increased pressure. This can easily cause permanent brain damage or death.
Excessive shaking causes the rupture of cortical and bridging veins in the brain, possibly resulting in subdural haematoma, or less frequently subarachnoid haematoma and brain oedema. Subdural haematoma is the most common intracranial pathology observed in cases of SBS, and it is seen in approximately 80% of children with this syndrome. In the United States 750–3750 cases of SBS are diagnosed each year, whereas in Estonia only 2–3 cases per year. The incidence rate of SBS is 40.5 cases per 100 000 children below one year of age in Estonia. The study performed by Talvik and co-authors revealed that the majority of the families of these children had economical difficulties (75% of the families received only social benefits, but no salary at the time of injury) (Talvik et al., 2002). These facts suggest that a poor socio-economic situation is one important factor contributing to violence against children. This is confirmed by the data from other research that the people who abuse children have frequently low educational status and more frequently drug and alcohol abusers.
A unique form of physical child abuse is Munchausen syndrome by proxy. In this situation, a parent will purposely either invent symptoms and falsify records (for example, fever) resulting in unnecessary tests, hospitalizations, and even surgical procedures. This psychiatric illness of the parent(s) requires a high index of suspicion, and its consideration is

part of the investigation of any child with recurrent complaints that are not supported by physical or laboratory findings.

3.2 Sexual abuse

Sexual abuse of children is forcing or persuading a child to participate in sexual acts without the child's understanding of the situation. It does not necessarily mean sexual intercourse or physical contact. It also includes incest, paedophilia, exhibitionism and molestation, but also sexual intercourse - urogenital, anogenital or vaginal intercourse with a child. It is difficult to determine how often child sexual abuse occurs, because it is more secret than physical abuse. Children are often scared to tell anyone about the abuse. Many cases of abuse are not reported.

Children become the victims of sexual violence usually at home and from people, who they actually know, most often stepfathers and fathers. Child sexual abuse occurs in all social and economic classes of people. It has the same type of risk factors as physical child abuse, including: alcohol and drug abuse and family troubles. Abusers often have a history of physical or sexual abuse themselves (Johnson, 2007).

In sexual abuse cases, the most important factor is a timely and correct gynaecological examination, but also a correctly taken analysis (sperm). The importance of interviewing the child cannot be underestimated, what they say should be recorded in their own words. When it is possible, the nature of sexual contact should be ascertained. All other parts of the examination are the same as in the case of physical abuse including a complete general examination, recording growth and sexual maturity.

The colposcopic investigation of the anogenital region in girls and anal region of boys is very important, as injuries to the mucosa are not easy to see and with the attached camera, it provides documentation of the examination's findings. The possibility to use a colposcope is available in all four forensic departments in Estonia. Both specialists (gynaecologist, forensic doctor) attend the examination if this is possible, but this is not mandatory. In Estonia forensic doctors are capable of carrying out gynaecological examinations without the presence of a gynaecologist.

If the child is less than 16 years the consent of the parent of carer is needed. If the parents want to have the examination but the child is against this, then the child's wish is taken into account. The child has the right to refuse or accept the parent's presence during the examination.

It is advised that the physical and gynaecological examination is performed by a forensic doctor, but if it is not possible, the doctor on duty has to do it following the same principals.

In cases of sexual abuse, cooperation between the police, social worker, paediatrician and the forensic doctor is very important.

Similarly to the data reported in published papers, the victims of sexual abuse in Estonia are usually younger than 12 years of age, most frequently between three and seven years of age, and two to three times more likely to be handicapped children (Kvam, 2000). During the past two years (2008-2009) Estonian forensic medical doctors performed in total 27 examinations on sexually abused children aged 0-14 years, and the majority of them were girls (girls vs. boys ratio 22 : 5). In Estonia the cases of vaginal and anogenital intercourse are the most frequent, and the cases of incest are also not uncommon. In the cases of sexual abuse it is often hard to evaluate the examination's findings, because injuries usually heal within a short time period and abnormal findings of the anogenital region may be caused by other factors (blunt force trauma, infection). The problem concerning Estonian forensic doctors is the small number of reported cases giving them very little experience of the problem.

4. External causes of death

In every single industrialized country, injury has now become the leading killer of children.Taken together, traffic accidents, intentional injuries, drownings, falls, fires, poisonings and other accidents kill more than 20 000 of 1–14-year-old children every year in the OECD countries.

Deaths from injury in Estonia form about one third of all deaths to children aged up to 14, this is considerably more than in neighbouring countries. The most pronounced difference between Estonia and other countries in child deaths resulting from injuries are in infant deaths. External causes of death form about one third of all deaths in children 0–14 years old in Estonia. The reduction in childhood mortality shows some progress has been achieved over the recent years.

Year	Injury deaths (V01–Y89)		All deaths,	Total mortality rate per
	N	%	N	1000
2001	56	28.6	196	0.82
2002	40	28.4	141	0.61
2003	44	27.5	160	0.71
2004	31	23.1	134	0.62
2005	40	30.1	133	0.64
2006	31	27.7	112	0.55
2007	29	23.2	125	0.63
2008	27	22.3	121	0.61
2009	17	12.5	87	0.43

Table 1. Total mortality rate per 1000 for all deaths (including injury related deaths) among children, 2001–2009 (Statistics Estonia, 2011)

The annual total mortality rate in Estonia was 0.62 in 2001–2009. During the last few years a decrease has been observed both in the general mortality and injury-related mortality of children (Table 1; Figure 1). In 2007–2009 injury mortality rate decreased from 14.9 to 4.9 per 100 000 among 10–14-year-old children children in Estonia (Figure 1).

From the beginning of 2006 infant mortality has decreased, but less significant progress has been observed for childhood and adolescent deaths. During 2001–2009, 391 children aged 0–14 were autopsied by forensic doctors at the Forensic Science Institute and 310 (79.2%) of causes of death were attributed to the external causes.

The primary external causes of child death in Estonia are various kinds of mechanical suffocation (strangulation, aspiration of foreign bodies or gastric content, drowning, compression). In Estonia asphyxia formed 40.3% of unintentional deaths, followed by mechanical injuries (transport and falls) and poisonings. Drowning and aspiration were the most frequent cause of asphyxia. Strangulation was registered as the cause of death in six cases, with an additional 18 other cases in which the intent was impossible to identify. This group included for example obstruction of the airways with a foreign body, being struck by a blunt object and others.

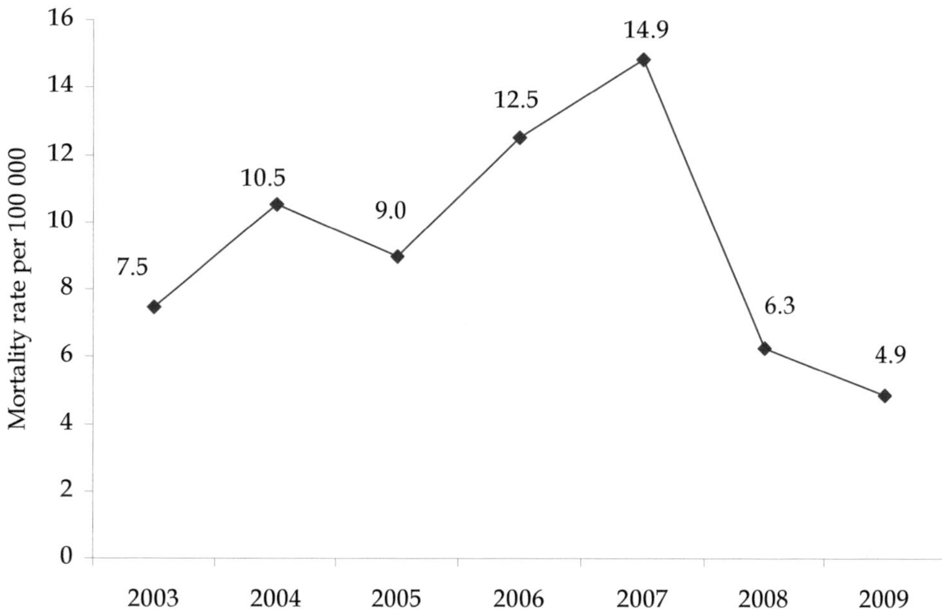

Fig. 1. Injury mortality rates per 100 000 among 10–14-year-old children, 2003–2009 (Statistics Estonia, 2011)

The major problem in Estonia is a high mortality rate from unintentional injuries (accidents) that formed 64.2% of all deaths of children aged 10–14 in 2001–2009 (Table 2).

Intent of death	**Number**	**Column %**
Disease	81	20.7
External causes (injuries)	310	79.3
Unintentional injuries	251	64.2
Asphyxia	125	32.0
Drowning	56	14.3
Aspiration	45	11.5
Strangulation	6	1.5
Other	18	4.6
Transport accidents	80	20.5
Poisoning	24	6.1
Intentional injuries	29	7.4
Homicides, suicides	16	4.1
Intent unknown	29	7.4
Total	**391**	**100.0**

Table 2. Deaths from diseases and injuries among 10–14-year-old children, 2001–2009 (Statistics Estonia, 2011)

Traffic accidents are the leading health threat to children in many countries (Törõ et al., 2011; Durkin et al., 1999). Although the number of traffic accidents has decreased considerably in Estonia in recent years, including also the number of accidents involving children, transport accidents still prevail among mechanical injuries, constituting 25.8% of external causes of death. Most of the victims were from the oldest age group (between 15 and 19 years of age), and 78% were passengers in motor vehicles, 19% pedestrians (most of the cases represent accidents in the home environment where the car reversed over a child) and only one child died as the result of a bike accident. Similar results were also reported in an article comparing the injuries to children who died from traffic accidents in three capital cities (Budapest, Vilnius, and Tallinn) (Törõ et al., 2011).

Poisonings constitute about 7.7 % of all cases of unintentional deaths, and they are mainly caused by carbon monoxide (CO) and medicinal products. Poisonings with medicinal products are usually observed in children one to four years of age who happen to get access to the drugs at home. These include three cases of poisoning with aethazine tablets, and poisoning with dimedrole and amitriptyline. In addition opiate poisoning occurred in a 14-year-old boy and one case of poisoning with unknown gas (presumably butane) was also registered. The rest of the cases represent poisoning with CO in association with fires (seven boys and ten girls).

When looking at the causes of unintentional death by age group, it can be concluded that the decrease in children's mortality has mainly occurred on account of the age group of children below one year of age (Figure 2). In 2005–2009 unintentional infant mortality rate decreased steadily from 85.1 to 31.6 per 100 000. Mortality rates in other age groups have not changed significantly. Analysing the cause of death and manners of death, the main causes of death in children below one year of age include head traumas and suffocation, although the manner of death remains unclear in many cases.

Unclear causes are also apparent in children aged one to four years, but the prevailing causes of death are accidents. The reason for this is a limited availability of accompanying data and therefore forensic doctors have not enough medical data to decide about the form of violence used.

Accidents prevail also in the age groups five to nine years and 10–14 years, the latter group also includes the occasional case of suicide. Similar to other countries a big problem in the case of deaths among children below one year of age is the high rate of deaths from an unknown cause.

Thus, 29 cases of death with an unknown cause were registered between 2001–2009, including nine cases of putrefaction, eight cases of suffocation, one case of poisoning, one fatality in a fire, and 10 cases of mechanical injury, including three unclear cases where the child died during birth.

The task of a forensic doctor is to try to find out whether the injuries detected at the autopsy represent intentional injuries, or whether the child could develop these as the result of an accident. Similar to other countries such accidents happen mostly at home. According to Sengoelge (Sengoelge et al., 2010) home injuries were the leading cause of injury death in children under five years of age in 16 European countries.

Brain traumas are prevailing among the cases of deaths of unknown manner (in nine cases out of ten and one case represented a combined head and chest trauma). In 2001–2009 brain traumas constituted 17.1% (63 cases) of all causes of death in children, first of all in children between one and five years of age.

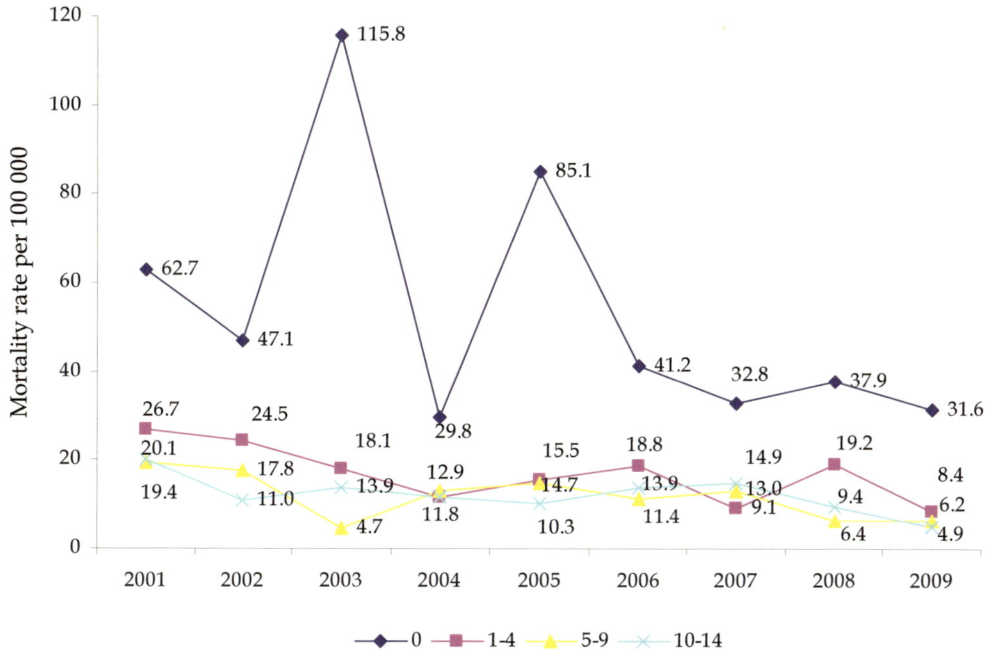

Fig. 2. Unintentional mortality rates per 100 000 by age group, 2001–2009 (Statistics Estonia, 2011)

Forensic doctors are usually able to find out the cause of death in the case of a head trauma, but this is not enough to establish the exact mechanism of injury. For example: A two-and-a-half month old infant was found in a pram, the forensic doctor has found an epidural and subdural haematoma. Question: could the child have fallen by itself?

Second example: a five-month-old infant: linear fractures of both temporal bones, comminuted fracture of the right occipital bone, epidural, subdural and subarachnoid haematoma. Question: mechanism of injury (beating)?

Third example: two-month-old infant: subarachnoidal haematoma in the right frontal lobe, cerebral contusion, major haematoma of the aponeurosis and haematomas of the face.

Question: mechanism of injury (caused by forceful blows with a wide-surfaced object, e.g. hands)?

Injuries from traffic accidents and those caused by blunt objects are commonly the cause of a brain trauma. A forensic doctor finds as the cause of death either asphyxia or head trauma, but this is not enough to establish the exact cause of the injury and determine the manner of death, because of insufficient preliminary data.

The number of youth suicides has decreased in recent years but Estonia still is among the countries with the highest risk of suicide in the world. Suicides were registered in 16 cases in the study years, and the majority of cases were boys (12 cases). Most of the children committing suicide were aged between 10–14 years, but some children were younger (Figure 3). In 2001–2009 the highest suicide mortality rate was 7.5 per 100 000 among 10–14-year-old girls in the first study year.

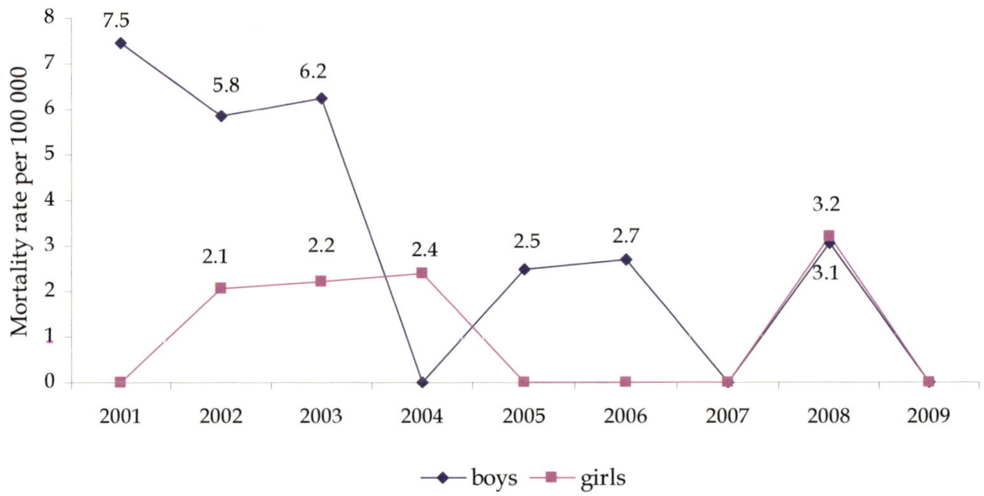

Fig. 3. Suicide mortality rates per 100 000 among 10–14-year-old boys and girls, 2001–2009 (Statistics Estonia, 2011)

The most common way of committing suicide was hanging, in addition to this one shooting injury and one case of jumping from height were registered. 13 cases of homicide were registered in the study years, and most of these were children below one year of age (eight cases). In 2001–2009, the highest homicide infant mortality rate was 15.4 per 100 000 in 2003 (Figure 4).

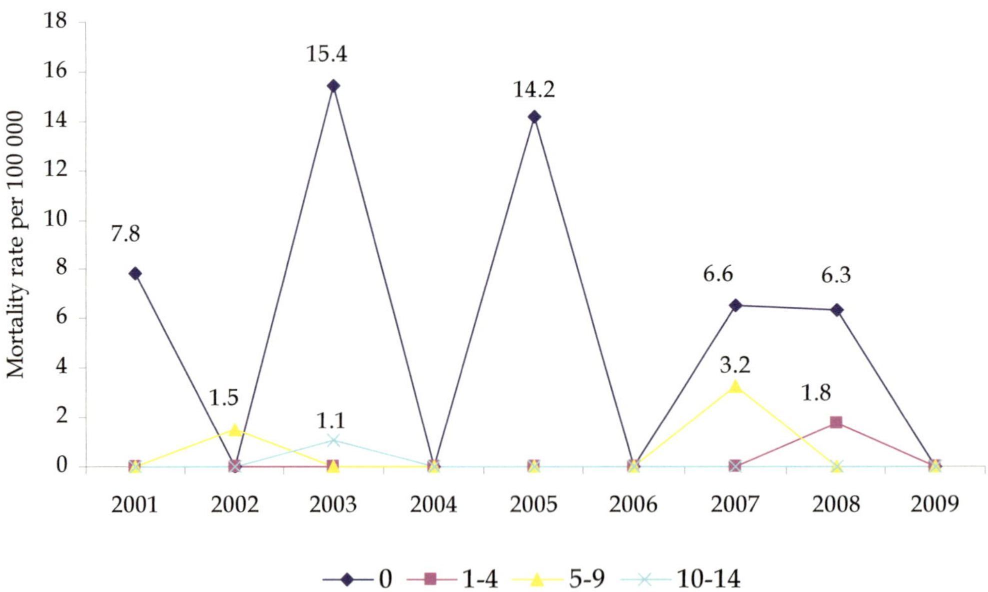

Fig. 4. Homicide mortality rates per 100 000 by age group, 2001–2009 (Statistics Estonia, 2011)

Head injury and choking were the main ways of carrying out the homicide. Two cases include knife injuries, where also the other members of the family were killed (father and one other relative in one case). One shooting injury occurred also in the study years.

5. Conclusion

Reduction of death through injury should be included in the current public health agenda and given a high priority in many countries, including Estonia. It is important to identify the potentially preventable cases and detect risk factors (single parents, young mothers, low educational level, bad living conditions etc), as well as to analyze the incidence and circumstances of different types of violence.

Deaths related to child abuse are preventable and it is therefore important to estimate the amount of such deaths, but also to study the circumstances leading to these deaths. Deaths related to child abuse occurred more often in families that had problems with alcohol abuse, unemployment etc. and/or mothers who had a low level of education.

More information is needed on the circumstances of the violent deaths among children. This would enable not only to correctly classify the manner of death in suspicious cases, but also to eventually reduce the numbers of violent deaths among children.

For adequate assessment of the level of child abuse, it is important to know, who and how evaluates the injuries inflicted on a child, as well as who are the members of the investigation team. Close cooperation between various specialists is essential for the correct diagnosis.

Rates of child mortality from injuries have fallen across Europe. In the former Soviet countries, this is likely to reflect improvements in living conditions since the transition. Child deaths from injuries are avoidable and measures to reduce them would have a significant impact upon the overall burden of child mortality in Europe.

It is important to identify the potentially preventable cases and detect risk factors (single parents, young mothers, low educational level, bad living conditions etc), as well as to analyze the incidence and circumstances of different types of violence. According to published figures more than 50% of cases can be prevented.

6. Acknowledgment

The study was supported by the Estonian Science Foundation (grants no 6592 and 8256).

7. References

Durkin, M.S., Laraque, D., Lubman, I. & Barlow, B. (1999). Epidemiology and the prevention of traffic injuries to urban children and adolescents. *Pediatrics,* Vol.103, No.6, pp. 1273–1274, ISSN 0031-4005

Johnson CF. Abuse and neglect of children. In: Kliegman RM, Behrman RE, Jenson HB, Stanton BF. (2007). *Nelson Textbook of Pediatrics*. 18th ed. Philadelphia, Pa: Saunders Elsevier, chap 36

Kvam, M.H. (2000). Is sexual abuse of children with disabilities disclosed? A retrospective analysis of child disability and the likelihood of sexual abuse among those attending Norwegian hospitals. *Child Abuse Negl,* Vol. 24, No. 8, pp. 1073–1084, ISSN 0145-2134

Lang, K., Pärna, K., Grjibovski, A.M. & Väli, M. (2010). Deaths of infants subject to a forensic autopsy in Estonia from 2001 to 2005: what can we learn from additional information? *Popul Health Metr,* Vol. 8, pp. 27, ISSN 1478-7954

Laursen, B. & Nielsen, J.W. (2008). Influence of sociodemographic factors on the risk of unintentional childhood home injuries. *Eur J Public Health,* Vol. 18, No. 4, pp. 366-370, SSN 1464-360X

Overpeck, M.D., Brenner, R.A., Trumble, A.C., Smith, G.S., MacDorman, M.F. & Berendes, H.W. (1999). Infant injury deaths with unknown intent: what else do we know? *Inj Prev,* Vol. 5, No. 4, pp. 272–275, ISSN 1475-5875

Sengoelge, M., Hasselberg, M. & Laflamme, L. (2011). Child home injury mortality in Europe: a 16-country analysis. *Eur J Public Health,* Vol. 21, No. 2, pp. 166–170, ISSN 1464-360X

Smith, S.L. & Andrus, P.K. (1998). Infant rat model of the shaken baby syndrome: preliminary characterisation and evidence for the role of free radicals in cortical hemorrhaging and progressive neuronal degeneration. *J Neurotrauma,* Vol. 15, No. 9, pp. 693–705, ISSN 0897-7151

Statistics Estonia. (2011). *Statistical database.* Available from http://www.stat.ee/ (16. March 2011, date last accessed).

Talvik, I., Vibo, R., Metsvaht, T., Männamaa, M., Jüri, P., Heidmets, L.-T., Hämarik, M. & Talvik, T. (2002). Raputatud lapse sündroom. *Eesti Arst,* Vol. 81, No. 1, pp. 23–29, ISSN 0235–8026

Törõ, K., Szilvia, F., György, D., Pauliukevicius, A., Caplinskiene, M., Raudys, R., Lepik, D., Tuusov, J. & Väli, M. (2011). Fatal Traffic Injuries Among Children and Adolescents in Three Cities (Capital Budapest, Vilnius, and Tallinn). *J Forensic Sci,* [Epub ahead of print], ISSN 1556-4029

Väli, M., Lang, K., Soonets, R., Talumäe, M. & Grjibovski, A.M. (2007). Childhood deaths from external causes in Estonia, 2001–2005. *BMC Public Health,* Vol. 7, pp. 158, ISSN 1478-7954

9

Sexual Assault in Childhood and Adolescence

Hakan Kar
Mersin University, Faculty of Medicine, Department of Forensic Medicine
Turkey

1. Introduction

1.1 Definition of sexual assault

Although definition of violence may vary in different societies and cultures, it can be defined as all behavior that affects bio-psycho-social status of individuals.

In the United Kingdom the Sexual Offences Act 2003 defines "sexual assault" as when a person (A)

1. intentionally touches another person (B),
2. the touching is sexual,
3. B does not consent to the touching, and
4. A does not reasonably believe that B consents (Official text of the Sexual Offences Act, 2003).

In the United States the definition of sexual assault varies widely between the individual states. The Rape, Abuse & Incest National Network defines "sexual assault" as unwanted sexual contact that stops short of rape or attempted rape. This includes sexual touching and fondling. (Rape, Abuse, and Incest National Network [RAINN], 2005) According to the U.S. Department of Health & Human Services, "sexual assault can be verbal, visual, or anything that forces a person to join in unwanted sexual contact or attention." Sexual assault is therefore somewhat of an umbrella term, and can describe many things, including:

- rape, including partner and marital rape
- unwanted sexual contact (touching or grabbing)
- unwelcome exposure of another's body, exhibitionism, or voyeurism
- child sexual abuse
- incest or molestation
- sexual harassment
- sexual exploitation of clients by therapists, doctors, dentists, or other professionals (U.S. Department of Health & Human Services,2011).

Sexual violence is described as sexually motivated behavior that exerted against one's privacy despite one's resistance. Furthermore, all sexually motivated behavior directed to low aged or mentally retarded individuals included in scope of the term of sexual violence (Christian et al., 2000; Chu&Tung, 2005; Herbert et al., 1992).

1.2 Incidance and prevelance sexual assault

Sexual assault is significantly underreported worldwide. Most of the rape victims do not disclose the assault because of being accused or exposed to repeated assaults.

Underreporting of sexual assault "might arise from the fear of being re-victimized in the criminal justice system, of not being believed, from self-blame and from failure by rape victims to equate their experience with the legal definition of rape."

Women may fear that they would be blamed for the assault, or believe that reporting would place them or their families in danger of retaliatory violence. A recent publication by the Open Society Institute's Network Women's Program states: “Rape goes largely unreported across the region. The act of rape is surrounded by pejorative stereotypes: women ask for it, they provoke it by their dress or behavior, or they cry rape to take revenge on a man; normal men do not commit rape, and so on. In addition, reporting procedures, at the police station and again in the courts, are complicated and degrading. In most cases, if a woman reports being raped, she is regarded with suspicion and rarely believed; she lacks any form of police or court protection, leaving her vulnerable to retaliation—either from the offender or, in some cases, from members of her family who feel she has brought them dishonor.”

Approximately 700.000 women in the reproductive age group are victims of sexual assault in the United States and, 25,000 women are raped per year in France. Unfortunately only 16% of rapes are reported to police, however 50% of victims of rape have expressed that, they would report the rape after a warranty of secrecy about their identity (Bechtel&Podrazik, 1999; Santiago et al., 1985). Most of the rape victims do not disclose the assault because of being accused or exposed to repeated assaults (Ledoux&Hazelwood, 1995, Crowley, 1999).

Despite this underreporting, available statistics indicate that sexual assault is a pervasive problem in all societies. Charlotte Bunch, in an article included in UNICEF's 1997 publication, The Progress of Nations, has stated that "statistics on rape from industrialized and developing countries show strikingly similar patters: Between one in five and one in seven women will be victims of rape in their lifetime."

Special Rapporteur on Violence Against Women, Radika Coomaraswamy, in her 1997 report on violence against women, detailed the following statistics:

- A Canadian study reports that 23.3% of women had been victims of rape or attempted rape.
- 22% of adult women in Seoul had been the victims of rape or attempted rape.
- In Jakarta, Indonesia, city police recorded 2,300 cases of sexual violence against women in 1992, 3,200 cases in 1993, and 3,000 in the first half of 1994.
- Out of 331,815 reported crimes against women in 1993 in the Russian Federation, 14,000 were rapes.
- A survey in the United Kingdom found that 19.4% of women had been victims of sexual violence.
- Adolescents constitute 20-50% of all rape victims in the United States.
- In a study conducted at a university in the United States, one of six female students reported having been the victim of rape or attempted rape in the past year. One out of fifteen men reported having committed rape or attempted to commit rape (Coomaraswamy, R. 1997).

According to estimates from the World Health Organization:

- In some countries, almost one in four women may experience sexual violence by an intimate partner, and that almost one-third of young girls report that their first sexual encounter was forced.

- The percentage of women who reporting having been sexual assaulted in the past five years in Tirana, Albania in 1996 was 6%.
- The percentage of women who reporting having been sexual assaulted in the past five years in Budapest, Hungary in 1996 was 2%.
- The percentage of women who reporting having been sexual assaulted in the past five years in Điauliai, Kaunas, Klaipeda, Panevežys, and Vilnius in Lithuania in 1997 was 4.8%.
- The percentage of women who reporting having been sexual assaulted in the past five years in Ulaanbaatar and Zuunmod, Mongolia in 1996 was 3.1%.
- In a survey of women in the Czech Republic, 11.6% of women reported experiencing forced sexual contact in their lifetime, and 3.4% reported that they had experienced this on more than one occasion. (World Health Organization [WHO], 2002)

2. Child Sexual Assault

2.1 Definition and classification

Child sexual abuse is a form of child abuse in which an adult or older adolescent uses a child for sexual stimulation. It is generally defined as contacts between a child and an adult or other person significantly older or in a position of power or control over the child, where the child is being used for sexual stimulation of the adult or other person. The World Health Organization has defined child sexual abuse and exploitation as the involvement of a child in sexual activity that he or she does not fully comprehend, is unable to give informed consent to, or for which the child is not developmentally prepared and cannot give consent, or that violates the laws or social taboos of society.

The United Nations Convention on the Rights of the Child (CRC) is an international treaty that legally obliges states to protect children's rights. Articles 34 and 35 of the CRC require states to protect children from all forms of sexual exploitation and sexual abuse. This includes outlawing the coercion of a child to perform sexual activity, the prostitution of children, and the exploitation of children in creating pornography. States are also required to prevent the abduction, sale, or trafficking of children (United Nations, 1989).

Forms of child sexual abuse include asking or pressuring a child to engage in sexual activities (regardless of the outcome), indecent exposure of the genitals to a child, displaying pornography to a child, actual sexual contact against a child, physical contact with the child's genitals (except in certain non-sexual contexts such as a medical exam), viewing of the child's genitalia without physical contact (except in nonsexual contexts such as a medical exam), or using a child to produce child pornography.

Child sexual abuse can be classified as:

- **Sexual assault** - a term defining offenses in which an adult touches a minor for the purpose of sexual gratification; for example, rape (including sodomy), and sexual penetration with an object. Most U.S. states include, in their definitions of sexual assault, any penetrative contact of a minor's body, however slight, if the contact is performed for the purpose of sexual gratification.
- **Sexual exploitation** - a term defining offenses in which an adult victimizes a minor for advancement, sexual gratification, or profit; for example, prostituting a child, and creating or trafficking in child pornography.

- **Sexual grooming** - defines the social conduct of a potential child sex offender who seeks to make a minor more accepting of their advances, for example in an online chat room. (APA Board of Professional Affairs , 1999; Child Welfare Information Gateway, 2009; Finkelhor & Ormrod, 2001; WHO, 1999)

2.2 Incidance and prevelance

Sexual assault is a sociological problem affecting individuals in all age groups. According to the Convention on the Rights of the Child, a child means every human being below the age of eighteen years unless under the law applicable to the child, majority is attained earlier (Office of the United Nations High Commissioner for Human Rights,1989).

Different studies reports different percentages of child and adolescent sexual assault. For example it's reported that % 43 of 766 cases of sexual assault were under 18 age in a study of Michigan State University (Jones et al., 2003). It's mentioned that 178 of 405 victims were adolescent in another research. Teenagers 16-19 are reported to be victims of rape or sexual assault more than twice as likely as any other age group in USA. Children and especially adolescent females are sexually assaulted more frequent comparatively to adults according to many studies (Navratil, 2003; Jones et al., 2003; Peipert&Domagalski, 1994). In author series most of the sexual assault victims (%87.65) were less than 18 years of age.

Estimates of child sexual abuse rates vary for many reasons. Less than 10 percent of set abuse is reported to the policed (Finkelhor et al,1988). Even in self-reporting surveys, abuse may be underreported because many people are afraid or ashamed to reveal victimization, have repressed memories of abuse, refuse to participate in studies or deny that what happened was "real" abuse.

Definitions of both abuse and the age of maturity affect frequency rates. Some researchers have estimated that over 50% of the female child population will experience some form of sexual abuse before the age of 18 (Russell, 1984; Wyatt, 1985), while others have reported rates of 11% and lower (Fritz et al., 1981; Kercher & McShane, 1984). Similarly, while a meta-analytic study by Rind and Tromovitch, (1998) reported mean prevalence rates of 17% and 28% for males and females respectively, the range for males was 3% to 37%, and for females 8% to 71%. The results of the systematic review of 11 studies on the prevalence of child sexual assault in Switzerland shows that the percentage of participants that ever experienced any form of child sexual assault, prevalence rates assessed by a single general item are considerably lower (up to 18.1% for girls and 3.0% for boys) than when rates were calculated on the basis of several items assessing specific forms of child sexual assault (up to 39.8% for girls and 10.9% for boys) (Schönbucher et al., 2011). Such wide variation in the prevalence rate is due to differences in the definition of child sexual abuse, the type of sample used, design, and measurement techniques.

Sarafino (1979) estimated the national incidence of reported and unreported child sexual abuse to be over 336,000 cases per year. Sarafino arrived at this figure by calculating the rates of reported sexual offences per 100,000 children in each of the four locales, and then applying this rate to the national total of 61 million children. This led to an estimated 74,725 cases of child sexual abuse in a one-year period. The rate of unreported cases was calculated by multiplying 74,725 by 3.5 (assuming that the number of unreported cases is at least 3 or 4 times higher than the reported cases as believed by several experts in the field). The number of reported cases was added to the estimated number of unreported cases. Consequently, it was estimated that approximately 336,200 sexual offences are committed against children every year in the United States.

In this respect, the prevalence of sexual assaults, especially among children and adolescent, is thought to be extremely higher than in literature.

2.3 Characteristic features of child sexual assault

Few people are aware of the true state of the science on child abuse. Instead, most people's beliefs have been shaped by common misconceptions and popular myths about this hidden crime. Societal acceptance of these myths assists sex offenders by silencing victims and encouraging public denial about the true nature of sexual assaults against children. Common Myths about Child Sexual Abuse:

- Child sexual abuse is a rare experience.
- Children make up stories or lie about sexual abuse.
- A child is most likely to be sexually abused by a stranger
- Child sexual abuse is always perpetrated by adults.
- Normal-appearing, well educated, middle-class people don't molest children
- Children who are being abused would immediately tell their parents.
- Boys can't be sexually abused.
- Sexual abuse of a child is usually an isolated, one-time incident.
- Child molesters are all, 'Dirty old men.

Boys abused by males are or will become homosexual

- Boys are less traumatized as victims of sexual abuse than girls
- Children will naturally outgrow the effects of sexual abuse or incest
- People are too quick to believe an abuser is guilty, even if there is no supporting evidence.
- Children who are being abused will show physical evidence of abuse.
- Acts like fondling, kissing, or touching, for example, are not really sexually abusive, and don't really harm the young person
- Children and youth are sexually abused because their parents/caregivers neglected to care for, or supervise them properly.
- Preschoolers do not need to know about child sexual abuse and would be frightened if educated about it.

However children of all ages, races, ethnicities, and economic backgrounds are vulnerable to sexual abuse. Child sexual abuse affects both girls and boys in all kinds of neighborhoods and communities, and in countries around the world.

Even the mean age of child sexual assault varies in different studies, most authors agree upon the reality of "children are sexually assaulted in every ages of childhood and adolescence". Many researches represent data about the age of child sexual assault between infancy and 18 years of age (De Jong et al., 1982; Mian et al., 1986; Riggs et al., 2000). Even sexual assault of girls especially adolescents are more frequent; boys are also at significant risk of sexual abuse, often at younger ages than girls. (De Jong et al., 1982)

Female dominancy of the victims is described in many descriptive researches which focused on child and adolescence sexual assault (Peipert&Domagalski, 1994; Jones et al.; 2003, Navratil, 2003). It was found 254 female (86%) and 40 male (14%) children in South Africa, 85.5% of the victims were female and 14.5% were male in Canada, 113 girls and 17 boys in Minessota, USA and 77% of girls and 23% of boys in England (Bentovim, 1987; Dubé& Hébert, 1988; Cox et al., 2007; Tilelli et al., 1980).

Most often, sexual assault victims are assaulted by an acquaintance not stranger. A number of studies revealed the percentages of acquaintance assailants as changing from 56% to 78% (Christian et al., 2000; Csorba et al., 2005; Dube&Hebert, 1988; Grossin et al., 2003; Lauritsen&Meldgaard, 2000; Muram et al., 1995; Peipert,&Domagalski, 1994; Sahu et al., 2005). Most children are abused by someone they know and trust, although boys are more likely than girls to be abused outside of the family (American Medical Association, 1992; Courtois, 1988 A study in three states found 96 percent of reported rape survivors under age 12 knew the attacker. Four percent of the offenders were strangers, 20 percent were fathers 16 percent were relatives and 50 percent were acquaintances or friends. Among women 18 or older, 12 percent were raped by a family member, 33 percent by a stranger and 55 percent by an acquaintance. (Langan&Harlow, 1994) In another study it was found that fifty-nine percent (398) of the children were sexually abused by an acquaintance, 21% (145) of the children were sexually abused by a relative, and 5% (33) of the children were sexually abused by a stranger. (Murphy et al., 2010) Abuse typically occurs within a long-term, on-going relationship between the offender and victim, escalates over time and lasts an average of four years. Offenders often develop a relationship with a targeted victim for months before beginning the abused (Courtois, 1988) In author's series 73 cases were acquaintance sexual assault, stranger assault were only in 4 cases. (Table 1)

Types of acquaintance ship / Age , sex	*Relative*	*Neighbor*	*Non Relative acquain-tance*	*Adjunct*	*Fiancé*	*Husband religiously but not registry married*	*Friend or beloved*	*Stranger*	*Step father*	*Total (%)*
M	1									
0-6										2
F		1								(2.6)
M		2	1					1		
7-12										11
F		3	1					2	1	(14.28)
M		1	1							
13-15										22
F	3		5			2	8	1	1	(28.58)
E										
16-18										42
K	1	7	8	1	2	5	18			(54.54)
Total (%)	5	14	16	1	2	7	26	4	2	77 (100)

Table 1. Relationship between victims and perpetrators with respect to sex and age groups

This finding might be connected with characteristics of these age groups such as physically weakness, low comprehension about the abusive acts.

The place of sexual assault are indoor especially victims own home and outdoor sexual assault is rare in most studies. The location of assault are reported as Own home inside 25%, other home inside 19%, own home outside 9%, other home outside 5%, other 11%, public place 6%, school 4%, unknown 21% in a study performed in South Africa. (Cox et al. 2007) The incidents most often took place in the victim's or assailant's home (76.7%). A total of 11.9% of the incidents occurred in another closed place, while 8.8% occurred in an open public place in another study (Dube&Hebert, 1988). The place of sexual assault was perpetrators' home in 39.74 % of the cases, followed by outdoor in only 23.08 % of the cases in authors' series.

Children are mostly assaulted during the day rather than night. In a study 60% of the cases were seen during the day, 34.9% between 18:00 and midnight, and 5.1% between midnight and 6:00 (Dube&Hebert, 1988). Another author mentioned that 49% of sexually assaults occur in broad daylight (Firsten, 1990).

Child abuser is young rather than an old person in generally. Adolescent sexual offenders report having approximately two paraphilias with onsetbetween ages 15 to 18 years of age (Abel et al., 1987). It is typical that they act upon these deviant impulses in adolescence. Nearly half of adult convicted rapists and child molesters committed their first offense between 8 and 18 years of age, with model age being 16 (Groth et al., 1982). The disparity between the age of victims' and perpetrators' was detected to be 1-2 years in 14.29% of the cases, 3-5 years in 25.97%, 6-10 years in 32.47%, and 11 years and over in 27.27% cases in authors' series.

More offenders are male than female, though the percentage varies between studies. The percentage of incidents of sexual abuse by female perpetrators that come to the attention of the legal system is usually reported to be between 1% and 4% (Denov, 2003). Other studies shows that women commit 14% to 40% of offenses reported against boys and 6% of offenses reported against girls (Dube et al., 2005; Finkelhor, 1994).

A number of studies have stated that, victims of child sexual assault are generally do not disclose the assault. However, most of victims applied to legal authorities disclose the assault because of secondary psychiatric problems and fear, and 55.6% of these had noticed to be assaulted many years before reporting (Safran, 1998; Jones et al., 2003). There are many factors that may have influenced the rate at which children were referred for medical care following the sexual abuse, including delayed disclosures. However, abuse by strangers is often treated with more seriousness by other disciplines than abuse by family members or others known to the child. Similarly, 76.92% of cases referred to sexual assault evaluation unit later than three days after assault, in authors' study. The main cause of delay in 19.23% of the cases explained the cause of delay as, they were anxious about being accused or punished, which support the idea of "victims might conceal the assault because of the fear of being accused, punished or injured by perpetrators".

The American Academy of Pediatrics Committee on Child Abuse and Neglect recommends forensic evidence collection when sexual abuse has occurred within 72 hours of the examination (Kellogg, 2005). Adams recommends evidence collection within 24 hours for prepubertal children (Adams, 2008; Christian et al., 2000) suggest that the best evidentiary material obtained from children post-abuse is found in the first 24 hours.

3. Forensic investigation of child sexual abuse victims

Anyone evaluating children for suspected sexual abuse must have an education and working knowledge of forensic interviewing, child bio-psycho-social development, prepubertal and postpubertal anatomy, and the ability to identify and interpret physical findings, including those which are normal, indicative of trauma, or unclear or uncertain (base on our understanding of these issues to date)

3.1 Forensic interviewing

First step of child sexual abuse evaluation is the interviewing the victim. Obtaining an unbiased history from a child who may have been sexually abused may be the most important part of the evaluation, particularly since diagnostic physical findings are frequently absent. Interviewing the child, steps must be taken by the examiner to prepare the child for the interview and examination, such as and to explain why.

The conversation should begin with topics that are interesting and not "threatening" for the child. The examiner spend enough time getting acquainted with the child before examination and should be patient and friendly in order to establish the desired level of relationship. Children are frightened by a hurried or demanding examiner, but they generally respond sufficiently to and cooperate with a pleasant one. It is not necessary for the examiner to wear a lab coat or other hospital and medical suit; such apparel may be frightening for younger children.

Then the history regarding concerns about sexual abuse should be obtained from the parent or caregiver separately from the child. Many parents are understandably worried and appreciate an opportunity to share their concerns privately. The history should be comprehensive and include the child's current and past medical problems, as well as social and family histories. Parents should be asked how the abuse came to light or, if the child has not disclosed abuse, why the parents suspect it.

The interview and examination room must be designed child-friendly. It would be helpful to perform this interview with multidisciplinary approach at once in sexual evaluation units for children to avoid retraumatization of the victim. The interview should be designed in multidisciplinary assessment involving skilled forensic interviewing of the child and a medical examination done by a medical provider with specialized training in sexual abuse. In order to minimize child interviews, these assessments are frequently held in settings such as child advocacy centers, where forensic interviewers and medical clinicians, child protective service workers, and police and district attorneys can work jointly to address the legal and protective issues in a coordinated fashion. Therefore Children's Advocacy Centers was found and have spread rapidly in USA. One of the primary goals of Children's Advocacy Centers (CACs) is to improve child forensic interviewing following allegations of child sexual abuse. They aim to coordinate law enforcement, child protective, medical, and other agencies, and typically use a single interviewer to provide information to every investigator involved in the case. Traditional methods for interviewing children have often been criticized as ineffective in assessing the truth and unnecessarily stressful for children. Three specific criticisms of these methods are that (1) investigation activities and decision-making are not coordinated across the multiple agencies involved, (2) children are interviewed too many times by too many interviewers and have to "tell their story over and over again," and (3) children are interviewed in stressful or compromising locations that disturb them further and make it difficult to talk. Sexual evaluation units or centers for children like CACs must aim to coordinate multiple investigations, to limit the number of interviews and interviewers children have, and to provide "child friendly" locations for interviews (Cross, 2007)

Interview should be structured and protocol-guided rather than standard interview practices. There are many useful structured interview protocols frequently used just like National Institute of Child Health and Human Development's Structured Interview Protocol or Investigative Interviewing Practice Guideline of American Professional Society on the Abuse of Children etc. Researchers examining the National Institute of Child Health and Human Development (NICHD) interview protocol, inparticular, have found that the recommended open-ended, free narrative questioning techniques are effective in eliciting information about abuse in forensic settings, at least with children who are forthcoming in disclosing the abuse. Lamb et al. (2003) also showed that open-ended invitations are just as effective with the younger as with the older children, although younger children report over all less information than older children (Lamb, 2003).

Children should be asked if they know why they have been brought to the doctor and to relate what happened to them. Open-ended questions such as "Has anyone ever touched you in a way that you didn't like or in a way that made you feel uncomfortable?" should be asked. The child's statement should be recorded in its own words. Whenever possible, the nature of the sexual contact, including pain, penetration and ejaculation, should be ascertained. Careful documentation of questions and responses is critical.

When an incident is disclosed, the following information must be obtained with a gentle and non-threatening manner, using language that the child can understand

- Who was the person who did this?
- With what part of his/her body?
- What part(s) of the patient's body was (were) touched?
- How many times was the child touched?
- When was the last time that it happened?
- At what location did the abuse occur?
- Was there any exposure to blood or body fluids?
- Did the child experience pain to the affected body part?
- For male assailants, was there ejaculation?
- Did the child tell anyone about the incident? (Adams, 2004)

The history must be recorded using the exact words used by the child to describe the event, particularly when such language is unique, for example, "He put his finger in my coochie." Words to describe the genitalia can be singular to the vocabulary of a child, giving credence to his or her testimony in a court of law (American Academy of Pediatrics. Committee on Child Abuse and Neglect., 1999; Giardiano, 2005; Sternberg, 2001).

3.2 Physical examination

3.2.1 Informed consent

Prior to physical examination, written, witnessed informed consent to examination, collection of specimens, release of information to authorities, and taking photographs should be obtained by parents, relatives or acquaintances. The law officer is not present at the examination.

Before examination some steps must be taken to prepare the child for the examination, such as explaining its comprehensive nature "The doctor will examine your entire body, including your private parts", to empower the child "Nothing will be done to hurt you, but if it does hurt or you feel uncomfortable, say stop and we will find another way", and to explain its purpose "I need to check you to make sure your body is okay".

3.2.2 Physical examination of the body

The first step is the complete physical examination of the body with careful recording of any trauma away from the genital area. There is a spectrum of injuries from incipient bruises, fresh abrasions and lacerations, up to evidence of prolonged physical abuse of the child with healing injuries of various types and ages and old scars. In some assaults, restraining force is severe enough to leave "fingertip" and other bruises on the limbs or strangling marks on the neck (Fig 1). Bite marks are common in sexual assaults and it is important to measure and photograph them carefully to allow matching or exclusion of the teeth of the alleged assailant (Fig 2). If there is a bite mark on the patient or if the patient gives a history of the perpetrator's licking a portion of her body (e.g., the nipples), these areas should be swabbed in an attempt to recover saliva. These swabs can then be analyzed for DNA. Positive DNA identification has been made in a number of cases from saliva on the body of the victim. After the swabbing of the bite mark, photographs should be taken. A metric ruler should be included in the photographs. Ideally, one should have a forensic odontologist on call so that they can examine and document the bite mark. They might take casts of the bite mark in addition to photographing it. The medical examiner should carefully search for fibers, hair, glass, paint, or any foreign material that might have been transferred to the victim's body from the assailant (Laraque, 2006)

All clothing also should be examined for stains, tears, missing buttons, dirt, gravel, grease, leaves, etc. The examiner should examine the hands to see if the fingernails are broken. Is the pubic hair matted? Are there any foreign hairs mixed with the patient's pubic hair? After examining the hands for trace evidence, the fingernails are clipped and placed in marked containers. The fingernail clippings and foreign materials or pubic hairs can subsequently be examined by the Crime Laboratory for foreign material that might have come from the assailant.

Oral cavity should be examined and should include evaluation for evidence of forced oral penetration such as bruising or petechiae of the hard or soft palate and/or tears of the frenulum.

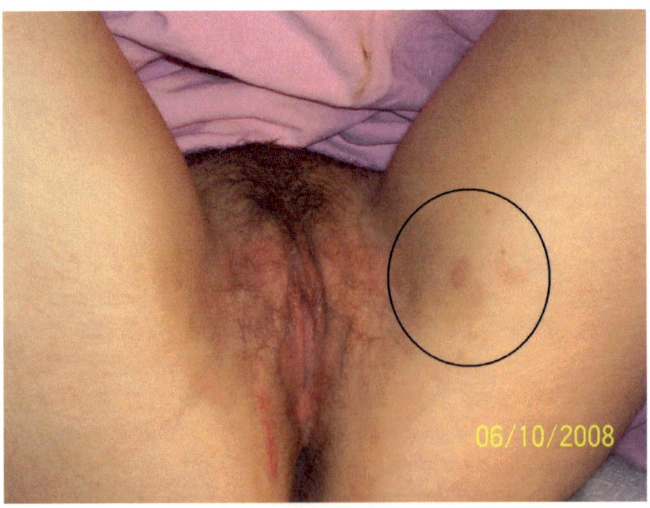

Fig. 1. Fingertips on the inner side of the thigh

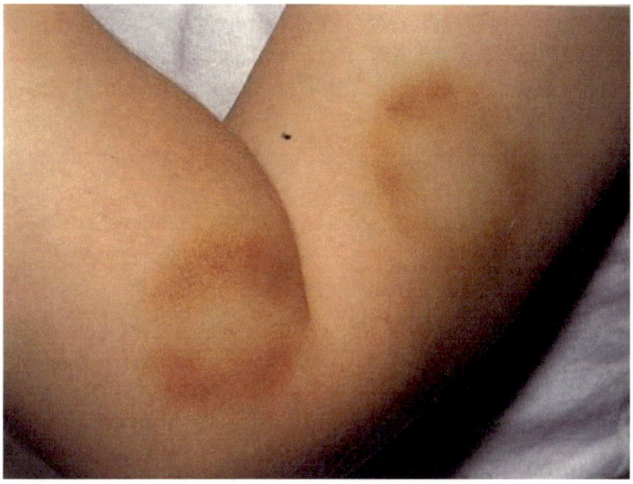

Fig. 2. Bite marks

3.2.3 Genital examination

Knowledge of normal ano-genital anatomy is crucial for all forensic examiners. This knowledge will provide a framework for understanding that a normal ano-genital examination does not negate the possibility of sexual abuse and most importantly will allow the examiner to recognize deviations from normal that may be concerning for sexual abuse. One of the most challenging aspects of the female genitalia examination is evaluation of the hymen. The appearance of the hymen changes with age and in response to hormonal influences. The prepubertal hymen is characterized as thin, translucent, and sensitive to touch. It becomes thickened, elastic, redundant, and accommodating in puberty, as the result of a physiologic increase in estrogen exposure (Fig 3). Common normal variations in the appearance of the hymen include imperforate, microperforate, cribriform, and septate forms.

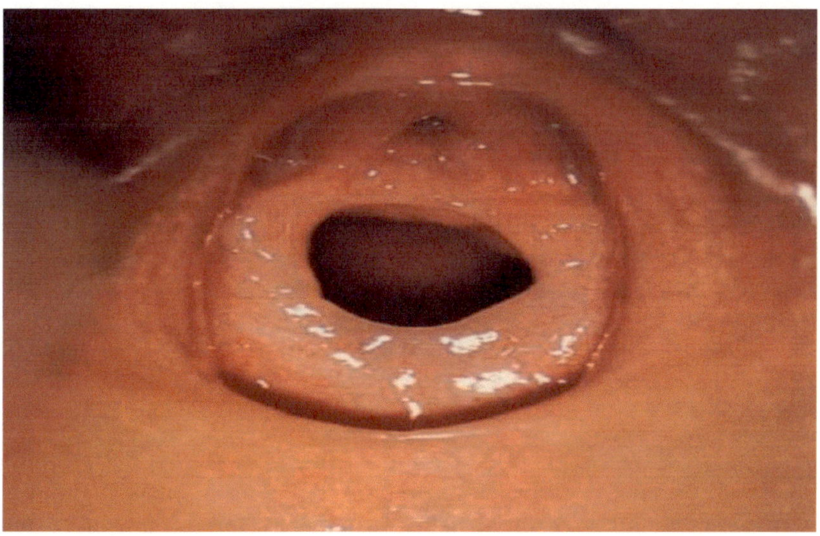

Fig. 3. Prepubertal hymen

An infant or a very young girl can be examined either on the examining table or while on a parent's lap. During the genital and anal examination, the mother positions the child and the assisting nurse separates the child's thighs so that the examiner can inspect the genital and the anal areas. The use of labial traction can greatly enhance visualization of the hymen. The labia majora are gently retracted between the thumb and forefinger with force applied downward and outward. Locations of abnormalities should be described as on a clock face with the urethra in the 12-O'clock position and the anus at the 6-O'clock position. In pubertal girls, estrogen causes the hymenal tissue to become thicker and more compliant; therefore, detection of trauma can be more challenging (Lahoti et al., 2001). Any abnormal findings should be confirmed in the knee-chest position. The examiner should take particular note of vulvar inflammations, eruptions, open lesions, tears, lacerations, pain, and discharge (Fig 4). The patency of the hymenal orifice is determined, the size of the introital opening measured, and the form and thickness of the hymen is recorded. In the prepubertal girl, vaginal penetration usually results in tearing of the hymen in the posterior 180°. These lacerations may be associated with bruising or abrasions both ventrally and towards to the posterior fourchette and lateral introital tissues. The colposcopy will improve injury detection and provide more details including small lacerations, inlamation and scars (Fig 5). If there is a discharge, the character, consistency, and color should be noted. The presence of any odor should also be recorded. If there is evidence of infection, dry smears for bacteriologic studies, cultures, and wet slide preparations should be prepared. Fresh wet smears must be examined for Trichomonas vaginalis, clue cells, and Candida albicans. A speculum examination may be necessary for pubertal adolescent females. The vaginal walls as well as the cervix should be visualized to detect any evidence of trauma and to obtain samples from fluid collections.

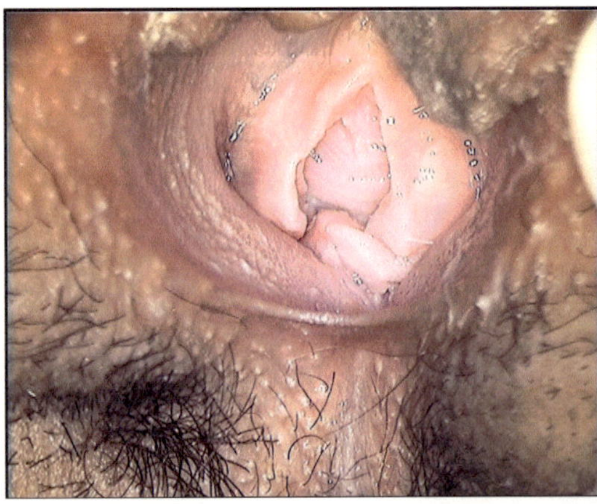

Fig. 4. Hymenal laseration at 7-O'clock position

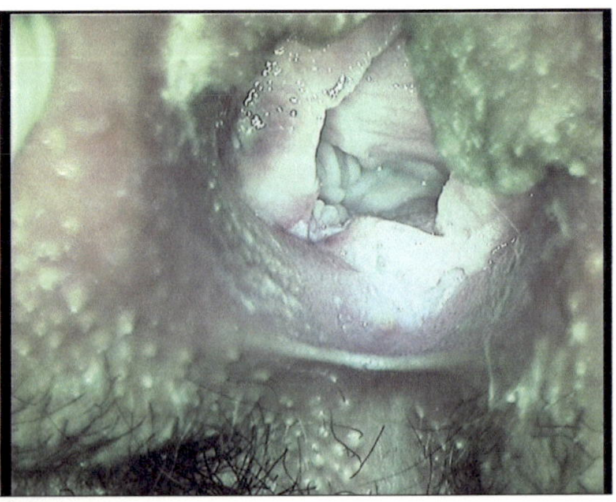

Fig. 5. Colposcopic filter view of Fig4 (Inflammation of the laceration wall and ecchymosis at 10-O'clock is obvious)

Clinical examination of the anus is often disappointing in the sense, first, that little is to be found and, secondly, that the correct interpretation of abnormalities remains a matter of serious debate. Vaginal injuries or abnormalities are more often recognized as possible signs of abuse, while anal and perianal injuries may be dismissed as being associated with common bowel disorders such as constipation or diarrhea. Penetration by a larger object may result in injury varying from a little swelling of the anal verge to gross tearing of the sphincter, or even bowel perforation. If lubrication is used and the sphincter is relaxed, perhaps no physical evidence will be found. Even penetration by an adult penis can occur without significant injury. After penetration, sphincter laxity, ecchymosis, swelling, and small mucosal tears of the anal verge may be observed as well as sphincter spasm (Fig 6, 7). Within a few days the swelling subsides and the mucosal tears heal. Skin tags can form because of the tears. Repeated anal penetration over a long period may cause a loose anal sphincter and an enlarged opening (Fig 8) Perianal region should also be examined for genital warts (Condyloma accuminata) (Fig 9). DNA typology of Human Papilloma Virus must be identified to compare with the suspected perpetrators.

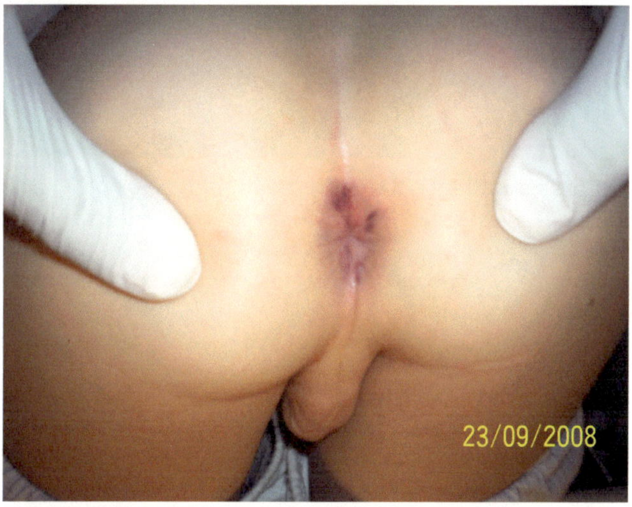

Fig. 6. Perianal ecchymosis

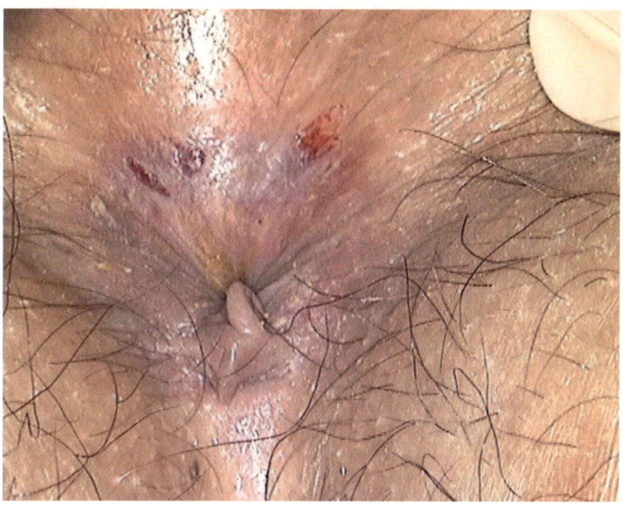

Fig. 7. Mucosal tears

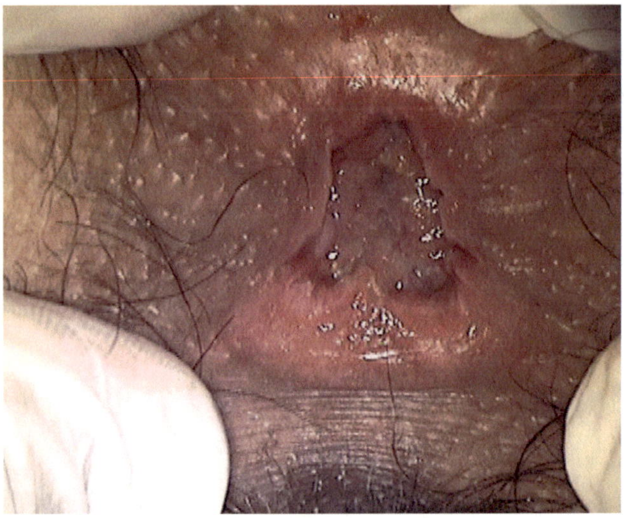

Fig. 8. A loose anal sphincter and an enlarged opening

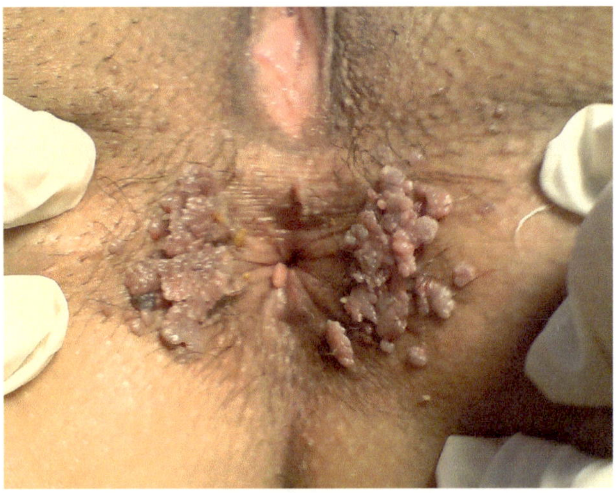

Fig. 9. Anal warts (Condyloma accuminata)

In performing an anal examination in children, the examiner carefully notes the symmetry and tone of the anus when the buttocks are separated. This can be performed with the child supine or in the more traditional lateral position. Again, positive findings need to be confirmed in the prone position. In addition to symmetry, the physician should note the presence of tags, fissures, or scars. With the exception of a bleeding laceration after are port of sodomy (Fig 10), the presence of anal tags, bumps, and scars may be nonspecific findings that do not confirm whether a child has been sexually abused unless they can be positively related to previously identified acute findings. Evidence of acute anal trauma may be seen if the child is evaluated soon after the assault; however, anorectal changes are rarely definitive indicators of abuse. Swelling of the anus with blue discoloration is suggestive of trauma and may be present up to 48 hours after the event. It is important not to confuse this finding with hemorrhoids. Perianal erythema is suspicious for trauma. It may also be seen in children with encopresis, poor hygiene, pinworms, or Group A streptococcal or staphylococcal infection. Documented anal injury after sexual assault is distinctively uncommon, and any injuries that do occur can heal quickly and often without visible residua (Hobbs&Wynne, 1989).

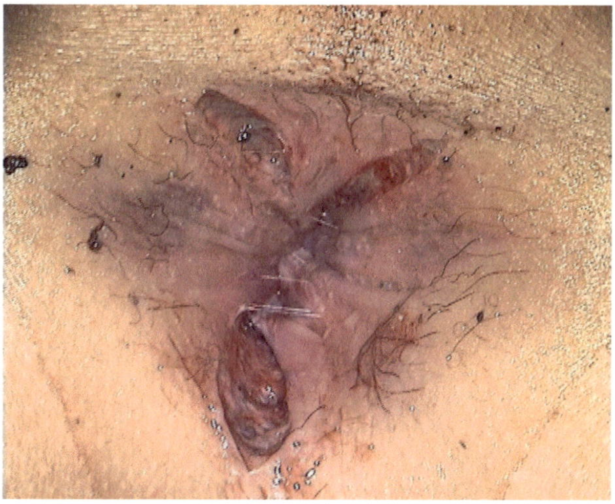

Fig. 10. Deep lacerations of the anus

The physician should examine the penis, testicles and perineum for bite marks, abrasions, bruising or suction ecchymosis in the anogenital examination of the male child victim. Evaluation of the anus may be performed with the patient in the supine, lateral recumbent or prone position with gentle retraction of the gluteal folds. The anal examination of the male is the same as in the female.

Current practice dictates that positive findings be recorded photographically or with video, and colposcopic or digital imaging should be of diagnostic quality. As it is clear that utilization of a colposcope improves injury detection colposcope should be the standard of care for examining children who may have been sexually abused.

The American Academy of Pediatrics Committee on Child Abuse and Neglect recommends forensic evidence collection when sexual abuse has occurred within 72 hours of the examination (Kellogg, 2005). Christian et al. (2000) suggest that the best evidentiary material obtained from children post-abuse is found in the first 24 hours. Adams et al.'s (1994) study showed a significantly higher incidence of abnormal genital findings in girls examined within 72 hours of the abuse as compared to those examined a month or more from the event.

Different studies repot various percentages of genital injuries depend on time of examination after assault. Percentage of anogenital injuries was reported 84%, and average interval of medical evaluation after assault is 17 hours in a study of Michigan State University (Jones et al., 2003). Some form of forensic evidence was identified in 24.9% of children, all of whom were examined within 44 hours and over 90% of children with positive forensic evidence findings were seen within 24 hours of their assault, presence of genital injury was %23 and in another child sexual assault series (Christian et al., 2000). Nongenital trauma was found in only 5.5% and anomalies were found in the genital examination of 25.4% of the victims in another review of 511 cases (Dubé&Hébert, 1988). However, the absence of these findings is common in girls who have suffered perceived genital penetration. For example, an observational study of 506 girls age 5 to 17 years, who disclosed penile-genital penetrative abuse, found that most girls did not have definitive physical findings of abuse regardless of the number of reported penetrations. Specifically, no findings were seen on expert review of photocolposcopy in all of the girls less than 10 years of age (N=74), 87 percent of girls ≥10 years of age with no history of consensual sex (358 of 410 patients), and 82 percent of girls ≥10 years of age with a history of consensual sex (18 of 22 patients) (Anderst, et al., 2009).

3.3 Forensic evidence sampling for laboratory examinations

Rates of recovery of forensic evidence from prepubertal children evaluated for sexual assault vary from 6 to 42%. Early clinical examination within 24 to 72 hours to assault is the key point in determining traumatic changes and forensic evidences. Forensic studies should be performed especially when the examination occurs within 72 hours of acute sexual assault or sexual abuse (Christian et al., 2000).

Forensic evaluation requires collection of numerous specimens. Providers should use evidence collection kits with careful attention to guidelines for specimen collection. Collected samples include

- The victim's clothing
- Swabs and smears from the buccal mucosa, vagina, and rectum and from other areas highlighted by ultraviolet light
- Combed specimens from the scalp and pubic hair
- Fingernail scrapings and clippings
- Control samples of the victim's scalp and pubic hair (ideally, at least 20 to 25 pulled hairs per site)
- Whole blood sample
- Saliva sample

Obviously the most important identifying element for the examiner and the pathologist is the documented presence of an ejaculate, so that the retrieval of the spermatozoa is more critical than ever. It should be stressed that the lack of evidence of ejaculation by no means refutes a complaint of sexual assault. Many of the men convicted for sexual assault may suffer from some form of sexual dysfunction that impaires their ability to ejaculate. If the abuse has occurred within the last 72 hours the presence of sperm should be investigated. Detection of acid phosphatase is another technique used to detect semen, acid phosphatase can, however, normally be found in very low levels in the adult female vagina, so quantification of the enzyme is important to verify ejaculation. The p30 protein is a semen glycoprotein of prostatic origin. The p30-enzyme is linked with an immunosorbent assay. This protein is semen-specific and is not found in vaginal fluids. It is thus a more sensitive and specific method of semen detection. Acid phosphatase and p30 protein test should be helpful when perpetrator is suffered from asospermia or aspermia (Stefanidou et al., 2005).

Identification of genetic markers in blood, saliva and serum (ABO typing and other blood enzyme systems) should be performed within 72 hours of acute sexual assault or sexual abuse. DNA fingerprinting can, nowadays, establish the identity of a perpetrator with a high degree of certainty.

The victim should also be evaluated for pregnancy and sexually transmitted infections by a gynecologist in multidisciplinary approach. The diagnosis of sexually transmitted diseases is important not only to the care of the victim but also in determining the fact of sexual contact. This evidence may be prima facie, or confirmatory. Gonorrhea or syphilis infections are diagnostic of sexual abuse after perinatal transmission has been ruled out. Herpes type 2, Chlamydia, Trichomonas, and condyloma infections are extremely unlikely to be due to anything but abuse, particularly in children beyond infancy. HIV, and herpes simplex virus type 2 should also be tested (Kawsar et al., 2008).

Finally, toxicological analysis of blood and urine should be performed in case that the child has been abused while under the influence of drugs.

3.4 Interpretation of findings

The interpretation of findings in children with suspected sexual abuse depends upon the constellation of historical, physical, and laboratory findings. The history is often the most important part of the evaluation. The provision by the child of a spontaneous, clear, consistent, and detailed description of sexual molestation is specific for sexual abuse and should be reported to legal authorities and/or child protective services.

Adams et. al. published a series of criteria about interpreting physical and laboratory findings in suspected child sexual abuse in 2007. (Table2).

A Product of an ongoing collaborative process by child maltreatment physician specialists, under the leadership of Joyce A. Adams, MD
Findings documented in newborns or commonly seen in non-abused children:
(The presence of these findings generally neither confirms nor discounts a child's clear disclosure of sexual abuse)
Normal variants
1. Periurethral or vestibular bands 2. Intravaginal ridges or columns 3. Hymenal bumps or mounds 4. Hymenal tags or septal remnants 5. Linea vestibularis (midline avascular area) 6. Hymenal notch/cleft in the anterior (superior) half of the hymenal rim (prepubertal girls), on or above the 3 o'clock - 9 o'clock line, patient supine 7. Shallow/superficial notch or cleft in inferior rim of hymen (below 3 o'clock - 9 o'clock line) 8. External hymenal ridge 9. Congenital variants in appearance of hymen, including: crescentic, annular, redundant, septate,cribiform, microperforate, imperforate 10. Diastasis ani (smooth area) 11. Perianal skin tag 12. Hyperpigmentation of the skin of labia minora or perianal tissues in children of color, such as Mexican-American and African-American children 13. Dilation of the urethral opening with application of labial traction 14. "Thickened" hymen (May be due to estrogen effect, folded edge of hymen, swelling from infection, or swelling from trauma. The latter is difficult to assess unless follow-up examination is done)

Findings commonly caused by other medical conditions:
15. Erythema (redness) of the vestibule, penis, scrotum or perianal tissues. (May be due to irritants, infection or trauma * 16. Increased vascularity ("Dilatation of existing blood vessels") of vestibule and hymen. (May be due to local irritants, or normal pattern in the non estrogenized state) 17. Labial adhesions. (May be due to irritation or rubbing) 18. Vaginal discharge. (Many infectious and non-infectious causes, cultures must be taken to confirm if it is caused by sexually transmitted organisms or other infections.) 19. Friability of the posterior fourchette or commissure (May be due to irritation, infection, or may be caused by examiner's traction on the labia majora) 20. Excoriations/bleeding/vascular lesions. These findings can be due to conditions such as lichen sclerosus, eczema or seborrhea, vaginal/perianal Group A Streptococcus, urethral prolapse, hemangiomas) 21. Perineal groove (failure of midline fusion), partial or complete 22. Anal fissures (Usually due to constipation, perianal irritation) 23. Venous congestion, or venous pooling in the perianal area. (Usually due to positioning of child, also seen with constipation) 24. Flattened anal folds (May be due to relaxation of the external sphincter or to swelling of the perianal tissues due to infection or trauma* 25. Partial or complete anal dilatation to less than 2 cm (anterior-posterior dimension), with or without stool visible. (May be a normal reflex, or may have other causes, such as severe constipation or encopresis, sedation, anesthesia, neuromuscular conditions,)
INDETERMINATE Findings: Insufficient or conflicting data from research studies: (May require additional studies/evaluation to determine significance. These physical/laboratory findings may support a child's clear disclosure of sexual abuse, if one is given, but should be interpreted with caution if the child gives no disclosure. In some cases, a report to child protective services may be indicated to further evaluate possible sexual abuse.)
Physical Examination Findings
26. Deep notches or clefts in the posterior/inferior rim of hymen in pre-pubertal girls, located between 4 and 8 o'clock, in contrast to transections (see 41) 27. Deep notches or complete clefts in the hymen at 3 or 9 o'clock in adolescent girls. 28. Smooth, non-interrupted rim of hymen between 4 and 8 o'clock, which appears to be less than 1 millimeter wide, when examined in the prone knee-chest position, or using water to "float" the edge of the hymen when the child is in the supine position. 29. Wart-like lesions in the genital or anal area. (Biopsy and viral typing may be indicated in some cases if appearance is not typical of Condyloma accuminata) 30. Vesicular lesions or ulcers in the genital or anal area (viral and/or bacterial cultures, or nucleic acid amplification tests may be needed for diagnosis) 31. Marked, immediate anal dilation to an anterior-posterior diameter of 2 cm or more, in the absence of other predisposing factors
Lesions with etiology confirmed: Indeterminate specificity for sexual transmission (Report to protective services recommended by AAP Guidelines[2] unless perinatal or horizontal transmission is considered likely)
31. Genital or anal Condyloma accuminata in child, in the absence of other indicators of

abuse. 32. Herpes Type 1 or 2 in the genital or anal area in a child with no other indicators of sexual abuse.
Findings Diagnostic of Trauma and/or Sexual contact (The following findings support a disclosure of sexual abuse, if one is given, and are highly suggestive of abuse even in the absence of a disclosure, unless the child and/or caretaker provide a clear, timely, plausible description of accidental injury. (It is recommended that diagnostic quality photo-documentation of the examination findings be obtained and reviewed by an experienced medical provider, before concluding that they represent acute or healed trauma. Follow-up examinations are also recommended.)
Acute trauma to external genital/anal tissues
33. Acute lacerations or extensive bruising of labia, penis, scrotum, perianal tissues, or perineum (May be from unwitnessed accidental trauma, or from physical or sexual abuse) 34. Fresh laceration of the posterior fourchette, not involving the hymen. (Must be differentiated from dehisced labial adhesion or failure of midline fusion. May also be caused by accidental injury or consensual sexual intercourse in adolescents
Residual (healing) injuries
(These findings are difficult to assess unless an acute injury was previously documented at the same location)
36. Perianal scar (Rare, may be due to other medical conditions such as Crohn's Disease, accidental injuries, or previous medical procedures) 37. Scar of posterior fourchette or fossa. (Pale areas in the midline may also be due to linea vestibularis or labial adhesions)
Injuries indicative of blunt force penetrating trauma (or from abdominal/pelvic compression injury if such history is given)
38. Laceration (tear, partial or complete) of the hymen, acute. 39. Ecchymosis (bruising) on the hymen (in the absence of a known infectious process or coagulopathy). 40. Perianal lacerations extending deep to the external anal sphincter (not to be confused with partial failure of midline fusion) 41. Hymenal transection (healed). An area between 4 and 8 o'clock on the rim of the hymen where it appears to have been torn through, to or nearly to the base, so there appears to be virtually no hymenal tissue remaining at that location. This must be confirmed using additional examination techniques such as a swab, prone knee-chest position or Foley catheter balloon (in adolescents), or prone-knee chest position or water to float the edge of the hymen (in prepubertal girls). This finding has also been referred to as a "complete cleft" in sexually active adolescents and young adult women. 42. Missing segment of hymenal tissue. Area in the posterior (inferior) half of the hymen, wider than a transection, with an absence of hymenal tissue extending to the base of the hymen, which is confirmed using additional positions/methods as described above.
Presence of infection confirms mucosal contact with infected and infective bodily secretions, contact most likely to have been sexual in nature:
43. Positive confirmed culture for gonorrhea, from genital area, anus, throat, in a child outside the neonatal period.

44. Confirmed diagnosis of syphilis, if perinatal transmission is ruled out. 45. Trichomonas vaginalis infection in a child older than 1 year of age, with organisms identified by culture or in vaginal secretions by wet mounts examination. by an experienced technician or clinician) 46. Positive culture from genital or anal tissues for Chlamydia, if child is older than 3 years at time of diagnosis, and specimen was tested using cell culture or comparable method approved by the Centers for Disease Control. 47. Positive serology for HIV, if perinatal transmission, transmission from blood products, and needle contamination has been ruled out.
Diagnostic of sexual contact
48. Pregnancy 49. Sperm identified in specimens taken directly from a child's body.

Table 2. Approach to Interpreting Physical and Laboratory Findings in Suspected Child Sexual Abuse. (Adams et. al., 2007)

4. Management of sexual abuse in children and adolescents

The management of sexual abuse involves prevention of sexually transmitted infections (STI) and pregnancy. Psychosocial support and anticipatory guidance should be offered to the victims and their nonoffending caregivers.

4.1 Sexually transmitted infections prophylaxis

A prepubertal child will acquire a sexually transmitted infection (STI) as the result of sexual abuse is low and varies according to the local prevalence of STIs. Thus asymptomatic children do not generally require STI prophylaxis. However, cultures must be obtained prior to treatment whenever prophylaxis is prescribed (Siegel et. al, 1995). For adolescents, STI prophylaxis is recommended for those who present within 72 hours of the event (because of the high prevalence of preexisting asymptomatic infection, the risk of pelvic inflammatory disease, and the possibility of loss to follow-up). For pubertal females who present after 72 hours, STI prophylaxis should be prescribed if the assailant is known to be infected, the victim has signs or symptoms of infection, or at the victim's request. (American Academy of Pediatrics, 2006).

4.2 Pregnancy prophylaxis

The highest risk of pregnancy occurs during the three days preceding and including ovulation. Knowing the timing of the event in relation to the patient's ovulatory period is helpful in further assessing risk. Emergency contraception (postcoital contraception) should be offered to all pubertal female patients and should be strongly advised to females at highest risk for pregnancy.

4.3 Psychological support

The child's physical and emotional well-being are of primary concern. The child should be reassured that what happened was not the child's fault and that he or she did nothing wrong. Children in whom sexual abuse is confirmed or suspected should be referred to a mental health professional for evaluation and counseling. The family of the victim may also need treatment and support to cope with the emotional trauma of their child's abuse

Short-term sequelae of sexual abuse include fear, disturbances in sleep and eating, phobias, guilt, shame, anger, depression, school problems, delinquency, aggression, hostility, antisocial behavior, inappropriate sexual behavior, and running away. Longer-term effects include depression, sleep problems, eating disorders, obesity, feelings of isolation, stigmatization, poor self-esteem, problems with interpersonal relationships, negative effect on sexual function, revictimization, substance abuse, and suicidal behavior. Psychosocial follow-up is the key point to avoid these short-term or longer-term sequelaes (Hymel& Jenny 1996)

4.4 Social support

Social support is one of the most important steps in the management of abused children. The case should be reported to the social services or child protective services after forensic investigation completed. Social support should be maintained to prevent further harm to children from sexual or other types of abuse or neglect. When the case is reported to social services, they must look into it if they think there is a real risk to the safety or well-being of the child. Social services will decide if the child needs protection and what needs to be done to protect them.

They must decide, or contribute to decision-making in some key areas. Is a child safe? Should a child remain at home, or be removed? What type and level of services does this child/family need? Can these services be offered while the child is living with the alleged abuser? Of the myriad problems presented by this family, which one(s) should be addressed, and which ones should be addressed first? How therapeutically accessible are the members of this family? At what stage of change are they? What is the level of future risk to the child (as opposed to immediate safety)?

- Social services accomplish all these services through:
- Assessing suspected cases of abuse and neglect
- Assisting the family in diagnosing the problem
- Providing in-home counseling and supportive services to help children stay at home with their families
- Coordinating community and agency services for the family
- Petitioning the court for removal of the child, if necessary
- Providing public information about child abuse, neglect, and dependency.

5. Conclusion

- Child Sexual Abuse defined as contacts between a child and an adult or other person significantly older or in a position of power or control over the child, where the child is being used for sexual stimulation of the adult or other person.
- The United Nations Convention on the Rights of the Child (CRC) is an international treaty that legally obliges states to protect children's rights. Articles 34 and 35 of the CRC require states to protect children from all forms of sexual exploitation and sexual abuse.
- The prevalence of sexual assaults, especially among children and adolescent, is thought to be extremely higher than in literature.
- Children and especially adolescent females are sexually assaulted more frequent comparatively to adults.
- Children are sexually assaulted in every ages of childhood and adolescence.

- Sexual assault victims are mostly female and assaulted by an acquaintance not stranger.
- Children are mostly assaulted indoor and during the day.

Most of the child abuser is male and young rather than an old person.

- Victims of child sexual assault generally do not disclose the assault.
- During forensic investigation, obtaining an unbiased history from a child who may have been sexually abused may be the most important part of the evaluation, particularly since diagnostic physical findings are frequently absent.
- In order to minimize child interviews, these assessments should be held in settings such as child advocacy centers, where forensic interviewers and medical clinicians, child protective service workers, and police and district attorneys can work jointly to address the legal and protective issues in a coordinated fashion.
- Prior to physical examination, written, witnessed informed consent to examination, collection of specimens, release of information to authorities, and taking photographs should be obtained by parents, relatives or acquaintances.
- All clothing, the body, oral cavity and genitalia should be examined for any evidences of sexual assault.
- Early clinical examination within 24 to 72 hours to assault is the key point in determining traumatic changes and forensic evidences.
- Examiners should use evidence collection kits which guidelines for specimen collection for laboratory analysis.

The interpretation of findings in children with suspected sexual abuse depends upon the constellation of historical, physical, and laboratory findings.

- The management of sexual abuse involves prevention of sexually transmitted infections (STI) and pregnancy. Psychosocial support and anticipatory guidance should be offered to the victims and their nonoffending caregivers.

6. Referances

Abel, G.G., Becker, J.V., Mittleman, M., Cunningham-Rathner, N., Rouleau, J.L., & Murphy, W.D. (1987). Self-reported sex crimes of non-incarcerated paraphiliacs (Final Report No. MH-33678). Washington, DC: PublicHealth Service

Adams, J. (2008). Guidelines for medical care of children evaluated for suspected sexual abuse: An update for 2008. *Current Opinion in Gynecology and Obstetrics*, 29(5),435–441.

Adams, JA., Kaplan, RA., Starling, SP., Mehta, NH., Finkel MA., Botash AS., Kellogg ND. & Shapiro RA. (2007). Guidelines for medical care of children who may have been sexually abused. *J Pediatr Adolesc Gynecol,* 20:163-72.

Adams, J.A., Harper, K., Knudson, S., & Revilla, J. (1994). Examination findings in legally confirmed child sexual abuse: It's normal to be normal. *Pediatrics*, 94(3), 310–317

Adams, JA. (2004). Medical evaluation of suspected child sexual abuse. *J Pediatr Adolesc Gynecol*, 17:191.

American Academy of Pediatrics. Sexually transmitted diseases in adolescents and children. In: Red Book 2006: The Report of the Committee on Infectious Diseases, 27rd ed, Pickering, LK (Ed), American Academy of Pediatrics, Elk Grove Village, IL 2006. p.166.

American Academy of Pediatrics. Committee on Child Abuse and Neglect. (1999) Guidelines for the Evaluation of Sexual Abuse of Children: Subject Review. *Pediatrics*, 103: 186-191

American Medical Association (1992) Diagnostic and Treatment Guidelines on Child Sexual Abuse. AMA. Chicago.

American Professional Society on the Abuse of Children. (1995). *Practice guidelines: descriptive terminology in child sexual abuse medical evaluations.* APSAC.Chicago, IL.

Anderst, J, Kellogg, N & Jung, I. (2009). Reports of repetitive penile-genital penetration often have no definitive evidence of penetration. *Pediatrics,* 124:e403.

APA Board of Professional Affairs, Committee on Professional Practice and Standards, (1999) Guidelines for psychological evaluations in child protection matters. *The American Psychologist* 54 (8): 586–93.

Bechtel, K. & Podrazik, M. (1999). Evaluation of the adolescent rape victim. Pediatr *Clin North Am.* 46(4):809-23

Bentovim, A., Boston, P. & van Elburg, A. (1987). Child sexual abuse--children and families referred to a treatment project and the effects of intervention. *Br Med J (Clin Res Ed).* 5;295(6611):1453-7

Child Welfare Information Gateway (2009). Definitions of Child Abuse and Neglect, Summary of State Laws, National Clearinghouse on Child Abuse and Neglect Information, U.S. Department of Health and Human Services. Retrieved 2011-03-25. Available from: http://www.childwelfare.gov/systemwide/laws_policies/statutes/define.pdf

Christian, C.W., Lavelle J.M., De Jong A.R., Loiselle J., Brenner L. & Joffe M. (2000). Forensic evidence findings in prepubertal victims of sexual assault. *Pediatrics,* 106(1 Pt 1):100-4.

Chu L.C. & Tung W.K. (2005) The clinical outcome of 137 rape victims in Hong Kong. *Hong Kong Med J.* 11(5):391-6

Coomaraswamy, R. (1997). Report of the Special Rapporteur on Violence Against Women, Alternative Approaches and Ways and Means Within the United Nations System for Improving the Effective Enjoyment of Human Rights and Fundamental Freedoms (E/CN.4/1997/47). Retrieved 2011-03-25. Available from: http://www.unhchr.ch/Huridocda/Huridoca.nsf/0/043c76f98a706362802566b1005e9219?Opendocument

Courtois, C. (1988). *Healing the Incest Wound: Adult Survivors in Therapy,* WW Norton & Co. ISBN: 0-393-70051-8. New York

Cox, S., Andrade, G., Lungelow, D., Schloetelburg, W. & Rode H. (2007). The child rape epidemic: Assessing the incidence at Red Cross Hospital, Cape Town, and establishing the need for a new national protocol. *SAMJ* (97)10: 950-955)

Cross, TP., Jones, LM., Walsh, WA., Simone, M. & Kolko, D. (2007). Child forensic interviewing in Children's Advocacy Centers: Empirical data on a practice model. *ChildAbuse&Neglect,* 31, 1031–1052

Crowley SR. (ed) (1999) *Sexual Assult. The Medical-Legal Examination.* McGraw-Hill/Appleton & Lange. Stamford, Connecticut.

Csorba, R., Aranyosi, J., Borsos, A., Balla, L., Major, T. and Poka, R. (2005). Characteristics of female child sexual abuse in Hungary between 1986 and 2001: a longitudinal, prospective study. *Eur J Obstet Gynecol Reprod Biol.* 120(2):217-21.

De Jong, AR., Emmett, GA. & Hervada, AA. (1982). Epidemiologic factors in sexual abuse of boys. Am J Dis Child. 136(11):990-3.

Denov, M. S. (2003). "The myth of innocence: sexual scripts and the recognition of child sexual abuse by female perpetrators". *The Journal of Sex Research* 40 (3): 303–314

Dubé, R & Hébert, M. (1988). Sexual abuse of children under 12 years of age: a review of 511 cases. Child Abuse Negl. 12(3):321-30

Dube, SR., Anda, RF., Whitfield, C.L, Brown, DW., Felitti, VJ., Dong, M. & Giles, WH. (2005). Long-term consequences of childhood sexual abuse by gender of victim. *American Journal of Preventive Medicine* 28 (5): 430–8

Finkelhor, D. (1994). Current information on the scope and nature of child sexual abuse. *The Future of Children* 4 (2): 31–53.

Finkelhor, D., Hotaling, G. & Yllo, K. (1988). *Stopping Family Violence: Research Priorities in the Coming Decade.* Sage Publications. ISBN: 0-8039-3215-4.Newbury Park

Finkelhor, D. & Ormrod, R. (2001). "Child Abuse Reported to the Police". *Juvenile Justice Bulletin* (U.S. Office of Juvenile Justice and Delinquency Prevention).

Firsten, T. (1990). *An Exploration of the Role of Physical and Sexual Abuse for Psychiatrically Institutionalized Women.* Toronto: Ontario Women's Directorate.

Fritz, G. S., Stall, K. & Wagner, N. N. (1981). A comparison of males and females who were sexually molested as children. *Journal of Sex and Marital Therapy*. 7, 54-59

Giardiano, AP. & Finkel, MA. (2005). Evaluating child sexual abuse. *Pediatr Ann*, 34: 382-394

Grossin, C., Sibille, I., Lorin de la Grandmaison, G., Banasr, A., Brion, F. & Durigon, M. (2003). Analysis of 418 cases of sexual assault. *Forensic Sci Int.* 131(2-3):125-30

Groth, A., Longo, R., & McFadin, B. (1982). Undetected recidivism among rapists and child molesters. *Crime and Delinquency*, 28, 450–458.

Harlow, CW. & Langan, P. (1994). "Child Rape Victims, 1992," Crime Data Brief, U.S. Department of Justice, Office of Justice Programs, Bureau of Justice Statistics. Retrieved 2011-03-25. Available from:
http://bjs.ojp.usdoj.gov/content/pub/pdf/CRV92.PDF

Herbert, CP., Grams, GD. & Berkowitz, J. (1992). Sexual assault tracking study: who gets lost to follow-up? *CMAJ* Oct 15;147(8):1177-84.

Hobbs, CJ. & Wynne, JM. (1989). Sexual abuse of English boys and girls: the importance of anal examination. *Child Abuse Negl*, 13:195.

Hymel, KP. & Jenny, C. (1996). Child sexual abuse. *Pediatr Rev*, 17:236.

Jones, JS., Rossman, L., Wynn, BN., Dunnuck, C. & Schwartz, N. (2003) Comparative analysis of adult versus adolescent sexual assault: epidemiology and patterns of anogenital injury. *Acad Emerg Med.* 2003 10(8):872-7.

Kawsar, M., Long, S. & Srivastava, OP. (2008). Child sexual abuse and sexually transmitted infections: review of joint genitourinary medicine and paediatric examination practice. *Int J STD AIDS*, 19:349-350.

Kellog, N. & Committee on Child Abuse and Neglect. (2005).The evaluation of sexual abuse in children. *Pediatrics*, 116, 506–512.

Kercher, G., & McShane, M. (1984). The prevalence of child sexual abuse victimization in an adult sample of Texas residents. *Child Abuse and Neglect*, 8, 495-501.

Lahoti, SL., McClain, N., Girardet, R., McNeese, M. & Cheung, K. (2001). Evaluating the child for sexual abuse. *Am Fam Physician*, 63: 883-892

Lamb, M.E., Sternberg, K.J., Orbach, Y., Esplin, P.W., Stewart, H., & Mitchell, S. (2003). Age differences in young children's responses to open-ended invitations in the course of forensic interviews. *Journal of Consulting and Clinical Psychology*, 71,926–934.

Laraque, D., DeMattia, A. & Low C. (2006). Forensic child abuse evaluation: a review. *Mt Sinai J Med, 73*: 1138-1147.

Lauritsen, AK., Meldgaard, K. & Charles, AV. (2000). Forensic examination of sexually abused children. *J Forensic Sci.* 45(1):115-7.

Ledoux J & Hazelwood R. (1995). *Police attitudes and beliefs concerning rape.* Rape Investigations, CRC Press, Boca Raton, pp:13-25.

Mian, M., Wehrspann, W., Klajner-Diamond, H., LeBaron, D. & Winder, C. (1986). Review of 125 children 6 years of age and under who were sexually abused. Child Abuse Negl. 10(2):223-9.

Muram, D., Hostetler, BR., Jones, CE. & Speck, PM. (1995). Adolescent victims of sexual assault. *J Adolesc Health.* 17(6):372-5.

Murphy, SB., Potter, SJ., Stapleton, JG., Wiesen-Martin, D. & Pierce-Weeks J. (2010). Findings from Sexual Assault Nurse Examiners (SANE): A case study of New Hampshire's pediatric SANE database. J Forensic Nurs.6(4):163-9.

Navratil, F. (2003). Sexual abuse in adolescence: patient assessment, necessity and meaning of the physical examination. Gynakol Geburtshilfliche Rundsch. 43(3):146-51.

Russell, D. E. H. (1984). Sexual exploitation: Rape, child sexual abuse, sexual harassment.: Sage. Beverly Hills, CA

Office of the United Nations High Commissioner for Human Rights (1989). Convention on the Rights of the Child. Retrieved 2011-03-25. Available from: http://www2.ohchr.org/english/law/crc.htm

Official text of the Sexual Offences Act, 2003 as amended and in force today within the United Kingdom, Retrieved 2011-03-25. Available from: UK Statute Law Database: http://www.legislation.gov.uk/ukpga/2003/42/contents

Peipert, JF. & Domagalski LR. (1984). Epidemiology of adolescent sexual assault. *Obstet Gynecol.* (5):867-71.

RAINN: Rape, Abuse, and Incest National Network. Stop Abuse For Everyone. Retrieved 2011-03-25. Available from: http://www.rainn.org/

Riggs, N., Houry, D., Long, G., Markovchick, V. & Feldhaus, KM. (2000). Analysis of 1,076 cases of sexual assault. Ann Emerg Med. 35(4):358-62.

Rind, B., & Tromovitch, P., (1997). A meta-analytic review of findings from national samples on psychological correlates of child sexual abuse. *The Journal of Sex Research,* 34, 237-255

Safran, N. (1998). Irza geçme mağdurlarına toplumun bakış açısı. Yüksek Lisans Tezi, I.U. Adli Tıp Ens. Istanbul (in Turkish)

Sahu, G., Mohanty, S. & Dash, JK. (2005). Vulnerable victims of sexual assault. *Med Sci Law.* 45(3):256-60.

Santiago, JM., Mc Call-Perez, F., Gorcey, M. & Beigal, A. (1985). Long-term psychological effects of rape in 35 rape victims. *Am J Psychiatry* Nov;142(11):1338-40.

Sarafino, E. P. (1979). An estimate of nationwide incidence of sexual offenses against children. *Child Welfare,* 58, 127-134

Schönbucher, V., Maier, T., Held, L., Mohler-Kuo, M., Schnyder, U. & Landolt, MA. (2011). Prevalence of child sexual abuse in Switzerland: a systematic review. *Swiss Med Wkly.* 20;140:w13123

Siegel, RM., Schubert, CJ., Myers, PA. & Shapiro, RA. (1995). The prevalence of sexually transmitted diseases in children and adolescents evaluated for sexual abuse in Cincinnati: rationale for limited STD testing in prepubertal girls. *Pediatrics,* 96:1090.

Stefanidou, M., Mourtzinis, D. & Spiliopoulou, C. (2005). Forensic identification of semen-a short communication. *Jura Medica,* 2: 357-365.

Sternberg, KJ., Lamb, ME., Orbach, Y., Esplin, PW. & Mitchell, S. (2001). Use of a structured investigative protocol enhances young children's responses to free-recall prompts in the course of forensic interviews. *J Appl Psychol.* 86(5):997-1005.

Tilelli, AJ., Turek, D. & Jaffe, AC. (1980). Sexual Abuse of Children — Clinical Findings and Implications for Management. *N Engl J Med.* 302:319-323

United Nations (1989). Convention on the Rights of the Child. Retrieved 2011-03-25. Available from: http://www.crin.org/resources/treaties/CRC.asp?catName=International+Treatie

U.S. Department of Health & Human Services. Injury and Violence Prevention. Retrieved 2011-03-25. Available from: http://www.hhs.gov/opa/pubs/hp2010/hp2010rh_sec2_ivp.pdf

World Health Organization (1999). Report of the consultation on child abuse prevention. Geneva, 1999.p.13-7. Retrieved 2011-03-25. Available from: http://whqlibdoc.who.int/hq/1999/aaa00302.pdf

World Health Organization (2002). First World Report on Violence and Health, 149-151 Retrieved 2011-03-25. Available from: http://whqlibdoc.who.int/hq/2002/9241545615.pdf

Wyatt, G. E. (1985). The sexual abuse of Afro-American and White-American women in childhood. *Child Abuse and Neglect*, 9, 507-519.

Young, KJ., Jones, JG., Worthington, T., Simpson, P. & Casey, PH. (2006). Forensic laboratory evidence in sexually abused children and adolescents. *Arch Pediatr Adolesc Med*, 160: 585-8.

10

Cannabinoids: Forensic Toxicology and Therapeutics

Helena M. Teixeira[1,2,3] and Flávio Reis[4]
[1]*National Institute of Legal Medicine – North Branch and CENCIFOR – Forensic Sciences Center, Portugal*
[2]*Medicine Faculty, University of Coimbra*
[3]*Medicine Faculty University of Porto*
[4]*Laboratory of Pharmacology and Experimental Therapeutics, IBILI, Medicine Faculty, University of Coimbra*
Portugal

1. Introduction

Marijuana, hashish and other psychoactive products obtained from *Cannabis sativa* are the most produced and trafficked illicit drugs around the world (CND, 2006).
It is difficult to estimate the moment when man began to use some of the preparations from *cannabis sativa*. Thus, the reported consumption of the plant and its derivatives appears as an ancient practice, in many parts of the globe, from India to China, extending from the Middle East (Persia, Asia Minor and Egypt) to Africa, through the Christian culture, until the West (Ellenhorn & Barceloux, 1988; Ladrón de Guevara & Moya Pueyo, 1995; Rodríguez-Vicente et al., 1995). The effects that these compounds have on an individual brain have been addressed in several instances, such as religious practice, or simply in the search of pleasurable sensations. *Cannabis sativa* has been used in China nearly for five thousand years, being its cultivation related to fiber, oil and seeds production (Camp, 1936). However, Asians also knew its narcotic action in the seventh century BC, incorporating *cannabis* in their religious rituals and as a therapeutic agent, in neurological and psychiatric diseases (Mechoulam, 1991).
Cannabis consumption came to the Iberian Peninsula across North Africa, once conquered by the Arabs. But its presence was ephemeral, not achieving a significant presence on all the Christian kingdoms (Nahas, 1982). Ramazzini, an eighteenth century physician, studied its potential toxic effects, but it was O'Shaughnessy, an Irish surgeon who lived in India as a British colonial army doctor, the first scientific researcher to carry out pharmacological studies with the plant and the promoter of its application in therapy (Nahas, 1973; O'Shaughnessy, 1842). Thus, in 1842, after reviewing its therapeutic use in India and after some experimental research on animals, he introduced *Cannabis* in Europe (Robson, 2001). Indeed, this doctor was impressed with the outstanding application of this drug as a muscle relaxant, anticonvulsant, analgesic and anti-emetic. However, due to its uncontrollable power, there was a rapid decline in its therapeutic value. Thus, in 1840, the French physician Jacques-Joseph Moreau, considered as the father of psychopharmacology, described in his book "*Du Haschisch et de l'alienation mentale, Psychologiques études*" (1845), the toxic effects of

hallucinogens, calling attention to the danger of its use, since it could produce individual and social deterioration, and also cause addiction. Since 1971, the use of *cannabis* was controlled by the so-called "Drug Abuse Act", which forbade the use of both medical herbs and their active constituents, cannabinoids. Its use had already been removed from medical practice since 1932, the year it was eliminated from the British Pharmacopoeia. Ten years later, it was removed from the United States and 34 years later, from the Indian Pharmacopoeia. The controversy over its hallucinogenic actions on the brain has eclipsed its possible medical uses (Evans, 1997).

Cannabis consumption as a drug of abuse begins to spread in some European countries in the 60's and was popularized in the '70s and '80s. It is estimated that, presently, *cannabis* world production mainly occurs in America (46%), followed by Africa (26%) and by Asia (22%) (UNODC, 2007).

2. Botany: Cannabis sativa L

The genus *Cannabis* is composed of a single plant species, *Cannabis sativa* Linn., classified by Linnaeus in 1753, based on specimens from India but with different shapes. The morphological characteristics, fiber production, oils or resins, and even the size, are so varied that botanical classification becomes very difficult (Astolfi et al., 1979; Ellenhorn & Barceloux, 1988; Rodríguez-Vicente et al., 1995). Some botanists argue for the existence of three species: *Cannabis sativa, Cannabis indica* and *Cannabis ruderalis*, while others admit the existence of only two. *Cannabis sativa*, hemp common name (*Cannabis* means hemp; *sativa* means sowing or cultivating), is a plant endemic to a geographic area between the Caspian and Black Seas, passing through Persia and India, growing up in the Far East since ancient times. Under normal conditions it can have one or two meters height reaching, in its highest development stage, up to four meters. *Cannabis sativa* has been cultivated, for centuries, due to the hemp present on the stems, seeds and oil and due to its biological active substance (Δ^9-Tetrahydrocannabinol) in the higher parts with flowers, varying its chemical composition according to the different parts of the plant. The plant growth favourable conditions are a moist soil with high nitrogen content, being the clayey soils the worse conditions to its growth (Wilsie & Reddy, 1946). This plant has been adapting to different climates, adaptation accompanied by morphological changes, especially related to the leaf (Eckler & Miller, 1912). In fact, plant cannabinoids chemistry is much more complicated than the pure Δ^9-THC and thus, multiple effects can be expected due to the additional cannabinoids presence as well as other chemicals (Turner et al., 1980).

3. Consumption patterns

The potency of *cannabis* products is determined by its Δ^9-THC content, usually given as a percentage of Δ^9-THC. ElSohly et al. (2000) estimated, in a study performed between 1980 and 1997 in confiscated *marijuana* samples, that Δ^9-THC percentage was between 1.5 and 4.2%, being, however, sometimes higher. The highest percentages were found in *marijuana* samples (29.9%), *hashish* (52.9%) and oil (47.0%). In 2005, the average or typical level of Δ^9-THC *Cannabis* resin at the retail level ranged between 1% and 17%, being this variation range difficult to explain given the common origin of most European resin.

Over the past 20 years, more modern farming methods and crops increasingly sophisticated have been developed, leading to increased potency on *Cannabis* products. In the so-called "flower power" days from the 60s and 70s, every *marijuana* cigarette contained about 10 mg of Δ^9-THC. Currently, a cigarette can have about 150 mg Δ^9-THC (Δ^9-THC between 6 and 20%, corresponding to 60-200 mg/cigarette) or 300 mg, if mixed with *hashish* oil. Thus, nowadays, a *cannabis* consumer is frankly exposed to higher doses than in previous 60 or 70 decades (Gold, 1991; Mendelson, 1987; Schwartz, 1991). However, the Δ^9-THC content also varies extraordinarily, depending on the different *Cannabis* sources and preparations. In fact, there are several *Cannabis* preparations, leading to different consumption forms and different names (even according to different countries), as well as different power degrees (Astolfi et al., 1979; Ellenhorn & Barceloux, 1988; Rodríguez-Vicente et al., 1995): the herb, consisting of several parts of the plant, presents a variable active ingredients quantity depending on the part of the plant used for its preparation. It is usually smoked alone, but it may be mixed with tobacco. It has different names according to the country (among others, in Portugal and in Mexico, *marijuana;* in Morocco and Spain, *grifa* or *marihuana;* in South Africa, *dagga;* in Great-Britain, *hemp;* in Brazil, *maconha*); the resin, also called *haxixe, hachis, hashis, hash, charas* or *chira,* is five to eight times more potent than the herb, being the product spontaneously secreted by plants in small drops, thus corresponding to the resin of the plant. It can also be extracted from the plant through organic solvents. It can be smoked in special pipes or in cigarettes, being the resin, after burning, mixed with tobacco; the hash oil, obtained by hot extraction of the plant or by hashish extraction with organic solvents and consequent evaporation, has, as a concentrated resin, a high power.

Class	N° compound in the plant	Class	N° compound in the plant
Cannabinoids	61	*Simple ketones*	13
Cannabigerol (CBG)	6	*Simple acids*	20
Cannabichromene (CBC)	4	*Fatty acids*	12
Cannabidiol (CBD)	7	*Simple esters and lactones*	13
$\Delta^{1(9)}$-THC	9	*Steroids*	11
$\Delta^{1(8)}$-THC	2	*Sugars and similar*	34
Cannabiciclol (CBL)	3	Monosaccharides	13
Cannabielsoin (CBE)	3	Disaccharides	2
Cannabinol (CBN)	6	Polysaccharides	5
Cannabinodiol (CBND)	2	Cyclitols	12
Cannabitriol (CBT)	6	Amino-sugars	2
Other Cannabinoids	13	Terpenes	103
Nitrogen compounds	20	Monoterpenes	58
Quaternary bases	5	Sesquiterpenes	38
Amides	1	Diterpenes	1
Amines	12	Triterpenes	2
Alkaloids spermidines	2	Mixture of terpenoid	4
Amino Acids	18	*Non-cannabinoid phenols*	16
Proteins, glycoproteins & enzymes	9	*Flavonoid glycosides*	19
Hydrocarbons	50	*Vitamins*	1
Simple alcohols	7	*Pigments*	2
Simple aldehydes	12	*Total*	421

Table 1. Compounds classes found in Cannabis sativa (Honório & Silva, 2006).

4. Chemical structure and properties

Cannabis sativa present a large number of different chemicals, as illustrated in Table 1, being cannabinoids the main class. These compounds vary in number and quantity, according to the climate, soil type, variety cultivated and the way the crop was performed.
The observed variations also depend on the part of the plant used for their extraction, the drugs preparation method for the consumption, as well as its storage conditions (Waller, 1971). *Cannabis* contains about 421 different chemical compounds, including 61 cannabinoids (Turner et al., 1980). During the consumption by smoking, more than 2000 compounds can be produced by pyrolysis. Eighteen different classes of chemicals, including nitrogen compounds, amino acids, hydrocarbons, sugars and fatty acids can contribute to the single known pharmacological and toxicological properties of cannabinoids (Huestis, 2002). The term "cannabinoid" was attributed to the compound's group with 21 carbon atoms present in *Cannabis sativa,* also added to their carboxylic acids, analogs and possible transformation products (Honório & Silva, 2006). They are usually formed by three rings, cyclohexene, benzene and tetrahidropiran. Some are the responsible for the power of the various psychoactive plant preparations (Mendelson, 1987).

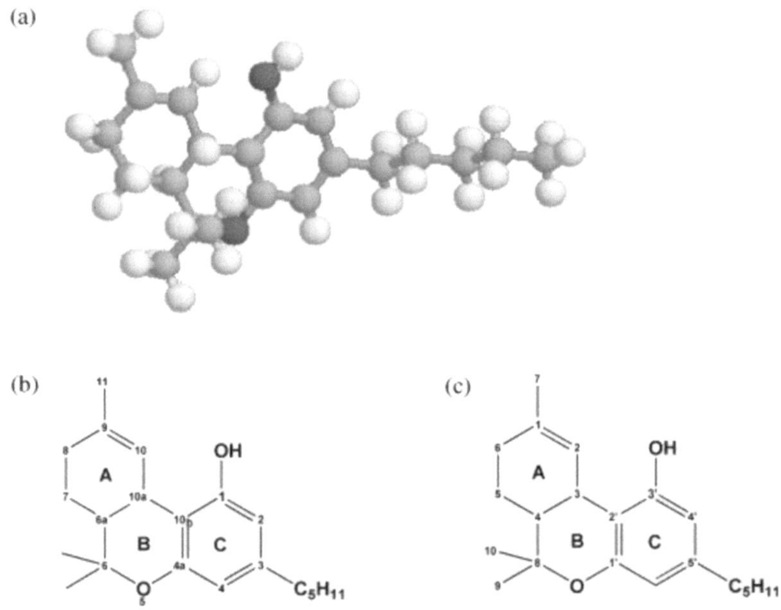

Fig. 1. Cannabinoid 3*D* chemical structure (a) and linear structures of two numbering systems used for cannabinoid compounds (b) and (c) (*Honório & Silva, 2006*).

The chemical structure of a cannabinoid type is shown in Figure 1, indicating the main numbering systems in the literature. The first report of proven isolation of the *cannabis* active ingredient in its pure form, Δ^9- Tetrahydrocannabinol or simply Δ^9-THC, dates from 1964, by Gaon and Mechoulam. Due to the great interest in the effects caused by the compounds extracted from *cannabis,* several studies have been conducted with the aim of identifying possible relationships between their chemical structure and their biological

activity. Cannabinol (CBN) was the first known cannabinoid, a phenolic compound resin obtained by Wood and collaborators in 1896. Canh, in 1932 got its cleansing in the crystalline acetate form, demonstrating that it is a phenolic derivative of dibenzopiran. Later, thanks to Cahn (1933) and Adams (1940), the structure of the CBN was established.
In 1940, Adams and Baker isolated another *cannabis* resin principle, which designated as Cannabidiol (CBD). Both CBN and CBD have lack active and enhancer effects. Later, in 1970, Mechoulam demonstrated that in the plant, there is a cannabinoids biosynthesis cycle that relates them, proving that the different components isolated by different authors were intermediate products. Although it is known that Δ^9-THC has six isomers (as an isomerization result), only the isomers Δ^9-THC e Δ^8-THC were isolated from the natural product. Of all the natural cannabinoids, Δ^9-THC is the most active compound, existing in the two forms mentioned above.

5. Cannabinoids properties

In fact, Δ^9-THC is the psychoactive cannabinoid with higher potency. Concerning the other cannabinoids present in the plant and about which there is some information:

i. Δ^8-THC presents a very similar pharmacological profile to that of Δ^9-THC, although lower, and thus, it has been studied for its possible use in drugs without psychoactive effects. This compound is only present is some plant varieties, being its concentration much lower when compared to Δ^9-THC (Mechoulam et al., 1992).

ii. CBN (Canabinnol) also has some psychoactive properties, among which are those related to the Δ^9-THC discriminative stimuli (Järbe & Mathis, 1992). This activity is, in animals, about one tenth of the described for Δ^9-THC. However, the results in humans have been quite contradictory, since some authors found that, by its intravenous administration, the CBN produces similar effects to those described for Δ^9-THC (Pérez-Reyes et al., 1973), contrary to those observed by Hollister (1974), who didn't detect any effect when administration was performed orally.

In fact, when comparing with Δ^9-THC, CBN has a higher affinity for the CB2 cannabinoid receptors than for the CB1 cannabinoid receptors (Munro et al., 1993). Being CB2 a peripheral receptor, CBN seems to participate in the immune system modulation, having been attributed, a long ago, to cannabinoids.
iii) CBD (Cannabidiol) is a cannabinoid practically devoid of psychoactive properties, since it is not capable to disconnect, from a CB1 receptor, neither an agonist nor an antagonist (Thomas et al., 1998). Since it is not a psychoactive substance, a detailed research has been developed in order to evaluate its possible clinical effects, and it has been described at least one case where its oral administration resulted in an effective long-term treatment of a psychosis framework (Zuardi et al., 1995).
We can, thus, say that cannabinoids properties depend on their chemical structure. Minimal variations in the THC molecule components can cause major changes in its activity.

6. Toxicokinetics

6.1 Absorption

Δ^9-THC absorption varies depending on the administration route. Inhalation is the most common administration route among *cannabis* consumers (smoke inhalation from water pipes or cigarettes), although there are also references to its use either orally (beverages or food ingestion) or parenteral, providing a rapid and efficient method for drug distribution in the body. *Cannabis sativa* preparations (*hashish, marijuana*) are mainly consumed in cigarettes, and approximately 30% of the Δ9-THC present in *marijuana* cigarettes or *hashish* are destroyed by pyrolysis during smoking (Huestis, 2002). The combustion heat leads to THC acids transformation to Δ9-THC, as well as Δ8-THC synthesis from CBD. Simultaneously, the existent Δ9-THC is largely destroyed by smoking, originating CBN. This suggests that the maximum amount of Δ9-THC absorbed during smoking does not exceed 70% of the Δ9-THC content existent in the cigarettes. The intense pleasure effects can be produced due to the almost immediate CNS exposure to the drug. In fact, after smoking, there is a rapid absorption of Δ9-THC through the respiratory tract into the bloodstream. However, about 18% of an inhaled Δ9-THC dose is absorbed (Ohlsson et al., 1980), being an oral dose significantly less effective (Nahas, 1979). Moreover, Δ9-THC bioavailability after inhalation is highly variable (Barnett et al., 1982, Lindgren et al. 1981; Ohlsson et al. 1980; Ohlsson et al., 1982, Pérez-Reyes et al., 1982), because it is affected, not only by the specific characteristics of the cigarette and its corresponding combustion, but also by the inhalation intensity, administration duration, among other factors. Experienced smokers inhale more efficiently than inexperienced people, being the Δ9-THC bioavailability, in a *marijuana* cigarette with approximately 1-2% of the drug, between 16 and 40% for chronic users and between 13 and 14% for occasional users (Ohlsson et al., 1982). Cannabinoids oral ingestion leads to lower plasma Δ9-THC levels than by inhalation, i.e., gastrointestinal absorption represents, approximately, one third of the achieved via inhalation. Orally, its bioavailability is reduced due to the gastric fluid acidity, the intestinal metabolism, as well as the first-pass enterohepatic system effect (Agurell et al., 1986). It has been observed that in acidic conditions (at a pH above 4.0), Δ9-THC isomerizes, giving rise to Δ8-THC or 9-hidroxihexahidrocanabinol. At a more acidic pH, the rupture of the pyran ring occurs, leading to the formation of several replaced cannabinoids. These changes could possibly explain the loss of Δ9-THC activity after oral administration due to the acidic pH of the stomach (Garret et al., 1978). However, large intra-and inter-individual differences may also contribute to uncertainty in the effective dose distribution (Agurell et al. 1986; Ohlsson et al., 1982).

Δ9-THC can be detected in plasma within seconds after inhaling the smoke of a *marijuana* cigarette ([a]Huestis et al., 1992), with plasma peak levels reached about 7 to 8 minutes after starting smoking, with euphoria and a maximum heart acceleration at about 20 minutes after (Perez-Reyes et al., 1982). However, after an oral administration, absorption is slow and irregular (Blaw et al. 1984; Ohlsson et al., 1980, Wall et al., 1983), reaching the highest Δ9-THC plasma levels about 45 minutes after ingestion and remaining relatively constant for 4 to 6 hours (Wall et al., 1983). The clinical effects begin 30-60 minutes after oral consumption, reaching a peak 2-3 hours after ingestion (Isbell et al., 1967) and it can hardly be correlated with plasma levels. Bioavailability is reduced in about 20-40% after oral administration (Ohlsson et al., 1980, Wall et al., 1983) due to the drug degradation within the gastrointestinal tract (Perez-Reyes et al., 1973). We can, thus, say that a greater oral amount of Δ9-THC is required to achieve the same physiological effects as by inhalation. Moreover, after oral administration, a gradual increase of its plasma concentration is produced and it can last for several hours, delaying the onset of their psychoactive effects (Cone and Huestis, 1993).

6.2 Distribution

Studies on Δ9-THC bioavailability showed considerable differences between pulmonary and oral routes. Smoking seems to be the most effective method for drug administration. Δ9-THC

entrance in the blood and its subsequent distribution to the tissues is very rapid, with very similar kinetics to the ones obtained after an intravenous administration.
Only 3% of the Δ9-THC detected in the blood is in its free form. About 97 to 99% is bound to plasma proteins, primarily (60%) to lipoproteins (α and β) (Hunt & Jones, 1980; Wall et al., 1983) and the remain to albumin at a 6: 4 ratio. For this reason, the free concentration in plasma is actually very low (Klansner et al., 1975), being in the erythrocytes in only about 10% (Garret & Hunt, 1974; Widman et al., 1974). With a large distribution volume (10L/Kg), high Δ9-THC lipid solubility leads to increased concentration and prolonged retention of the drug in fatty tissues ([a]Johansson *e col.*, 1989), like the nervous tissue. Indeed, concerning its effective distribution in the tissues, Δ9-THC is pulled out from the plasma to the tissues in about 70% (Hunt and Jones, 1980), although the distribution (which only occurs for the free fraction) is limited by the low concentration of its free form in the blood. Therefore, this distribution will depend on each organ blood flow. Consequently, given the greater distribution through more vascularized organs, and due to its high lipid solubility, brain is the organ where higher Δ9-THC concentrations are achieved: 3 to 6 times higher than in plasma and just in 30 minutes.
Initial studies in animals, after Δ9-THC administration, marked with ^{14}C, showed that Δ9-THC concentrations in the tissues (in many cases of Δ9-THC and metabolites) were higher in the lung, liver, kidney, heart, stomach, spleen, fat gray, placenta, thyroid, pituitary and mammary gland, when compared with brain or blood (Kreuz & Axelrod, 1973; Leighty, 1973; Ryrfeldt et al., 1973, Siemens et al., 1979). Later studies in rabbits also suggested that the highest Δ9-THC concentrations can be detected in fat and in the heart, but not in the brain (Leuschner et al., 1986). The relatively low Δ9-THC levels found in the brain can be, mainly due to its strong irrigation and consequent rapid and constant Δ9-THC transportation from the blood into and out of the brain. Afterwards, it distributes by adipose tissue, which is, together with the spleen, its major deposit, three days after administration (Rawich et al., 1979). Several weeks are needed for the drug to be completely eliminated, even after discontinuing the administration (Kreuz & Axelrod, 1973). A slow cannabinoids release from fatty tissues and a significant enterohepatic recirculation contributes to the long half-life in plasma, which has been estimated to be around 4 days, or even more in chronic *marijuana* users (Johansson et al., 1988). Moreover, cannabinoids may remain the double of the time, in the plasma of regular smokers (Mason et al., 1983). In fact, this gradual cannabinoids release from the tissues to the bloodstream extends its presence in the blood and subsequent entry into the brain, being this one possible explanation for the absence of a withdrawal syndrome when the administration is suspended (Agurell et al., 1986).

6.3 Metabolism

Only a minimal amount of Δ9-THC is eliminated from the body in its original form (with less than 1% excreted by the kidneys in its unchanged form), and most appear as metabolites in faeces (68%) or in urine (12%). The drug is also present in other tissues and biological fluids such as saliva, hair and sweat. Δ9-THC is almost completely metabolized in the liver, although metabolism can also occur in the lung and intestine (Agurell et al., 1986).
In man, Δ9-THC metabolism involves allylic oxidation, epoxidation, aliphatic oxidation, decarboxylation and conjugation reactions. The allylic oxidation at C-8 and C-11 and aliphatic oxidation at the side chain lead to the formation of hydroxylated metabolites. The mono- and di-hydroxy metabolites are then oxidized to form acids and hydroxy acids.

Thus, in studies performed in vivo and in vitro, it was been shown that Δ^9-THC is primarily metabolized in its hydroxylated compound by the hepatic microsomal enzymes (cytochrome P450) by allylic hydroxylation at carbon 11. Δ^9-THC is metabolized in 11-hydroxy-Δ^9-tetrahydrocannabinol (Δ^9-THC-OH) (Iribarne et al., 1996, Matsunaga et al., 1995), considered to be his true active metabolite (Lemberger et al., 1970). Similarly, Δ^8-THC follows a very comparable degradation pathway (Agurell et al., 1981), being rapidly hydroxylated to 11-hydroxy-Δ^8-tetrahydrocannabinol in the liver (Matsunaga et al., 1995).
Hydroxylation at position 11 is the most important Δ^9-THC metabolism reaction in most species, including humans. The 11-hydroxy-Δ^9-tetrahydrocannabinol (Δ^9-THC-OH) has a similar pharmacological activity and potency than Δ^9-THC. Δ^9-THC-OH is quantifiable in plasma 10 minutes after a Δ^9-THC intravenous administration. However, by oral administration, the relationship between this metabolite and the main drug is about 5 times higher than the one measured after an intravenous administration (Lemberger et al., 1971). Even so, plasma concentrations achieved after oral administration can range from 50 to 100% when compared to the detected Δ^9-THC concentrations (Wall et al., 1983). After smoking *marijuana*, the detected Δ^9-THC-OH concentrations are lower, about 10% of the Δ^9-THC concentrations ([a]Huestis et al., 1992; Wall et al., 1983), reaching the maximum Δ^9-THC - OH peak (Cmax) in approximately 13 minutes after smoking, with maximum concentrations of, around, 7 ng/ml, after a single *marijuana* cigarette.
After Δ^9-THC administration, its psychological effects begin to occur about 10 to 20 minutes after, although the effects caused by Δ^9-THC-OH are only evident about 3-5 minutes later (Lemberger et al., 1973). This difference may be due to their pharmacokinetic properties, particularly different distribution and transfer into the nervous system, since their effects are equivalent. This can also explain the fact that, after an oral administration, the pharmacodynamic effects are higher than those induced with the same Δ^9-THC concentration, but reached after smoking (Ohlsson et al., 1980). However the biotransformation process continues, and the active metabolite Δ^9-THC-OH may oxidize, giving rise to the corresponding carboxylic acid (Δ^9-THC-COOH) or return to hydroxylate itself. In this second case, it converts to 8, 11-dihydroxy-Δ^9-THC, i.e., 11-hydroxy derivative transformation occurs in the liver into dihydroxy-Δ^9-THC. These compounds are then transformed into other hydroxylated metabolites, more polar, inactive, which are then excreted in urine and faeces. The Δ^9-THC-OH oxidation leads to the production of an inactive metabolite, 11-nor-9-carboxy-Δ^9-tetrahydrocannabinol (Δ^9-THC-COOH) (Lemberger et al., 1972), identified in plasma, urine and faeces (Wall & Perez-Reyes, 1981, Wall et al., 1983). Subsequently, conjugation with the glucuronic acid can occur, being Δ^9-THC-COOH and its glucuronide conjugates the main end biotransformation products in many species, including humans (Halldin & Widman, 1983). Renal clearance of these polar metabolites is always slow due to its extensive plasma protein binding (Hunt & Jones, 1980). After smoking, Δ^9-THC-COOH plasma concentrations gradually increase, becoming higher than Δ^9-THC concentrations shortly after smoking, whereas Δ^9-THC plasma concentrations decrease very rapidly ([a]Huestis et al., 1992). Hence, the Δ^9-THC-COOH detection time is much higher than for Δ^9-THC or for Δ^9-THC-OH. The CBD (Cannabidiol) metabolism is quite complex, with the possible production of almost 83 metabolites (Harvey, 1991). The proportions of these compounds also vary between species (Harvey & Mechoulam, 1990).
The metabolism of CBN (cannabinol) is less complex than for other cannabinoids. In most species, the hydroxylation at C-11 predominates, although there is also an important side

chain hydroxylation. The excreted metabolites are mainly 11-hydroxy-CBN, the CBN acid-11-oic acid and its hydroxylated side chain analogues (Brown and Harvey, 1990).

6.4 Elimination

Over 65% of the drug is excreted in faeces (68%), with approximately 13% excreted in urine (Wall et al., 1983). A total of 80-90% is excreted in 5 days, mainly in the hydroxylated and carboxylated metabolites forms. Only minimal amounts are excreted in their free forms (Hunt & Jones, 1980, Wall et al., 1983). Therefore, we can say that both Δ^9-THC and Δ^8-THC are not eliminated in their free form but in the form of metabolites (THC-OH and/or THC-COOH) or by glucuronic acid conjugation, producing different glucuronides. This process takes place in the liver involving several enzymes. The glucuronides formed are highly hydrophilic and therefore easily eliminated in the urine. Δ^9-THC-COOH metabolite has been detected in either urine or faeces (Wall & Perez-Reyes, 1981), while Δ^9-THC-OH predominates in the faeces. In fact, biliary excretion, and the consequent elimination through the faeces is the major route of unconjugated metabolites elimination (Wall et al., 1983), although most of the metabolites are reabsorbed from the gut. This enterohepatic circulation, which leads to more than 15% of the metabolites (Nahas, 1979), is responsible for the delay in the final active metabolites disposition, contributing to a prolonged excretion and to its accumulation among different body tissues.

In urine a total of 20 Δ^9-THC metabolites were identified, two glucuronic acid and 18 unconjugated acids forms. Indeed, the Δ^9-THC-COOH glucuronide conjugate is the primary urinary metabolite formed (Williams & Moffat, 1980). All other unconjugated acids metabolites identified in urine, excepting the 11-nor-9-Δ^9-THC-COOH, undergo oxidation or are degraded, forming varied carboxylated or hydroxylated metabolites. The average life of the inactive metabolites is about seven days, staying in the body for up to thirty days (Sutheimer et al., 1985). Some authors even accept the metabolites presence in urine within 72 days after use (Ellis et al., 1985), despite having an estimated Δ^9-THC plasma elimination time of 4 days ([a]Johansson et al., 1989).

7. Action mechanism

For a long time ago, some hypotheses had been proposed to explain Δ^9-THC action mechanism, suggesting that Δ^9-THC may exert its actions through a nonspecific drug interaction with cell membranes and intracellular organelles (Hillard et al., 1985; Martin, 1986). However, it is notoriously difficult to delineate the precise action mechanisms of cannabinoids, given the evident Δ^9-THC activity in several places, including the receptors for opiates and benzodiazepines, as well as marked effects on prostaglandins synthesis and protein metabolism (Burstein et al. 1982; Welch & Eads, 1999). Cannabinoids inhibit macromolecular metabolism according to the dose, presenting a wide effects range on the enzyme systems, neurotransmitters and hormone secretion (Bloom, 1982, Chakravarty et al. 1975; Dalterio et al. 1977; Dalterio et al. 1987; Dill & Howlett, 1988; Pertwee, 1988). These numerous and diffuse effects supported the hypothesis of a nonspecific interaction. However, with cannabinoids pharmacology knowledge advance, it became obvious that some structural aspects would be required for the cannabinoids activity, including the receptor binding in the target cells (Mechoulam, 1991).

7.1 Cannabinoid receptors

Nowadays it is clearly known that cannabinoids act through its interaction with specific endogenous receptors, discovered by Devane et al. (1988) and later colonized. Indeed, a specific protein receptor was discovered, named CB1 (central receptors) (Matsuda et al., 1990, Munro et al., 1993), in the mouse nerve cells, being now known that it can also be found in the brain of the mouse, guinea pig, dog, monkey, pig and man, and peripheral nerves. The biology and behaviour associated with brain areas are consistent with the behavioural effects produced by cannabinoids (Table 2). The highest density of receptors is found in the basal ganglia cells, involved in coordinating body movements.

A) - Brain regions where cannabinoid receptors are abundant	
Brain regions	*Tasks associated with the region*
Basal ganglia	Motion control
Cerebellum	Coordination of body movements
Hippocampus	Learning, memory, stress
Cerebral Cortex	Cognitive functions
B) - Brain regions where cannabinoid receptors are moderately concentrated	
Brain regions	*Tasks associated with the region*
Hypothalamus	Maintenance of body functions (temperature, electrolyte balance, reproductive function)
Amygdale	Emotional response, fear
Backbone	Peripheral sensation, including pain
Brainstem	Sleep, temperature regulation, motor control

Table 2. Brain regions where cannabinoid receptors are abundant or moderately concentrated and functions associated with these areas *(Honório & Silva, 2006)*.

CB1 receptors mediate the majority of the cannabinoids responses in the central nervous system (CNS), being abundant in the cerebral cortex, hippocampus, amygdale, basal ganglia, cerebellum, and thalamus (Ashton, 2001; Robson, 2001). The high receptors density in the caudate nucleus and cerebellum are consistent with the marked cannabinoids effects in motor behaviour (Romero et al. 1995; Sanudo-Pena et al., 2000). The significant link within the cerebral cortex and hippocampus explains the marked cannabinoids effects on perception, cognitive aspects, memory, learning, endocrine function and body temperature regulation (Chait & Perry, 1994, Compton et al. 1993; Hampson & Deadwyler, 1999).

The CB1 receptors location in the hippocampus supports that cannabinoids play an import role in appetite and energy regulation. This supposition is strengthened by its presence in important peripheral organs, as the GI tract, liver, skeletal muscle and adipose tissue.

Despite being primarily viewed as a central receptor (presence in the nervous tissue) (Herkenham et al., 1990), this CB1 receptor was also found in the adipose tissue (Bensaid et al., 2003), myocardium (Bonz et al. 2003), vascular endothelium (Liu et al., 2000) and in sympathetic nerve terminals (Ishac et al., 1996).

In 1993, Munro et al. identified a second cannabinoid receptor, the CB2 receptor, present, preferentially, in the immune system cells, outside the CNS (peripheral receptor). Efforts have been made to improve the chemical manipulation of cannabinoids, to maximize the selectivity for these receptors CB2, avoiding the psychoactive effects (Robson, 2001). This distinctive peripheral cannabinoid receptor seems to play a major role in immunomodulation (Lynn & Herkenham, 1994; Reggio et al., 1997), showing a significant anti-inflammatory and immunosuppressive activity. It has already been postulated the existence of a third receptor - CB_3 - (Fride et al., 2003), but the receptor itself has not been colonized yet. It is believed now that the two cannabinoid receptors - CB1 e CB2 - are responsible for many biochemical and pharmacological effects produced by the majority of cannabinoid compounds (Matsuda et al., 1990). The functional differences existent between the two receptors types are still not known, but structural differences raise that possibility.

In 1986, Howlett et al. showed that Δ^9-THC inhibited the intracellular enzyme adenylyl cyclase (AC) and that this inhibition occurred only in the presence of a G-protein complex, this is, in the presence of a cannabinoid receptor, which is a typical member of the largest known receptors family: G-coupled protein, containing seven transmembrane domains (Glass & Northup, 1999; Howlett et al., 1991). The body's cells respond in different ways when a ligand interacts with the cannabinoid receptor. The receptor intracellular surface interacts with G proteins that regulate effectors' proteins such as AC, or calcium and potassium channels, and via a protein kinase activated by mitogen (Bayewitch et al. 1996; Bidaut-Russell et al. 1990).

7.2 Endogenous cannabinoids

The cannabinoid receptors discovery prompted the search for an endogenous ligand to which the receptors naturally interact. For each biological receptor (in this case, a brain receptor) there is probably an endogenous agonist, i.e., a compound naturally produced by the body that interact with the receptor. The first endogenous cannabinoid discovered was arachidonoylethanolamine known as anandamide, derived from the Sanskrit word ananda, meaning "happiness." This substance was isolated from pig brain, by Devane et al. (1992), and these authors observed that, being chemically distinct from the cannabinoid plant, compared with Δ^9-THC, it has a moderate affinity for CB1 receptors, but with most of the Δ^9-THC actions, although having a short action period. In general, the affinity of anandamide for cannabinoid receptors is only ¼ to ½ the affinity displayed by Δ^9-THC, these differences being related to the cells or tissues used in those studies as well as with the other experimental conditions (Smith et al. , 1994). Anandamide mimics Δ^9-THC action since it binds to both receptor subtypes, CB1 and CB2, and has a similar pharmacological activity, despite having little power to exert some effects (Fride & Mechoulam, 1993; Howlett , 1995; Mechoulam & Hanus, 1996; Pertwee 1995). This ligand was found in several regions of the human brain (hippocampus, striatum and cerebellum) where CB1 receptors are abundant, suggesting the involvement of endogenous cannabinoids in the brain functions controlled by these areas. However, substantial concentrations of anandamide are also found in the thalamus, a brain area with few CB1 receptors (Di Marzo et al., 1994). An interesting fact is that anandamide was also found in small amounts in other parts of the body such as the spleen, where there are high concentrations of CB2 receptors, and heart (Ameri, 1999; Fowler, 2003; Howlett, 1998; Pop, 1999). It may, therefore, be concluded that the molecule anandamide has both central and peripheral impact (Di Marzo et al., 2000). Although Deutsch and Chin (1993) have proposed a biosynthetic pathway for anandamide, it appears that this gets rid of cell membranes followed by depolarization due to a calcium influx (Di Marzo, 1998, Evans et al., 1992). Also Sugiura et al. (1995) examined the effects of anandamide and another endogenous compound, 2-araquidonil glycerol (2-AG) in connection with a specific cannabinoid receptor, assuming that the latter substance can also be an endogenous ligand with relevant role in the brain. Under normal conditions, the endocannabinoid system appears to be tonically active; instead, the endocannabinoids are produced as needed, act locally and are rapidly inactivated by cellular uptake and enzymatic hydrolysis (Giuffrida et al., 2001).

In addition to the identification of these ligands there were also synthesized some specific CB1 receptors antagonists (Rinaldi-Carmona, 1994) and CB2 (Portier et al., 1999). The SR141716 (now under the name of Rimonabant) was the first specific CB1 antagonist receptor, with high affinity, blocking the acute effects of Δ^9-THC and other CB1 agonists in vitro and in animals (Adams et al. 1998; Rinaldi-Carmona, 1994). In 2001, Huestis et al., conducting the first clinical studies on the pharmacokinetic and pharmacodynamic effects of Rimonabant, administered orally, in combination with *cannabis* smoking, demonstrated that *cannabis* administration alone produced the expected physiological responses with the consequent intoxication reflection and, when combined with Rimonabant, a dose-dependent blocking effect of *cannabis* was observed. Significant advances in cannabinoid research have opened new frontiers leading to an increasing interpretation of their effects and the role of endogenous cannabinoids in man.

8. Pharmacodynamic effects

Due to their action mechanism, cannabinoids exert multiple conducts, acting in almost all biological systems. Its activity is multiple and complex due to the variety of psychoactive products present in the plant whose toxic and pharmacological actions may overlap or be additive. The main factors influencing the toxicity of these substances are: dose, administration route, individual's personality, dependence degree, concomitant administration of other substances and chronological stage of the administration.

The behavioural and physiological cannabinoids effects have been increasingly reported over the recent decades (Adams & Martin, 1996; Dewey, 1986; Jones, 1987), including euphoria and relaxation feelings, times reaction changes, lack of concentration, learning and memory changing or mood states (such as panic reactions and paranoia). The spectrum of cannabinoids behavioural effects is unique, leading to a consequent classification of these drugs as stimulants, tranquilizers, or hallucinogenic (Benowitz et al. 1979; Hollister, 1986; Law et al., 1984). Other common physiological effects include increased appetite, dry mouth, vasodilation and decreased respiratory rate. Cannabinoids may affect the immune and endocrine systems, producing lung damage and influencing neonatal and child development of (Chandler et al., 1996, Day et al., 1991, Fried et al. 1999; Fried & Smith, 2001; Tashkin et al., 1991). The physiological effects of cannabinoids are most relevant for the main systems are:

a. Effects on Cardiovascular System

The Δ^9-THC effects of on the cardiovascular system depend on the dose, with a decrease in heart rate with low doses and increased at higher doses (which may exceed 160 beats/min). This substance may also lead to a decrease in contractile force and lead to progressive reduction in coronary blood flow (Tashkin et al., 1978). Acute administration of cannabinoids in humans produces vasodilation and tachycardia, resulting in an overall effect on systemic blood pressure (Huestis et al., 1992). However, the unrelenting use of Δ^9-THC results in hypotension mediated by CB1 receptors and bradycardia (Benowitz et al., 1975, Lake et al., 1997). Endocannabinoids induce vasodilation by acting, directly, on CB1 receptors located in the arterial smooth muscle of the brain (Gebremedhin et al., 1999). Moreover, the same occurs at other vessels, through an increased synthesis of nitric oxide (NO) endothelium-dependent (Deutsch et al., 1997). These and many other effects on CV can be an increased risk for individuals with pre-existing heart disease (especially in patients with heart failure and coronary), as already reported, for example, in acute cardiac accidents cases, often fatal for *Cannabis* consumers (Ashton, 2001).

b. Metabolic Effects

The endocannabinoid system appears to play a crucial role in regulating metabolism and body composition. The appetite stimulation (especially for sweets) and dry mouth due to decreased salivary secretion are usually adverse reactions produced in *cannabis* consumers. The consequent weight loss may suppose that there is a changing in glucose metabolism. However, several studies show that there is no agreement on the glucose levels change (Hollister et al. 1968; Lindemann, 1933, Weil et al., 1969). However, its effect on other metabolic processes is of great significance. Thus, control of food intake and body composition results from complex interactions between the adipocytes, the mesolimbic system, hypothalamus and gastrointestinal tract. The hunger feeling often existent in consumers is mediated by an intestinal hormone, ghrelin, which is produced in most circumstances of weight loss. Moreover, leptin, an endogenous hormone, can reduce food intake. The serum concentration of this hormone is directly proportional to the degree of adiposity, but obese people have lower sensitivity to the hormone. A protein produced in adipose tissue, adiponectin stimulates fatty acid oxidation and body weight decrease, being its concentration lower in obese individuals (Considine et al., 1996, Cummings et al. 2002; Fruebis et al. 2001).

Both cannabinoid receptors and their endocannabinoids ligands are present in tissues related to food intake. The concentration of endocannabinoids in the hypothalamus decreases after leptin administration (Di Marzo et al., 2001). Studies in animals (rodents) showed that the CB1 receptor agonists are potent inducers of hyperphagia (Jamshidi et al., 2001, Kirkham et al., 2002, Williams et al., 1999), while their antagonists prevent such effect (Di Marzo et al., 2001). In another study, it was found that mice do not express CB1 receptors resulting in spontaneous calories reduction (Cota et al., 2003). For all these interferences at the cannabinoid system, metabolic modulation of this pathway has been considered to be a greater possibility for therapeutic intervention in obesity (Feliciano et al. 2007; Francischetti et al., 2006).

c. Effects on Pulmonary System

Inhaling the smoke of *marijuana* cigarettes (or Δ^9-THC) produces acute bronchodilation in healthy subjects and asthmatics, bronchodilation that may last at least one hour (Tashkin et al. 1977; Vachon et al., 1973). It is important to note that *cannabis* smokers have a higher lung cancer risk than tobacco consumers because of the high aromatic hydrocarbons content in *marijuana* smoke, which has higher concentrations of irritant substances, such as sterols, terpenes, among others (Fehr and Kalant, 1972). Comparing a normal about five times tobacco cigarette with a *marijuana* cigarette, it is estimated that the latter produces more carboxyhemoglobin, with consequent maintenance increase in the respiratory tract (Benson & Bentley, 1995, Wu et al., 1988). Chronic use of *cannabis* cigarettes is associated with bronchitis and emphysema. It is estimated that 3-4 *cannabis* cigarettes per day equals more than 20 tobacco cigarettes a day, with subsequent evidence of acute and chronic bronchitis (Benson and Bentley, 1995).

d. Effects on Vision
The administration of *cannabis* cigarettes in normal individuals causes a slight constriction of the pupil, preserving light reflection, marked congestion of conjunctiva vessels, tearing and intraocular pressure reduction related to dose. In fact, vasodilatation and redness of the conjunctiva is a characteristic sign of *cannabis* use (Paton & Pertwee, 1973). Other changes include colour perception and light adaptation changes (Ohlsson et al., 1980).

9. Cannabinoids and driving influence

Experimental studies have been repeatedly demonstrating Δ^9-THC effects on an individual cognitive function and psychomotor skills, influencing learning and information acquisition, changing the individual's memory capacity, coordination and reaction times (Chait & Pierri, 1992; Kurzthaler et al. 1999; Leire et al., 1989). The biggest concern with cannabinoids acute effects is related to road traffic or labour accidents (Hall, 2001). Indeed, Δ^9-THC acute effects on cognitive function and psychomotor skills have been subject of extensive study, noting that, at doses between 40 and 300 mg/kg, cannabinoids can cause a dose-dependent reduction in tasks that require memory use, reaction times, in motor functions and coordination (Ameri, 1999; Curran et al. 2002; D 'Souza et al. 2004; Hall & Solowij 1998; Hampson & Deadwyler 1999; Lewek et al. 1998; Lichtman et al. 2002; Ramaekers et al., 2004).
The impaired state induced by cannabinoids has been studied by several authors in tests performed on drivers (Lamers & Ramaekers, 2001; Ramaekers et al., 2000), demonstrating that their driving risk effects increase with the dose, being more extensive and persistent in activities that require more careful attention. There is an enormous concern, both in the European Union and in the United States of America (USA) regarding the link between cannabinoids consumption and traffic accidents. However, from a legal standpoint, the evaluation and interpretation of the corresponding accuracy is still a big challenge, since the association between Δ^9-THC levels and the accidents risk is not perfectly clear. Currently, some authors claim that there is very little scientific evidence demonstrating that Δ^9-THC or Δ^9-THC-COOH detection in body fluids can be used as impairment evidence in any circumstance. They assume, for example, that Δ^9-THC or its metabolite can be detected in the body for days after smoking *cannabis* and thus, their presence may be indicative of a previous consumption and not of a recent use, not being certain that the presence of the drug in the body indicates an impairment state (Drummer et al., 2003). Papafotiou et al. (2005), through experimental studies in volunteers, acknowledged that the negative relationship between driving performance and Δ^9-THC levels found in blood is due to the fact that the Δ^9-THC peak concentrations are achieved in the CNS a few time after being achieved in blood. Similarly to what occurs with benzodiazepines, where the maximum influenced state is observed one hour after peak plasma concentrations are reached (Rush & Griffiths, 1996), the maximum influenced state after Δ^9-THC consumption occurs after achieving the maximum blood concentration. On the other hand, it has been shown that the influence and accident risk due to recent *cannabis* increases with dose, with an influenced state already present at low doses, being even worse at higher concentrations (Ramaekers et al., 2004). Note, however, that it is not perfectly acknowledged how to correlate the plasma Δ^9-THC levels variation with driver's behaviour, although this relationship has been simulated in experimental behavioural cannabinoid pharmacodynamics and pharmacokinetics studies. Ramaekers et al. (2006) developed, thus, a study in *cannabis* consumers, concluding that the impairment sate was progressively higher with increasing

Δ⁹-THC concentrations. They admitted that already with Δ⁹-THC concentrations between 2 and 5 ng/ml there was significant influence state; when Δ⁹-THC was detected between 5 and 10 ng/ ml, about 75 to 90% of the individuals were under the influence and over 30 ng/ml, there was a were 100% influence. Cone and Huestis (1993) also conducted a similar research and concluded that the ability to drive may be influenced one hour after consumption, during the Δ⁹-THC elimination phase, even when the concentrations decrease to 13 ng/ml. Berghaus et al. (1995) go even further, stating that with 6 ng/ml of Δ⁹-THC the information processing is already affected, with attention and vision changes at 9 ng/ml and 12 ng/ml, respectively. They demonstrated that the Δ⁹-THC driving influence is mainly evident in the first two hours after consumption, leading to performance changes, with higher prevalence on attention, psychomotor and cognitive capacities.

10. Therapeutic perspectives of the endocannabinoid system modulation

Endocannabinoids (EC) are involved in several physiological functions, among which, special attention has been given to the regulation of appetite by central mechanisms and its influence on obesity (van Thuijl et al., 2008; Kirkham, 2009). Considering these innovative findings, the research for new pharmacological agents has drastically increased and the discovery of rimonabant, a synthetic antagonist of CB1 receptors, has confirmed the important role of endocannabinoid system on the modulation of food ingestion and energetic balance (Butler et al., 2009). These facts led to the first clinical studies using rimonabant as a new tool against obesity and its associated metabolic disorders. However, psychiatricside-effects, namely central, which include increased risk of depression and even suicide, US Food and Drug Administration declined permission for rimonabant, and in October 2008, rimonabant was also suspended across the EU. After rimonabant withdrawal, other CB1 antagonist drugs have also tested, including the taranabant, which was associated with weight loss in rats and in humans (Fong et al., 2007; Addy et al., 2008). However, due also to central side effects, including anxiety and depression, the clinical trials were stopped in October 2008 (EMEA. The European Medicines Agency recommends suspension of the marketing authorisation of Acomplia: http://www.emea.europa.eu 2008).

Although several other different influences of endocannabinoids have been discussed during the last years, including in inflammation, diabetes, cancer, affective and neurodegenerative diseases, and epilepsy (Izzo et al., 2009), the most recent findings are related to their cardiovascular actions (Durst & Lotan, 2011), which seem to be very ample bust also complex. *In vivo* experiments with rats have demonstrated the action of anandamide and 2-AG on the development of atherosclerotic plaque, as well as an effect on heart rate, blood pressure, vasoactivity and energy metabolism (action in dyslipidemia and obesity). Recent studies with an antagonist of CB1 receptors showed that the modulation of ECS can play an important role in reducing cardiovascular risk in obese and dyslipidemic patients. Similarly, studies in rats have demonstrated the action of CB2 receptors in adhesion, migration, proliferation and function of immune cells involved in the atherosclerotic plaque formation process. The ECS have been implicated in hypotensive stages associated with hemorrhagic chock, both endotoxic and cardiogenic, and even to advanced liver cirrhosis; on the other hand, recent evidence suggests that ECS plays an important role in cardiovascular regulation associated with hypertension, as well as a protective role in ischemia grafting. The development of atherosclerotic plaque and the metabolic stages associated to obesity are also matter of study of possible ECS pharmacomodulation.

Effects on myocardial ischemia/reperfusion and preconditioning

Initial studies used isolated preparations of heart to study the role of ECS in myocardial ischemia/reperfusion (I/R) and preconditioning. The involvement of ECS in preconditioning induced by the endotoxin (lipopolysaccharide: LPS) against the injury induced by I/R on myocardium has been implicated for the first time in 2001, based on the hypothesis that LPS could increase the production of endocannabinoids in inflammatory cells (Varga et al., 1998). A 90 minutes of low flow ischemia followed by 60 minutes of reperfusion with normal flow in isolated rat hearts pretreated with LPS was compared with a saline solution. The pretreatment with LPS reduced the infarct size and improved functional recovery after reperfusion when compared with control group, which could be attenuated by SR144528 (CB2 antagonist), but not by rimonabant (CB1 antagonist), suggesting the involvement of myocardium CB2 in the cardioprotection induced by LPS (Lagneux & Lamontagne, 2001). In a subsequent study, in which the preconditioning was triggered by heat stress, the SR144528 also abolished the effect of reducing the infarct size, unlike rimonabant (Joyeux et al., 2002).

These early studies suggested that the protection created by the preconditioning induced by heat stress or by LPS was mediated by the action of endocannabinoids in the CB2 receptors. In contrast, when preconditioning was induced by a brief period of ischemia (5 minutes), the blockade of CB1 and CB2 receptors did not raise the abolition of protection, and both receptors have been implicated in preserving endothelium-dependent vasodilatation induced by serotonin (Bouchard et al., 2003). The palmitoylethanolamide or the 2-AG, but not anandamide, when added to perfused isolated rat hearts offer protection against ischemia by reducing myocardial damage and infarct size and by improving the functional recovery of myocardium (Lepicier et al., 2003). The SR144528 completely blocked the cardioprotective effect of palmytoylethanolamide and 2-AG, whereas rimonabant only inhibited, partially, the effect of 2-AG (Lepicier et al., 2003). Similarly, ACEA and JWH015 (CB1 and CB2 agonists) also reduced the size of the infarct in this model (Lepicier et al., 2003). In contrast, it was found that anadamida's effect of reducing infarct area could also be antagonized by CB1 and CB2 antagonists; however, the same could not be mimicked by selective CB1 and CB2 agonists, suggesting an involvement of a different site of CB1 and CB2 receptors. Another recent study, which used a model of delayed preconditioning in rats, induced by transdermal treatment of nitroglycerin (as an NO donor) for 24 hours, suggested that the protective effect of nitroglycerin against myocardial infarction is mediated trough CB1 receptors. Nitroglycerin increased the concentration of 2-AG in myocardium, but did not increase anandamide (Wagner et al., 2006). These pioneer studies implicated a possible contribution of CB2 functional receptors in cardiomyocytes and the endothelial cells responsibility, at least in part, on the protective effects of preconditioning. Indeed, subsequent studies showed the presence of CB2 receptors in myocardium, in cardiomyoblast cells and in endothelial cells with different origins ((Mukhopadhyay et al., 2003; Blazquez et al., 2003). Concurrently with the beneficial effect of the activation of CB2 receptors in cardiomyocytes, a recent study showed that THC protected cardiomyoblast cells H9c2 submitted to hypoxia *in vitro*, presumably trough the activation of CB2 receptors and increased NO production (Shmist et al., 2006).

In an ischemia/reperfusion injury model in rats, both anandamide and HU-210 decreased the incidence of ventricular arrhythmias and reduced the size of the infarct, presumably trough the activation of CB2 receptors but not CB1 receptors (Krylatov et al., 2001). In an myocardic I/R injury model induced by ligation of coronary artery in rats, the reduction of the second myocardic injury depending on leucocytes subsequent to the initial I/R injury was attributed to the activation of CB2 receptors, since the protection given by WIN 55.212-2 could be prevented by AM630, but not by AM251 (a CB1 antagonist) (Di Filippo et al., 2004). Two recent studies in myocardial infarct models, acute and chronic, in rats, showed that cannabinoids contribute to hypotension and cardiac depression associated to cardiogenic acute shock, which could be attenuated by antagonists of CB1 receptors (Wagner et al., 2003).

Overall, despite the role of CB1 receptors and of endocannabinoids in the protection given by the preconditioning against myocardic I/R, the issue remains controversial, recommending further investigation namely using mice with deletion of genes and more selective agonists of CB2 receptors. However, the findings that imply CB2 receptors' importance, presumably in both endothelial and inflammatory cells and perhaps in cardiomyocytes, are quite encouraging.

Cerebral ischemia/reperfusion (cerebrovascular accident)

The ECS may constitute an essential mechanism of neuroprotection, in both acute forms of neuronal injury, such as stroke or brain trauma, and in several chronic neurodegenative disorders, including multiple sclerosis, Parkinson's disease, Hungtington's disease, Alzheimer's disease and amyotrophic lateral sclerosis (Pacher et al., 2006a). Although the exact mechanisms of this neuroprotection are not yet completely understood, several processes dependent and independent of CB receptors seem to be involved: 1) modulation of the immune responses and release of inflammatory mediators by CB1, CB2 and not CB1/not CB receptors in neurons, astrocytes, microglia, macrophages, neutrophils and lymphocytes (Klein, 2005); 2) modulation of synaptic plasticity and excitatory glutamatergic transmissions via presynaptic CB1 receptors (Freund et al., 2003); 3) activation of cytoprotective signaling pathways (Pacher et al., 2006a); 4) modulation of calcium homeostasis and excitability trough interactions with calcium channels, potassium and sodium, gap junctions and intracellular calcium reserves, and with NMDA receptors (Freund et al., 2003); 5) central hypothermia mediated by CB1 receptors, presumably by the reduction of the metabolic rate of needed oxygen; 6) antioxidant properties of cannabinoids (Hampson et al., 2000); 7) modulation of endothelial activity and inflammatory response, leucocytes mobilization, adhesions to the endothelium, transmigration and activation presumably through CB2 receptors. The first evidence of a neuroprotective effect of cannabinoids has emerged in research studies on cerebrovascular accident, in which was used the non psychoactive cannabinoid dexanabinol/HU-211 that exerts its effect through CB1/CB2 independent mechanisms, in cerebral ischemia models *in vivo* in rats and gerbils (Pacher et al., 2006a). Further studies also investigated the neuroprotective effects of CB1 receptors stimulation with synthetic agonists. The synthetic cannabinoid WIN 55.212-2 attenuated the neurological damage in the hypothalamus resulting from cerebral global and transient ischemia in rats and reduced infarct size after permanent focal cerebral ischemia induced by cerebral middle artery occlusion, when it was administrated 40 minutes before or 30 minutes after occlusion, in a dependent way from CB1 receptors, since the protective effect was prevented by rimonabant (Nagayama et al., 1999). WIN 55.212-2, as well as anandamide and 2-AG, did also confer protection to cultured cortical neurons submitted to hypoxia and glucose deprivation *in vitro*, but these effects proved to be insensitive to antagonists of CB1 and CB2 receptors (Nagayama et al., 1999).

In models of cerebral middle artery occlusion in rats, the agonist BAY38-7271 reduced the size of the infarct, even when administered intravenously 4 hours after the occlusion (Mauler et al., 2002). The pre-treatment with rimonabant partially attenuated the effect of HU-210, indicating the involvement of CB1 receptor. However, the protective effect of HU-210 could be completely abolished by warming the animals' body until the controls temperature, showing that hypothermia mediated by CB1 receptors was responsible for the beneficial effects observed (Leker et al., 2006). Similarly, hypothermia mediated by CB1 receptors was responsible for the neuroprotective effects of THC in a model of cerebral ischemic injury in rats (Hayakawa et al., 2004), and in a model of global cerebral ischemia injury in rats (Louw et al., 2000). Concurrently with the neuroprotection mediated by CB1 receptors, mice without CB1 receptors showed an increased neurotoxicity to NMDA and high mortality levels in permanent focal cerebral ischemia, and an increased infarct area, with neurological deficits more severe after transient focal cerebral ischemia and decreased blood flow in brain in ischemic penumbra during reperfusion, when compared with controls under the same aggressions (Parmentier-Batteur et al., 2002). In contrast, several recent studies do not support the neuroprotective role of endocannabinoids in the activation of CB1 receptors. In fact, rimonabant and LY320135 (CB1 receptors antagonist) reduced the size of the infarct and improved the neurological function in a cerebral ischemia model in rats, induced by brain middle artery occlusion (Muthian et al., 2004), while low doses of WIN 55,212-2 showed no protective effects (Muthian et al., 2004). Recent studies have evaluated the effect of selective CB2 agonists (O-3853, O-1966) in a model of cerebrovascular accidents. CB2 agonists significantly decreased cerebral infarct and improved motor function after cerebral middle artery occlusion for one hour, followed by 23 hours of reperfusion in rats, by attenuation of the increased mobilization of leucocytes and their adherence to vascular endothelial cells induced by transient ischemia (Zhang et al., 2007). The role of CB2 receptors in I/R injury was also supported by the increased accumulation of CB2-positive macrophages derived from resident microglia and/or from invading monocytes resulting from I/R cerebral injury (Ashton et al., 2007).

In general, it seems clear that both agonists and antagonists of CB1 receptors may play a neuroprotective effect on cerebral I/R injury. The reason for the contradictory effects of the pharmacological blockade versus genetic "knockout" of CB1 receptors is still unclear, but could be related with effects that are independent from CB1 antagonists, and that's the reason why this subject requires further clarification. In the case of CB2 agonists, the most likely protection mechanism is the reduction of increased leukocyte infiltration, mobilization and adhesion to vascular endothelial cells and consequent activation, in a process induced by I/R transient injury.

Circulatory shock (organ/body ischemia and/or ischemia/reperfusion)

In addition to its well-known immunologic and neurobehavioral actions, cannabinoids and their synthetic endogenous analogs exert complex cardiopressant and vasodilator effects, which were implicated in the mechanisms underlying hypotension associated to hemorrhagic shock, cardiogenic and septic, advanced liver cirrhosis, cirrhotic cardiomyopathy, heart failure induced by doxorubicin and shock associated to necrotizing pancreatitis (Lamontagne et al., 2006; Ashton & Smith, 2007; Ribuot et al., 2005; Moezi et al., 2008; Sarzani, 2008). These depressant effects of the cardiovascular system could be prevented or reversed by the pretreatment with CB1 receptor antagonists, and they have been analyzed in many recent studies. CB receptors antagonists (eg. rimonabant, AM281,

AM251 and SR144528) prolonged the survival in septic shock or in necrotizing pancreatitis (Varga et al., 1998), increasing mortality in hemorrhagic (Wagner et al., 1997) and cardiogenic (Wagner et al., 2001) shock, despite the increase in blood pressure. One possible explanation for this intriguing controversy is the hypothesis that vasodilatation mediated by endocannabinoids can provide a survival value by increasing tissues oxygenation, neutralizing the excessive sympathetic vasoconstriction triggered by hemorrhage or by myocardium infarct, which could be avoided by blocking CB1 receptors. In contrast, the blockade of CB1 receptors could increase survival in endotoxic shock by preventing the primary hypotensive response to LPS (Pacher et al., 2006a). Even more complicated is the fact that, in hemorrhagic shock, both cardiogenic and septic, UH-210, WIN 55,212-2 and THC (CB agonists) are able to improve endothelial function and/or survival (Varga et al., 1998). Since cardiovascular failure and dysfunction in many of the cited studies are triggered by I/R injury and/or ischemia, and consequently oxidative/nitrosative stress and inflammatory response associated to the activation of several cell death pathways downstream (Pacher et al., 2007), another explanation for the different beneficial effects of agonists and antagonists in circulatory shock could reside in their various anti-inflammatory and/or antioxidant properties (Klein, 2005). These could be attributed to their inverse agonist properties or to mechanisms independent from CB1 and CB2 receptors (Pertwee, 2006).

In global terms, it seems clear that both cannabinoids and antagonists of CB receptors may exert several beneficial effects in shock models in rats; however, the specificity of these effects and their importance for the circulatory shock in humans requires further investigation.

Role of endocannabinoid system in hypertension

The potential use of cannabinoid ligands as antihypertensive agents was even considered since 1970 (Archer, 1974; Birmingham, 1973), and were further reviewed (Sarzani, 2008; Pacher et al., 2005). Cannabinoids decrease blood pressure in hypertensive rodents primarily because of decrease cardiac contractility, suggesting that could have a therapeutic role on hypertension and cardiac hypertrophy. Rimonabant, the CB(1) receptor blocker induced a significant increase in cardiac contractility and blood pressure in hypertensive rats but, on the contrary, contributed to decrease blood pressure in weight-loss clinical trials especially in obese patients with hypertension, which suggests that the overactivation of the ECS in intra-abdominal obesity could be a deleterious effect, in particular from a cardiometabolic opinion (Sarzani, 2008). In addition to the studies in animal models that were already mentioned, it was found that inhalation of THC causes a greater and more lasting fall in blood pressure in hypotensive subjects when compared with normotensive subjects (Crawford et al., 1979). Although the mechanism underlying this increased sensitivity is not cleared yet, it suggests a role of endocannabinoid system in the regulation of cardiovascular functions in hypertension. In a recent study, using three different experimental models of hypertension to explore this possibility, the authors found a significant endocannabinergic tone in hypertension that limits the blood pressure rise and cardiac contractility through the activation of cardiac and vascular CB1 receptors (Bátkai et al., 2004b). It was also found, that over-regulation of these same receptors contributes to potentiate of this tone, maybe trough the inhibition of the activation of endogenous anandamide, stabilizing blood pressure and the contractility of the heart in hypertension.

These findings contribute to the interesting possibility of using inhibitors of fatty acid amide hydrolase in the treatment of hypertension. More clinical studies will be needed to clarify this interesting possibility in a near future.

Role of endocannabinoid system in atherosclerosis

Cannabinoids, endogenous and synthetic, have complex cardiovascular actions through the activation of CB1 receptors (vascular and myocardial) (Steinberg et al., 2007). The decline of cardiac function associated with age and the changes in inflammation genes expression, nitrative stress and apoptosis in rats FAAH-/- compared with wild type rats was analyzed (Batkai et al., 2007; Mach & Steffens, 2008). The authors found that increased levels of anandamide in FAAH-/- rats have a protective effect, which is consistent with the protective role of cannabinoids in inflammatory disorders, such as atherosclerosis. Besides that, anandamide demonstrated its capacity to attenuate, in a dose-dependent manner, the expression of ICAM-1, induced by TNF-α, and of VCAM-1 in endothelial cells of human coronary arteries, and also THP-1 monocytes adhesion in a process dependent on CB1 and CB2 receptors (Batkai et al., 2007). Contrary to the potential beneficial effect in cardiovascular disease, the endocannabinoids may exhibit some prothrombotic effects. In fact, both anandamide and 2-AG were described as activators of human and rodent platelets. The platelets are cellular anucleated fragments that circulate on blood stream. Besides their recognized role in homeostasis and in thrombus formation, platelets may also have proinflammatory properties and be growth regulators, contributing to the progression of atherosclerosis (Leite et al., 2009). Endothelial cells, macrophages and platelets may, by itself, increase their synthesis of endocannabinoids during the formation of atherosclerotic plaque, leading to the activation of platelets. Alternatively, these cells are able to metabolize 2-AG and anandamide, which can offset the increased levels of cannabinoids. CB1 blockade with rimonabant, besides reduce weight and abdominal adiposity, improves cardiometabolic profile, due to multiple influences, including increased levels of high density lipoprotein (HDL)-cholesterol and reduced triglycerides (Despres et al., 2005; Van Gaal et al., 2005). A possible role for CB2 receptors on the progression of atherosclerosis was suggested in an experimental model. The authors found that oral low-doses THC treatment could inhibit the development of atherosclerostic plaque, which was reversed using SR144528, an antagonist of CB2 receptors (Klein et al., 2003). The progression of atherosclerosis was associated with a reduced infiltration of macrophages in the atherosclerotic lesions. The mobilization, adhesion and trans-endothelial migration of leukocytes are triggered by the local production of chemokines, its receptors and adhesion molecules (Braunersreuther & Mach, 2006). Cannabinoids, endogenous or synthetic, have shown to modulate the migration of several cell types, including immune cells trough activation of CB2 receptors (Miller & Stella, 2008). In overall, despite some interesting findings, a specific role of endocannabinoid signaling during atherosclerosis remains to be better elucidated.

New therapeutic opportunities of ECS in cardiovascular disorders

Obesity remains a continuous healthy problem and research issue, which is explained by the serious consequences associated with it, as well as by the increasing incidence of type 2 diabetes and associated obesity, including in younger individuals. In this way, the ECS, due to its well known properties of weight control and energy balance, appeared as a promising target for the treatment of obesity, namely by blocking its receptors. The blockade of these receptors was effectively done by rimonabant, which was viewed as a promising drug for the treatment of obesity. Besides its action on obesity, rimonabant has also proved to be efficient in controlling vascular diseases in several clinical trials and, therefore, this drug was presented as an effective therapeutic approach for treating obesity and cardiovascular disease. However, despite the proven effectiveness in weight loss, rimonabant clinical use was associated with several side effects, which mainly includes the following three groups: the first one includes psychiatric disorders such as depression and anxiety; the second one is associated with gastrointestinal disturbances such as nausea; and finally the third group with regard to neurological changes that are reflected in headaches and vertigo. Despite these adverse effects, which originated its removal from the marker, since the blockade of CB1 receptors continues to prove an asset in the management of obesity and its associated risks (such as reduction of lipogenesis, decreased waist circumference, insulin resistance and dyslipidemia), research in the modulation of the ECS has continued.

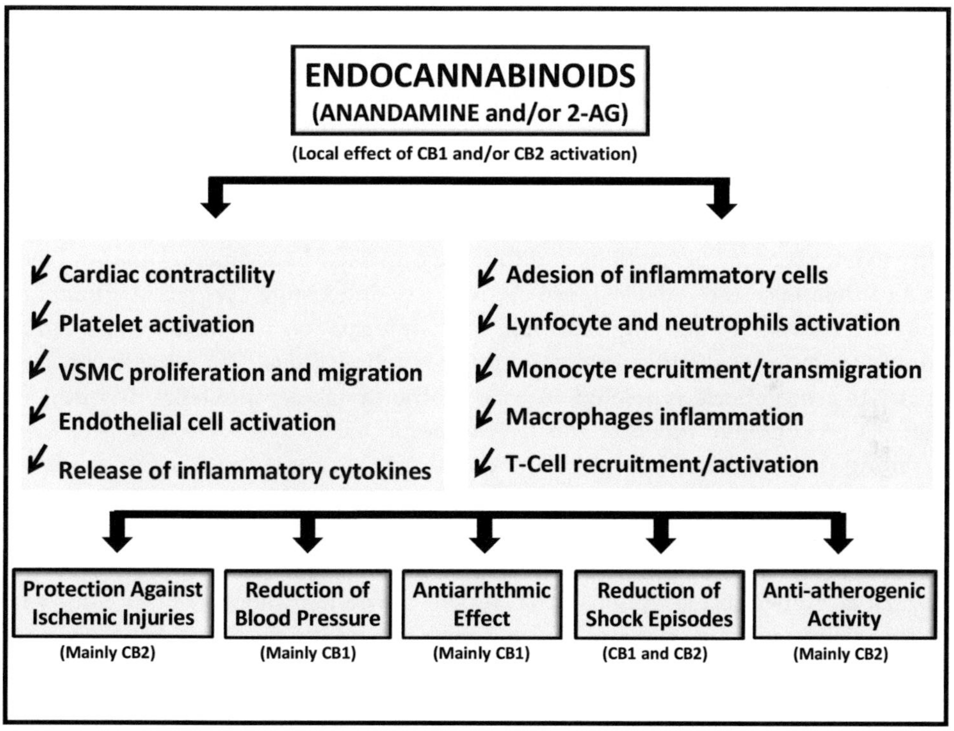

Fig. 3. Endocannabinoids pleiotropic effects on cardiovascular physiology, demonstration protection activity on several tissues, together with positive impact on various other cells that contribute to cardiovascular/atherosclerotic pathologies, such as the monocytes, macrophages, lymfocyttes, leucocytes, neutrophils and other inflammatory cells.

Although CB1 receptors seem to be the main target for new therapeutic interventions, CB2 receptors are also involved in several mechanisms and, since they are present in immune cells and are, apparently, involved in modulating immune responses, they are extremely important and may be seen as a therapeutic target as well. Several line of evidences have been clearly suggesting that cannabinoids and their endogenous and synthetic analogs can promote important cardiac effects, which includes hypotension and cardiodepression. The actions seem to be mediated by complex mechanisms, including both direct and indirect effects both on the vasculature and on the myocardium. Furthermore, the ECS, including endocannabinoids and cannabinoid receptors, have been implicated in the myocardial and cerebral ischemia/reperfusion, in hypotensive state associated with hemorrhagic, endotoxic and cardiogenic shock, and in advanced liver cirrhosis. There is also promising evidences hypothesizing a key role for the endocannabinergic system in the cardiovascular regulation in hypertension, as well as a beneficial action on atherosclerotic plaque. Resuming, cannabinoids are able to modulate a countless number of physiologic functions, demonstration a pleiotropic protective action on the cardiovascular physiology (Figure 3) and therefore, endocannabinoid system is a potential target for the treatment of several diseases and the research about this subject still have a long way to go. The evidence so far gathered shows that the modulation of ECS (as agonism or antagonism of its receptors) is an enormous potential field for research and intervention in multiple areas of human pathophysiology. The development of selective drugs for the CB1 and CB2 receptors may open a door to new therapeutic regimens, in particular in several cardiovascular disorders.

11. Conclusion

The recreational use of the plant *Cannabis sativa* and the attempt to exploit their potential therapeutic use have been described over the centuries. The popularity of *marijuana*, one of the most common forms of consumption as a recreational substance and as a drug, reflects its ability to later sensory perceptions and to reduce anxiety. Experimental studies have been repeatedly demonstrated Δ^9-THC effects on an individual cognitive function and psychomotor skills, influencing learning and information acquisition, changing the individual's memory capacity, coordination and reaction times. The biggest concern with cannabinoids acute effects is related to road traffic or labour accidents. Indeed, Δ^9-THC acute effects on cognitive function and psychomotor skills have been subject of extensive study, noting that, at doses between 40 and 300 mg/kg, cannabinoids can cause a dose-dependent reduction in tasks that require memory use, reaction times, in motor functions and coordination. It has been shown that the influence and accident risk due to recent *cannabis* increases with dose, with an influenced state already present at low doses, being even worse at higher concentrations. Δ^9-THC plasma concentrations can be very variable, with values between 1 and 35 ng/ml in suspected impaired drivers and between 1 and 100 ng/ml in fatal road traffic drivers.

Non-psychoactive actions of *marijuana*, like pain relief, were also described in ancient texts. However, the biochemical and pharmacological study of this substance has a fairly recent start. Endocannabinoids are involved in several physiological functions, among which, special attention has been given to the regulation of appetite by central mechanisms and its influence on obesity. Considering these innovative findings, the research for new pharmacological agents has drastically increased and the discovery of rimonabant, a synthetic antagonist of CB1 receptors, has confirmed the important role of endocannabinoid system on the modulation of food ingestion and energetic balance. Although several other different influences of EC have been discussed during the last years, including in inflammation, diabetes, cancer, affective and neurodegenerative diseases, and epilepsy, the most recent findings are related to their cardiovascular actions, which seem to be very ample bust also complex. The ECS, which includes the endocannabinoids and its receptors, have been implicated in hypotensive stages associated with hemorrhagic chock, both endotoxic and cardiogenic, and even to advanced liver cirrhosis; on the other hand, recent evidence suggests that ECS plays an important role in cardiovascular regulation associated with hypertension, as well as a protective role in ischemia grafting. The development of atherosclerotic plaque and the metabolic stages associated to obesity are also matter of study of possible ECS pharmacomodulation.

The continued approach of biophysics and molecular characterization of ligands for the cannabinoid receptor will contribute decisively to the success of cross-level research of ECS. Those advances will be pivotal for the development and definition of the profile of new chemical entities as therapeutic endocannabinoid modulators. They may also facilitate the identification of new dynamics of the ECS to be used as predictive and/or diagnostic orientation biomarkers for the patients, as well as therapeutic based on ECS pharmacomodulation. The therapeutic approach of cardiovascular system starting from the modulation of ECS appears to be a promising and multidisciplinary issue of study that is still in its early stages but that could be a field for better therapeutic intervention in several disorders, including of cardiovascular and cardiometabolic nature.

12. References

Adams IB, Compton DR, Martin BR. Assessment of anandamide interaction with the cannabinoid brain receptor: SR141716 antagonism studies in mice and autoradiographic analysis of receptor binding in rat brain. *J Pharmacol Exp Ther.* 1998; 284: 1209-17.

Adams IB, Martin BR. Pharmacology and toxicology in animals and humans. *Addiction.* 1996; 91: 1585-614.

Adams R., Baker B.R. Structure of cannabidiol VII. A method of synthesis of a tetrahydrocannabinol which possesses *marijuana* activity. *J Am Chem Soc* 1940; 62: 2405-08.

Addy C, Wright H, Van Laere K, et al. The acyclic CB1R inverse agonist taranabant mediates weight loss by increasing energy expenditure and decreasing caloric intake. *Cell Metab* 2008; 7: 68–78.

Agurell S, Carlsson S, Lindgren JE, Ohlsson A, Gillespie H, Hollister L. Interactions of 1-tetrahydrocannabinol with cannabinol and cannabidiol following oral administration in man. Assay of cannabinol and cannabidiol by mass fragmentography. *Experientia.* 1981; 37: 1090-1.

Agurell S, Halldin M, Lindgren JE, Ohlsson A, Widman M, Gillespie H, Hollister L. Pharmacokinetics and meta-bolism of delta 1-tetrahydrocannabinol and other cannabinoids with emphasis on man. *Pharmacol Rev.* 1986; 38: 21-43.

Ameri A. The effects of cannabinoids on the brain. *Prog Neurobiol.* 1999; 58: 315-48.

Archer RA. The cannabinoids: therapeutic potentials. *Annu Rev Med Chem.* 1974; 9:253–259.

Ashton CH. Pharmacology and effects of *cannabis*: a brief review. *Br J Psychi.* 2001; 178: 101-16.

Ashton JC, Rahman RM, Nair SM, Sutherland BA, Glass M, Appleton I. Cerebral hypoxia-ischemia and middle cerebral artery occlusion induce expression of the cannabinoid CB2 receptor in the brain. *Neurosci Lett* 2007; 412: 114–117.

Ashton JC, Smith PF. Cannabinoids and cardiovascular disease: the outlook for clinical treatments. *Curr Vasc Pharmacol.* 2007; 5(3): 175-85.

Astolfi E, Gotelli C, Kiss J, López-Bolado J, Maccagno A, Poggi VL. *Toxicomanias*. Editorial Universidad, Buenos Aires (1979).

Barnett G, Chiang CN, Perez-Reyes M, Owens S.M. Kinetic study of smoking *marijuana*. *J Pharmacokinet Biopharm.* 1982; 10: 495-506.

Bátkai S, Pacher P, Osei-Hyiaman D, et al. Endocannabinoids acting at CB1 receptors regulates cardiovascular function in hypertension. *Circulation* 2004b; 110(14): 1996–2002.

Batkai S, Rajesh M, Mukhopadhyay P, et al. Decreased age-related cardiac dysfunction, myocardial nitrative stress, inflammatory gene expression, and apoptosis in mice lacking fatty acid amide hydrolase. *Am J Physiol Heart Circ Physiol* 2007; 293: H909–H918.

Bayewitch M, Rhee MH, Avidor-Reiss T, Breuer A, Mechoulam R, Vogel Z. Delta-9-tetrahydrocannabinol antagonizes the peripheral cannabinoid receptor-mediated inhibition of adenylyl cyclase. *J Biol Chem.* 1996; 271: 9902-05.

Benowitz NL, Jones RT. Cardiovascular effects of prolonged delta-9-tetrahydro-cannabinol ingestion. *Clin Pharmacol Ther.* 1975; 18(3): 287-97.

Benowitz NL, Rosenberg J, Rogers W, Bachman J, Jones RT. Cardiovascular effects of intravenous delta-9-tetrahydro-cannabinol: autonomic nervous mecha-nisms. *Clin Pharmacol Ther.* 1979; 25: 440-6.

Bensaid M, Gary-Bobo M, Esclangon A, Maffrand JP, Le Fur G, Oury-Donat F, Soubrié P. The cannabinoid CB1 receptor antagonist SR141716 increases Acrp30 mRNA expression in adipose tissue of obese fa/fa rats and in cultured adipocyte cells. *Mol Pharmacol.* 2003; 63(4): 908-14.

Benson MK, Bentley AM. Lung disease induced by drug addiction. *Thorax.* 1995; 50: 1125-7.

Berghaus G, Scheer N, Schmidt P. Effects of *cannabis* on psychomotor skills and driving performance - a meta-analysis of experimental studies. In: *Alcohol, Drugs and Safety - T95.* Kloeden CN, McLean AJ (Eds.), NHMRC Road Accident Research Unit, Adelaide, 1995, pp. 403-9.

Bidaut-Russell M, Devane WA, Howlet AC. Cannabinoid receptors and modulation of cyclic AMP accumulation in the rat brain. *J Neurochem.* 1990; 55:21-6.

Birmingham MK. Reduction by 9-tetrahydrocannabinol in the blood pressure of hypertensive rats bearing regenerated adrenal glands. *Br J Pharmacol.* 1973; 48(1): 169-71.

Blazquez C, Casanova ML, Planas A, et al. Inhibition of tumor angiogenesis by cannabinoids. *FASEB J* 2003; 17: 529–531.

Bloom AS. Effect of delta-9-tetra-hydrocannabinol on the synthesis of dopamine and norepinephrine in mouse brain synaptosomes. *J Pharmacol Exp Ther.* 1982; 221: 97-103.

Bonz A, Laser M, Küllmer S, Kniesch S, Babin-Ebell J, Popp V, Ertl G, Wagner JA. Cannabinoids acting on CB1 receptors decrease contractile performance in human atrial muscle. *J Cardiovasc Pharmacol.* 2003; 41(4): 657-64.

Bouchard JF, Lepicier P, Lamontagne D. Contribution of endocannabinoids in the endothelial protection afforded by ischemic preconditioning in the isolated rat heart. *Life Sci* 2003; 72: 1859–1870.

Braunersreuther V, Mach F. Leukocyte recruitment in atherosclerosis: potential targets for therapeutic approaches? *Cell Mol Life Sci* 2006; 63: 2079–2088.

Brown NK, Harvey DJ. Comparative in vitro metabolism of cannabinol in rat, mouse, rabbit, guinea pig, hamster, gerbil and cat. *Eur J Drug Metab Pharmacok.* 1990; 15: 253-8.

Burstein S, Hunter SA, Sedor C, Shulman S. Prostaglandins and *cannabis*. IX. Stimulation of prostaglandin E2 synthesis in human lung fibroblasts by delta-1-tetrahydrocannabinol. *Biochem Pharmacol.* 1982; 31: 2361-5.

Butler H, Korbonits M. Cannabinoids for clinicians: the rise and fall of the cannabinoid antagonists. *Eur J Endocrinol.* 2009; 161(5): 655-62.

Camp W.H. The antiquity of hemp as an economic plant. *J NY Bot Gard.* 1936; 37: 110-14.

Chait LD, Perry JL. Acute and residual effects of alcohol and *marijuana*, alone and in combination, on mood and performance. *Psychopharmacology* (Berlin) 1994; 115: 340-9.

Chait LD, Pierri J. Effects on smoked *marijuana* on human performance: A critical review. In: *Marijuana/Cannabinoids: Neurobiology and neurophysiology.* L.Murphy, A. Bartke, eds. CRC Press, Boca Raton, Florida, 1992, pp. 387-423.

Chakravarty I, Sheth AR, Ghosh JJ. Effect of acute delta9-tetrahydrocannabinol treatment on serum luteinizing hormone and prolactin levels in adult female rats. *Fertil Steril.* 1975; 26(9): 947-8.

Chandler LS, Richardson GA, Gallagher JD, Day NL. Prenatal exposure to alcohol and *marijuana*: effects on motor development of preschool children. *Alcohol Clin Exp Res.* 1996; 20: 455-61.

CND (2006), *World drug situation with regard to drug trafficking: Report of the Secretariat,* Comissão das Nações Unidas sobre os Estupefacientes, Nações Unidas, Conselho Económico e Social, Viena.

Compton DR, Rice KC, De Costa BR, Razdan RK, Melvin LS, Johnson MR, Martin BR. Cannabinoid structure activity relationships: correlation of receptor binding and in vivo activities. *J Pharmacol Exp Ther.* 1993; 265: 218-26.

Cone EJ, Huestis MA. Relating blood concentrations of tetrahydrocannabinol and metabolites to pharmacologic effects and time of marihuana usage. *Ther Drug Monit.* 1993; 15: 527-32.

Considine RV, Sinha MK, Heiman ML, Kriauciunas A, Stephens TW, Nyce MR, Ohannesian JP, Marco CC, McKee LJ, Bauer TL, et al. Serum immuno-reactive-leptin concentrations in normal-weight and obese humans. *N Engl J Med.* 1996; 334(5): 292-5.

Cota D, Marsicano G, Tschöp M, Grübler Y, Flachskamm C, Schubert M, Auer D, Yassouridis A, Thöne-Reineke C, Ortmann S, Tomassoni F, Cervino C, Nisoli E, Linthorst AC, Pasquali R, Lutz B, Stalla GK, Pagotto U. The endogenous cannabinoid system affects energy balance via central orexigenic drive and peripheral lipogenesis. *J Clin Invest.* 2003; 112(3): 423-31.

Crawford WJ, Merritt JC. Effects of tetrahydrocannabinol on arterial and intraocular hypertension. *Int J Clin Pharmacol Biopharm* 1979; 17:191–196.

Cummings DE, Weigle DS, Frayo RS, Breen PA, Ma MK, Dellinger EP, Purnell JQ. Plasma ghrelin levels after diet-induced weight loss or gastric bypass surgery. *N Engl J Med.* 2002; 346(21): 1623-30.

Curran HV, Brignell C, Fletcher S, Middleton P, Henry J. Cognitive and subjective dose-response effects of acute oral delta-9-tetrahydrocannabinol (THC) in infrequent *cannabis* users. *Psychopharmacology.* 2002; 164: 61-70.

D' Souza DC, Perry E, MacDougall L, Ammerman Y, Cooper T, Wu YT, Braley G, Gueorguieva R, Krystal JH. The psychotomimetic effects of intravenous delta-9-tetrahydrocannabinol in healthy individuals : implications for psychosis. *Neuro psychopharmacology.* 2004; 29 : 1558-72.

Dalterio S, Bartke A, Burstein S. Cannabinoids inhibit testosterone secretion by mouse testes in vitro. *Science.* 1977; 196: 1472-3.

Dalterio S, Bernard S, Esquivel C. Acute delta-9-tetrahydrocannabinol ex-posure alters Ca^{2+} ATPase activity in neuroendrine and gonadal tissues in mice. *Eur J Pharmacol.* 1987; 137: 91-100.

Day N, Sambamoorthi U, Taylor P, Richardson G, Robles N, Jhon Y, Scher M, Stoffer D, Cornelius M, Jasperse D. Prenatal *marijuana* use and neonatal outcome. *Neurotoxicol Teratol.* 1991; 13: 329-34.

Despres JP, Golay A, Sjostrom L. Effects of rimonabant on metabolic risk factors in overweight patients with dyslipidemia. *N Engl J Med* 2005; 353: 2121–2134.

Deutsch DG, Chin SA. Enzymatic synthesis and degradation of anandamide, a cannabinoid receptor agonist. *Biochem Pharmacol.* 1993; 46: 791-6.

Deutsch DG, Goligorsky MS, Schmid PC, Krebsbach RJ, Schmid HH, Das SK, Dey SK, Arreaza G, Thorup C, Stefano G, Moore LC. Production and physiological actions of anandamide in the vasculature of the rat kidney. *J Clin Invest.* 1997; 100(6): 1538-46.

Devane WA, Dysarz FA, Johnson MR, Melvin LS, Howlett AC. Determination and characterization of a cannabinoid receptor in rat brain. *Molec Pharmacol.* 1988; 34: 605-13.

Devane WA, Hanus L, Breuer A, Pertwee RG, Stevenson LA, Griffin G, Gibson D, Mandelbaum A, Etinger A, Mechoulam R. Isolation and structure of a brain constituent that binds to the cannabinoid receptor. *Science.* 1992; 258: 1946-9.

Dewey WL. Cannabinoid Pharmacolo-gy. *Pharmacol Rev.* 1986; 38: 151-78.

Di Filippo C, Rossi F, Rossi S, D'Amico M. Cannabinoid CB2 receptor activation reduces mouse myocardial ischemia–reperfusion injury: involvement of cytokine/chemokines and PMN. *J Leukoc Biol* 2004; 75: 453–459.

Di Marzo V, Breivogel CS, Tao Q, Bridgen DT, Razdan RK, Zimmer AM, Zimmer A, Martin BR. Levels, metabolism, and pharmacological activity of anandamide in CB(1) cannabinoid receptor knockout mice: evidence for non-CB(1), non-CB(2) receptor-mediated actions of anandamide in mouse brain. *J Neurochem.* 2000; 75: 2434-44.

Di Marzo V, Fontana A, Cadas H, Schinelli S, Cimino G, Schwartz JC, Piomelli D. Formation and inactivation of endogenous cannabinoid anandamide in central neurons. *Nature.* 1994; 372: 686-91.

Di Marzo V, Goparaju SK, Wang L, Liu J, Bátkai S, Járai Z, Fezza F, Miura GI, Palmiter RD, Sugiura T, Kunos G. Leptin-regulated endocannabinoids are involved in maintaining food intake. *Nature.* 2001; 410(6830): 822-5.

Di Marzo V. "Endocannabinoids" and other fatty acid derivatives with cannabimimetic properties: biochemistry and possible physiopathological relevance. *Biochim Biophys Acta.* 1998; 1392: 153-75.

Dill JA, Howlett AC. Regulation of adenylate cyclase by chronic exposure to cannabimimetic drugs. *J Pharmacol Exp Ther.* 1988; 244: 1157-63.

Drummer OH, Gerostamoulos J, Batziris H, Chu M, Caplehorn JRM, Robertson MD, Swann P. The incidence of drugs in drivers killed in Australian road traffic crashes. *Forens Sci Int.* 2003; 134: 154-64.

Durst R, Lotan C. The potential for clinical use of cannabinoids in treatment of cardiovascular diseases. *Cardiovasc Ther.* 2011; 29(1): 17-22.

Eckler C.R., Miller F.A. A study of American grown *Cannabis* in comparison with samples from various other sources. *Am J Pharm.* 1912, 84: 488-95.

Ellenhorn MJ, Barceloux DG. Alternative testing matrices. In: *Ellenhorn's Medical Toxicology: Diagnosis and Treatment of Human Poisoning*. M.J. Ellenhorn, ed. Baltimore: CRC Press, Boca Raton, 1997, pp. 25-49.

Ellis GM, Mann MA, Judson BA, Scramm NT, Tashchian A. Excretion patterns of cannabinoid metabolites after last use in a group of chronic users. *Clin Pharmacol Ther.* 1985; 38: 572-8.

ElSohly MA, Arafat ES, Jones AB. Analysis of the major metabolites of Δ^9-THC in urine. III. A GC/ECD *procedure, J Anal Toxicol.* 1984; 8: 7-9.

Evans DM, Johnson MR, Howlett AC. Ca(2+)-dependent release from rat brain of cannabinoid receptor binding activity. *J Neurochem.* 1992; 58: 780-2.

Fehr K., Kalant A. Analysis of *cannabis* smoke obtained under different combustion conditions. *Can J Physiol Pharmacol.* 1972; 50: 761-67.

Feliciano JE, Mmendivil CO, Sierra ID. Sistema Endocanabinóide: su utilidad clinica. Em: *Hacia el manejo práctivo de las dislipidemias.* 2ª Ed. 2007; Bogotá, Colómbia.

Fong TM, Guan XM, Marsh DJ, et al. Antiobesityefficacy of a novel cannabinoid-1 receptor inverse agonist,N-[(1S,2S)-3-(4-chlorophenyl)-2-(3-cyanophenyl)- 1-methylpropyl]-2-methyl-2-[[5-(trifluoromethyl)pyridin-2- yl]oxy]propanamide (MK-0364), in rodents. *J Pharmacol Exp Ther* 2007; 321: 1013–1022.

Fowler CJ. Plant-derived, synthetic and endogenous cannabinoids as neuroprotective agents. Non-psychoactive cannabinoids, 'entourage' compounds and inhibitors of N-acyl ethanolamine breakdown as therapeutic strategies to avoid pyschotropic effects. *Brain Res Rev.* 2003; 41: 26-43.

Francischetti EA, Sanjuliani AF, francischetti A, Genelhu VA. The role of the endocannabinoid system in the management of cardiometabolic risck factors and obesity. *Int J Atheroscler* 2006; 1(3): 211-20.

Freund TF, Katona I, Piomelli D. Role of endogenous cannabinoids in synaptic signalling. *Physiol Rev* 2003; 83: 1017–1066.

Fride E, Foox A, Rosenberg E, Faigenboim M, Cohen V, Barda L, Blau H, Mechoulam R. Milk intake and survival in newborn cannabinoid CB1 receptor knockout mice: evidence for a "CB3" receptor. *Eur J Pharmacol.* 2003 Feb 7; 461(1): 27-34.

Fride E, Mechoulam R.. Pharma-cological activity of the canna-binoid receptor agonist, anandamide, a brain constituent. *Eur J Pharmacol.* 1993; 231: 313-4.

Fried PA, Smith AM. A literature review of the consequences of prenatal marihuana exposure. An emerging theme of a deficiency in aspects of executive function. *Neurotoxicol Teratol.* 2001; 23: 1-11.

Fried PA, Watkinson B, Gray R. Growth from birth to early adolescence in offspring prenatally exposed to cigarettes and *marijuana. Neurotoxicol Teratol.* 1999; 21: 513-25.

Fruebis J, Tsao TS, Javorschi S, Ebbets-Reed D, Erickson MR, Yen FT, Bihain BE, Lodish HF. Proteolytic cleavage product of 30-kDa adipocyte complement-related protein increases fatty acid oxidation in muscle and causes weight loss in mice. *Proc Natl Acad Sci U S A.* 2001; 98(4): 2005-10.

Garret ER, Gouyette AJ, Roseboom H. Stability of tetrahydrocannabinoids II. *J Pharm Sci.* 1978; 67: 27-32.

Garret ER, Hunt CA. Physicochemical properties, solubility, and protein binding of delta-9-tetrahydrocannabinol. *J Pharm Sci.* 1974; 63: 1056-64.

Gebremedhin D, Lange AR, Campbell WB, Hillard CJ, Harder DR. Cannabinoid CB1 receptor of cat cerebral arterial muscle functions to inhibit L-type Ca2+ channel current. *Am J Physiol.* 1999; 276(6 Pt 2): H2085-93.

Giuffrida A, Beltramo M, Piomelli D. Mechanisms of endocannabinoid inacti-vation: biochemistry and pharmacology. *J Pharmacol Exp Ther.* 2001 Jul;298(1):7-14.

Glass M, Northup JK. Agonist selective regulation of G proteins by cannabinoid CB1 and CB2 receptors. *Mol Pharmacol.* 1999; 56: 1362-9.

Gold MS. *Marijuana.* In: *Comprehensive handbook of alcohol and drug addiction.* Miller NS, ed. Nova Iorque: Marcel Decker, 1991, pp 353-76.

Hall W, Solowij N. Adverse effects of *cannabis*. *Lancet.* 1998; 352: 1611-5.

Hall W. Reducing the harms caused by *cannabis* use: the policy debate in Australia. *Drug Alcohol Depend.* 62: 163-74 (2001)

Halldin MM, Widman M. Glucuronic acid conjugate of delta 1-tetrahydro-cannabinol identified in the urine of man. *Arzneimittelforschung*. 1983; 33: 177-8.

Hampson AJ, Grimaldi M, Lolic M, Wink D, Rosenthal R, Axelrod J. Neuroprotective antioxidants from *marijuana*. *Ann NY Acad Sci* 2000; 899: 274–282.

Hampson RE, Deadwyler SA. Cannabinoids, hippocampal function and memory. *Life Sci.* 1999; 65: 715-23.

Harvey DJ, Mechoulam R. Metabolites of cannabidiol identified in human urine. *Xenobiotica.* 1990; 20: 303-20.

Hayakawa K, Mishima K, Abe K, et al. Cannabidiol prevents infarction via the non-CB1 cannabinoid receptor mechanism. *Neuroreport* 2004; 15: 2381–2385.

Herkenham M, Lynn AB, Little MD, Johnson MR, Melvin LS, de Costa BR, Rice KC. Cannabinoid receptor localization in brain. *Proc Natl Acad Sci U S A.* 1990; 87(5): 1932-6.

Hillard CJ, Campbell WB. Biochemistry and pharmacology of arachidonylethanolamide, a putative endogenous cannabinoid. *J Lipid Res.* 1997; 38: 2383-98.

Hillard CJ, Harris HR, Bloom AS. Effects of the cannabinoids on physical properties of brain membranes and phospholipid vesicles: fluorescence studies. *J Pharmacol Exp Ther.* 1985; 232: 579-88.

Hollister LE, Richaros R.K., Gillespie B.A. Comparision of THC and Synhexil in man. *Clin Pharmacol Ther* 1968; 9: 783-91.

Hollister LE. Health aspects of *cannabis*. *Pharmacol Rev.* 1986; 38: 1-20.

Honório KM, Silva AA. Aspectos terapêuticos de compostos da planta *Cannabis sativa*. *Quim. Nova.* 2006; 29:318-25.

Howlett AC, Champion-Dorow TM, McMahon LL, Westlake TM. The cannabinoid receptor: biochemical and cellular properties in neuroblastoma cells. *Pharmacol Biochem Behav.* 1991; 40: 565-9.

Howlett AC. Pharmacology of canna-binoid receptors. *Ann Rev Pharmacol Toxicol.* 1995; 35: 607-34.

Howlett AC. The CB1 cannabinoid receptor in the brain. *Neurobiol. Dis.* 1998; 5: 405-16.

Huestis MA, Gorelick DA, Heishman SJ, Preston KL, Nelson RA, Moolchan ET, Frank RA. Blockade of effects of smoked *marijuana* by the CB1-selective cannabinoid receptor antagonist SR-141716. *Arch Gen Psychiat.* 2001; 58:322-8.

Huestis MA, Henningfield JE, Cone EJ. Blood cannabinoids. I. Absortion of THC and formation of 11-OH-THC and THCCOOH during and after smoking *Marijuana. J Anal Toxicol.* 1992a; 16: 276-82.

Huestis MA, Sampson AH, Holicky BJ, Henningfield JE, Cone EJ. Characterization of the absorption phase of *marijuana* smoking. *Clin Pharmacol Ther.* 1992; 52:31-41.

Huestis MA. *Cannabis (Marijuana)* - Effects on human behaviour and performance. *Forensic Sci Rev.* 2002; 14: 16-60.

Hunt CA, Jones RT. Tolerance and disposition of tetrahydrocannabinol in man. *J Pharmacol Exp Ther.* 1980; 215: 35-44.

Iribarne C, Berthou F, Baird S, Dréano Y, Picart D, Bail JP, Beaune P, Ménez JF. Involvement of cytochrome P450 3A4 enzyme in the N-demethylation of methadone in human liver microsomes. *Chem Res Toxicol.* 1996; 9: 365-73.

Ishac EJ, Jiang L, Lake KD, Varga K, Abood ME, Kunos G. Inhibition of exocytotic noradrenaline release by presynaptic cannabinoid CB1 receptors on peripheral sympathetic nerves. *Br J Pharmacol.* 1996; 118(8): 2023-8.

Izzo AA, Borrelli F, Capasso R, Di Marzo V, Mechoulam R. Non-psychotropic plant cannabinoids: new therapeutic opportunities from an ancient herb. *Trends Pharmacol Sci.* 2009; 30(10): 515-27.

Jamshidi N, Taylor DA. Anandamide administration into the ventromedial hypothalamus stimulates appetite in rats. *Br J Pharmacol.* 2001 Nov;134(6):1151-4.

Järbe TUC, Mathis DA. Dissociative and discriminative stimulus functions of cannabinoids/cannabimi-metics. In: *Marihuana/Cannabinoids: Neurobiology and Neurophysiology*, Bartke A., Murphy L.L., eds. Florida: CRC Press, Boca Raton, 1992, pp. 459-524.

Johansson E, Agurell S, Hollister LE, Halldin MM Prolonged apparent half-life of delta-1-tetrahydrocannabinol in plasma of chronic *marijuana users J Pharm Pharmacol.* 1988; 40: 374-5.

Johansson E, Norén K, Sjövall J, Halldin MM Determination of delta-1-tetrahydrocannabinol in human fat biopsies from marihuana users by gas chromatography-mass spectrometry. *Biomed Chromatogr.* 1989a; 3: 35-8.

Jones RT. Drug of abuse profile: *cannabis. Clin Chem.* 1987; 33 (11 Suppl):72B-81B.

Joyeux M, Arnaud C, Godin-Ribuot D, Demenge P, Lamontagne D, Ribuot C. Endocannabinoids are implicated in the infarct size-reducing effect conferred by heat stress preconditioning in isolated rat hearts. *Cardiovas Res* 2002; 55: 619–625.

Kirkham TC, Williams CM, Fezza F, Di Marzo V. Endocannabinoid levels in rat limbic forebrain and hypothalamus in relation to fasting, feeding and satiation: stimulation of eating by 2-arachidonoyl glycerol. *Br J Pharmacol.* 2002; 136(4): 550-7.

Kirkham TC. Cannabinoids and appetite: food craving and food pleasure. *Int Ver Psychiatry.* 2009; 21(2): 163-71.

Klansner HA, Wilcox HG, Dingell JV. The use of zonal ultracentrifugation in the investigation of the binding of delta-9-THC by plasma lipoproteins. *Drug Metab Dispos.* 1975; 3: 314-9.

Klein TW, Newton C, Larsen K, et al. The cannabinoid system and immune modulation. *J Leukoc Biol* 2003; 74: 486–496.

Klein TW. Cannabinoid-based drugs as anti-inflammatory therapeutics. *Nat Rev Immunol* 2005; 5: 400–411.

Kreuz D.S., Axelrod J. Delta-9-tetrahydrocannabinol: localization in body fat. *Science.* 1973; 179: 391-3.

Krylatov AV, Ugdyzhekova DS, Bernatskaya NA, et al. Activation of type II cannabinoid receptors improves myocardial tolerance to arrhythmogenic effects of coronary occlusion and reperfusion. *Bull Exp Biol and Med* 2001; 131: 523–525.

Kurzthaler I, Hummer M, Miller C, Sperner-Unterweger B, Gunther V, Wechdorn H, Battista HJ, Fleischhacker WW. Effect of *cannabis* use on cognitive functions and driving ability. *J Clin Psychiatry*: 1999; 60: 395-9.

Ladrón de Guevara J, Moya Pueyo V. *Toxicología Médica*: Interamericana-McGraw-Hill., Madrid 1995, pp. 638-41.

Lagneux C, Lamontagne D. Involvement of cannabinoids in the cardioprotection induced by lipopolysaccharide. *Br J Pharmacol* 2001; 132: 793–796.

Lake KD, Compton DR, Varga K, Martin BR, Kunos G. Cannabinoid-induced hypotension and bradycardia in rats mediated by CB1-like cannabinoid receptors. *J Pharmacol Exp Ther.* 1997; 281(3): 1030-7.

Lamers CT, Ramaekers JG. Visual search and urban driving under the influence of *marijuana* and alcohol. *Hum Psychopharmacol.* 2001; 16: 393-401.

Lamontagne D, Lepicier P, Lagneux C, Bouchard JF. The endogenous cardiac cannabinoid system: a new protective mechanism against myocardial ischemia. *Arch Mal Coeur Vaiss* 2006; 99: 242–246.

Law B, Mason PA, Moffat AC, Gleadle RI, King LJ. Forensic aspects of the metabolism and excretion of cannabinoids following oral ingestion of *cannabis* resin. *J. Pharm Pharmacol.* 1984b; 36: 289-94.

Law B, Mason PA, Moffat AC, King LJ, Marks V. Passive inhalation of *cannabis* smoke. *J Pharm Pharmacol.* 1984; 36: 578-81.

Leighty E.G. Metabolism and distribution of cannabinoids in rats after different methods of administration. *Biochem Pharmac.* 1973; 22: 1613-21.

Leirer VO, Yesavage JA, Morrow DG. *Marijuana*, aging, and task difficulty effects on pilot performance. *Aviat Space Environ Med.* 1989; 60: 1145-52.

Leite C, Mocelin C, Peterson G, Leal M, Thiesen F. Rimonabant: na antagonist drug of the endocannabinoid system for the treatment of obesity. *Pharmacological Reports* 2009; 61: 217-224.

Leker RR, Gai N, Mechoulam R, Ovadia H. Drug-induced hypothermia reduces ischemic damage: effects of the cannabinoid HU-210. *Stroke* 2003; 34: 2000–2006.

Lemberger L, Crabtree RE, Rowe HM. 11-hydroxy-delta-9-tetrahy-drocannabinol: pharmacology, disposition and metabolism of a major metabolite of *marijuana* in man. *Science.* 1972; 177: 62-4.

Lemberger L, Martz R, Rodda B, Forney R, Rowe H. Comparative pharmacology of Δ^9-tetrahydrocannabinol and its metabolite, 11-OH-Δ^9-tetrahydrocannabinol. *J Clin Invest*: 1973; 52: 2411-7.

Lemberger L, Tamarkin NR, Axelrod J, Kopin IJ. Δ^9-tetrahydrocannabinol: Metabolism and disposition in long-term *marijuana* smokers. *Science*: 1971; 173: 72-4.

Lemberger L., Silberstein S.D., Axelrod J., Kopin I.J. Marihuana: studies on the disposition and metabolism of delta-9-tetrahydrocannabinol in man. *Science*: 1970; 170: 1320-2.

Lepicier P, Bouchard JF, Lagneux C, Lamontagne D. Endocannabinoids protect the rat isolated heart against ischaemia. *Br J Pharmacol* 2003; 139: 805–815.

Leuschner JT, Harvey DJ, Bullingham RE, Paton WD. Pharmacokinetics of delta-9-tetrahydro-cannabinol in rabbits following single or multiple intravenous doses. *Drug Met Dispos.* 1986; 14: 230-8.

Leweke M, Kampmann C, Radwan M, Dietrich DE, Johannes S, Emrich HM, Munte TF. The effects of tetrahydrocannabinol on the recognition of emotionally charged words: an analysis using event-related brain potentials. *Neuropsychobiology* 1998; 37: 104-11.

Lichtman AH, Varvel SA, Martin BR. Endocannabinoids in cognition and dependence. *Prostaglandins Leukot Essent Fatty Acids.* 2002; 66: 269-85.

Lindemann E. The neurophysiological effects on intoxicating drugs. *Am J Psychiat*: 1933; 90: 1007-37.

Lindgren JE, Ohlsson A, Agurell S, Hollister LE, Gillespie H. Clinical effects and plasma levels of *cannabis*. *Psychopharmacology*. 1981; 74: 208-12.

Liu J, Gao B, Mirshahi F, Sanyal AJ, Khanolkar AD, Makriyannis A, Kunos G. Functional CB1 cannabinoid receptors in human vascular endothelial cells. *Biochem J*. 2000 15; 346 Pt 3: 835-40.

Louw DF, Yang FW, Sutherland GR. The effect of delta-9-tetrahydrocannabinol on forebrain ischemia in rat. *Brain Res* 2000; 857: 183–187.

Lynn AB, Herkenham M. Localization of cannabinoid receptors and nonsaturable high-density cannabinoid binding sites in peripheral tissues of the rat: implications for receptor-mediated immune modulation by cannabinoids. *J Pharmacol Exp Ther*. 1994; 268: 1612-23.

Mach F, Steffens S. The Role of the Endocannabinoid System in Atherosclerosis. *J Neuroendocrinol* 2008; 20 (Suppl. 1): 53–57.

Martin BR. Cellular effects of canna-binoids. *Pharmacol Rev*. 1986; 38: 45-74.

Mason AP, Perez-Reys M, McBay RJ, Foltz RL. Cannabinoid concentrations in plasma after passive inhalation of *marijuana* smoke. *J Anal Toxicol*. 1983; 7: 172-7.

Matsuda LA, Lolait SJ, Brownstein MJ, Young AC, Bonner TI. Structure of a cannabinoid receptor and functional expression of the cloned cDNA. *Nature*. 1990; 346: 561-4.

Matsunaga T, Iwawaki Y, Watanabe K, Yamamoto I, Kageyama T, Yoshimura H. Metabolism of delta-9-tetrahydro-cannabinol by cytochrome P450 isozymes purified from hepatic microsomes of monkeys. *Life Sci*. 1995; 56: 2089-98.

Mauler F, Mittendorf J, Horvath E, De Vry J. Characterization of the diarylether sulfonylester (_)-(R)-3-(2-hydroxymethylindanyl-4-oxy)phenyl-4,4,4-trifluoro-1-sulfonate (BAY 38-7271) as a potent cannabinoid receptor agonist with neuroprotective properties. *J Pharml Exp Ther* 2002; 302: 359–368.

Mechoulam R, Devane WA, Glaser R. Cannabinoid geometry and biological activity. In: *Marihuana/Cannabinoids: Neurobiology and Neurophysiology*, Bartke A, Murphy LL, eds. Florida: CRC Press, Boca Raton, 1992, pp. 1-34.

Mechoulam R, Hanus L. Endogenous cannabinoid ligands - Chemical and biological studies. *J Lipid Mediat Cell Signal*. 1996; 14: 45-9.

Mechoulam R. A random walk through a *cannabis* field. *Pharmacol Biochem Behav*. 1991; 40: 461-4.

Mechoulam R. Marihuana chemistry. *Science*. 1970; 168: 1159-66.

Mechoulam R. *Marijuana, chemistry, pharmacology, metabolism and clinical effects*. Academic Press, New York, 1973, 101-36.

Mechoulam R. The pharmacohistory of *Cannabis sativa*. In: *Cannabinoids as therapeutic agents*. Mechoulam R., ed. Florida: CRC Press, Boca Raton, 1986, pp. 1-19.

Mendelson JH. Marihuana. In: *Psychopharmacology: The third generation of progress*, Meltzer HY, ed. Nova Iorque: Raven Press, 1987, pp. 1565-8.

Miller AM, Stella N. CB2 receptor-mediated migration of immune cells: it can go either way. *Br J Pharmacol* 2008; 153: 299–308.

Moezi L, Gaskari SA, Lee SS. Endocannabinoids and liver disease. V. endocannabinoids as mediators of vascular and cardiac abnormalities in cirrhosis. *Am J Physiol Gastrointest Liver Physiol*. 2008; 295(4): G649-53.

Mukhopadhyay P, Batkai S, Rajesh M, et al. Pharmacological inhibition of cannabinoid receptor-1 protects against doxorubicin-induced cardiotoxicity. *J Am Coll Cardiol* 2007; 50: 528–536.

Munro S, Thomas K, Abu-Shaar M. Molecular characterization of a peripheral receptor for cannabinoids. *Nature*. 1993; 365: 61-5.

Muthian S, Rademacher DJ, Roelke CT, Gross GJ, Hillard CJ. Anandamide content is increased and CB1 cannabinoid receptor blockade is protective during transient, focal cerebral ischemia. *Neuroscience* 2004; 129: 743–750.

Nagayama T, Sinor AD, Simon RP, et al. Cannabinoids and neuroprotection in global and focal cerebral ischemia and in neuronal cultures. *J Neurosci* 1999; 19: 2987–2995.

Nahas GG. Botany: The unstabilized species. In: *Marihuana – Deceptive Weed*, Raven Press, NY, 1973, pp. 59-84.

Nahas GG. Current status of *marijuana* research. *JAMA*. 1979; 242: 2775-8.

Nahas GG. Hashish and Islam: 9th to 18th century. *Bull NY Acad Med*. 1982; 58: 814-31.

O'Shaughnessy W.B. On the preparation of Indian hemp or gunjah. *Trans Med Phys Soc Bombay*. 8: 421-61 (1842)

Ohlsson A, Lindgren JE, Wahlén A, Agurell S, Hollister LE, Gillespie HK. Single dose kinetics of deuterium labelled delta-1-tetrahydrocannabinol in heavy and light *cannabis* users. *Biomed Mass Spectrom*. 1982; 9: 6-10.

Ohlsson A, Lindgren JE, Whalen A, Agurell S, Hollister LE, Gillespie HK. Plasma delta-9-tetrahydrocannabinol con-centrations and clinical effects after oral and intravenous administration and smoking. *Clin Pharmacol Ther*. 1980; 28: 409-16.

Pacher P, Bátkai S, Kunos G. Blood pressure regulation by endocannabinoids and their receptors. *Neuropharmacology*. 2005; 48(8): 1130-8.

Pacher P, Batkai S, Kunos G. The endocannabinoid system as an emerging target of pharmacotherapy. *Pharmacol Rev* 2006a; 58: 389–462.

Pacher P, Beckman JS, Liaudet L. Nitric oxide and peroxynitrite in health and disease. *Physiol Rev* 2007; 87: 315–424.

Papafotiou K, Carter JD, Stough C. The relationship between performance on the standardised field sobriety tests, driving performance and the level of Δ9-tetrahydrocannabinol (THC) in blood. *Forens Sci Int.* 2005; 155: 172-8.

Parmentier-Batteur S, Jin K, Mao XO, Xie L, Greenberg DA. Increased severity of stroke in CB1 cannabinoid receptor knock-out mice. *J Neurosci* 2002; 22: 9771–9775.

Paton WD, Pertwee RG. The action of *cannabis* in man. In: *Marijuana: Chemistry, pharmacology, metabolism and clinical effects*. R. Mechoulam, ed., Londres: Academic Press, 1973, pp. 288-334

Pérez-Reyes M, Di Giuseppi S, Davis KH, Schindler VH, Cook CE.Comparison of effects of marihuana cigarettes to three different potencies. *Clin Pharmacol Ther.* 1982; 31: 617-24.

Pérez-Reyes M., Timmons M.C., Davis K.H., Wall E.M. A comparison of the pharmacological activity in man of intravenously administered delta9-tetrahydrocannabinol, cannabinol, and cannabidiol. *Experientia.* 1973; 29: 1368-9.

Pertwee RG (2006). The pharmacology of cannabinoid receptors and their ligands: an overview. Int J Obes 2006; 30: S13–8.

Pertwee RG. Pharmacological, physiological and clinical implications of the discovery of cannabinoid receptors: an overview. In: *Cannabinoid receptors,* Pertwee R ed., Harcourt Brace, 1995, pp. 1-34.

Pertwee RG. The central neurophar-macology of psychotropic cannabinoids. *Pharmacol Ther.* 1988; 36: 189-261.

Pop E. Cannabinoids, endogenous ligands and synthetic analogs. *Curr Opin Chem Biol.* 1999; 3:418-25.

Portier M, Rinaldi-Carmona M, Pecceu F, Combes T, Poinot-Chazel C, Calandra B, Barth F, Le Fur G, Casellas P. SR 144528, an antagonist for the peripheral cannabinoid receptor that behaves as an inverse agonist *J Pharmacol Exp Ther.* 1999; 288: 582-9.

Raes E, Verstraete A, Wennig R Drugs and driving. *Forensic Science Handbook of Analytical Separations.* Bogusz MJ, Smith R, Eds, Elsevier vol. 6, 2007, pp. 617-57.

Ramaekers JG, Berghaus G, van Laar M, Drummer OH. Dose related risk of motor vehicle crashes after *cannabis* use. *Drug Alcohol Depend.* 2004; 73: 109-19.

Ramaekers JG, Moeller MR, van Ruitenbeek P, Theunissen EL, Schneider E, Kauert G. Cognition and motor control as a function of Δ^9-THC concentration in serum and oral fluid: limits of impairment. *Drug Alcohol Depend.* 2006; 85: 114-22.

Ramaekers JG, Robbe HW, O'Hanlon JF. *Marijuana,* alcohol and actual driving performance. *Hum Psychopharmacol.* 2000; 15: 551-8.

Rawich B, Roher G, Vardaris RM. Δ9-tetrahydrocannabinol uptake by adipose tissue; preferential accumulation in gonadal fat organs. *Gen Pharmacol.* 1979; 10: 525-34.

Reggio PH, Wang T, Brown AE, Fleming DN, Seltzman HH, Griffin G, Pertwee RG, Compton DR, Abood ME, Martin BR. Importance of the C-1 substituent in classical cannabinoids to CB2 receptor selectivity: synthesis and characterization of a series of O,2-propano-delta-8-tetrahydrocannabinol analogs. *J Med Chem.* 1997; 40: 3312-8.

Ribuot C, Lamontagne D, Godin-Ribuot D. Cardiac and vascular effects of cannabinoids: toward a therapeutic use? *Ann Cardiol Angeiol* (Paris). 2005; 54(2): 89-96.

Rinaldi-Carmona M, Barth F, Heaulme M. Shire D, Calandra B, Congy C, Martinez S, Maruani J, Neliat G, Caput D, Ferrara P, Soubrie P, Breliere JC, Le Fur G. SR141716A, a potent and selective antagonist of the brain cannabinoid receptor. *Fed Eur Biochem Soc Letters*. 1994; 350: 240-4.

Robson P. Therapeutic aspects of *cannabis* and cannabinoids. *Br J Psychi*. 2001; 178: 107-15.

Rodríguez-Vicente MC, Sanz P, Repetto M. Estado actual de la toxicología del *cannabis*. In: *Toxicologia Avanzada,* Repetto M ed., Díaz de Santos, SA, Madrid, 1995, pp. 477-516.

Romero J, Garcia L, Cebeira M, Zadrozny D. Fernandez-Ruiz J.J.., Ramos, J.A. The endogenous cannabinoid receptor ligand, anandamide, inhibits the motor behavior: role of nigrostriatal dopaminergic neurons. *Life Sci*. 1995; 56: 2033-40.

Rush C, Griffiths. Zolpidem, triazolam and temazepam: behavioral and subject-rated effects in normal volunteers. *J Clin Psychopharmacol*. 1996; 16: 146-57.

Ryrfeldt A, Ramsay CH, Nilsson IM, Widman M, Agurell S. Whole-body autoradiography of delta-1-tetrahydro-cannabinol and delta-8-tetrahydro-cannabinol in mouse. *Acta Pharm Suec*. 1973; 10: 13-28.

Sanudo-Pena MC, Romero J, Seale GE, Fernandez-Ruiz JJ, Walker JM. Activational role of cannabinoids on move-ment. *Eur J Pharmacol*. 2000; 391: 269-74.

Sarzani R. Endocannabinoids, blood pressure and the human heart. *J Neuroendocrinol*. 2008; 20 Suppl 1: 58-62.

Schultes RE. Random thoughts and queries on the botany of *cannabis*. In: *The Botany and Chemistry of Cannabis*, Joyce CRB, Curry SH, eds., J&A Churchill, Londres, 1970, pp. 11-38.

Schwartz RH. Heavy *marijuana* use and recent memory impairment. In: *Physiopathology of illicit drugs: Cannabis, Cocaine, Opiates*, Nahas GG, Latour C, eds., Pergamon Press, Oxford, 1991, pp. 13-21.

Shmist YA, Goncharov I, Eichler M, et al. Delta-9-tetrahydrocannabinol protects cardiac cells from hypoxia via CB2 receptor activation and nitric oxide production. *Mol Cell Biochem* 2006; 283: 75–83.

Smith PB, Compton DR, Welch SP, Razdan RK, Mechoulam R, Martin BR. The pharmacological activity of anandamide, a putative endogenous cannabinoid, in mice. *J Pharmacol Exp Ther*. 1994; 270: 219-27.

Steinberg B, Cannon C. Cannabinoid-1 Receptor Blockade in Cardiometaolic Risk Reduction; Safety, Tolerability, and Therapeutic Potential. *Am J Cardiol* 2007; 100: 27P-32P.

Sugiura T, Kondo S, Sukagawa A, Nakane S, Shinoda A, Itoh K, Yamashita A, Waku K. 2-arachidonoylycerol: A possible endogenous cannabinoid receptor ligand in brain. *Biochem Biophys Res Commun*. 1995; 215: 89-97.

Sutheimer CA, Yarborough R, Hepler BR, Sunshine I. Detection and confirmation of urinary cannabinoids. *J Anal Toxicol*. 1985; 9: 156-60.

Tashkin DP, Gliederer F, Rose J, Change P, Hui KK, Yu JL, Wu TC. Effects of varying *marijuana* smoking profile on deposition of tar and absorption of CO and delta-9-THC. *Pharmacol Biochem Behav*. 1991; 40: 651-6.

Tashkin DP, Reiss S, Shapiro BJ. Bronchial effects of aerosolized Δ^9-Tetra-hydrocannabinol in healthy and asthmatic subjects. *Am Rev Respir Dis*. 1977; 115: 57-65.

Tashkin DP, Soures JR, Helper RS. *Cannabis*. *Ann Intern Med*. 1978; 89: 539-49.

Thomas BF, Gilliam AF, Burch DF, Roche MJ, Seltzman HH. Comparative receptor binding analyses of cannabinoid agonists and antagonists. *J Pharmacol Exp Ther.* 1998; 285: 285-92.

Turner CE, ElSohly MA, Boeren EG. Constituents of *cannabis sativa* L. XVII. A review of the natural constituents. *J Nat Prod.* 1980; 43: 169-234.

UNODC. *2007 World drug report* [Relatório mundial sobre a droga 2006], Gabinete das Nações Unidas contra a Droga e o Crime, Viena, 2007.

Vachon L, Fitzgeral MX, Solliday NH. Single dose effect of *marijuana* smoke. Bronchial dynamics and respiratory center sensitivity in normal subjects. *N Engl J Med.* 1973; 288: 985-9.

Van Gaal LF, Rissanen AM, Scheen AJ, Ziegler O, Rossner S. Effects of the cannabinoid-1 receptor blocker rimonabant on weight reduction and cardiovascular risk factors in overweight patients: 1-year experience from the RIO-Europe study. *Lancet* 2005; 365: 1389–1397.

van Thuijl H, Kola B, Korbonits M. Appetite and metabolic effects of ghrelin and cannabinoids: involvement of AMP-activated protein kinase. *Vitam Horm.* 2008; 77: 121-48.

Varga K, Wagner JA, Bridgen DT, Kunos G. Platelet and macrophage-derived endogenous cannabinoids are involved in endotoxin-induced hypotension. *FASEB J* 1998; 12: 1035–1044.

Wagner JA, Abesser M, Harvey-White J, Ertl G. 2-Arachidonylglycerol acting on CB1 cannabinoid receptors mediates delayed cardioprotection induced by nitric oxide in rat isolated hearts. *J Cardiovasc Pharmacol* 2006; 47: 650–655.

Wagner JA, Hu K, Bauersachs J, et al. Endogenous cannabinoids mediate hypotension after experimental myocardial infarction. *J Am Coll Cardiol* 2001; 38: 2048–2054.

Wagner JA, Hu K, Karcher J, et al. CB(1) cannabinoid receptor antagonism promotes remodelling and cannabinoid treatment prevents endothelial dysfunction and hypotension in rats with myocardial infarction. *Br J Pharmacol* 2003; 138: 1251–1258.

Wagner JA, Varga K, Ellis EF, Rzigalinski BA, Martin BR, Kunos G. Activation of peripheral CB1 cannabinoid receptors in haemorrhagic shock. *Nature* 1997; 390: 518–521.

Wall ME, Perez-Reyes M. The metabolism of delta-9-tetrahydrocannabinol and related cannabinoids in man. *J Clin Pharmacol.* 1981; 21: 178s-89s.

Wall ME, Sadler BM, Brine D, Taylor H, Pérez-Reyes M. Metabolism, disposition and kinetics of delta-9-tetrahydrocannabinol in men and women. *Clin Pharmacol Ther.* 1983; 34: 352-63.

Waller CW. Chemistry of marihuana. *Pharmacol Rev.* 1971; 23: 265-71.

Weil AT, Zinberg NE, Nelsen JM. Acute effects of marihuana on speech. *Nature.* 1969; 222: 434-37.

Welch SP, Eads M. Synergistic interactions of endogenous opioids and cannabinoid systems. *Brain Res.* 1999; 848: 183-90.

Widman M, Agurell S, Ehrnebo M, Jones G. Binding of (+) and (-)-delta-1-tetrahydrocannabinols and (-)-7-hydroxy-delta-1-tetrahydrocannabinol to blood cells and plasma proteins in man. *J Pharm Pharmacol.* 1974; 26: 914-6.

Williams CM, Kirkham TC. Anandamide induces overeating: mediation by central cannabinoid (CB1) receptors. *Psychopharmacology (Berl).* 1999; 143(3): 315-7.

Williams PL, Moffat AC. Identification in human urine of delta-9-tetrahydrocannabinol-11-oic glucuronide - A tetrahydrocannabinol metabolite. *J Pharm Pharmacol.* 1980; 32: 445-8.

Wilsie CR, Reddy CS. Seed treatment experiments with hemp. *J Am Soc Agron.* 1946; 38: 693-701.

Wu TC, Tashkin DP, Djahed B, Rose JE. Pulmonary hazards of smoking *marijuana* as compared with tobacco. *N Engl J Med.* 1988; 318: 347-51.

Zhang M, Martin BR, Adler MW, Razdan RK, Jallo JI, Tuma RF. Cannabinoid CB(2) receptor activation decreases cerebral infarction in a mouse focal ischemia/reperfusion model. *J Cereb Blood Flow Metab* 2007; 27: 1387–1396.

Zuardi AW, Morais SL, Guimarães FS. Mechoulam R. Antipsychotic effects of cannabidiol. *J Clin Psychiatry.* 1995; 56: 485-6.

11

Pharmacogenetics Role in Forensic Sciences

Loredana Buscemi and Adriano Tagliabracci
Institute of Legal Medicine, Department of Neuroscience, Università Politecnica delle Marche, Ancona, Italy

1. Introduction

The completion of Human Genome Project and advancement of analytical technology with the large-scale identification of genome polymorphisms have contributed to the field of forensic science, especially in the studies on genetic basis of most important inherited arrhythmia syndromes responsible to sudden cardiac death, a major cause of death worldwide, and of individual differences in response to potential toxicants, with a new emerging area of interest, the so called pharmacogenetics.

The term pharmacogenetics was first used in the late 1950s (Clayman, 1952) and can be defined as the study of variability in drug responses as a function of genetic differences among individuals; applied to nontherapeutic foreign substances, collectively referred to as xenobiotics, the equivalent term toxicogenetics is used (Nebert, 1999; Mancinelli, 2000; Park and Pirmohamed, 2001; Roses, 2002; Wolf, 2000). The later coined term 'pharmacogenomics' usually refers to changes in gene expression as a consequence of drug exposure. However, the two terms, pharmacogenetics and pharmacogenomics, are often used synonymously.

One of the goals of pharmacocogenetics is the identification of the molecular genetic bases for interindividual variations in susceptibility to the anticipated effects of a drug or of xenobiotics (Pirmohamed and Park, 1999). If we want to provide a modern interpretation of the famous assertion of Paracelsus (1493-1541), it is true that "the dose makes the poison", but in different degrees, depending on the genetic characteristics of individuals.

There is no doubt that adverse drug reactions (ADRs) are a common cause of morbidity and mortality, despite extensive and well-regulated registration processes for proving drug efficacy and drug safety, and are associated with substantial costs of medical care (Lazarou, 1998; Pirmohamed, 1999).

Genetic studies could also clarify the origins of addictions, a diverse set of common, complex diseases, that are to some extent tied together by shared genetic and environmental etiological factors (Goldman, 2005; Kendler, 2003). The use and abuse of legal and illegal substances is a worldwide public health priority with repercussions extending from the level of the individual to the family, community, and society.

This chapter will focus on: a) adverse drug reactions; b) drug addiction; c) variability in the human genome; d) pharmacogenetic variability in drug response; e) genetic approaches to understand the individual differences in susceptibility to drugs/xenobiotics responses; f) ethical issues relating to the collection of genetic data.

2. Adverse drug reactions

Any substance that is capable of producing a therapeutic effect can also produce unwanted or adverse effects; the risk of such effects ranges from near zero to high (Edwards, 2000). An adverse drug reaction (ADR), according to the World Health Organization definition, is "a response to a drug that is noxious, unintended, and undesired effect of a drug, which occurs at doses used in man for prophylaxis, diagnosis, or therapy of disease, or for modification of physiological function". This definition excludes therapeutic failures, intentional and accidental poisoning (ie, overdose), and drug abuse. Also, this does not include adverse events due to errors in drug administration or non-compliance (taking more or less of a drug than the prescribed amount); using this narrow definition avoids overestimating the ADR incidence (Lazarou, 1998). The terms adverse reaction and adverse effect are interchangeably, but must be kept in mind that is the "drug" that has an adverse effect whereas it is the "patient" that experience an adverse reaction. However, the two terms must be distinguished from "adverse event", that is an averse outcome that occurs while a patient is taking a drug, but is not necessarily attributable to it (Edwards, 2000).

The interest in ADRs was stimulated by the thalidomide tragedy in the 1960s and, over the past several years, ADRs have gained worldwide attention: the Food and Drug Administration (FDA) has planned a system of pharmacovigilance to be followed by regulatory agencies, pharmaceutical companies, and individual health care providers (U.S. Department of Health and Human Services Food and Drug Administration, 2005).

The occurrence of ADRs is associated with morbidity and mortality and substantial costs of medical care. Numerous studies provide a wide range of epidemiological data regarding adverse drug reactions. ADRs are one of the top ten causes of death in the United States, causing over 100 000 deaths annually; approximately 2–5% of all hospital admissions can be attributed to adverse drug reactions (Lazarou, 1998). In a study performed in 1999 in emergency departments of French public hospitals, out of a total of 1937 patients consulting, 328 (21%) of these patients consulted an physician because of an ADR (Queneau, 2007). During the year 2000, a prospective Italian study was performed in two observational periods of 10 days each in 22 Italian emergency departments: on 18 854 enrolled patients, 629 (3.3%) were affected by ADR and among these, 244 (38.8% of ADR patients) reported a serious event (Trifirò G, 2005). In a prospective Scandinavian study with 13.992 patients of internal medicine, the incidence of lethal ADR was estimated to be 0.95% (Ebbesen, 2001). Another prospective study conducted in the UK demostrated that about 6.5% of hospital admissions were ADR related in 18.820 patients (Pirmohamed, 2004). In a nationwide study in Spain, during a six-year period (2001-2006), the total number of hospitalized patients with ADR diagnosis was 350 835, 1.69% of all acute hospital admissions (Carrasco-Garrido, 2010); in The Netherlands, in 2001, 12 249 hospitalisations were coded as ADR related, 1.83% of all acute hospital admissions (van der Hooft, 2010).

Unfortunately, many physicians still consider adverse drug reactions to be an exception, rather than a primary diagnosis and adverse drug reactions have become cases of medical professional liability, with great increase of lawsuits (Wooten, 2010).

The classification of ADRs distinguished dose-related and non-dose related reactions, named type A and type B, respectively; type A reactions are common, predictable and therefore potentially preventable, based on the drug's pharmacological action, while type B reactions are more troublesome, uncommon and unpredctable. More recently, additional types were added, such as chronic (type C) and delayed (type D) effects, as well as withdrawal or end of use syndromes (type E) and therapeutic failures (type F) (Edwards, 2000).

Different subjects with the same diagnosis could respond differently to the same drug administered at the same dose, with a diminished, absent or excessive response or interaction with other drugs (Mancinelli, 2000; Meyer, 2004). Potential risk factors for ADRs include patients' age, sex, race, nutritional status, organ function, especially of liver and kidneys, co-morbidities, co-medication, as well as some lifestyle variables (smoking habits, concomitant use of alcohols and drugs) and, of course, genetics. Some ADRs caused by genetic variation, previously considered unpredictable, may now be preventable. In general, genetic factors are estimated to account for 15-30% of interindividual differences in drug metabolism and response, but for certain drugs this can be as high as 95% (Evans, 2004; Weinshilboum, 2003)

ADRs may be reduced by means of the introduction of "personalized medicine", which anticipates the screening of patients for polymorphisms associated with a drug response, usually performed prior to the initiation of therapy. Despite significant progress in this field, only few drugs, such as cetuximab, dasatinib, maraviroc and trastuzumab, require a pharmacogenetic test before being prescribed: there are several gaps that limit the application of pharmacogenetics based upon the complex nature of the drug response itself (Gervasini, 2010).

This kind of policy foresees the introduction of new sophisticated tests, especially in the field of genetics, like DNA microarrays or DNA chips.

3. Drug addiction

Drug addiction is a chronic, relapsing disorder in which compulsive drug-seeking and drug-taking behavior persists despite serious negative consequences; continued use induces adaptive changes in the central nervous system that lead to tolerance, physical dependence, sensitization, craving, and relapse (Goodman, 2008). This mental health disorder imposes a significant burden on those directly affected, health care systems, and society in general, since it is associated with considerable morbidity and mortality, violence, and legal issues.

According to World Health Organization (WHO) figures, about 2 billion people worldwide consume alcoholic beverages, 1.3 billion nicotine and 185 million illegal drugs. In Europe the use of alcohol, nicotine and illicit substances is responsible for respectively 10%, 12% and 2% of the total cost of illness. (WHO, 2002).

Polydrug use of psychoactive substances, legal and illegal, characterizes and defines the style of consumption prevailing more and more common among younger subjects. There is another emerging market worldwide for an increasing number of psychoactive substances whose compositions are not well known and whose effects have not yet been recorded by physicians and they are difficult to recognize, delaying the diagnosis and treatment of patients themselves.

In addition there is another phenomenon in recent years: it is a marked shift in the marketing of licit and illicit drugs through online pharmacies, without requiring a prescription. The new generations are particularly vulnerable to this risk because they are very prone to use new technologies.

The nonmedical use of a prescription or over-the-counter (OTC) medication is another significant international emerging problem. OTC medications are pharmaceuticals that do not require a prescription and are sold on the shelves of markets, stores and pharmacies.

The several classes of medications that are commonly abused include: analgesics opioids, which are most often prescribed to treat severe pain (morphine, oxycodone, hydrocodone, hydromorphone, codeine); central nervous system depressants, commonly prescribed to treat anxiety and sleep disorders (barbiturates and benzodiazepines); stimulants, which are used primarily to treat attention deficit disorder, attention deficit hyperactivity disorder (ADHD) and narcolepsy (dextroamphetamine and methylphenidate). The OTC medicines, such as certain cough suppressant (dextromethorphan), sleep aids (doxylamine), antihistamines (diphenhydramine), decongestants and others can be abused for their psychoactive effects (Lessenger, 2008).

According to figures reported by NIDA, in 2009 approximately 7 million (M) reported past month non-medical use of psychotherapeutic drugs (2.8 percent of the U.S. population). The medications most commonly abused are: pain relievers (5.3 M), tranquilizers (2.0 M), stimulants (1.3 M), sedatives (0.4 M). The abuse of drugs is particularly problematic in adolescents, shows that in boys aged 12 to 17 years 8,3% reported abuse of Vicodin (hydrocodone) and 5% of Oxicontin (oxycodone hydrochloride) (NIDA, 2010).

All substances that are abused have ability to induce dependence and withdrawal.

The current challenge is to transfer the important increase of the knowledges of addiction's neurobiology in patients with addiction problems and to identify specific genes responsible for the particular vulnerability or resistance to addiction. Some schools of thought contend that addiction is entirely preventable through proper legislative action and individual choice, and claim that genetic research in this field is to assume a role as a low priority (Merikangas, 2003). Genetic research, however, plays a very important role, since the origins of addiction susceptibility are complex and wide-ranging; the underlying genetic factors need to be identified to solve the puzzle of what causes these pervasive and relatively intractable disorders (Goldman, 2005).

Both genetic and environmental variables contribute to the initiation of use of addictive agents and to the transition from use to addiction (Bevilacqua, 2009). Evidence from twin and adoption studies suggest that 40-60% of the risk of developing substance abuse disorders is due to genetic factors, with the percentage depending on the substance (Nestler, 2000). The addiction are complex disorders involving multiple genes and environment interaction (G x E). The genetic influences are more prominent in the later phases of individuals' progression toward substance dependence; this variation could add to allelic variations that could produce effects on addiction susceptability phenotypes by other routes that could include: differences in pharmacokinetic characteristics of the substance such as metabolism and biodistribution; differences in drug's rewarding properties; differences in traits manifest by the addict, including personality differences; differences in addict's psychiatric comorbidities (Uhl, 2004). This suggests two broad types of genetic predisposition to addiction: genetic profiles that make people more likely to find the acute effect of drugs rewarding and genetic profiles that make people more or less likely to developing addiction if they use drugs (EMCDDA, 2009). Finally, evidence indicates that there is a genetic predisposition that is shared between the different substance use disorders; nearly 25-36% of the genetic influences of alcohol, nicotine and cannabis problem use is attributable to overlapping factors (Young, 2006).

The inheritance of addictions has been evaluated in many ways, including studies on families and adoptees, but the main reference of our knowledge comes from the patterns of correlations in monozygotic (MZ) and dizygotic (DZ) twins. The overall genetic influence for substance use disorders has proved to be consistent and heritabilities for most substance use disorders are estimated to be moderate to high (Wong, 2008). This moderate to high inheritance may seem paradoxical: addiction depends initially on individual choice to use an additive agent. Cocaine and opiates, among the most addictive of substances, are among the most heritable; in contrast, hallucinogens, are among the least addictive, and are also the least heritable (Bevilacqua, 2009).

The genes involved in the of the condition are very numerous (Kreek, 2005).

The phenotype for addiction to drugs is not well defined, and the heritability of addiction to drugs of abuse is far from clear. Knowledge of genetic factors in etiology and treatment response may enable the individualization of prevention and treatment, as well as the identification of new therapeutic targets (Buckland, 2008).

4. Variability in the human genome

Individuals are all different from each other and much of this difference has a genetic basis. Two unrelated human beings also share 99.9% of their genomic sequence, and could be considered genetically almost identical: the difference has been estimated to be of 0.1% overall, but still, this means that there are at least several million nucleotide differences per individual. There are, on average, three million genetic differences between any two people; the human genome contains approximately 3 billion base pairs of DNA and the variability of genetic material between any two individuals averages approximately one variation for every 1,000.

This genetic diversity in most cases have no functional significance, but in some cases have important consequences (Marchant, 2003). The most dramatic examples are seen with inherited disorders, where small alterations in gene sequence can result in premature death or severe disability (Alberts, 2002; Habener and Williams, 2002; King, 2002). It is also responsible of the phenotypic diversity, which results in the heterogeneous capacity of each individual to respond to exogenous substances, such as drugs and xenobiotics, and in the different susceptibility to induce adverse health effects.

The types of genetic variations used in these studies have changed in the past 25 years and can be classified into five major classes: RFLP (restriction fragment length polymorphism), VNTR (variable number of tandem repeat), STR (short tandem repeat), SNP (single-nucleotide polymorphism) and CNV (copy-number variation); furthermore, construction of the international SNP database and recent development of high-throughput SNP typing platforms enabled us to perform genome-wide association studies, which have identified genes or genetic variations susceptible to common diseases or those associated with drug responses (Nakamura, 2009).

SNPs are found at a frequency of about 1:1000 bases in humans and they are changes in a single base at a specific position in the genome, in most cases with two alleles. By definition, the more rare allele should be more abundant than 1% in the general population; if the variant is rare, with a frequency below 0.1%, it is referred to as a mutation. More than 99% of these genetic variations are biologically silent, while some polymorphisms can affect biological function according to their position within the genome.

Following the scheme of Orphanides and Kimber (2003), it is possible to distinguish:

1. SNPs that fall within the coding region of a gene can give rise to a protein that has an amino acid substitution, or is truncated, causing a change in activity, localization, or stability;

2. SNPs that induce shifts in translational reading frames will lead to the synthesis of proteins with altered aminoacid sequence and, perhaps, activity;
3. nucleotide alterations in the regulatory regions of a gene can also have a significant impact on the integrity of protein function;
4. polymorphisms in promoter regions may change the regulation and level of expression of a protein, whereas those that fall near intron-exon junctions may cause alterations in mRNA splicing;
5. more dramatic polymorphisms involving larger segments of the genome include gene deletions, gene conversions, and gene duplications (Orphanides and Kimber, 2003).

5. Pharmacogenetic variability in drug response

Gene polymorphisms account for the polymodal distribution of the frequency of response to a drug in a non-homogeneous population, i.e. one encompassing multiple genetic profiles capable of affecting response.
Current pharmacogenetic studies are exploring individual responses to drugs in relation to the genetic variations in the proteins involved in pharmacokinetics (absorption, distribution, metabolism and excretion) and pharmacodynamics (receptors, ion channels and other enzymes) (Roses A, 2000; Nebert, 2008) (figure 1).

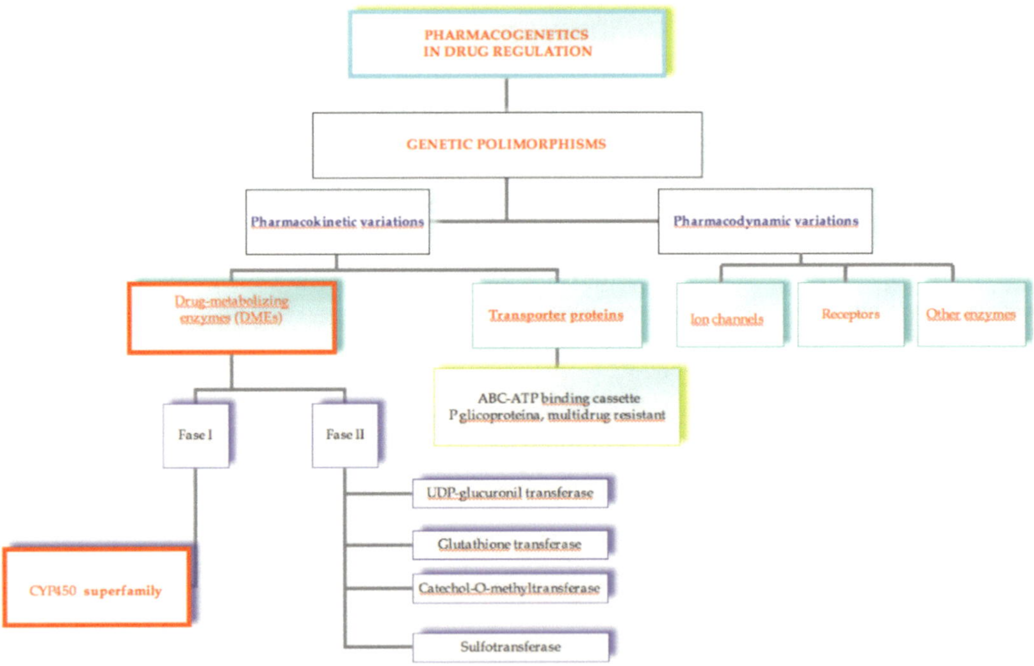

Fig. 1. Pharmacogenetic variations affecting the individual response to a drug

Drug-metabolizing enzymes (DMEs) play a key pharmacokinetic role (Meyer, 1997). Drugs are turned to metabolites in the liver, by transformation of functional groups (phase I reactions) and subsequent conjugation with endogenous lipophilic substances to form inactive compounds (phase II reactions) for ready excretion in urine or bile. Oxidative drug metabolism is mainly catalyzed by the enzymes of the large CYP450 gene family, that contains 57 functional genes and 58 pseudogenes playing an important role in the metabolism of therapeutic drugs and other xenobiotics. CYP450 are so named because they are bound to membranes within a cell (cyto) and contain a heme pigment (chrome and P) that absorbs light at a wavelength of 450 nm when exposed to carbon monoxide. The corresponding genes are highly polymorphic and genetic variability underlies interindividual differences in drug response. CYP2D6, 2C19, and 2C9 polymorphisms account for the most frequent variations, since almost 80% of drugs in use today are metabolized by these enzymes (Danielson, 2002; Ingelman-Sundberg, 1999; Nebert, 2002; Nelson, 1999; Zhou, 2009). The polymorphisms of CYP2D6 significantly affect the pharmacokinetics of about 50% of the drugs in clinical use (De Gregori M, 2010).

The CYP450 enzimes convert the substances into electrophilic intermediates, which are then conjugated by phase II enzymes, of which the most important are the highly polymorphic UDP-glucuronil transferase, sulfotransferase, catechol-O-methyltransferase (COMT) and glutathione transferase, to facilitate substrate excretion by turning them into more water-soluble forms.

All these factors determine the trend of concentration over time and therefore the effectiveness of drugs and duration of effect. DME genetic variations result in marked phenotypic consequences; these range from poor metabolizers (where toxic drug effects may arise due to the absence of the gene product) to ultrarapid metabolizers (where therapeutic failure may be induced by the indicated dosage, with the risk of achieving high plasma concentrations and concentration-dependent side effects due to gene overexpression). The resulting phenotypes are poor (PMs), intermediate (IMs), extensive (EMs) and ultrarapid (UMs) metabolizers.

To leave the cell, some drugs are actively transported by membrane transporter proteins. The major transporter enzymes are MDR1 (multidrug resistance proteins), MRP (multidrug resistance-associated proteins) and OATP (organic anion-transporting polypeptides), where several genetic polymorphisms have been demonstrated. MDRs are transmembrane transporters of the large ABC protein family: P-glycoprotein (P-gp, or MDR1/ABCB1), the best known, is highly polymorphic. It can influence substrate absorption at the level of the blood brain barrier; high P-gp concentrations can limit entry of the required amount of drug, whereas low levels may result in abnormal accumulation. Recently, allele frequencies and findings regarding functional variants in drug transporter systems were reported in an interesting review (Kroetz, 2010).

Pharmacodynamic processes mediate the biochemical and physical effects of drugs on the organism. Variations in the sequence of the genes encoding the primary therapeutic target, such as receptors and ion channels, are capable of inducing protein forms with different functional characteristics. This can account for abnormal drug responses, which may also underpin some adverse reactions.

Recently, researchers are focusing on most important genetic variations that could contribute to the initiation of use of addictive agents and to the transition from use to addiction. The complex genetic constitution is partly accounted for by heterogeneity and polygenicity: the first assumes that a single or a few genetic variation(s) determine vulnerability and resiliency, but different alleles would lead to the same clinical presentation in different individuals; the second, on the other hand, assumes that a phenotype is a result of simultaneous function of multiple genetic variants (Goldman, 2005; Wong, 2008).

Pharmacogenetic studies can assess the effects of genetic variation on the risk for particular phenotypes for addiction, for example being an alcoholic (Onori, 2010; Buscemi, 2011). In recent years abundant evidence has accumulated demonstrating that alcoholism, a major health and social issue, being one of the most frequent disease and cause of premature death, is a multifaceted disease of the brain, caused by numerous genetic, neurobiological, environmental factors that are still not yet fully understood. Numerous genes are up- and/or down-regulated by alcohol exposure: the ethanol-responsive genes mainly encode functional proteins such as proteins involved in nucleic acid binding, transcription factors, selected regulatory molecules, and receptors. Currently there are only three medications approved by the U.S. Food and Drug Administration (FDA) for use in the treatment of alcohol abuse and alcohol dependence: the aldehyde dehydrogenase inhibitor disulfiram, the micro opioid receptor antagonist naltrexone, and the N-methyl-D-aspartate (NMDA) receptor inhibitor acamprosate (Wang, 2010).

6. Pharmacogenetic approaches

Pharmacogenetic studies can be categorized into two methodologic approaches: genome-wide linkage analysis and candidate gene approach.

Linkage analysis is applied to families with several affected individuals, to establish whether specific alleles of marker genes are found more often in individuals with the disease than in healthy subjects. The whole genome is analysed using markers that are uniformly distributed on all chromosomes, seeking chromosome regions that could contain genes involved in complex disorder susceptibility. The linkage is sought only in recent ancestors. Since only a small number of recombination events are involved, the gene regions detected by linkage analysis are likely to be large and to encompass hundreds or even thousands of genes. Genetic association studies assess correlations between genetic variants and trait differences on a population scale and they have been used widely to identify regions of the genome and candidate genes that contribute to complex disease.

A disease-associated SNP that falls within a gene can provide information on the mechanistic basis for disease, while a SNP that is in linkage disequilibrium with a genetic allele that confers disease predisposition may be used to identify susceptible individuals, and naturally this can include those genetic variations that influence relative susceptibility or resistance to toxicants (Roses, 2000). The common errors encountered in association studies of complex diseases are the small sample size, subgroup analysis and multiple testing, random error, poorly matched control group, failure to attempt study replication and to detect linkage disequilibrium with adjacent loci, overinterpreting results and positive publication bias, unwarranted candidate gene declaration after identifying association in arbitrary genetic region (Cardon, 2001). Despite these known limitations, the power of association analysis to detect genetic contributions to complex disease can be much greater than that of linkage studies (Risch, 2000).

Association studies can be distinguished into family-based, which use the transmission disequilibrium test, and population-based, which use case-control testing. Case-control studies compare genes from two groups of individuals, healthy and diseased. Ideally, the two groups should be homogeneous, with subjects matching for measures like age, ethnicity, years of education, and marital status, and differing only in terms of the disease studied. The allele frequency of the gene markers (e.g. SNPs) in or close to the genes are analysed and frequency differences between the groups taken to indicate that the gene contributes to the disease.

Association studies draw from historic recombination so disease-associated regions are extremely small in outbred random mating populations, encompassing only one gene or gene fragment. As the disease mutation is transmitted from one generation to the next, recombination will separate it from the alleles of its original haplotype.
A specific genetic profile, or haplotype, i.e. the combination of allelic states in a set of polymorphic markers found on the same chromosome, could be identified by association studies by analyzing a number of markers of a given chromosome region in a group of affected subjects and in a control group (case-control study). Different haplotypes can be found in a population as a result of mutation or genetic recombination. The recombination is principally determined by the genetic distance between markers and by the propierties of the locus where they are found (recombination hotspots). Markers that do not undergo recombination are characterized by linkage disequilibrium (LD). The tendency of some alleles at distinct loci to be co-inherited, due to reduced rates of, or absent, genetic recombination may lead to their association in a population, i.e. to LD. Recent LD studies by analysis of SNP haplotypes have suggested a block structure, at least in some portions of the genome. Haplotype blocks appear as regions made up of consecutive alleles that are co-inherited. Given the limited haplotype diversity within blocks, several SNPs will be redundant, enabling a minimum number of informative markers to be used to identify the common haplotypes in each block: these markers are called tag-SNPs. Different block structures can be found in different populations, with significant implications for association studies, since the tag-SNPs identified in a population will be useless in another if they are found in different blocks.

7. Ethical issues

It is necessary to make a reflection on how informations from the human genome will be used. The collection of genetic data has attracted much public attention for the possible ethical, moral and political issues relating to the use of these informations.
Genome-wide association studies trying to identify genes that contribute a small risk to common diseases can only be performed on an international scale; meanwhile, it is becoming more and more clear that genomic information is hard to hide. Thus the traditional promise in research that privacy will be protected appears to be less realistic. The deciphering of the genetic code may pose a threat to the protection of one's privacy; some variants that predict drug response are also markers for disease predisposition. This may subsequently lead to medico-legal implications, such as the issue of data confidentially: whether employers and insurance companies should given rights to assess the genetic data (Koo, 2006). Access to genetic might lead to discrimination of individuals with an unfavourable genetic constitution; for example, individuals who have a genetic predisposition for a certain condition, or who would only tolerate expensive drugs, might be charged higher insurance premiums (Vijverberg, 2010).
Most European countries have adopted genetic anti- discrimination legislation; Belgium was the first in 1990, and many countries followed. After a 13-year battle in Congress-longer than it took to map the human genome-the Genetic Information Nondiscrimination Act (GINA) was passed into law on 21 May 2008. Francis Collins, the director of the National Human Genome Research Institute, said that the success of personalized medicine hinged on the passing of the legislation.
Van Hoyweghen and Horstman state that many European genetic non-discrimination laws only provide the illusion of protection and the protection against potential risks of

discrimination based on predictive medical information is still so far. Some insurance companies may still use genetic test results or genetic information derived from physician records or insurance questionnaires (Van Hoyweghen, 2008). This practice is mainly caused by ignorance, confusion and misunderstanding, but also due to the lack of clear legal definitions of 'genetic data' and 'genetic tests'(Vijverberg, 2010). The definitions of genetic testing used by 65 organisations and entities, including genetics professional organisations, insurance organisations, pharmaceutical companies, and legal organisations, was reviewed; it was found that the definitions used were extremely variable; ranging from DNA testing solely, to any source that can provide unambiguous genetic information, including family history (Sequeiros, 2005).

It has been suggested that potential problems with the ethical use of this kind of genetic data can be minimized by selecting SNPs that are of pharmacogenetic and toxicogenetic value, while avoiding those that predict genetic disease (Roses, 2002).

Toxicogenetics can learn from the forensic sciences: the widely used technique of "genetic fingerprinting" uses a small number of highly polymorphic, unlinked genetic markers that have no known implications to the health of an individual (Orphanides and Kimber, 2003).

8. Conclusion

The potential of pharmacogenetics to improve the clinical practice is only at the very beginning but will present an important biomedical tool in the post-genomic era. The aim is to aid physicians in the prescription of the right medicine to a person in an attempt to obtain maximum efficacy and minum toxicity based on a genetic test, according the new strategy named "personalized medicine": prescribing the right drug in the right dose to the right patient according to specific health needs and individual characteristics.

Advanced diagnostic analyses, genetic counselling, and interdisciplinary and multidisciplinary approach, involving neurobiological, genetical, toxicological, psychological, and social sciences, should be integral parts of forensic practice.

Although a relatively novel concept in the forensic context, pharmacogenetics has the capability to assist in the interpretation of drug related deaths, particularly in unintentional drug poisonings where the cause of death remains unclear (Pilgrim, 2010). The recommendation number eleven of the report from the National Academy of Sciences (NAS) titled "Strengthening Forensic Science in the United States: A Path Forward" is concerned with improving medicolegal death investigations: "Best practices should include the utilization of new technologies such as laboratory testing for the molecular basis of diseases".

The forensic science community, however, has not yet fully received this directive and only few studies to date have been able to ascertain a correlation between genotype and phenotype for a limited number of drugs and to establish a link with the death (Koski, 2006; Koski, 2007; Launiainem, 2010; Levo, 2003).

The correlation between genotype and phenotype still remains a limitation in a molecular autopsy ant it is complicate for a number of reason. Only individuals completely lacking the enzyme activity (PMs) are highly correlated with the expected phenotype. There is substantial overlap in activity within and between the other phenotypic classes: subjects with identical genotypes may also exhibit different phenotypic activities which may be explained by population-specific factors, such as unidentified genetic, such as other enzyme and proteins, and non-genetic factors, such as diet. In addition, the funtional consequence of the genetic variation may be substrate (e.g. drug or its metabolite) specific (Gaedigk, 2008; Sajantila, 2010).

The new opportunities, offered by pharmacogenetics, to analyse the genetic variations related to the risk of ADRs or to susceptibility to drug addiction are of considerable interest to forensic scientists, for their role in the evaluation of drug addiction in its various phases of development, from beginning to end stage. A better understanding of genetic susceptibility to addiction may be also useful for ascertaining the causes and circumstances of death. Some gene variants may, in fact, determine in some individuals more sensitive to the substance, with an increased risk of toxic effects, even death.

9. References

Alberts, B.; Johnson, A.; Lewis, J.; Raff, R.; Roberts, K. & Walker, P. (2002). *Molecular Biology of the Cell*, 4 th ed., Garland Publishing, ISBN 978-0815332183, New York

Bevilacqua, L. & Goldman, D. (2009). Genes and Addictions. *Clinical Pharmacology & Therapeutics*, Vol.4, No.85, (April 2009), pp. 359-361, ISSN 0009-9236

Buckland, P.R. (2008). Will we ever find the genes for addiction? *Addiction*, No.103, (April 2008), pp. 1768-1776, ISSN 0965-2140

Buscemi, L. & Turchi, C. (2011). An overview of the genetic susceptibility to alcoholism. *Medicine, Science & the Law*, in press, ISSN 0025-8024

Cardon, L.R. & Bell, J.I. (2001). Association study designs for complex diseases. *Nature Genetics*, Vol.2, No.2, (February 2001), pp. 91-99, ISSN 1061-4036

Carrasco-Garrido, P.; De Andrés, L.A.; Barrera, V.H.; De Miguel, G.A. & Jiménez-García, R. (2010). Trends of adverse drug reactions related-hospitalizations in Spain (2001-2006). *BMC Health Services Research*, Vol.10, No.287, (October 2010), ISSN 1472-6963

Clayman, C.B.; Arnold, J.; Hockwald, R.S.; Yount, E.H.Jr.; Edgcomb, J.H. & Alving, A.S. (1952). Toxicity of primaquine in Caucasians. *The Journal of the American Medical Association*, Vol.17, No.149, (August 1952), pp. 1563-1568, ISSN 0098-7484

Danielson, P.B. (2002). The cytochrome p450 superfamily: biochemistry, evolution, and drug metabolism in humans. *Current Drug Metabolism*, Vol.6, No.3, (December 2002), pp. 561-597, ISSN 1389-2002

De Gregori, M.; Allegri, M.; De Gregori, S.; Garbin, G.; Tinelli, C.; Regazzi, M.; Govoni, S. & Ranzani, G.N. (2010). How and why to screen for CYP2D6 interindividual variability in patients under pharmacological treatments. *Current Drug Metabolism*, Vol.3, No.11, (March 2010), pp. 276-282, ISSN 1389-2002

Dressler, L.G. & Terry, S.F. (2009). How will GINA influence participation in pharmacogenomics research and clinical testing? *Clinical Pharmacology & Therapeutics*, Vol.5, No.86, (November 2009), pp. 472-475, ISSN 0009-9236

Ebbesen, J.; Buajordet, I.; Erikssen, J.; Brørs, O.; Hilberg, T.; Svaar, H. & Sandvik L. (2001). Drug-related deaths in a department of internal medicine. *Archives of Internal Medicine*, Vol.19, No.161, (October 2001), pp. 2317-2323, ISSN 0003-9926

Edwards, I.R. & Aronson, J.K. (2000). Adverse drug reactions: definitions, diagnosis, and management. *Lancet*, Vol.9237, No.356, (October 2000), pp. 1255-1259, ISSN 0140-6736

Eichelbaum, M.; Ingelman-Sundberg, M. & Evans, W.E. (2006). Pharmacogenomics and individualized drug therapy. *Annual Review of Medicine,* No.57, (February 2006), pp.119-137, ISSN 0066-4219

EMCDDA Monographs (2009). Genetic susceptibility to addiction, In: Addiction neurobiology: ethical and social implications, A. Carter, B. Capps, W. Hall (Ed.), 47-50, Luxembourg, ISBN 978-92-9168-347-5. Available from http://www.emcdda.europa.eu/publications/monographs/neurobiology

Evans, W.E. & Relling, M.V. (2004). Moving towards individualized medicine with pharmacogenomics. *Nature,* Vol.6990, No.429, (May 2004), pp. 464-468, ISSN 0028-0836

Gaedigk, A.; Simon, S.D.; Pearce, R.E.; Bradford, L.D.; Kennedy, M.J. & Leeder, J.S. (2008). The CYP2D6 activity score: translating genotype information into a qualitative measure of phenotype. *Clinical Pharmacology & Therapeutics,* Vol.2, No.83, (February 2008), pp. 234-42, ISSN 0009-9236

Gervasini G.; Benítez J. & Carrillo J.A. (2010). Pharmacogenetic testing and therapeutic drug monitoring are complementary tools for optimal individualization of drug therapy. *European Journal of Clinical Pharmacology,* Vol.8, No.66, (August 2010), pp. 755-774, ISSN 0031-6970

Goldman, D.; Gabor, O. & Ducci, F. (2005). The genetics of addiction: uncovering the genes. *Nature Reviews Genetics* Vol.7, No.6, (July 2005), pp. 521-532, ISSN 1471-0056 .

Goodman, A. (2008). Neurobiology of addiction. An integrative review. *Biochemical Pharmacology,* Vol.1, No.75, (January 2008), pp. 266-322, ISSN 0006-2952

Habener, J.F. & Williams, G. H. (2002). *Metabolic Basis of Common Inherited Diseases,* 1 st ed. W.B. Saunders, (Ed.), ISBN 978-072-1686-78-3

Ingelman-Sundberg, M.; Oscarson, M. & McLellan, R.A. (1999). Polymorphic human cytochrome P450 enzymes: An opportunity for individualized drug treatment. *Trends in Pharmacological Sciences,* Vol.8, No.20, (August 1999), pp. 342–349, ISSN 0165-6147

Kendler, K.S.; Jacobson, K.C.; Prescott, C.A. & Neale, M.C. (2003). Specificity of genetic and environmental risk factors for use and abuse/dependence of cannabis, cocaine, hallucinogens, sedatives, stimulants, and opiates in male twins. *American Journal of Psychiatry,* Vol.4, No.160, (April 2003), pp. 687-695, ISSN 0002-953X

King, R.A.; Rotter, J.I. & Motulsky, A.G. (2002). *The Genetic Basis of Common Diseases,* 2 nd ed. (Oxford monographs on medical genetics, 44). Oxford University Press, ISBN 0-1951-2582-7, Oxford, UK

Koo, S.H. & Lee, E.J. (2006). Pharmacogenetics approach to therapeutics. *Clinical and Experimental Pharmacology and Physiology,* Vol.5-6, No.33, (May-June 2006), pp. 525-532, ISSN 0305-1870

Koski, A., Sistonen, J., Ojanperä, I., Gergov, M., Vuori, E., Sajantila, A (2006). CYP2D6 and CYP2C19 genotypes and amitriptyline metabolite ratios in a series of medicolegal autopsies. *Forensic Sciences International,* Vol.2-3, No.158, (May 2006), pp. 177-183, ISSN 0379-0738

Koski, A., Ojanperä, I., Sistonen, J., Vuori, E., Sajantila, A. (2007). A fatal doxepin poisoning associated with a defective CYP2D6 genotype. *The American Journal of Forensic Medicine and Pathology,* Vol.3, No.28, (September 2007), pp. 259-261, ISSN 0195-7910

Kreek, M.J.; Nielsen, D.A.; Butelman, E.R. & LaForge, K.S. (2005). Genetic influences on impulsivity, risk taking, stress responsivity and vulnerability to drug abuse and addiction. *Nature Neuroscienze,* Vol.11, No.8, (November 2005), pp. 1450-1457, ISSN 1097-6256

Kroetz, D.L.; Yee, S.W. & Giacomini, K.M. (2010). The pharmacogenomics of membrane transporters project research as the interface of genomics and transporter pharmacology. *Clinical Pharmacology & Therapeutics,* Vol.1, No.87, (January 2010), pp. 109-116, ISSN 0009-9236

Lazarou, J.; Pomeranz, B.H. & Corey, P.N. (1998). Incidence of adverse drug reactions in hospitalized patients: a meta-analysis of prospective studies. *The Journal of the American Medical Association,* Vol.15, No.279, (April 1998), pp. 1200-1205, ISSN 0098-7484

Lessenger, J.E. & Feinberg, S.D. (2008). Abuse of Prescription and Over-The-Counter Medications. *Journal of American Board Family Medicine,* Vol.1, No.21, (January-February 2008), pp. 45-54, ISSN 1557-2625

Levo, A.; Koski, A.; Ojanperä, I.; Vuori, E. & Sajantila, A. (2003). Post-mortem SNP analysis of CYP2D6 gene reveals correlation between genotype and opioid drug (tramadol) metabolite ratios in blood. *Forensic Sciences International,* Vol.1, No.135, (July 2003), pp. 9-15, ISSN 0379-0738

Mancinelli, L.; Cronin, M. & Sadèe, W. (2000). Pharmacogenomics: the promise of personalized medicine. *AAPS PharmSci,* Vol.1, No.2, ISSN 1522-1059

Marchant, G.E. (2003). Genomics and Toxic Substances: Part II-Genetic Susceptibility to Enviromental Agents. *Environmental Law Review,* Vol.9, No.33, (September 2003), pp. 10641-10667

Meyer, U.A. & Zanger, U.M. (1997). Molecular mechanisms of genetic polymorphisms of drug metabolism. *Annual Review of Pharmacology and Toxicology,* No.37, pp. 269-296, ISSN 0362-1642

Meyer, U.A. (2000). Pharmacogenetics and adverse drug reactions. *Lancet* Vol.9242, No.356, (November 2000), pp. 1667-1671, ISSN 0140-6736

Meyer, U.A. (2004). Pharmacogenetics-five decades of therapeutic lessons from genetic diversity. *Nature Review Genetics,* Vol.9, No.5, (September 2004), pp. 669-676, ISSN 1471-0056

Merikangas, K.R. & Risch, N. (2003). Genomic priorities and public health. *Science,* Vol.5645, No.302, (October 2003), pp. 599-601, ISSN 0036-8075

National Research Council (2009). *Strengthening Forensic Science in the United States: A Path Forward.* In: National Academies Press (Ed.), ISBN: 0-309-13131-6, Washington D.C.

Available from http://www.nap.edu/catalog/12589.html

Nakamura, Y. (2009). DNA variations in human and medical genetics: 25 years of my experience. *Journal of Human Genetics,* Vol.1, No.54, (January 2009), pp. 1-8, ISSN 1434-5161

Nebert, D.W. (1999). Pharmacogenetics and pharmacogenomics: Why is this relevant to the clinical geneticist? *Clinical Genetics,* Vol.4, No.56, (October 1999), pp. 247–258, ISSN 0009-9163

Nebert, D.W. & Russell, D.W. (2002). Clinical importance of the cytochromes P450. *Lancet,* Vol.9340, No.360, (October 2002), pp. 1155–1162, ISSN 0140-6736

Nebert, D.W.; Zhang, Ge. & Vesell, E.S (2008). From human genetics and genomics to pharmacogenetics and pharmacogenomics: past lessons, future directions. *Drug Metabolism Reviews,* Vol.2, No.40, pp. 187-224, ISSN 0360-2532

Nelson, D.R. (1999). Cytochrome P450 and the individuality of species. *Archives of Biochemistry and Biophysics,* Vol.1, No.369, (September 1999), pp. 1–10, ISSN 0003-9861

Nestler, E.J. (2000). Genes and addiction. *Nature Genetics, Vol.3, No* 26, (November 2000), pp. 277-281, ISSN 1061-4036

NIDA (2010). Prescription drug abuse. In: *Topics in brief,* Available from http://www.nida.nih.gov/tib/prescription.html

Onori, N.; Turchi, C.; Solito, G.; Gesuita, R.; Buscemi, L. & Tagliabracci, A. (2010). GABRA2 and alcohol use disorders: no evidence of an association in an Italian case-control study. *Alcoholism: Clinical and Experimental Research,* Vol.4, No.34, (April 2010), pp. 659-668, ISSN 0145-6008

Orphanides, G. & Kimber, I. (2003). Toxicogenenetics: applications and opportunites. *Toxicological Sciences,* Vol.1, No.75, (September 2003), pp. 1-6, ISSN 1096-6080

Park, B. K. & Pirmohamed, M. (2001). Toxicogenetics in drug development. *Toxicoogy Letters,* Vol.1-3, No.120, (March 2001), pp. 281–291, ISSN 0378-4274

Pilgrim, J.L.; Gerostamoulos, D. & Drummer, O.H. (2010). Review: Pharmacogenetic aspects of the effect of cytochrome P450 polymorphisms on serotonergic drug metabolism, response, interactions, and adverse effects. *Forensic Science, Medicine and Pathology, electronic only,* (November 2010), ISSN 1547-769X

Pirmohamed, M. & Park, B.K. (1999). The adverse effects of drugs. *Hospital Medicine,* Vol.5, No.60, (May 1999), pp. 348-352, ISSN 1462-3935

Pirmohamed, M.; James S.; Meakin S.; Green C.; Scott A.K.; Walley T.J.; Farrar K.; Park B.K. & Breckenridge A.M. (2004). Adverse drug reactions as cause of admission to hospital: prospective analysis of 18 820 patients. *British Medical Journal.* Vol.7456, No.329, (July 2004), pp. 15–19, ISSN 0959-8138

Queneau, P.; Bannwarth, B.; Carpentier, F.; Guliana, J.M.; Bouget, J.; Trombert, B.; Leverve, X.; Lapostolle, F.; Borron, S.W.; Adnet, F. & Association Pédagogique Nationale pour l'Enseignement de la Thérapeutique (APNET) (2007). Emergency department visits caused by adverse drug events: results of a French survey. *Drug Safety,* Vol1, No.30, pp. 81-88, ISSN 0114-5916

Risch, N.J. (2000). Searching for genetic determinants in the new millennium. *Nature,* Vol.6788, No.405, (June 2000), pp. 847–856, ISSN 0028-0836

Roses, A.D. (2000). Pharmacogenetics and the practice of medicine. *Nature,* Vol.6788, No.405, (June 2000), pp. 857–865, ISSN 0028-0836

Roses, A.D. (2002). Genome-based pharmacogenetics and the pharmaceutical industry. *Nature Review Drug Discovery,* Vol.7, No.1, (July 2002), pp. 541–549, ISSN 1474-1776

Sajantila, A.; Palo, J.U.; Ojanperä, I.; Davis, C. & Budowle, B. (2010). Pharmacogenetics in medico-legal context. *Forensic Science International,* Vol.1-3, No.203, (December 2010), pp. 44-52, ISSN 1872-4973

Sequeiros, J. & Guimarães B. *Definitions of genetic testing, 3rd draft.* EuroGentest. 2005. Available from http://www.eurogentest.org/web/files/public/unit3/DefinitionsGeneticTesting-3rdDraf18Jan07.pdf (accessed February 2009).

Trifiro, G.; Calogero, G.; Ippolito, F.M.; Cosentino, M.; Giuliani, R.; Conforti, A.; Venegoni, M.; Mazzaglia, G. & Caputi, A.P. (2005). Adverse drug events in emergency department population: a prospective Italian study. *Pharmacoepidemiol and Drug Safety,* Vol.5, No.14, (May 2005), pp. 333-340, ISSN 1053-8569

Uhl, G.R. (2004). Molecular genetic underpinnings of human substance abuse vulnerability: likely contributions to understanding addiction as a mnemonic process. *Neuropharmacology,* No.47, Suppl.1, pp. 140-147. ISSN 0028-3908

U.S. Department of Health and Human Services Food and Drug Administration (March, 2005). Good Pharmacovigilance Practices and Pharmacoepidemiologic Assessment. In: *Guidance for Industry,* 1.03.2010, Available from http://www.fda.gov/cber/guidelines.htm

Van der Hooft, C.S.; Sturkenboom M.C.; van Grootheest K.; Kingma H.J. & Stricker B.H. (2006). Adverse drug reaction-related hospitalisations: a nationwide study in The Netherlands. *Drug Safety,* Vol.2, No.29, pp. 161-168, ISSN 0114-5916

Van Hoyweghen, I., Horstman, K. (2008). European practices of genetic information and insurance: lessons for the genetic information nondiscrimination act. *The journal of the American Medical Association,* Vol.3, No.300, (July 2008), pp. 326-327, ISSN 0098-7484

Vijverberg, S.J.H.; Pieters, T. & Cornel, M.C. (2010). Ethical and Social Issues in Pharmacogenomics Testing. *Current Pharmaceutical Design,* Vol.2, No.16, pp. 245-252, ISSN 1381-6128

Wang, L.L.; Yang, A.K.; He, S.M.; Liang, .J; Zhou, Z.W.; Li Y. & Zhou, S.F. (2010). Identification of molecular targets associated with ethanol toxicity and implications in drug development. *Current Pharmaceutical Design,* Vol.11, No.16, pp. 1313-55, ISSN 1381-6128

WHO (2002). The global burden. In: *Management of substance abuse,* Available from http://www.who.int/substance_abuse/facts/global_burden/en/index.html)

Wolf, C.R.; Smith, G. & Smith, R. L. (2000). Science, medicine, and the future: Pharmacogenetics. *British Medical Journal,* Vol.7240, No.320, (April 2000), pp. 987–990, ISSN 0959-8138

Wong, C.C.Y, Schumann. G. (2008). Genetics of addiction: strategies for addressing heterogeneity and polygenicity of substance use disorders. *Philosophical transactions of the Royal Society of London. Series B, Biological sciences,* Vol.1507, No.363, (october 2008), pp. 3213-3222, ISSN 0962-8436

Wooten, J. M. (2010). Adverse Drug Reaction: Part I. *Southern Medical Journal,* Vol.10, No.103, (October 2010), pp. 1025-1028, ISSN 0038-4348

Young, S.E.; Rhee, S.H.; Stallings, M.C.; Corley, R.P. & Hewitt, J.K. (2006). Genetic and enviromental vulnerabilities underlying adolescent substance use and problem use: general or specific? *Behavior Genetics,* Vol.4, No.36, (July 2006), pp. 603-615, ISSN 0001-8244

Zhang, K.; Qin, Z.S.; Liu, J.S.; Chen T.; Waterman M.S. & Sun F. (2004). Haplotype block partitioning and Tag SNP selection using genotype data and their applications to association studies. *Genome Research,* Vol.5, No.14, (May 2004), pp. 908-916, ISSN 1088-9051

Zhou, S.F.; Liu, J.P. & Chowbay, B. (2009). Polymorphism of human cytochrome P450 enzymes and its clinical impact. *Drug Metabolism Reviews,* Vol.2, No.41, pp. 89-295, ISSN 0360-2532

12

Forensic Pharmacogenetics

Susi Pelotti and Carla Bini
University of Bologna, Section of Legal Medicine
Italy

1. Introduction

Pharmacogenetics and *pharmacogenomics* are gaining importance both in the clinical setting and in forensic pathology to investigate causes of death where no findings emerge from autopsy, and in the medical liability arena where scientific issues meet the justice system (Pilgrim et al., 2011). Generally speaking, *Pharmacogenetics* is the study of how genetic variations give rise to differences in drug response, while *pharmacogenomics (PGx)* is the application of genomic technologies to the discovery of new therapeutic targets (Evans & Relling, 1999). Nevertheless, there is a diversity of opinion regarding the definitions and benefits of pharmacogenetics and pharmacogenomics. Depending on the purpose, pharmacogenetics can be used to define applications of single gene sequences or a limited set of multiple gene sequences, but not gene expression or genome-wide scans, to study variations in DNA sequences related to drug action and disposition. Pharmacogenomics can be used to define applications of genome-wide single-nucleotide polymorphism (SNP) scans and genome-wide gene expression analyses to study variations influencing drug action (Lesko et al., 2003). Some authors use a very broad definition of pharmacogenomics including the study of inter-individual variations in whole-genome or candidate gene single nucleotide polymorphisms (SNP maps), haplotype markers and alterations in gene expression or inactivation that might be correlated with pharmacological function and therapeutic response. Pharmacogenetics is narrower in definition and refers to the study of inter-individual variations in DNA sequence related to drug absorption and disposition (pharmacokinetics) or drug action (pharmacodynamics), including polymorphic variation in genes encoding transporters, drug-metabolizing enzymes, receptors and other proteins (Lesko & Woodcock, 2004). With the accumulating knowledge of human genomic variation, the Human Genome Project offers the opportunity to develop personalized medicine, decreasing adverse drug reactions and increasing the efficacy of drug treatment (Weinshilboum & Wang, 2004). Historically, Johansson & Ingelman-Sundberg (Johansson & Ingelman-Sundberg, 2011) consider that inter-individual variation in response to a xenobiotic was probably described first by Pythagoras in 510 BC when he noted that some individuals developed hemolytic anemia after ingestion of fava beans. Then, they record that at the beginning of the last century, Garrod and Oxon suggested the involvement of a genetic component in biochemical processes where the cause of inter-individual differences in adverse reactions was because of enzyme deficiencies (Garrod, 1902, as cited in Johansson & Ingelman-Sundberg, 2011). Observations implying that genetic variation was responsible for the diversity in some drug responses was established nearly 50 years ago, with the discovery that deficiency in glucose-6-phosphate dehydrogenase (G6DP) results in hemolytic anemia following ingestion of the anti-malarial primaquine (Beutler, 1959). Another example is succinylcholine, which is administered as an adjunct to anesthesia and can induce prolonged apnea due to altered kinetics of a pseudocholinesterase (Lehmann & Ryan, 1956). In 1959, Vogel coined the term of pharmacogenetics to describe inherited differences in drug response (Vogel, 1959). The best-known example of a genetic defect in drug biotransformation is the acetylation polymorphism in tuberculosis therapy with Isoniazid characterized by mutations in *N*-acetyltransferase-2 (*NAT2*) on chromosome 8 (Evans et al., 1960). Alvan et al. (Alvan et al., 2001) remember the case of debrisoquine, an antihypertensive agent inducing orthostatic hypotension in a small percentage of individuals. The reason for the exaggerated effect was found to be the lack of an enzyme almost exclusively responsible for the metabolic elimination of debrisoquine and the affected subjects were classified as poor metabolizers of debrisoquine (Mahgoub, 1977, as cited in Alvan et al, 2001). The enzyme named "debrisoquine hydroxylase" is now known as CYP2D6. The oxidation of sparteine was found to be catalyzed by the same enzyme (Eichelbaum, 1975, 1979 as cited in Alvan et al, 2001). Now it is well-established that the therapeutic failure of drugs, and adverse side-effects in individuals may also have a genetic component due to genetic variations in the receptors, ion channels, transporter, enzymes and regulatory proteins involved in drug metabolism that may influence pharmacodynamics (e.g. the binding and functional capacity of the receptor or regulatory proteins) and pharmacokinetics, consisting in drug bio-availability at the level of metabolic enzymes and transporters. Most studies have focused on single nucleotide polymorphisms (SNPs) in genes encoding important metabolizing enzymes, like the cytochrome P450 enzyme superfamily, revealing an association with clinical phenotypes of drug efficacy/toxicity (Bishop & Ellingrod, 2004; Korkina et al., 2009; Mellen & Herrington, 2005; Wilkinson, 2005; Yang et al., 2010). One of the goals of pharmacogenetics is to develop predictive genetic tests to reduce the risks associated with drug administration (de Leon et al., 2006, 2009). According to the World Health Organization (WHO), adverse drug reactions (ADRs) are any harmful, unintended reactions to medicines that occurs at doses normally prescribed for prophylaxis, diagnosis and therapy and in some cases can lead to death (Edwards & Aronson, 2000). ADRs represent a significant clinical and economic problem: a prospective study conducted in the United Kingdom showed that 6.5% of hospital admissions are related to ADRs (Pirmohamed et al., 2004). According to the Food and Drug Administration (FDA), the frequency of reported serious and fatal adverse drug events increased 2.6 fold from 1998 through 2005 (Moore et al., 2007). Moreover, it has been estimated that ADRs were between the fourth and sixth leading causes of death in the world due to treatment with drugs like anti-inflammatories, analgesics, antidepressants, sedatives, anticoagulants and antibiotics (Carleton et al., 2009; Lazarou et al., 1998). Given the association between response to treatment and genetic variability on the basis of clinical trials, the European Medicines Agency (EMEA) and the FDA currently recommend the use of biomarkers in informing prescribing decisions for certain drugs (Frueh et al., 2008). Moreover, growing information is available on biomarkers indicating whether a therapy could work on a particular individual. In 2004, a "Personalized Medicine Coalition" was launched in the USA, giving strong input to the US Senate bill on the Patient-Centered

Outcome Research Act. But questions arise, including: Will pharmacogenetics in general be accepted by physicians and patients? "Safe and effective medicines for all" is a vision that will not come true in general. Furthermore, even if its outcome and cost-effectiveness have to be proven, personalized medicine can currently contribute to solving the problems of lack of efficacy, drug resistance and adverse effects in some indications, and this opportunity should be used (Cascorbi, 2010). The scientific literature highlights the magnitude of this public health problem at different levels and point of views and illustrates the need for improved systems to select the appropriate drug dosage to achieve the optimal therapeutic response, avoid therapeutic failure and minimize side-effects and toxicity (Davies et al., 2009). Recently, Sim et al. (2011) emphasize the need of updated databases for providing guidance to both scientists, physicians, regulatory agencies, and industries to cope with this major problem in human health. The medico-legal implications are evident both for medical liability issues and in forensic death investigation.

2. Genetic polymorphism of Cytochrome P450 (P450 or CYP)

The primary site of drug metabolism is the liver, where enzymes chemically change drug components into substances known as metabolites that are then bound to other substances for excretion mainly through the kidneys, lungs or bodily fluids or by intestinal re-absorption. Some drugs do not change chemical structure and are removed from the body as such. Drug pharmacokinetics and pharmacodynamics are regulated by complex chemical reactions with the participation of numerous proteins encoded by different genes, deputies for the transport and metabolism of drugs, or involved in their mechanism of action (Weinshilboum, 2003). Two different types of metabolic reactions are involved: in *phase 1* molecules are characterized by oxidation, reduction and hydrolysis reactions, in *phase 2* drugs are conjugated with other compounds and then discarded (Johansson & Ingelman-Sundberg, 2011; Zhou et al., 2008). If two or more polymorphic genes regulate drug metabolism and transport inside a cell, the variability in the response to treatment depends on the interaction of these gene variants. The cytochrome P450 enzyme system plays a central role in phase I oxidative metabolism of the vast majority of prescribed drugs and also of endogenous substances (Bertz & Granneman, 1997). The genes coding for these enzymes are called *CYP*. The Human Genome Project identified 57 human *CYPs* divided into families and subfamilies based on structural similarity in amino acid sequence of the enzymes. Enzymes in families 1 to 3 are involved in the detoxification of exogenous chemicals, whereas the remaining groups are mainly active in the metabolism of endogenous compound like steroids, fatty acids and bile acids (Ingelman-Sundberg & Sim, 2010). Many of the genes involved in drug metabolism are highly polymorphic and all researchers specify the different *CYP* variants as reported at the Human CYP allele nomenclature web site www.cypallele.ki.se (Oscarson & Ingelman-Sundberg, 2002). Sim et al. (Sim et al, 2011) describe that the main purpose of the *CYP*-allele website is the management of new allele designations based on recognized nomenclature guidelines, facilitation of rapid publication, as well as providing a readily available summary of alleles and their associated effects. In addition they summarize the inclusion criteria of the new alleles in the website: submission of new alleles is achieved by contacting the Webmaster of the *CYP*-allele Website, whereby the data characterizing the allele is reviewed for potential allele name designation. All information is kept confidential and a manuscript in preparation can often serve as a good basis for review and discussion between the author and the Webmaster. Designation of allele names outside the *CYP*-allele nomenclature committee is not advised, due to the apparent risk of confusion in the literature. Submissions with respect to additional functional in vivo and in vitro characterization of alleles listed are also highly relevant, and aids in keeping the *CYP*-allele Website up to date.

2.1 P 450 genes family: From genotype to phenotype

Of all the isoforms of the P450 gene family, *CYP2D6, CYP2C19, CYP3As, CYP2C9, CYP2B6, CYP2C8, CYP2A6* and *CYP1A2* are the most important and polymorphic enzymes and are responsible for several phase I metabolism xenobiotics (Anzenbacher & Anzenbacherová, 2001; Daly, 2003; Ingelman-Sundberg, 2004). In particular, CYP2D6, characterized by a high inter-individual variability in catalytic activity mainly caused by genetic polymorphisms, will be described in depth. The genetic bases of the polymorphism are single nucleotide polymorphisms, insertions/deletions and gene copy number variations (Ingelman-Sundberg et al., 1999). Because of such variability, individuals could be classified into four different phenotypes: ultra-rapid metabolizers (UM) with more than two active gene copies on the same allele or increased expression of a single gene, extensive metabolizers (EM) carrying two functional alleles, intermediate metabolizers (IM) with one defective allele or two partially defective alleles, and poor metabolizers (PM) lacking functional enzymes due to defective or deleted genes. PM and UM are the most clinically important phenotypes: PM individuals are at risk of having a higher than expected serum concentration in relation to the drug dose and hence more side-effects, especially in the case of drugs with a narrow therapeutic index (White, 2010; Prandota, 2010). Instead, UMs may require higher doses and more frequent administration of a drug in an active form to achieve optimal therapeutic concentrations. However, when an inactive "pro-drug" must be converted to the active metabolite (e.g. codeine and tamoxifen), the therapy will be ineffective in PM subjects and UMs will metabolize it quickly with accumulation of the metabolite and consequent toxicity. As a result, drug toxicity is related to metabolizer status (Ingelman-Sundberg et al., 1999; van der Weide & Steijns, 1999). Moreover, the phenomenon of *phenocopying* must be taken into account where EM individuals turn into apparent PM or IM phenotypes because of drug-drug interactions (Owen et al., 2009). Many drugs also inhibit or induce the activity of CYPs and knowledge of CYP–drug relations is therefore essential to recognize incompatible drug combinations and allows individualized therapies (Mishra et al., 2010). For this purpose, a user-friendly platform for researchers and health professionals was developed where each drug was attributed to those CYPs involved in drug metabolism as substrate, inhibitor or inducer. The SuperCYP database contains 1170 drugs with more than 3800 interactions including references (Preissner et al., 2010). Nevertheless, epigenetics, defined as heritable phenotypic changes not involving alteration in nuclear DNA, promises answer to interindividual variability in drug response not associated to genetic polymorphism (Ingelman-Sundberg & Gomez, 2010). Indeed, the CYPs expression can be influenced by diet, lifestyle and environmental pollutants. Update of P450 epigenetics knowledge and its relevance for cancer risk and treatment is reported in a recent review: *CYP1A1, CYP1A2, CYP1B1, CYP2E1, CYP2W1, CYP2A13* have been shown to have epigenetics component in their expression regulation (Rodriguez-Antona et al., 2010).

2.2 CYP2D6

CYP2D6 is the most extensively studied drug metabolizing enzyme in humans and its polymorphism was the first among polymorphic P450s to be characterized at the molecular level. About 20-25% of clinically used drugs are metabolized by this enzyme including beta-blockers, antiarrhythmics, antidepressants, neuroleptics, analgesics and anti-cancer drugs. Most of them are metabolized to the inactive form; others like codeine, tramadol and tamoxifen are bio-activated. CYP2D6 is the only drug metabolizing CYP which is not inducible and therefore genetic variation plays a major role in the inter-individual variation in enzyme activity (Ingelman-Sundberg et al., 2007). The gene, located near two cytochrome P450 pseudogenes on chromosome 22q13.1, is highly polymorphic and more than 80 allelic variants related to the gene activity have been described (Zhou, 2009). The wild type allele is *CYP2D6*1* and major variants associated with decreased and abolished enzyme catalytic activity are *CYP2D6*2, CYP2D6*4, CYP2D6*5, CYP2D6*10, CYP2D6*17* and *CYP2D6*41*. Multiple active gene copies are responsible for ultra-rapid metabolizer individuals. CYP2D6 phenotypying is characterized in vivo by the ratio of urinary amounts of parent compound relative to oxidative metabolite. The most commonly used probe substrates have been debrisoquine, sparteine and dextromethorphan. On the basis of the urinary metabolic ratio (MR), PM, UM, EM and IM phenotypes have been classified, but *CYP2D6* genotyping to predict metabolic status is considered a valid alternative to traditional phenotyping methods because genetic characteristics remain unchanged throughout life and are not influenced by environmental and physiologic factors (Gaedigk et al., 2003; Zanger et al., 2004). One of the most commonly used methods for *CYP2D6* genotyping consists in a combination of a first long-PCR (polymerase chain reaction) step designed to amplify the entire *CYP2D6* gene in a single fragment of about 5 kb followed by minisequencing, a multiplex PCR by SNP genotyping method (Fig. 1), screening the 11 most important polymorphic positions of the gene (Sistonen et al., 2005). The inferring phenotype from *CYP2D6* genotype information is based on different approaches including the conventional classification in PM, IM, EM and UM, established on the assumption of dominance, in which the phenotype is determined by the most efficient allele (Sistonen et al., 2007). However, this method does not consider inter-individual variability in urinary metabolic ratio-based phenotypes of subjects with identical genotype and the complexity of allele combinations. For this reason, the "activity score" (AS) system has been evaluated to translate genotype into a qualitative measure of phenotype and to overcome the difficulties of interpretation and comparison of different studies on CYP2D6 activity. For each variant allele a value is assigned based on CYP2D6 activity: "1" to the fully functional alleles and "0" to non-functional alleles, "0.5" or "0.75" to reduced activity alleles and double the value to duplicated genes. The AS is the sum of the individual allele values (Gaedigk et al., 2008).

2.2.1 Distribution of CYP2D6 polymorphism

Inter-ethnic differences in the distribution of *CYP2D6* genotypes have been described (Bernard et al., 2006; Gaedigk et al., 1999, 2002; Gaedigk & Coetsee, 2008; Griese et al., 2001; Kitada, 2003; Leathart et al., 1998; Luo et al., 2004; Wan et al., 2001; Zhou et al., 2009). In a worldwide survey (Sistonen et al., 2007) 5-10% of Europeans are PMs with the highest frequency of *CYP2D6*4* variant, while the UMs are most represented in North Africa and Oceania (40% and 26% respectively) due to the high percentage of gene duplication. In Asian populations alleles with absent CYP2D6 activity are very rare, but the **10* allele, causing a decreased enzyme function, occurs quite frequently leading to a high percentage of IMs. The **1* and **2* variants are the most represented in all population groups and their

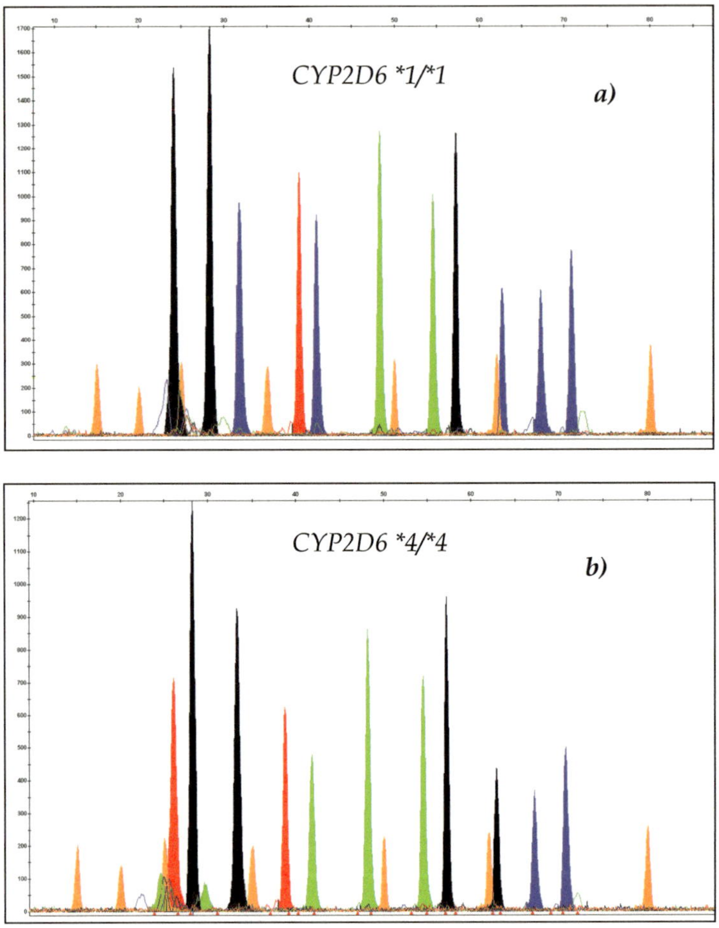

Fig. 1. Electropherograms of the multiplex PCR by SNP genotyping method (minisequencing) of two different individuals. Peaks correspond to 11 polymorphic positions (100C>T, 1023C>T, 1661G>C, 1707delT, 1846G>A, 2549delA, 2613-15delAGA, 2850C>T, 4180G>C, 2988G>A, 3183G>A) of the *CYP2D6* gene. *a*) Electropherogram of a homozygous *CYP2D6*1/*1* wild type genotype and *b*) Electropherogram of a homozygous *CYP2D6*4/*4* genotype

homogeneous geographic distribution could be regarded as the result of a long-term selective pressure maintaining the high frequency of alleles coding for a full-function enzyme. However, few rarely region-specific alleles associated with an altered enzymatic activity are observed and seem to be geographically dispersed over all four continents (Gaedigk et al., 2006, 2007, 2009, 2010; Luo et al., 2005). Ethnic specificity has become an integral part of pharmacogenetics research but caution is required against the use of continental labels to lump together heterogeneous populations. The Asian category, for example, is applied to individuals of distinct ethnicity and/or living in different countries or regions of the vast continent of Asia. Not surprisingly, significant variation in the distribution of pharmacogenetics polymorphism is detected among Asians (Suarez-Kurtz, 2008). Nevertheless, with increasing global migration, admixture gains relevance as an additional challenge to the successful worldwide implementation of pharmacogenetics in clinical practice. The Brazilian population, with tri-hybrid ancestral roots in Amerindian, European and African groups and five centuries of extensive inter-ethnic mating, provides a valuable model for studying the impact of admixture on the conceptual development and clinical implementation of pharmacogenetics-informed prescription. Recognition of this fact is important in the design and interpretation of pharmacogenetics clinical trials in Brazilians, but does not imply that pharmacogenetics-informed drug prescription requires investigation of individual ancestry. Rather, individual genotyping should be directed to polymorphisms of proven clinical utility, irrespective of biogeographical ancestry (Suarez-Kurtz, 2010).

2.3 CYP2C9

CYP2C9 accounts for approximately 20% of total hepatic CYP content and metabolizes approximately 15% of clinically used drugs including S-warfarin, tolbutamide, phenytoin, losartan, diclofenac and celecoxib (Goldstein, 2001). To date, at least 33 variants of *CYP2C9* (**1B* through to **34*) have been identified (Yasar et al., 1999, 2002). *CYP2C9*2* and *CYP2C9*3* differ from the wild-type *CYP2C9*1* by a single point mutation: *CYP2C9*2* is characterised by a 430C>T exchange in exon 3 resulting in an Arg144Cys amino acid substitution, whereas *CYP2C9*3* shows an exchange of 1075A>C in exon 7 causing an Ile359Leu substitution in the catalytic site of the enzyme (Wang et al., 2009). The *CYP2C9* polymorphism is clinically highly significant and also substrate-dependent (Rosemary & Adithan, 2007; Xie et al., 2001). Marked inter-racial differences have been reported: *CYP2C9*2* and *CYP2C9*3* were both found with highest frequencies in Northern African and European populations. The frequency of *CYP2C9*2* decreases rapidly when moving from Europe toward the east, and it is practically zero in Eastern Asian populations. *CYP2C9*3* occurs more evenly in different geographic regions. (Sistonen, et al., 2009). The polymorphism in admixed populations was studied in the context of warfarin dose requirements. Variant alleles *CYP2C9*5, CYP2C9*6, CYP2C9*8* and *CYP2C9*11* occur in Africans but are rare or absent in Europeans. Genotyping of the six polymorphisms could be justified in Brazilians and, most likely African-Americans, but not Europeans, in whom only *CYP2C9*2, CYP2C9*3* might be adequate for predicting the *CYP2C9* polymorphism (Suarez-Kurtz, 2010). Candidate-gene association studies for warfarin response have identified *CYP2C9* and *VKORC1*, which codes for warfarin's target, vitamin K epoxide reductase, responsible for most of the genetic effect. VKORC1 is a key enzyme of the vitamin K cycle and molecular target of coumarin anticoagulants. Among whites and Asians, *VKORC1* polymorphisms have shown a consistently significant influence on warfarin response, accounting for 11% to 32% of dose variability. Among North American blacks, *VKORC1* polymorphisms account for 4% to 10% of the variability in dose. Given that genetic diversity is known to be greater in persons of African descent, investigators have hypothesized that other *VKORC1* polymorphisms, or combinations of multiple polymorphisms (haplotypes), may better explain the variation in dose in this group (Limdi et al., 2010).

2.4 CYP2C19

The metabolism of tricyclic antidepressants, benzodiazepines and proton pump inhibitors is catalyzed mainly by *CYP2C19*. The most common genetic variation, designated *CYP2C19*2* (c.G681A), leads to a splicing defect that functionally affects the enzyme. Other alterations have also been reported such as loss-of-function: *CYP2C19*3* (c.G636A; stop codon), *CYP2C19*4* (c.A1G; transition in the initiation codon), and *CYP2C19*5* (c.C1297T; amino acid substitution) (Santos et al., 2011). A variant defining an ultra-rapid metabolizer has been identified (Sim et al., 2006). Pronounced ethnic differences exist in the frequencies of the non-functional alleles: a low frequency of up to 5% in the Caucasian and African populations, higher in Oriental populations (23%). *CYP2C19*2* and *CYP2C19*3* are together responsible for the majority of PM alleles, of which *CYP2C19*3* is mainly found in Asians (Chen et al., 2008; Xie et al., 2001).

2.5 CYP1A2 and CYP2A6

CYP2A6 is an inducible enzyme primarily expressed in the liver and was first recognized for its involvement in the metabolism of coumarin. The *CYP2A6* gene locus spans a region of 6kbp and has been physically mapped to the long arm of chromosome 19. Thirteen allelic variants have been discovered due to point mutation, deletion, and gene conversion, and several of these result in altered enzyme activity. CYP2A6 is involved in the metabolism of nicotine, some procarcinogens and several toxins. Variants may affect smoking, cancer and the treatment of cigarette smoking. (Xu et al., 2002). CYP1A2 metabolizes clozapine, tacrine, tizanidine and theophylline, a number of procarcinogens like benzo[*a*]pyrene and aromatic amines, and several important endogenous compounds (e.g., steroids). CYP1A2 is subject to reversible and/or irreversible inhibition by a number of drugs, natural substances and other compounds. The *CYP1A* gene cluster has been mapped on chromosome 15q24.1, with a close link between *CYP1A1* and *1A2* sharing a common 5′-flanking region. More than 15 variant alleles and a series of subvariants of the *CYP1A2* gene have been identified and some of them have been associated with altered drug clearance and response and disease susceptibility (Zhou et al., 2010).

2.6 CYP2B6 and CYP2C8

CYP2B6, mapped to the *CYP2* gene cluster on chromosome 19, plays a major role in the biotransformation of several therapeutically important drugs including cyclophosphamide, ifosfamide, tamoxifen, ketamine, artemisinin, nevirapine, efavirenz, bupropion, sibutramine and propofol. This enzyme also metabolizes arachidonic acid, lauric acid, 17β-estradiol, estrone, ethinylestradiol and testosterone (Mo et al., 2009). Genetic polymorphisms in *CYP2B6* are defined in terms of 29 allelic variants many of which are associated with increased, decreased or abolished enzyme activity (Watanabe et al., 2010). Overall, there is a marked inter-individual variability in CYP2B6 activity, but current pharmacogenetic knowledge is not sufficient to provide efficient tools to predict the specific capacity for metabolism of CYP2B6 substrates (Ingelman-Sundberg et al., 2007). CYP2C8 is a polymorphic phase I drug-metabolizing enzyme involved in the metabolism of several therapeutic drugs including paclitaxel, amodiaquine, troglitazone, amiodarone and verapamil, and has also been implicated in the activation of procarcinogenic compounds (Totah & Rettie, 2005). The gene is located on chromosome 10q24 in a cluster with *CYP2C19* and *CYP2C18* and 14 different allelic variants have been reported (http://www.cypalleles.ki.se/cyp2c8.htm). The main *CYP2C8* polymorphisms code for the amino acid changes I269F, R139K, K399R and I264M. These single nucleotide polymorphisms define three main non-wild-type alleles, *CYP2C8*2* (I269F), *CYP2C8*3* (R139K and K399R) and *CYP2C8*4* (I264M). The *CYP2C8*2* allele has been found in black populations with an allele frequency of 18% but is very rare in white subjects (Dorado et al., 2008).

2.7 CYP3A

The CYP3A drug-metabolizing enzymes facilitate the metabolism and elimination of a wide range of structurally different xenobiotics and of 50% of all clinically used therapeutic drugs. In addition, they participate in the metabolism of key endogenous substrates, such as retinoic acid, steroid hormones and bile acids (Domanski et al., 2001; Ingelman-Sundberg et al., 2007; Thummel & Wilkinson, 1998). The four *CYP3A* genes lie within a 218 kb region of chromosome 7q22.1 in the following order: *CYP3A5, CYP3A7, CYP3A4,* and *CYP3A43* (Lamba et al., 2002; Westlind et al., 2001). More than 30 SNPs have been identified in the *CYP3A4* gene (Du et al., 2006; Garsa et al., 2005). Generally speaking, variants in the coding regions of *CYP3A4* occur at allele frequencies <5% and appear heterozygous with the wild-type allele. These coding variants may contribute, but are unlikely to be the major cause of inter-individual differences in CYP3A-dependent clearance, because of the low allele frequencies and limited alterations in enzyme expression or catalytic function (Eiselt et al., 2001). The most common variant, *CYP3A4*1B*, is an A-392G transition in the 5'-flanking region with an allele frequency ranging from 0% in Chinese and Japanese to 45% in African-Americans. Studies have not linked *CYP3A4*1B* with alterations in CYP3A substrate metabolism (Garcia-Martin et al., 2002; Lamba et al., 2002). *CYP3A5* is polymorphically expressed in adults with readily detectable expression in about 10–20% in Caucasians, 33% in Japanese and 55% in African-Americans. The primary causal mutation for its polymorphic expression (*CYP3A5*3*) confers low CYP3A5 protein expression and its allele frequency varies from approximately 50% in African-Americans to 90% in Caucasians (Adler et al., 2009; Lamba et al., 2002). CYP3A7 is considered to be the major fetal liver CYP3A enzyme. Three of the mutations represent SNPs (*CYP3A7*1B, *1D* and **1E*) and occurs in regions outside those associated with the regulation of CYP3A transcription. The fourth mutation (*CYP3A7*1C*) consists of the replacement of 60 bp from the CYP3A4 gene with the corresponding sequence from the *CYP3A7* gene (Lamba et al., 2002).

3. Personalized therapy: ethical and legal issues

Current prescribing practice involves administration of a standard "one size fits all" starting dose and is often a process of trial and error, varying the prescription until the most suitable treatment is found (Sadee, 1998). However, such a procedure exposes the patient to possible side-effects. In fact, around 21% of all outpatients suffer some kind of adverse reaction to drugs prescribed by their physician (Queneau et al., 2007). By investigating drug metabolism related to individual genetic polymorphism, pharmacogenetics has a significant impact on the clinical setting so that forensic implications may arise throughout the public health sector. The concept of "therapy with the right drug at the right dose in the right patient" was highlighted just about ten years ago (Mancinelli et al., 2000) and pharmacogenetic tests are now available for a number of drugs by biotechnology companies, some with FDA approval, as reported in Wong et al., (2010): Luminex xTag® (Luminex Corporation, TK, USA), Roche AmpliChip® (Roche, Basel, Switzerland), Affymetrix DMET® chip (Affymetrix, CA, USA), Autogenomics INFINITI™ Analyzer (Autogenomics, CA, USA), Osmetech eSensors® (WA, USA), ParagonDx (NC, USA), and ABI PRISM® SNaPshot™ (Applied Biosystems, CA, USA) and TaqMan® assays (Applied Biosystems). In addition, the Authors underlined the limitations: existing evidence to demonstrate significant and medically relevant correlations for many disease-causing genes and variants, limited detection of genetic variants within the context of each testing platform, clinical interpretation of genotype results including environmental factors, and transplanted organs interfering with testing. Nevertheless, SNP arrays covering 5 million SNPs will soon become a reality and the cost for whole-genome sequencing is rapidly decreasing (Sim & Ingelman-Sundberg, 2011). The influence of genetic polymorphism on drug failure or toxicity can be illustrated by some significant examples.

3.1 Moving to clinical practice: significant examples

An increasing number of studies on psychiatric patients have shown that genetic variation of *CYP2D6* and *CYP2C19* affects the metabolism of antidepressants and antipsychotics, thereby explaining the different therapeutic effects in different patients (Kirchheiner & Seeringer, 2007). Of the patients treated with antidepressants 10-20% react adversely and 25-35% do not respond to the medication. This can lead to treatment for patients being selected in what has been described as a "trial and error" fashion, as physicians try different pharmacological agents with their patients in order to select the best treatment (Morley & Hall, 2004). Given their selective mechanism of action, selective serotonin reuptake inhibitors (SSRIs) replaced tryciclic antidepressants and monoamino oxidase inhibitors, but because of their inhibitory effects on various CYP enzymes, SSRIs may be associated with clinically relevant pharmacokinetic interactions with other medications (Spina et al., 2008). In dementia, approximately 10-15% of direct costs are attributed to pharmacological treatment and only 10-20% of the patients are moderate responders to conventional anti-dementia drugs, with questionable cost-effectiveness (Cacabelos, 2008). Pharmacogenetic and pharmacogenomic factors are reported to be responsible for 75-85% of the therapeutic response in Alzheimer's disease (AD) patients treated with conventional drugs. Cholinesterase inhibitors of current use in AD, such as donepezil, tacrine and galantamine, are metabolized via CYP-related enzymes. EMs and IMs are the best responders, and PMs and UMs are the worst responders to pharmacologic treatments in AD. At this early stage of the development of pharmacogenomic/pharmacogenetic procedures in AD therapeutics, it seems very plausible that the pharmacogenetic response in Alzheimer's disease depends on the interaction of genes involved in drug metabolism and genes associated with Alzheimer's disease pathogenesis (Cacabelos, 2007). Paracetamol and tramadol were the most popular analgesics among individuals taking warfarin. A recent study supports clinical evidence of the significance of the adverse warfarin-paracetamol interaction, although the mechanism responsible for the interaction is not clear. Some case reports of warfarin tramadol interactions have been published and a CYP2D6-related mechanism has been proposed (Launiainen et al., 2010). Warfarin (4-hydroxy coumarin), the most frequently prescribed oral anticoagulant, has a narrow therapeutic index and a wide inter-individual variability in dose requirement: an increase or decrease in anticoagulant activity are associated with the risk of hemorrhagic or thrombotic events (Kamali & Wynne, 2010). Variants in the cytochrome P450 2C9 (*CYP2C9*) and vitamin K epoxide reductase (*VKOR*) genes have been shown to have a significant effect on warfarin dose requirement. Warfarin pharmacogenetics has become a case study for personalized medicine. Algorithms incorporating selected SNPs in two genes, *CYP2C9* and *VKORC1*, show improved dose prediction compared with algorithms based solely on clinical and demographic factors. However, the performance of these algorithms differs among racial groups, with a higher proportion of variability in dose explained in whites than in Asians or blacks. The first comprehensive assessment of the influence of six common *VKORC1* SNPS and haplotypes on warfarin dose among Asians, blacks and whites with the use of the largest racially diverse cohort captured the influence of common genetic variation in *VKORC1* on variability in warfarin dose by a single polymorphism (either -1639G>A or 1173C>T) across all racial groups. Incorporation of additional *VKORC1* SNPs or haplotypes did not improve dose prediction. Therefore, current evidence supports the use of -1639G>A (or 1173C>T) to capture dose variability related to *VKORC1*. Both *VKORC1* and *CYP2C9* influenced warfarin dose among individual patients in all three racial groups studied (Limdi et al., 2010). The case of tamoxifen is well-documented in the management of women with hormone receptor (HR) positive breast cancer (Hoskins et al., 2009). Tamoxifen is a pro-drug that is metabolized to its main active metabolite endoxifen by the cytochrome P450 2D6. Null or reduced enzyme activity in women treated with tamoxifen results in worse outcomes in terms of cancer relapse and lower event-free survival rates compared to extensive metabolizers. Addition data are required for a mandatory use of a *CYP2D6* genetic test, considering the demonstrated potential effect of *CYP2C19* polymorphism on relapse risk during tamoxifen treatment (Sim & Ingelman-Sundberg, 2011). In addition, selective serotonin reuptake inhibitor antidepressant drugs such as paroxetine and fluoxetine have also been used to manage tamoxifen-induced hot flushes. These drugs potently inhibit the metabolism of tamoxifen by CYP2D6 and thus potentially may lessen the efficacy of tamoxifen (Singh et al., 2011). Recently, it has been pointed out that there is sufficient reason to be aware of the real possibility of herbal products inhibiting cytochrome P450 enzymes. Considering that self-administration of complementary products is an increasingly common trend worldwide, the interactions may significantly increase the risk of ADR (Sevior et al., 2010). The picture that emerges highlights the crucial role of the physician to understand when to order the pharmacogenetics test and how to use the results in clinical decision-making (Robertson et al., 2002). The authors emphasized that if the risk of side-effects from a drug is great, a physician who failed to order the test indicative of toxicity could be found to have been negligent and future lawsuits for failure to give a test or properly interpret it will ensue, both reflecting and reinforcing acceptance of pharmacogenetic testing as an ordinary part of medical practice.

3.2 Legal and ethical issues

The development of pharmacogenetics has important implications in the medico-legal and forensic field because the classic topics of informed consent, shared genetic information, privacy and data base collection arise (Vaszar et al., 2002). Nevertheless the problem of orphan patients, non-responders for all available drug options, might have unforeseen consequences to avoid the label "hard to treat" (Robertson, 2001). Some patients might not want to be tested for pharmacogenetics profiles and this leads to the question of what a physician should do if a patient refuses to be genotyped. The responsibility of health care professionals will need to be defined as to who (doctors, pharmacist, clinical chemists) is responsible for the application of new technologies (genotyping) and what kind of patient counseling is needed (van Delden et al., 2004). A recent paper (Hamburg & Collins, 2010) highlighted that today about 10% of labels for FDA-approved drugs contain pharmacogenomic information – a substantial increase since the 1990s. Furthermore, there has been an explosion in the number of validated markers but relatively little independent analysis of the validity of the tests used to identify them in biologic specimens. The National Institute of Health (NIH) and the FDA will invest in advancing translational and regulatory science, and will better define regulatory pathways for coordinated approval of co-developed diagnostics and therapeutics, develop risk-based approaches for appropriate review of diagnostics to assess their validity and clinical utility more accurately, and make information on tests readily available. As the field advances, they expect to see more efficient clinical trials based on a more thorough understanding of the genetic basis of disease. The impact on the medico-legal field is evident. But, there are two schools of thought on how tort liability may affect personalized medicine, i.e., whether fear of lawsuits will tend to accelerate progress or slow it down. Tort suits include product liability suits against manufacturers and negligence suits against physicians and other providers of health-related services (Evans, 2007). Recently, Wong et al. (2010) stressed that personalized medicine by means of pharmacogenomics may have a dramatic impact on the justice system in ways we are only beginning to understand. They stated that if personalized medicine has already entered the curricula of well-regarded medical schools such as that of Johns Hopkins University (MD, USA), law schools offer no analogue. For example, "The FDA relabelled some drugs such as warfarin with CYP2C9 and vitamin K epoxide reductase complex 1 to reduce bleeding. If pharmacogenetics retrospectively reveals that the warfarin patient was at high risk and testing was not initially performed, litigation may follow. Indeed, some lawyers advertise on the Internet for cases involving warfarin-related errors. Consequently, pharmacogenomics may become part of defensive medicine". An important issue for legal and ethical use of pharmacogenetic tests arises from the evidence of genetic polymorphism distribution in different ethnic groups. *CYP2D6* gene polymorphism shows that the distribution of PMs, IMs and UMs varies in different ethnic groups so inter-ethnic differences in drug response highlight the need to evaluate the genetic makeup of individuals before prescribing drugs, also considering that the recent demographic movements and back migration of populations are reshaping the picture of genetic diversity within the native population (Suarez-Kurtz, 2010). A recent review by McNamara (McNamara, 2008) discusses investigations of pharmacogenomics in heart failure and the challenge of converting genomic heterogeneity into a usable clinical tool, concluding that investigators are beginning to delineate the genomic basis for differences in drug efficacy between black and white heart failure cohorts. The influence of *CYP2C9* and *VKORC1* genotypes on warfarin dose requirements has been demonstrated in diverse racial and ethnic patient groups and to choose a warfarin starting dose, dosing algorithms have been developed that incorporate clinical, demographic and genetic information. Because of these significant issues, the Journal of Health & Life Sciences Law explored personalized or patient-tailored medicine addressing the relevance of genetic information, and how race and genetics have affected and may impact on the development of medicines, pharmacogenomics and personalized medicine in the United States (Braff et al., 2008). A second part discussed current and proposed federal and state laws and regulations intended to protect individuals from the misuse of genetic information, including uses that discriminate based on genetic predispositions (Braff et al., 2009). It was recently pointed out (Nebert et al., 2008) that numerous reasons exist to show that an "unequivocal genotype" or even an "unequivocal phenotype" is virtually impossible to achieve in current limited-size studies of human populations. The problem of insufficiently stringent criteria leads to a decrease in statistical power and consequently an equivocal interpretation of most genotype-phenotype association studies. It remains unclear whether personalized medicine or individualized drug therapy will ever be achievable by DNA testing alone. The authors ask "Where are we, today, in our understanding of the role of human genetics and genomics in drug toxicity, efficacy and therapeutic failure? Few high-prevalence predominantly monogenic genes that do make a difference in metabolism of various drug substrates (e.g.,

CYP2D6, NAT2, TPMT, CYP2C19) might contribute perhaps 15% to 20% to the (EM or PM) phenotype, whereas a contribution of 90% or more is expected for the gene responsible for a monogenic human disease. If we know that dozens or hundreds of additional downstream genes might affect the ultimate outcome of a particular drug, how can we integrate and assemble this knowledge into a diagram or equation?" A recent paper discussed the possible application of genotyping for depression, cardiovascular diseases and thromboembolic disorders, gastric ulcer, malignant diseases and tuberculosis (Tomalik-Scharte et al., 2008). The authors noted that thousands of manuscripts addressing pharmacogenetic questions in *in vitro* studies and clinical trials have been published, but it seems that the way to a broader use of pharmacogenetics approaches at the patients' bedside is quite laborious. The unknown exact relationship between the genotype and phenotype, although in many cases the genotype explains most of the inter-individual variability, the lack of prospective clinical studies in large patient cohorts and no reliable data on the cost effectiveness of screening procedures explain the slow progress in clinical pharmacogenetics/pharmacogenomics. In this respect, Zhou (Zhou, 2009) wrote that the functional impact of most *CYP2D6* alleles has not been systematically assessed for most clinically important drugs that are mainly metabolized by CYP2D6, though some initial evidence has been identified for a very limited number of drugs. The majority of reported *in vivo* pharmacogenetic data on CYP2D6 are from single-dose and steady-state pharmacokinetic studies of a small number of drugs. Pharmacodynamic data on CYP2D6 polymorphisms are scanty for most drug studies. Given that genotype testing for *CYP2D6* is not routinely performed in clinical practice and there is uncertainty regarding genotype-phenotype, gene-concentration and gene-dose relationships, further prospective studies on the clinical impact of CYP2D6-dependent metabolism of drugs are warranted in large cohorts. The expectation is that this research field will provide both the industry and clinicians with useful pharmacogenomic biomarkers that can aid in procedures for drug development and specific drug treatment in order to optimize the results and improve human health. The process is slow, and for a solid basis for decisions on mandatory biomarkers to be used further large prospective clinical studies are required. One fruitful manner in which this can be achieved is a closer collaboration between industry and academics (Johansson & Ingelman-Sundberg, 2011).

4. Forensic investigation

In the forensic context, pharmacogenetics can assist in the interpretation of drug-related deaths, especially accidental drug poisonings or cases of sudden death with "nearly normal autopsy "(Karch, 2007), called "white autopsy" in Italy. The author claims that the ability to identify "invisible diseases" with post-mortem genetic testing has become a reality far more quickly than anyone had ever imagined and this development is not without irony: "at the same time that many clinicians are expressing frustration about the lack of tangible gains provided by the Human Genome Project and pathologists are wondering about the viability of their field, DNA technology is about to reshape the field of forensic pathology". The role of pharmacogenetic analysis in forensic investigation has already been emphasized as the holistic approach of molecular analysis connected to macroscopic, microscopic and toxicological observations, constituting an integral part of modern medico-legal study of death (Koski et al., 2007). Nevertheless, the area of medico-legal investigation also involves occupational medicine due to the consequences on toxic-exposed workers. In this field the role of *CYP2D6* genotype in determining parkinsonism resulting from pesticide exposure may play an important role (Elbaz et al., 2004). Pesticide exposure significantly increases the risk for Parkinson's disease even when the poor metabolizer allele is in the heterozygote state. Interestingly, poor metabolizers are less common in the Parkinson's disease group in rarely exposed subjects (Deng et al., 2004). Pharmacogenetics also plays an important role in drug-addiction studies: methadone is metabolized through the liver by cytochrome P450 enzymes CYP3A4, CYP2D6 and CYP1A2 and buprenorphine is mainly metabolized by CYP3A4 enzyme. A recent review reported that Caucasians who lack CYP2D6 function appear to be protected from oral opioid dependence since this genotype is under-represented in the opiate-addicted population and these poor metabolizers are satisfied with the withdrawal and anticraving relief provided by methadone treatment. Ultra-rapid metabolizer heroin-dependent patients have felt dissatisfied with methadone therapy and can do well using buprenorphine because it is not significantly metabolized by CYP2D6 (Haile et al., 2008). In a limited number of cases of methadone toxicity, Wong et al. (2003) showed that the prevalence of poor metabolizers was higher but not significantly different from that of a control group (n=23). They concluded that *CYP2D6* mutations may not yet be directly associated with methadone toxicity, and pharmacogenomics, complementing other case findings in molecular autopsy, is considered an adjunct in interpreting the methadone toxicity of poor and intermediate metabolizers.

4.1 Post mortem analysis

Genetic variation and its effects on metabolism can be applied to post-mortem analysis to help resolve cases initially believed to be suicide or classified as sudden unexplained deaths especially in cases where poisoning, incapacitation, inebriation or certain diseases where pharmacotherapy is an essential treatment (such as epilepsy, depression, cardiac diseases or diabetes) are factors in the cause of death. An additional benefit is that pharmacogenetics analysis may provide health information (certainly only via proper ethical disclosure practices) to at-risk relatives (Budowle & van Daal, 2009). As reported recently, the medico-legal community has yet to fully exploit genetic variation as a parameter in determining the causes of death as done by the National Academy of Science in recognizing the underutilization of molecular autopsies (Sajantila et al., 2010). The authors of this valuable review stressed that an individual's pathophysiological phenotype affecting drug efficacy depends on genetic constitution and several other factors such as developmental stage, physiological and environmental factors, association with disease or specific conditions. Hence, some of these studies may be ethically unacceptable or practically impossible to perform in the clinical setting, but may be more readily performed post-mortem as part of the cause of death investigation or retrospectively with proper authorization. Therefore they recommend that serious consideration and support be given to studies of medico-legal genetics not just because of the impact on death investigation but because of the tremendous value such information can have for personalized medicine. From this point of view and due to the increasing attention paid to sudden cardiac death, the role of pharmacogenetics is now studied in more depth considering that cytochrome P450 enzymes in acquired Q-T prolongation are more prevalent than the congenital form. Several risk factors have been identified with use of Q-T prolonging drugs as the most frequent cause (van Noord et al., 2010). The CYP2D6 hydroxylation capacity has already been implicated in causing elongation of the Q-T interval: patients treated with thioridazine that inhibits CYP2D6 activity itself, may be prone to an increased risk of death due to sudden arrhythmia such as "torsades de pointes" (Llerena et al., 2002). In general, fatal drug toxicity has been associated with either slow or ultra-rapid CYP2D6 metabolism depending on the substrate activation or inactivation. Sallee et al., (2000) described the clinical course of a nine-year-old boy diagnosed with attention-deficit hyperactivity disorder, obsessive-compulsive disorder and Tourette's disorder and treated with a combination of methylphenidate, clonidine and fluoxetine. After experiencing signs and symptoms suggestive of metabolic toxicity marked by bouts of gastrointestinal distress, low-grade fever, incoordination and disorientation for more than ten months, the patient presented generalized seizures, lapsed into status epilepticus followed by cardiac arrest and subsequently expired. At autopsy, blood, brain and other tissue concentrations of fluoxetine and norfluoxetine were several-fold higher than expected based on literature reports for overdose situations. The medical examiner's report indicated death caused by fluoxetine toxicity. As the child's adoptive parents controlled medication access, they were investigated by social welfare agencies. Further genetic testing of autopsy tissue revealed a gene defect at the cytochrome P450 *CYP2D6* locus, resulting in poor metabolism of fluoxetine. As a result of this and other evidence, the investigation of the adoptive parents was terminated. One of the first demonstrations that genetic variation in drug metabolizing enzyme can be analyzed in post-mortem blood was performed studying the *CYP2D6* gene variations correlated to the tramadol metabolite ratio in blood in 33 Finnish autopsy cases where tramadol was found (Levo et al., 2003). A series of fatal poisonings due to amitriptyline (AT) abuse not all due to suicides was reported in Finland in 2005 (Prahlow & Landrum, 2005). In view of this, Koski et al. (2006) investigated the genetic variation at *CYP2D6* and *CYP2C19* genes with the metabolic ratio of the drug in post-mortem samples. No cases of fatal poisoning due to a combination of AT treatment and poor metabolizer phenotypes was found, with the exception of one case of female suicide with a very high concentration of AT and homozygous null alleles at *CYP2D6*. The authors emphasized the role of confounding factors in the interpretation of pharmacogenetics results such as age and enzyme inhibition by drugs. The pharmacogenetics analysis in a post-mortem forensic setting to reveal the cause and manner of death demonstrated doxepin poisoning associated with a completely non functional *CYP2D6* genotype, considering that CYP2D6 is a major factor involved in the large inter-individual variation in doxepin metabolism (Koski et al., 2007). However, ultrarapid metabolizer for duplication in *CYP2D6* may also be responsible for fatal toxicities. The risk of opioid poisoning to breast-fed neonates whose mothers had been prescribed codeine was studied after a fatal case. Neonatal morphine plasma concentrations were simulated for various combinations of *CYP2D6* genotype and morphine clearance. Neonates of mothers with the ultrarapid *CYP2D6* genotype and neonates of mothers who are extensive metabolizers have comparable risks of opioid poisoning (Willmann et al., 2009). A tragic case was reported in 2006 when a 13-day-old baby died from morphine poisoning. Review of the medical records revealed that the mother had been prescribed Tylenol® 3 (codeine 30 mg and acetaminophen 500 mg) in the immediate post-partum period. Initially she took two tablets twice daily, but she halved the dose on post-partum day two owing to somnolence and constipation. Following the development of poor neonatal feeding, the mother expressed milk and stored it in a freezer. Analysis of the milk for morphine using a specific enzyme-linked immunosorbent assay method for morphine revealed a concentration of 87 ng/mL. The mother was later classified as a UM of CYP2D6 substrates, carrying one extra copy of a functional *CYP2D6* gene (Madadi et al., 2007). Since 2007, the FDA has required the manufacturers of prescription codeine products to include information on the label to inform prescribing doctors about these risks and to help prevent morphine overdose in breast-fed infants. Recently, the death of a ten-month-old boy found dead in the bed after exposure to-ethylmorphine was reported. The morphine-to ethylmorphine ratio in blood from the deceased was higher than expected for the exclusive ingestion of ethylmorphine. The explanations considered that the metabolism of ethylmorphine involves both the de-ethylation to morphine by CYP2D6 and the conjugation to glucuronide by the glucuronosyltransferase UGT2B7. The activity of the enzymes varies for genetic reasons and is influenced by age. Infants have lower glucuronidation capabilities than adults and CYP2D6 activity may exceed adult levels in infancy. The *CYP2D6* genotyping excluded the hypothesis of an ultra-rapid phenotype (Helland et al., 2010). Nevertheless, the genetic variability of *CYP2D6* and possibly in *UGT2B7* was studied in a large number of women receiving codeine for obstetric pain while breast-feeding. Breast-fed infants of mother who were *CYP2D6* UM combined with *UGT2B7* *2/*2 are at increased risk of potentially life-threatening central nervous system depression (Madadi et al., 2009). Molecular autopsy research was also performed on fentanyl that is clinically used as an adjunct to surgical anaesthesia or for chronic pain management and its toxicity may be partially due to *CYP 3A4*1B* and *3A5*3* variant alleles, resulting in variable fentanyl metabolism. The study of 25 fentanyl-related deaths by the analysis of fentanyl and norfentanyl in post-mortem blood samples showed the first scientific evidence of *CYP3A5* involvement in fentanyl metabolism: homozygous *CYP3A5*3* causes impaired metabolism of fentanyl, and *CYP3A4*1B* and *3A5*3* variants may help to certify the fentanyl toxicity (Jin et al., 2005). Furthermore, pharmacogenetic analysis has gained burgeoning interest in suicidal cases both for the correlation with antidepressant therapy and in researching endogenous serotonin metabolism. A study of the genetic profile of individuals in relation to the presence of *CYP2D6* and *CYP2C19* genes in 242 fatal intoxications, 262 suicides and 212 natural deaths showed that those dying from suicide (including hanging, shooting, sticking/cutting or jumping from a height) included a higher number carrying more than two active *CYP2D6* genes. A possible explanation was the lower concentration level of prescribed medication in these ultra-rapid metabolizers resulting in ineffective treatment, but no information was available on the medical history of the suicide cases (Zackrisson et al., 2010). Discussing the results of Isacsson et al. (Isacsson et al., 2009) and the treatment of depression with antidepressants, mainly SSRI, in preventing suicide, Bertilsson (2010) recently reported that the data seem to indicate that serotonergic mechanisms are involved in the etiology of suicidal behaviour. An alternative explanation to the overrepresentation of *CYP2D6* gene duplication among suicide cases was based on the presence of the CYP2D6 enzyme in the human brain where its distribution follows that of dopamine nerve terminals, demonstrating several endogenous substrates of CYP2D6 among which of special interest is the O-demethylation of 5-methoxytryptamine to serotonin. The author reported that serotonin might then be synthesized in dopaminergic neurons by CYP2D6 and act as a false transmitter in wrong (inhibitory?) neurons.

5. Conclusion

Current pharmacogenetics research in the clinical and medico-legal settings provides new options for disease treatment and prevention of ADR avoiding correlated death, and for screening interactions with the polymorphic P450 enzymes early on in drug development. The ensuing information will be translated into routine clinical practice in the years to come benefitting millions of patients worldwide (Ingelman-Sundberg & Sim, 2010). In the future, the research in relatively new fields such as epigenetics and small nuclear RNA mediated mechanisms will increase the number of useful biomarkers for personalized therapy. Indeed, epigenetics providing answers to interindividual variability in drug response not associated to genetic polymorphism, could represent the bridge that connects the environment to the genome (Gomez & Ingelman-Sundberg, 2009). In this respect, the area of pharmacoepigenomics has a promising future (Ingelman-Sundberg & Gomez, 2010). In medico-legal setting, molecular autopsy is becoming a reality also considering that robust techniques suitable for implementation in forensic laboratories are broadening the genetic analysis of P450 gene polymorphism. But we agree with Sajantila et al. (2010) that "in some ways this situation now confronting medico-legal geneticists is similar to the early years of the DNA level human identification era. The societal and judicial systems sought the technology and scientists had serious challenges to cope with demands. Like DNA-based identification at that time, fundamental pharmacogenetic research needs to be performed so that our knowledge is sufficient to render valid and reliable interpretations related to medico-legal genetic findings". Significantly, Wong et al. (2010) state that personalized justice complements personalized medicine, but "personalized justice" in a firm foundation should be based on sound legal principles as well as reliable and valid evidence-based studies, not on 'junk' science and unsubstantiated case reports. Furthermore, the American Academy of Forensic Sciences supports the National Academy of Science's 13 recommendations (National Academy of Sciences, 2009, as cited in Wong et al., 2010) and the following principles: the need for strong scientific foundations; laboratory accreditation; certification of technicians; the standardization of terminology; ethical protocols; governmental oversight; and the education of legal professionals, including judges, in forensic scientific methods and principles.

6. References

Adler, G.; Łoniewska, B.; Parczewski, M.; Kordek, A. & Ciechanowicz, A. (2009). Frequency of common CYP3A5 gene variants in healthy Polish newborn infants. *Pharmacol Rep.* Vol. 61, No.5, pp.947-951

Alvan, G.; Bertilsson, L.; Dahl, M.L.; Ingelman-Sundberg, M. & Sjöqvist, F. (2001). Moving toward genetic profiling in patient care: the scope and rationale of pharmacogenetic/ecogenetic investigation. *Drug Metab Dispos.* Vol.29, No.4, pp.580-585

Anzenbacher, P. & Anzenbacherová, E. (2001). Cytochromes P450 and metabolism of xenobiotics. *Cell Mol Life Sci.* Vol.58, No.5-6, pp.737-747

Bernard, S.; Neville, K.A.; Nguyen, A.T. & Flockhart, D.A. (2006). Interethnic differences in genetic polymorphisms of CYP2D6 in the U.S. population: clinical implications. *Oncologist.* Vol.11, No.2, pp.126-135

Bertilsson, L. (2010). CYP2D6, serotonin, and suicide-a relationship? *Clin Pharmacol Ther.* Vol.88, No.3, pp.304-305

Bertz, R.J. & Granneman, G.R. (1997). Use of in vitro and in vivo data to estimate the likelihood of metabolic pharmacokinetic interactions. *Clin Pharmacokinet.* Vol.32, No.3, pp.210-258

Beutler, E. (1959). The hemolytic effect of primaquine and related compounds: a review. *Blood.* Vol.14, No.2, pp.103-139

Bishop, J.R. & Ellingrod, V.L. (2004). Neuropsychiatric pharmacogenetics: moving toward a comprehensive understanding of predicting risks and response. *Pharmacogenomics.* Vol.5, No.5, pp.463-477

Braff, J.P.; Chatterjee, B.; Hochman, M.; Kelton, T.; Kennington, J.; Kolavala, C.; Layman, K.; Parver, C.; Selby, M.C.; Washlick, J.R. & Wolf, R. (2008). Patient-tailored medicine, Part one: the impact of race and genetics on medicine. *J Health Life Sci Law.* Vol.2, No.1, pp.1-3, 5-36.

Braff, J.P.; Chatterjee, B.; Hochman, M.; Kennington, J.; Kolavala, C.; Layman, K.; Parver, C.; Rice, C.S.; Selby, M.C.; Washlick, J.R. & Wolf, R. (2009). Patient-tailored medicine, part two: personalized medicine and the legal landscape. *J Health Life Sci Law.* Vol.2, No.2, pp.1-3, 5-43

Budowlc, B. & van Daal, A. (2009). Extracting evidence from forensic DNA analyses: future molecular biology directions. *Biotechniques.* Vol.46, No.5, pp.339-350

Cacabelos, R. (2008). Pharmacogenomics and therapeutic prospects in dementia. *Eur Arch Psychiatry Clin Neurosci.* Vol.258, No.1, pp.28-47

Cacabelos, R.; Llovo, R.; Fraile, C. & Fernández-Novoa, L. (2007). Pharmacogenetic aspects of therapy with cholinesterase inhibitors: the role of CYP2D6 in Alzheimer's disease pharmacogenetics. *Curr Alzheimer Res.* Vol.4, No.4, pp.479-500

Carleton, B.; Poole, R.; Smith, M.; Leeder, J.; Ghannadan, R.; Ross, C.; Phillips, M. & Hayden, M. (2009). Adverse drug reaction active surveillance: developing a national network in Canada's children's hospitals. *Pharmacoepidemiol Drug Saf.* Vol.18, No.8, pp.713-721

Cascorbi, I. (2010). Safe and effective medicines for all: is personalized medicine the answer? *Expert Rev Clin Pharmacol.* Vol.3, No.5, pp.697-637

Chen, L.; Qin, S.; Xie, J.; Tang, J.; Yang, L.; Shen, W.; Zhao, X.; Du, J.; He, G.; Feng, G.; He, L. & Xing, Q. (2008). Genetic polymorphism analysis of CYP2C19 in Chinese Han populations from different geographic areas of mainland China. *Pharmacogenomics.* Vol.9, No.6, pp.691-702

Daly, A.K. (2003). Pharmacogenetics of the major polymorphic metabolizing enzymes. *Fundam Clin Pharmacol.* Vol.17, No.1, pp.27-41

Davies, E.C.; Green, C.F.; Taylor, S.; Williamson, P.R.; Mottram, D.R. & Pirmohamed, M. (2009). Adverse drug reactions in hospital in-patients: a prospective analysis of 3695 patient-episodes. *PLoS One.* Vol.4, No.2, e4439

de Leon, J.; Susce, M.T. & Murray-Carmichael, E. (2006). The AmpliChip CYP450 genotyping test: Integrating a new clinical tool. *Mol Diagn Ther.* Vol.10, No.3, pp.135-151

de Leon, J.; Susce, M.T.; Johnson, M.; Hardin, M.; Maw, L.; Shao, A.; Allen, A.C.; Chiafari, F.A.; Hillman, G. & Nikoloff, D.M. (2009). DNA microarray technology in the clinical environment: the AmpliChip CYP450 test for CYP2D6 and CYP2C19 genotyping. *CNS Spectr.* Vol.14, No.1, pp.19-34

Deng, Y.; Newman, B.; Dunne, M.P.; Silburn, P.A. & Mellick, G.D. (2004). Further evidence that interactions between CYP2D6 and pesticide exposure increase risk for Parkinson's disease. *Ann Neurol.* Vol.55, No.6, pp.897

Domanski, T.L.; Finta, C.; Halpert, J.R. & Zaphiropoulos, P.G. (2001). cDNA cloning and initial characterization of CYP3A43, a novel human cytochrome P450. *Mol Pharmacol.* Vol.59, No.2, pp.386–392

Dorado, P.; Cavaco, I.; Cáceres, M.C.; Piedade, R.; Ribeiro, V. & Llerena, A. (2008). Relationship between CYP2C8 genotypes and diclofenac 5-hydroxylation in healthy Spanish volunteers. *Eur J Clin Pharmacol*. Vol.64, No.10, pp.967-970

Du, J.; Xing, Q.; Xu, L.; Xu, M.; Shu, A.; Shi, Y.; Yu, L.; Zhang, A.; Wang, L.; Wang, H.; Li, X.; Feng, G. & He, L. (2006). Systematic screening for polymorphisms in the CYP3A4 gene in the Chinese population. *Pharmacogenomics*. Vol.7, No.6, pp.831-841

Edwards, I.R. & Aronson, J.K. (2000). Adverse drug reactions: definitions, diagnosis, and management. *Lancet*. Vol.7, No.356, pp.1255-1259

Eiselt, R.; Domanski, T.L.; Zibat, A.; Mueller, R.; Presecan-Siedel, E.; Hustert, E.; Zanger, U.M., Brockmoller, J.; Klenk, H.P.; Meyer, U.A.; Khan, K.K.; He, Y.A.; Halpert, J.R. & Wojnowski, L. (2001). Identification and functional characterization of eight CYP3A4 protein variants. *Pharmacogenetics*. Vol.11, No.5, pp.447–458

Elbaz, A.; Levecque, C.; Clavel, J.; Vidal, J.S.; Richard, F.; Amouyel, P.; Alpérovitch, A.; Chartier-Harlin, M.C. & Tzourio, C. (2004). CYP2D6 polymorphism, pesticide exposure, and Parkinson's disease. *Ann Neurol*. Vol.55, No.3, pp.430-434

Evans, B.J. (2007). Finding a liability-free space in which personalized medicine can bloom. *Clin Pharmacol Ther*. Vol.82, No.4, pp.461-465

Evans, DA; Manley, KA & Mckusick, VA. (1960). Genetic control of isoniazid metabolism in man. *British Medical Journal*. Vol.13, No.2, pp.485-491

Evans, W.E. & Relling, M. V. (1999). Pharmacogenomics: Translating Functional Genomics into Rational Therapeutics. *Science*. Vol.286, No.5439, pp.487-491

Frueh, F.W.; Amur, S.; Mummaneni, P.; Epstein, R.S.; Aubert, R.E.; DeLuca, T.M.; Verbrugge, R.R.; Burckart, G.J. & Lesko, L.J. (2008). Pharmacogenomic biomarker information in drug labels approved by the United States food and drug administration: prevalence of related drug use. *Pharmacotherapy*. Vol.28, No.8, pp.992-998

Gaedigk, A.; Gotschall, R.R.; Forbes, N.S.; Simon, S.D. & Leeder, J.S. (1999). Optimization of cytochrome P4502D6 (CYP2D6) phenotype assignment using a genotyping algorithm based on allele frequency data. *Pharmacogenetics*. Vol.9, pp.669-682

Gaedigk, A.; Bradford, L.D.; Marcucci, K.A. & Leeder, J.S. (2002). Unique CYP2D6 activity distribution and genotype-phenotype discordance in African Americans. *Clin Pharmacol Ther*. Vol.72, pp.76-89

Gaedigk, A.; Ryder, D.L.; Bradford, L.D. & Leeder, J.S. (2003). CYP2D6 poor metabolizer status can be ruled out by a single genotyping assay for the -1584G promoter polymorphism. *Clin Chem*. Vol.49, pp.1008-1011

Gaedigk, A.; Bradford, L.D.; Alander, S.W. & Leeder, J.S. (2006). CYP2D6*36 gene arrangements within the cyp2d6 locus: association of CYP2D6*36 with poor metabolizer status. *Drug Metab Dispos*. Vol.34, No.4, pp.563-569

Gaedigk, A.; Eklund, J.D.; Pearce, R.E.; Leeder, J.S.; Alander, S.W.; Phillips, M.S.; Bradford, L.D. & Kennedy, M.J. (2007). Identification and characterization of CYP2D6*56B, an allele associated with the poor metabolizer phenotype. *Clin Pharmacol Ther*. Vol.81, No.6, pp.817-820

Gaedigk, A. & Coetsee, C. (2008). The CYP2D6 gene locus in South African Coloureds: unique allele distributions, novel alleles and gene arrangements. *Eur J Clin Pharmacol*. Vol.64, No.5, pp.465-475

Gaedigk, A.; Simon, S.D.; Pearce, R.E.; Bradford, L.D.; Kennedy, M.J. & Leeder, J.S. (2008). The CYP2D6 activity score: translating genotype information into a qualitative measure of phenotype. *Clin Pharmacol Ther.* Vol.83, No.2, pp.234-242

Gaedigk, A.; Frank, D. & Fuhr, U. (2009). Identification of a novel non-functional CYP2D6 allele, CYP2D6*69, in a Caucasian poor metabolizer individual. *Eur J Clin Pharmacol.* Vol.65, No.1, pp.97-100

Gaedigk, A.; Isidoro-García, M.; Pearce, R.E.; Sánchez, S.; García-Solaesa, V.; Lorenzo-Romo, C.; Gonzalez-Tejera, G. & Corey, S. (2010). Discovery of the nonfunctional CYP2D6 31 allele in Spanish, Puerto Rican, and US Hispanic populations. *Eur J Clin Pharmacol.* Vol.66, No.9, pp.859-864. Erratum in: (2011). *Eur J Clin Pharmacol.* Vol.67, No.1, pp.101

García-Martín, E.; Martínez, C.; Pizarro, R.M.; García-Gamito, F.J.; Gullsten, H.; Raunio, H. & Agúndez, J.A. (2002). CYP3A4 variant alleles in white individuals with low CYP3A4 enzyme activity. *Clin Pharmacol Ther.* Vol.71, No.3, pp.196-204

Garsa, A.A.; McLeod, H.L. & Marsh, S. (2005). CYP3A4 and CYP3A5 genotyping by Pyrosequencing. *BMC Med Genet.* Vol.9, pp.6:19

Goldstein, J.A. (2001). Clinical relevance of genetic polymorphisms in the human CYP2C subfamily. *Br J Clin Pharmacol.* Vol.52, No.4, pp.349-355

Gomez, A. & Ingelman-Sundberg M. (2009). Epigenetic and microRNA-dependent control of cytochrome P450 expression: a gap between DNA and protein. *Pharmacogenomics.* Vol. 10, No.7, pp.1067-1076

Griese, E.U.; Ilett, K.F.; Kitteringham, N.R.; Eichelbaum, M.; Powell, H.; Spargo, R.M.; LeSouef, P.N.; Musk, A.W. & Minchin, R.F. (2001). Allele and genotype frequencies of polymorphic cytochromes P4502D6, 2C19 and 2E1 in aborigines from western Australia. *Pharmacogenetics.* Vol.11, No.1, pp.69-76

Haile, C.N.; Kosten, T.A. & Kosten, T.R. (2008). Pharmacogenetic treatments for drug addiction: alcohol and opiates. *Am J Drug Alcohol Abuse.* Vol.34, No.4, pp.355-381

Hamburg, M.A. & Collins, F.S. (2010). The path to personalized medicine. *N Engl J Med.* Vol.363, No.4, pp.301-304

Helland, A.; Isaksen, C.V. & Slørdal, L. (2010). Death of a 10-month-old boy after exposure to ethylmorphine. *J Forensic Sci.* Vol.55, No.2, pp.551-553

Hoskins, J.M.; Carey, L.A. & McLeod, H.L. (2009). CYP2D6 and tamoxifen: DNA matters in breast cancer. *Nat Rev Cancer.* Vol.9, No.8, pp.576-86

Ingelman-Sundberg, M. & Gomez A. (2010). The past, present and future of pharmacoepigenomics. *Pharmacogenomics.* Vol.11, No.5, pp.625-627

Ingelman-Sundberg, M. & Sim, S.C. (2010). Pharmacogenetic biomarkers as tools for improved drug therapy; emphasis on the cytochrome P450 system. *Biochem. Biophys Res Commun* Vol.396, pp.90-94

Ingelman-Sundberg, M. (2004). Pharmacogenetics of cytochrome P450 and its applications in drug therapy: the past, present and future. *Trends Pharmacol Sci.* Vol.25, No.4, pp.193-200

Ingelman-Sundberg, M.; Oscarson, M. & McLellan, R.A. (1999). Polymorphic human cytochrome P450 enzymes: an opportunity for individualized drug treatment. *Trends Pharmacol Sci.* Vol.20, No.8, pp.342-349

Ingelman-Sundberg, M.; Sim, S.C.; Gomez A. & Rodriguez-Antona C. (2007). Influence of cytochrome P450 polymorphisms on drug therapies: pharmacogenetic, pharmacoepigenetic and clinical aspects. *Pharmacol Ther.* Vol.116, pp. 496-526

Isacsson, G.; Holmgren, A.; Osby, U. & Ahlner, J. (2009). Decrease in suicide among the individuals treated with antidepressants: a controlled study of antidepressants in suicide, Sweden 1995-2005. *Acta Psychiatr Scand.* Vol.120, No.1, pp.37-44

Jin, M.; Gock, S.B.; Jannetto, P.J.; Jentzen, J.M. & Wong, S.H. (2005). Pharmacogenomics as molecular autopsy for forensic toxicology: genotyping cytochrome P450 3A4*1B and 3A5*3 for 25 fentanyl cases. *J Anal Toxicol.* Vol.29, No.7, pp.590-598

Johansson, I. & Ingelman-Sundberg, M. (2011). Genetic polymorphism and toxicology-with emphasis on cytochorome p450. *Toxicol Sci.* Vol.120, pp.1-13

Kamali, F. & Wynne, H. (2010). Pharmacogenetics of Warfarin. *Annu Rev Med.* Vol.61, pp.63–75

Karch, S.B. (2007). Changing times: DNA resequencing and the "nearly normal autopsy". *J Forensic Leg Med.* Vol.14, No.7, pp.389-397

Kirchheiner, J. & Seeringer, A. (2007). Clinical implications of pharmacogenetics of cytochrome P450 drug metabolizing enzymes. *Biochimica et Biophysica Acta.* Vol. 1770, pp. 489–494

Kitada, M. (2003). Genetic polymorphism of cytochrome P450 enzymes in Asian populations: focus on CYP2D6. *Int J Clin Pharmacol Res.* Vol.23, No.1,pp.31-35

Korkina, L.; Scordo, M.G.; Deeva, I.; Cesareo, E. & De Luca, C. (2009). The chemical defensive system in the pathobiology of idiopathic environment-associated diseases. *Curr Drug Metab.* Vol.10, No.8, pp.914-931

Koski, A.; Ojanperä, I.; Sistonen, J.; Vuori, E. & Sajantila, A. (2007). A fatal doxepin poisoning associated with a defective CYP2D6 genotype. *Am J Forensic Med Pathol.* Vol.28, No.3, pp.259-261

Koski, A.; Sistonen, J.; Ojanperä, I.; Gergov, M.; Vuori, E. & Sajantila, A. (2006). CYP2D6 and CYP2C19 genotypes and amitriptyline metabolite ratios in a series of medicolegal autopsies. *Forensic Sci Int.* Vol.158, No.2-3, pp.177-183

Lamba, J.K.; Lin, Y.S.; Thummel, K.; Daly, A.; Watkins, P.B.; Strom, S.; Zhang, J. & Schuetz, E.G. (2002). Common allelic variants of cytochrome P4503A4 and their prevalence in different populations. *Pharmacogenetics.* Vol.12, No.2, pp.121-132

Launiainen, T.; Sajantila, A.; Rasanen, I.; Vuori, E. & Ojanperä, I. (2010). Adverse interaction of warfarin and paracetamol: evidence from a post-mortem study. *Eur J Clin Pharmacol.* Vol.66, No.1, pp.97-103

Lazarou, J.; Pomeranz, B.H. & Corey, P.N. (1998). Incidence of adverse drug reactions in hospitalized patients: a meta-analysis of prospective studies. *JAMA.* Vol.279, No.15, pp.1200-1205

Leathart, J.B.S.; London, S.J.; Steward, A.; Adams, J.D.; Idle, J.R. & Daly, A.K. (1998). CYP2D6 phenotype-genotype relationships in African-Americans and Caucasians in Los Angeles. *Pharmacogenetics.* Vol.8, pp.529-541

Lehmann, H & Ryan, E. (1956). The familial incidence of low pseudocholinesterase level. *Lancet.* Vol. 21, No.271, pp.124

Lesko, L.J. & Woodcock, J. (2004). Translation of pharmacogenomics and pharmacogenetics: a regulatory perspective. *Nat Rev Drug Discov.* Vol.3, No.9, pp.763-769

Lesko, L.J.; Salerno, R.A.; Spear, B.B.; Anderson, D.C.; Anderson, T.; Brazell, C.; Collins, J.; Dorner, A.; Essayan, D.; Gomez-Mancilla, B.; Hackett, J.; Huang, S.M.; Ide, S.; Killinger, J.; Leighton, J.; Mansfield, E.; Meyer, R.; Ryan, S.G.; Schmith, V.; Shaw, P.; Sistare, F.; Watson, M. & Worobec, A. (2003). Pharmacogenetics and pharmacogenomics in drug development and regulatory decision making: report of the first FDA-PWG-PhRMA-DruSafe Workshop. *J Clin Pharmacol.* Vol.43, No.4, pp.342-358

Levo, A.; Koski, A.; Ojanperä, I.; Vuori, E. & Sajantila, A. (2003). Post-mortem SNP analysis of CYP2D6 gene reveals correlation between genotype and opioid drug (tramadol) metabolite ratios in blood. *Forensic Sci Int.* Vol.135, No.1, pp.9-15

Limdi, N.A.; Wadelius, M.; Cavallari, L.; Eriksson, N.; Crawford, D.C.; Lee, M.T.; Chen, C.H.; Motsinger-Reif, A.; Sagreiya, H.; Liu, N.; Wu, A.H.; Gage, B.F.; Jorgensen, A. & Pirmohamed, M.; Shin, J.G.; Suarez-Kurtz, G.; Kimmel, S.E.; Johnson, J.A.; Klein, T.E. & Wagner, M.J. International Warfarin Pharmacogenetics Consortium. (2010). Warfarin pharmacogenetics: a single VKORC1 polymorphism is predictive of dose across 3 racial groups. *Blood.* Vol.6, No.115, pp.3827-3834

LLerena, A.; Berecz, R.; de la Rubia, A. & Dorado, P. (2002). QTc interval lengthening is related to CYP2D6 hydroxylation capacity and plasma concentration of thioridazine in patients. *J Psychopharmacol.* Vol.16, pp.361-364

Luo, H.R.; Aloumanis, V.; Lin, K.M.; Gurwitz, D. & Wan, Y.J. (2004). Polymorphisms of CYP2C19 and CYP2D6 in Israeli ethnic groups. *Am J Pharmacogenomics.* Vol.4, No.6, pp.395-401

Luo, H.R.; Gaedigk, A.; Aloumanis, V. & Wan, Y.J. (2005). Identification of CYP2D6 impaired functional alleles in Mexican Americans. *Eur J Clin Pharmacol.* Vol.61, No.11, pp.797-802

Madadi, P.; Koren, G.; Cairns, J.; Chitayat, D.; Gaedigk, A.; Leeder, J.S.; Teitelbaum, R.; Karaskov, T. & Aleksa, K. (2007). Safety of codeine during breastfeeding: fatal morphine poisoning in the breastfed neonate of a mother prescribed codeine. *Can Fam Physician.* Vol.53, No.1, pp.33-35

Madadi, P.; Ross, C.J.; Hayden, M.R.; Carleton, B.C.; Gaedigk, A.; Leeder, J.S. & Koren, G. (2009). Pharmacogenetics of neonatal opioid toxicity following maternal use of codeine during breastfeeding: a case-control study. *Clin Pharmacol Ther.* Vol.85, No.1, pp.31-35

Mancinelli, L.; Cronin, M. & Sadée, W. (2000). Pharmacogenomics: the promise of personalized medicine. *AAPS PharmSci.* Vol.2, No.1, Article 4

McNamara, D.M. (2008). Emerging role of pharmacogenomics in heart failure. *Curr Opin Cardiol.* Vol.23, No.3, pp.261-268

Mellen, P.B. & Herrington, D.M. (2005). Pharmacogenomics of blood pressure response to antihypertensive treatment. *J Hypertens.* Vol.23, No.7, pp.1311-1325

Mishra, N.K.; Agarwal, S. & Raghava, G.P. (2010). Prediction of cytochrome P450 isoform responsible for metabolizing a drug molecule. *BMC Pharmacol.* Vol.16, No.10, pp.8

Mo, S.L.; Liu, Y.H.; Duan, W.; Wei, M.Q.; Kanvar, J.R.; Zhou, S.F. (2009). Substrate specificity, regulation, and polymorphism of human cytochrome P450 2B6. *Curr Drug Metabol.* Vol. 10, pp. 730-753

Moore, T.J.; Cohen, M.R. & Furberg, C.D. (2007). Serious adverse drug events reported to the Food and Drug Administration, 1998-2005. *Arch Intern Med.* Vol.167, pp.1752-1759

Morley, K.I. & Hall, W.D. (2004). Using pharmacogenetics and pharmacogenomics in the treatment of psychiatric disorders: some ethical and economic considerations. *J Mol Med.* Vol.82, pp.21-30

Mwinyi, J.; Cavaco, I.; Yurdakok, B.; Mkrtchian, S. & Ingelman-Sundberg M. (2011). The ligands of the estrogen receptor {alpha} regulate cytochrome P4502C9 (CYP2C9) expression. *J Pharmacol Exp Ther.* doi: 10.1124/jpet.110.175075

Nebert, D.W.; Zhang, G. & Vesell, E.S. (2008). From human genetics and genomics to pharmacogenetics and pharmacogenomics: past lessons, future directions. *Drug Metab Rev.*Vol.40, No.2, pp.187-224

Oscarson, M. & Ingelman-Sundberg, M. (2002). CYPalleles: a web page for nomenclature of human cytochrome P450 alleles. *Drug Metab Pharmacokinet.* Vol.17, No.6, pp.491-495.

Owen, R.P.; Sangkuhl, K.; Klein, T.E. & Altman, R.B. (2009). Cytochrome P450 2D6. *Pharmacogenet Genomics.* Vol.19, pp.559-562

Pilgrim, J.L.; Gerostamoulos, D. & Drummer, O.H. (2011). Review: Pharmacogenetic aspects of the effect of cytochrome P450 polymorphisms on serotonergic drug metabolism, response, interactions, and adverse effects. *Forensic Sci med Pathol.* Vol.7, No.2, pp.162-184

Pirmohamed, M.; James, S.; Meakin, S.; Green, C.; Scott, A.K.; Walley, T.J.; Farrar, K.; Park, B.K. & Breckenridge, A.M. (2004). Adverse drug reactions as cause of admission to hospital: prospective analysis of 18.820 patients. *BMJ.* Vol.329, pp.15–19

Prahlow, J.A. & Landrum, J.E. (2005). Amitriptyline abuse and misuse. *Am J Forensic Med Pathol.* Vol.26, No.1, pp.86-88

Prandota, J. (2010). Advances of molecular clinical pharmacology in gastroenterology and hepatology. *Am J Ther.* Vol.17, No.5, e137-162

Preissner, S.; Kroll, K.; Dunkel, M.; Goldsobel, G.; Kuzmann, D.; Senger, S.; Günther, S.; Winnenburg, R.; Schroeder, M. & Preissner, R. (2010). SuperCYP: a comprehensive database on Cytochrome P450 enzymes including a tool for analysis of CYP-drug interactions. *Nucleic Acids Res* 38 (Database issue) D237-43. Available from http://bioinformatics.charite.de/supercyp *Psychiatry Clin Neurosci.* Vol.258, Suppl 1, pp.28-47

Queneau, P.; Bannwarth, B.; Carpentier, F.; Guliana, J.M.; Bouget, J.; Trombert ,B.; Leverve, X.; Lapostolle, F.; Borron, S.W.; Adnet, F. & Association Pédagogique Nationale pour l'Enseignement de la Thérapeutique (APNET). (2007). Emergency department visits caused by adverse drug events: results of a French survey. *Drug Saf.* Vol.30, No.1, pp.81-88

Robertson, J.A. (2001). Consent and privacy in pharmacogenetic testing. *Nat Genet.* Vol. 28, pp. 207–209

Robertson, J.A.; Brody, B.; Buchanan, A.; Kahn, J. & McPherson, E. (2002). Pharmacogenetic challenges for the health care system. *Health Aff (Millwood).* Vol.21, No.4, pp.155-167

Rodriguez-Antona, C.; Gomez, A.; Karlgren, M.; Sim, S.C. & Ingelman-Sundberg, M. (2010). Molecular genetics and epigenetics of the cytochrome P450 gene family and its relevance for cancer risk and treatment. *Hum Genet* Vol.127, No.1, pp.1-17

Rosemary, J. & Adithan, C. (2007). The pharmacogenetics of CYP2C9 and CYP2C19: ethnic variation and clinical significance. *Curr Clin Pharmacol.* Vol.2, No.1, pp.93-109

Sadee, W. (1998). Finding the right drug for the right patient. *Pharm Res.* Vol. 15, pp.959-963

Sajantila, A.; Palo, J.U.; Ojanperä, I.; Davis, C. & Budowle, B. (2010). Pharmacogenetics in medico-legal context. *Forensic Sci Int*. Vol.203, No.1-3, pp.44-52

Sallee, F.R.; DeVane, C.L. & Ferrell, R.E. (2000). Fluoxetine-related death in a child with cytochrome P-450 2D6 genetic deficiency. *J Child Adolesc Psychopharmacol*. Vol.10, No.1, pp.27-34

Santos, P.C.; Soares, R.A.; Santos, D.B.; Nascimento, R.M.; Coelho, G.L.; Nicolau, J.C.; Mill, J.G.; Krieger, J.E. & Pereira, A.C. (2011). CYP2C19 and ABCB1 gene polymorphisms are differently distributed according to ethnicity in the Brazilian general population. *BMC Med Genet*. Vol.19, pp.12:13

Sevior, D.K.; Hokkanen, J.; Tolonen, A.; Abass, K.; Tursas, L.; Pelkonen O. & Ahokas, J. T. (2010). Rapid screening of commercially available herbal products for the inhibition of major human hepatic cytochorome P450 enzymes using the N-in-one cocktail. *Xenobiotica*. Vol. 40, No.4, pp 245-254.

Sim, S.C.; Risinger, C.; Dahl, M.L.; Aklillu, E.; Christensen, M.; Bertilsson, L. & Ingelman-Sundberg, M. (2006). A common novel CYP2C19 gene variant causes ultrarapid drug metabolism relevant for the drug response to proton pump inhibitors and antidepressants. *Clin Pharmacol Ther*. Vol.79, No.1, pp.103-113

Sim, S.C. & Ingelman-Sundberg, M. (2011). Pharmacogenomic biomarkers: new tools in current and future drug therapy. *Trends Pharmacol Sci*. Vol.32, No.2, pp.72-81

Sim, S.C.; Altman, R.B. & Ingelman-Sundberg M. (2011). Databases in the area of pharmacogenetics. *Hum Mutat*. Vol.32, No.5, pp.526-531

Singh, M.S.; Francis, P.A. & Michael, M. (2011). Tamoxifen, cytochrome P450 genes and breast cancer clinical outcomes. *Breast*. Vol.20, No.2, pp.111-118

Sistonen, J.; Fuselli, S.; Levo, A. & Sajantila, A. (2005). CYP2D6 genotyping by a multiplex primer extension reaction. *Clin Chem*. Vol.51, pp.1291-1295

Sistonen, J.; Fuselli, S.; Palo, J.U.; Chauhan, N.; Padh, H. & Sajantila, A. (2009). Pharmacogenetic variation at CYP2C9, CYP2C19, and CYP2D6 at global and microgeographic scales. *Pharmacogenet Genomics*. Vol.19, No.2, pp.170-179

Sistonen, J.; Sajantila, A.; Lao, O.; Corander, J.; Barbujani, G. & Fuselli, S. (2007). CYP2D6 worldwide genetic variation shows high frequency of altered activity variants and no continental structure. *Pharmacogenet Genomics*. Vol.17, pp.93-101

Spina, E.; Santoro, V. & D'Arrigo, C. (2008). Clinically relevant pharmacokinetic drug interactions with second-generation antidepressants: an update. *Clin Ther*. Vol.30, No.7, pp.1206-1227

Suarez-Kurtz, G. (2008). The implications of population admixture in race-based drug prescription. *Clin Pharmacol Ther*. Vol.83, No.3, pp.399-400.

Suarez-Kurtz, G. (2010). Pharmacogenetics in the Brazilian population. *Front Pharmacol*. Vol.1, pp.118

Thummel, K.E. & Wilkinson, G.R. (1998). In vitro and in vivo drug interactions involving human CYP3A. *Annu Rev Pharmacol Toxicol*. Vol.38, pp.389–430

Tomalik-Scharte, D.; Lazar, A.; Fuhr, U. & Kirchheiner, J. (2008). The clinical role of genetic polymorphisms in drug-metabolizing enzymes. *Pharmacogenomics J*. Vol.8, No.1, pp.4-15

Totah, R.A. & Rettie, A.E. (2005). Cytochrome P450 C8: substrates, inhibitors, pharmacogenetics, and clinical relevance. *Clin Pharmacol Ther* . Vol.77, pp.341–352 van Delden, J.; Bolt, I.; Kalis, A.; Derijks, J. & Leufkens, H. (2004). Tailor-made pharmacotherapy: future developments and ethical challenges in the field of pharmacogenomics. *Bioethics*. Vol.18, No.4, pp.303-321

van der Weide, J. & Steijns, L.S. (1999). Cytochrome P450 enzyme system: genetic polymorphisms and impact on clinical pharmacology. *Ann Clin Biochem*. Vol.36, pp.722-729

van Noord, C.; Eijgelsheim, M. & Stricker, B.H. (2010). Drug- and non-drug-associated QT interval prolongation. *Br J Clin Pharmacol*. Vol.70, No.1, pp.16-23

Vaszar, L.T.; Rosen, G.D. & Raffin, T.A. (2002). Pharmacogenomics and the challenge to privacy. *Pharmacogenomics J*. Vol.2, No.3, pp.144-147

Vogel, F. (1959). Moderne problem der humangenetik. *Ergeb Inn Med U Kinderheilk*. Vol.12, 52–125.

Wan, Y.J.; Poland, R.E.; Han, G.; Konishi, T.; Zheng, Y.P.; Berman, N. & Lin, K.M. (2001). Analysis of the CYP2D6 gene polymorphism and enzyme activity in African-Americans in southern California. *Pharmacogenetics*. Vol.11, No.6, pp.489-499

Wang, B.; Wang, J.; Huang, S.Q.; Su, H.H. ; Zhou, S.F. (2009). Genetic polymorphism of the human cytochorome P450 2C9 gene and its clinical significance. *Curr Drug Metab*. Vol. 10, pp. 781-834

Watanabe, T.; Sakuyama, K.; Sasaki, T.; Ishii, Y.; Ishikawa, M.; Hirasawa, N. & Hiratsuka, M. (2010). Functional characterization of 26 CYP2B6 allelic variants (CYP2B6.2-CYP2B6.28, except CYP2B6.22). *Pharmacogenet Genomics*. Vol.20, No.7, pp.459-462

Weinshilboum, R. & Wang, L. (2004). Pharmacogenomics: bench to bedside. *Nat Rev Drug Discov*. Vol.3, No.9, pp.739-748

Weinshilboum, R. (2003). Inheritance and drug response. *N Engl J Med*. Vol.348, No.6, pp.529-537

Westlind, A.; Malmebo, S.; Johansson, I.; Otter, C.; Andersson, T.B.; Ingelman-Sundberg, M. & Oscarson, M. (2001). Cloning and tissue distribution of a novel human cytochrome P450 of the CYP3A subfamily, CYP3A43. *Biochem BiophysRes Commun*. Vol.281, No.5, pp.1349–1355

White, P.J. (2010). Patient factors that influence warfarin dose response. *J Pharm Pract*. Vol.23, No.3, pp.194-204

Wilkinson, G.R. (2005). Drug metabolism and variability among patients in drug response. *N Engl J Med*. Vol.352, No.21, pp.2211-2221

Willmann, S.; Edginton, A.N.; Coboeken, K.; Ahr, G. & Lippert, J. (2009). Risk to the breast-fed neonate from codeine treatment to the mother: a quantitative mechanistic modeling study. *Clin Pharmacol Ther*. Vol.86, No.6, pp.634-643

Wong, S.H.; Happy, C.; Blinka, D.; Gock, S.; Jentzen, J.M.; Donald Hon, J.; Coleman, H.; Jortani, S.A.; Lucire, Y.; Morris-Kukoski, C.L.; Neuman, M.G.; Orsulak, P.J.; Sander, T.; Wagner, M.A.; Wynn, J.R.; Wu, A.H. & Yeo, K.T. (2010). From personalized medicine to personalized justice: the promises of translational pharmacogenomics in the justice system. *Pharmacogenomics*. Vol.11, No.6, pp.731-737

Wong, S.H.; Wagner, M.A.; Jentzen, J.M.; Schur, C.; Bjerke, J.; Gock, S.B. & Chang, C.C. (2003). Pharmacogenomics as an aspect of molecular autopsy for forensic pathology/toxicology: does genotyping CYP2D6 serve as an adjunct for certifying methadone toxicity? *J Forensic Sci*. Vol.48, No.6, pp.1406-1415

Xie, H.G.; Kim, R.B.; Wood, A.J. & Stein, C.M. (2001). Molecular basis of ethnic differences in drug disposition and response. *Annu Rev Pharmacol Toxicol*. Vol.41, pp.815-850

Xu, C.; Goodz, S.; Sellers, E.M.; Tyndale, R.F. (2002). CYP2A6 genetic variation and potential consequences. *Advanced Drug Delivery Review*. Vol.54, pp.1245-1256

Yang, X.; Zhang, B.; Molony, C.; Chudin, E.; Hao, K.; Zhu, J.; Gaedigk, A.; Suver, C.; Zhong, H.; Leeder, J.S.; Guengerich, F.P.; Strom, S.C.; Schuetz, E.; Rushmore, T.H.; Ulrich, R.G.; Slatter, J.G.; Schadt, E.E.; Kasarskis, A. & Lum, P.Y. (2010). Systematic genetic and genomic analysis of cytochrome P450 enzyme activities in human liver. *Genome Res*. Vol.20, No.8, pp.1020-1023

Yasar, U.; Aklillu, E.; Canaparo, R.; Sandberg, M.; Sayi, J.; Roh, H.K. & Wennerholm, A. (2002). Analysis of CYP2C9*5 in Caucasian, Oriental and black-African populations. *Eur J Clin Pharmacol*. Vol.58, No.8, pp.555-558

Yasar, Ü.; Eliasson, E.; Dahl, M.L.; Johansson, I.; Ingelman-Sundberg, M. & Sjöqvist, F. (1999). Validation of methods for CYP2C9 genotyping: frequencies of mutant alleles in a Swedish population. *Biochem Biophys Res Commun*. Vol.254, No.3, pp.628-631. Erratum in: (1999). *Biochem Biophys Res Commun*. Vol.258, No.1, pp.227

Zackrisson, A.L.; Lindblom, B. & Ahlner, J. (2010). High frequency of occurrence of CYP2D6 gene duplication/multiduplication indicating ultrarapid metabolism among suicide cases. *Clin Pharmacol Ther*. Vol.88, No.3, pp.354-359

Zanger, U.M.; Raimundo, S. & Eichelbaum, M. (2004). Cytochrome P450 2D6: overview and update on pharmacology, genetics, biochemistry. *Naunyn Schmiedebergs Arch Pharmacol*. Vol.369, No.1, pp.23-37.

Zhou, Q.; Yu, X.M.; Lin, H.B.; Wang, L.; Yun, Q.Z.; Hu, S.N. & Wang, D.M. (2009). Genetic polymorphism, linkage disequilibrium, haplotype structure and novel allele analysis of CYP2C19 and CYP2D6 in Han Chinese. *Pharmacogenomics J*. Vol.9, No.6, pp.380-394

Zhou, S.F.; Di, Y.M.; Chan, E.; Du, Y.M.; Chow, V.D.; Xue, C.C.; Lai, X.; Wang, J.C.; Li, C.G.; Tian, M. & Duan, W. (2008). Clinical pharmacogenetics and potential application in personalized medicine. *Curr Drug Metab*. Vol.9, No.8, pp.738-784

Zhou, S.F. (2009). Polymorphism of human cytochrome P450 2D6 and its clinical significance: Part I. *Clin Pharmacokinet*. Vol.48, No.11, pp.689-723

Zhou, S.F. (2009). Polymorphism of Human Cytochrome P450 2D6 and Its Clinical Significance: Part II. *Clin Pharmacokinet*. Vol. 48, No. 12, pp. 761-804

Zhou, S.F.; Wang, B.; Yang, L.P. & Liu, J.P. (2010). Structure, function, regulation and polymorphism and the clinical significance of human cytochrome P450 1A2. *Drug Metabolism Reviews*. Vol. 42, No. 2, pp. 268-354

13

Forensic Microbiology

Herbert Tomaso and Heinrich Neubauer
Friedrich-Loeffler-Institut, Federal Research Institute for Animal Health, Institute of Bacterial Infections and Zoonoses, Jena, Germany

1. Introduction

Biocrime or bioterrorism is the threat or use of microorganisms, toxins, pests, prions, or their associated ancillary products to commit acts of crime or terror. Microorganisms can malevolently be used as biological warfare agents, in bioterrorist acts, and in crimes without political intentions. Such actions can be directed against humans and animals and can lead to outbreaks of infections with high morbidity and mortality. In recent years microbial forensics has been established as a new scientific discipline to strengthen the law enforcement response especially in a bioterrorism event (3). These tools can also be applied to investigate the transmission of pathogenic microorganism caused by sexual abuse and other physical offenses (1).

The aim of this review is to describe the corner stones of microbial forensics as a novel type of forensic analysis defined as "the detection of reliably measured molecular variations between microbial strains and their use to infer the origin, relationships, or transmission route of a particular isolate" (10).

Several microorganisms are a severe threat to human and/or animal health and a country's agricultural economy. Their malevolent use can have a major socio-economic impact. A number of these pathogens can affect both humans and animals (zoonoses), can contaminate the environment for decades, or may establish new enzootic foci. The World Organisation for Animal Health (OIE) lists several of these agents as diseases of importance to international trade with serious export restrictions for countries where the diseases are endemic.

Biological warfare agents to be used against humans and animals were developed and weaponized in the fifties of the last century in several countries including the USA, the former Soviet Union and the United Kingdom. An international arms control and disarmament treaty, the Biological Weapons Convention (BWC), banned the use of biological weapons in 1972 (http://www.opbw.org/convention/documents/btwctext.pdf). Today only few states are under suspicion of having biological warfare programs. Politically-binding confidence building measures provide a permanent transparency tool for building confidence in compliance with the BWC.

In the aftermath of the anthrax letters attacks in October 2001 that killed five people it has become evident that biocrimes can only be solved when genomic information can be used to identify the source of an organism. Evidence in a criminal investigation must be collected within the constraints of legal rules to ensure that any prosecution based upon that evidence can withstand judicial review in a court. Therefore, first responders must learn how to secure evidence and preserve the chain of custody (34). Quality-assurance and –control procedures have to assure that reliable evidence can be presented in court (3). Laboratories that have been officially accredited will be able to provide all relevant documents regarding quality control and assurance, proficiency test results, qualification of laboratory personnel etc. Also case specific material like photographs of gels, benchnotes, validation studies, and controls will usually be adequately documented. Evidence collection, transport, and storage need more attention than is usually needed for clinical routine samples. Test procedure will be according to standard operating procedures (SOPs) and any deviation of protocols will have to be documented. The final report should contain information about the specificity and accuracy of the applied tests and provide an interpretation of the result and its limitations.

Nucleic amplification and molecular-epidemiological techniques are essential tools in clinical microbiology for identifying pathogens and in outbreak investigations. Various typing tools have been developed for phylogenetic and phylogeographic studies. In forensic microbiology these methodologies can be used to detect and trace back the spread of microorganisms in the context of a crime. Whole-genome sequencing provides the most comprehensive, reliable and reproducible information about a strain, but until recently this technique was expensive and time consuming. The subsequent annotation of sequences was also a major endeavor. Nowadays this technique has become affordable and reference genomes for all select agents have been sequenced. They can be used to clarify the relationship of suspicious isolates with reference genomes.

Centralized reporting and surveillance systems on the national and international level are essential as single cases may be regarded as sporadic although they are part of a larger transboundary outbreak. Surveillance systems have already been established that store and provide DNA fingerprints of microbes being major causes of hospital-acquired or food borne infections.

Descriptive epidemiological data have to be analyzed with caution. Natural outbreaks can be difficult to discriminate from intentional use of microorganisms, especially if the organisms are endemic. Only molecular-epidemiological tools can corroborate the chain of infection.

This review will discuss the value of diagnostic and molecular-epidemiological tools developed for select agents and will provide examples of investigations focused on for example *Bacillus anthracis, Francisella tularensis*, and *Yersinia pestis*. The critical role of sample collection, packaging, transport, and storage will be highlighted.

2. Sample collection

Laboratories involved in forensic microbiology analysis must be prepared to deal with chain-of-custody documentation, secure storage of evidence, tracking of individual items of evidence and their derivatives and all the legal requirements for handling evidence. Chain-of-custody protocols document the unbroken chain of records showing who had handled the evidence, where and under which conditions (temperature, time etc.) the material had been stored and whether access to the samples was restricted (27). The NATO document AEP-10 "Handbook for Sampling and Identification of Biological and Chemical Agents (SIBCA)", 2007, 5th Edition, Procedures and Techniques, Volume 1 (STANAG 4329) provides practical guidelines how to sample select agents in the field even in a contaminated environment. These guidelines are used by NATO and Partnership for Peace (PFP) countries. Countries may have different national requirements, but general principles can be a guideline for Civilian-Military Cooperation (CIMIC) or purely civilian operational and forensic investigation teams. The European Guideline on Principles of Field Investigation "Biological Incident Response and Environmental Sampling" was published by the EU Commission, DG Health and Consumer Protection, Health Threats Unit in October 2006 and "describes the principles of response in the initial phase of a biological incident where the goal is to identify what has happened in order to initiate appropriate countermeasures". These documents underline the necessity of planning and pre-mission briefings as the environment may be life-threatening. Moreover, the quality of primary samples is critical for subsequent analyses. The personal protective equipment is also affecting personnel by limiting mobility, flexibility, and time available to work at the scene (2).

3. Sample matrix analysis

In clinical microbiology the sample matrix is important to decide, whether the analyses requested by the clinician are appropriate and which tests should be performed. Unfortunately, requests are not always justified by the clinical presentation and the sample matrix is sometimes conflicting. For example a microscopical inspection of sputum samples will indicate, if the quality of the specimens is adequate. In forensic microbiology the same rules apply, but more detailed investigations may be necessary to obtain relevant information about the history of a specimen, environmental conditions, chemical and physical constitution of the matrix, presence of pollen etc. (2).
This can be achieved by particle sizing, electron microscopy, analytical chemistry, isotope analysis, and other techniques. However, several analyses will have to be performed outside appropriate laboratory safety containment (e.g. BSL-3 for *Y. pestis*) and therefore, specimens will have to be inactivated. Especially when anthrax spores have to be killed the inactivation with chemical or physical techniques is quite aggressive. This treatment does not only denature the pathogens but will also cause changes of the matrix. It has to be demonstrated for each method that the inactivation process does not interfere with the subsequent tests.

4. Biological agents

The Centers for Disease Control (CDC) in Atlanta have evaluated the priority of agents according to their relevance for national security due to ease of dissemination and transmission from person to person, high mortality rates, the potential for major public health impact, risk of public panic and social disruption, and the requirement of special action for public health preparedness. Category A includes the most dangerous agents: *Variola* major virus (smallpox), *Bacillus anthracis* (anthrax), *Yersinia pestis* (plague), *Clostridium botulinum* toxin (botulism), *Francisella tularensis* (tularemia), and viral hemorrhagic fever viruses (33).

4.1 Microbe identification by classical microbiology

The identification of microbial agents - as defined by the SIBCA handbook - can be provisional (presumptive), when immunological methods, nucleic acid detection or cultivation and metabolic assays have been tested positive. Identification is confirmed by the combination of at least two of the above mentioned criteria. Unambiguous identification

requires cultivation and *in vivo* studies (animal models) that prove the pathogenicity of the agent. However, animal models should be avoided for ethical reasons whenever possible.
Biological agents can be difficult to cultivate due to sample contamination, low number of bacteria or pretreatment of patients with antibiotics. Some bacteria are fastidious (*F. tularensis, Brucella* spp.) and require special nutrient media, and some need prolonged cultivation times (*Brucella* spp.). Phenotypical characteristics such as antibiotic susceptibility and biochemical reaction profiles, susceptibility to specific phages, colony morphology and others are not always reliable. Mutations of agents can be induced or engineered, but naturally occurring atypical strains have also been found e.g. among *Bacillus anthracis* and *Yersinia pestis* isolates which can result in misidentification and treatment failure (52). Commercial biochemical identification systems are not optimized for these agents and can result in misidentification. Multiple antimicrobial resistances can occur through natural horizontal gene transfer or by genetic manipulation. Natural resistance to a multitude of antimicrobials is typical for *Burkholderia pseudomallei. Francisella tularensis* is naturally resistant to penicillins and cephalosporines. A very dangerous multidrug resistant strain of *Yersinia pestis* has been isolated from a patient with bubonic plague in Madagascar. This strain carries a self-transmissible plasmid with a genetic backbone also prevalent among *Escherichia coli, Klebsiella* spp. and *Salmonella* spp. conferring high-level resistance to streptomycin, tetracyclin, chloramphenicol, and sulfonamides (50). These facts underline the importance of cultivation and the assessment of antimicrobial susceptibility in addition to more rapid diagnostic tools. A polyphasic approach for identification and typing will help to avoid problems due to atypical genotype and phenotype, inhibition, or lack of specificity or sensitivity of assays.
Handling of select agents is highly dangerous and cumbersome and restricted to laboratories with biosafety-level 3 containment. Biosafety-level 3 laboratories have to be operated according to special regulations that require e.g. a sophisticated ventilation system and personal protective equipment (e.g. FFP3 masks, overalls, face shields, gloves etc.).

4.2 Nucleic acid amplification techniques

Many real-time PCR assays are highly specific and sensitive and shorten the time required to establish a diagnosis in comparison with conventional PCR protocols, cultivation, and biochemical identification methods. Therefore, real-time PCR assays have been developed for the identification of *Bacillus anthracis, Brucella* spp., *Burkholderia mallei* and *Burkholderia pseudomallei, Francisella tularensis* and *Yersinia pestis* (21). PCR results can be false negative due to inadequate quality of clinical samples, low number of bacteria in samples, DNA degradation, inhibitory substances and inappropriate DNA preparation.

4.3 Serology

Seroconversion may prove the exposure to a certain agent in the past. However, seroconversion can be expected only after several days or weeks and is of little use for rapidly diagnosing infections caused by highly pathogenic agents. It will be difficult to organize serological investigations (including follow-up tests) when a terrorist attack causes mass casualties that need medical treatment or when the situation is complicated by civil unrest, war or natural catastrophes at the same time.
Various immunological assays have also been used to identify pathogens in samples of patients and environmental samples. Hand-held test kits can be used as bed-side tests and

are useful under field conditions, but clinical validations hardly exist and most tests are "for scientific use only". Immunochromatographic lateral-flow assays have been developed e.g. for brucellosis, tularemia, and plague (4; 29; 37; 44). Limitations of these immunological assays are that they are frequently not available commercially, not specific enough, or have not been validated and licensed for use in humans or animals. Moreover, cross-reactions may cause false positives and modified or missing antigenic structures can cause false negatives.

5. Typing and strain identification

Differences among microbes have to be assessed to determine whether strains are from the same source or lineage or from a different origin. The accuracy and precision will depend on the typing method, expected mutation rates, and other characteristics of the organism. In court scientists may need to quantify the reliability of a relationship among strains determined using molecular phylogenetic analyses. This will establish the probability of association to a certain source of infection (16).

Techniques for forensic microbiology can be very similar to those being used for phylogenetic and epidemiological investigations e.g. for food-borne outbreaks.

Molecular-epidemiological tools used for genotyping are most promising and have been applied in the past to elucidate the origin of biological agents. Especially whole genome sequencing and bioinformatic tools for comparison of genomes are potent tools, but technical complexity and costs are still prohibitive for routine application.

In several chapters of the highly recommendable book "Microbial Forensics" by Bruce Budowle and many other "founders" of this new scientific discipline it was demonstrated that only highly specialized knowledge of microbial genetics will allow an assessment of the relevance of typing results obtained by Multi-locus Sequence Typing (MLST), Variable Number of Tandem Repeats (VNTR), Single Nucleotide Polymorphisms (SNPs) analysis or other typing tools ("Microbial Forensics" B. Budowle. ISBN 978-0-12-382006-8). Validation of typing assays and data of large collections of strains from all over the world are crucial for microbial forensic investigations. Typing methods should be reproducible, stable during the study period, applicable to every isolate, discriminating among isolates, and discrimination should be concordant with the epidemiological picture (46). DNA sequence-based data are robust, portable, easy to compare, and amenable to computerised analysis for phylogeographical and epidemiological studies. However, the quality of open access sequence databases depends on the accuracy of submitted sequences and is consequently sometimes not reliable.

6. Select agents

6.1 Anthrax

Bacillus (B.) anthracis is the causative agent of anthrax and a member of the *Bacillus cereus* group. This group includes *B. anthracis, B. cereus, B. thuringiensis, B. weihenstephanensis,* and *B. mycoides*. These closely related bacteria can be discriminated by using phenotypic characteristics. *B. anthracis* is typically non-motile, susceptible to penicillin, lysed by the gamma phage, and colonies are non-hemolytic with a typical morphology. However, more than 24 hours are required to assess these characteristics and misidentification can occasionally occur due to variations of the phenotype. Natural infections result mostly in

cutaneous anthrax. Anthrax caused by inhalation is rare, but the spores of *B. anthracis* can easily be disseminated in aerosols. The spores are very stable and persist in the environment especially in soil for many years or even decades (35).
In the fall of 2001 an attack with "anthrax letters" resulted in 22 cases including five deaths in the USA. This incident was investigated using VNTR analysis as described by Keim (22) and sequencing of *pag A* coding for the protective antigen which is one of the toxin genes of the bacterium. The obtained *B. anthracis* strains were all identical and could be identified as the Ames strain (18; 31). The Ames strain was originally isolated from cattle in Jim Hogg County, Texas, in 1981 (47). Whole genome sequencing revealed Ames specific SNPs and real-time PCR assays using TaqMan MGB probes were designed to rapidly identify the strain that was used in the bioterrorist attacks (47). This was a novel microbial forensic tool for differentiating natural outbreaks from an attack. However, in 2001 the CDC used MLVA for subtyping isolates and in a future attack other strains might be used which would require fast adaptation of this methodology. Massively parallel sequencing (MPS) technology will allow rapid whole-genome characterization (9).

6.2 Plague

Plague is caused by the gram-negative bacterium *Yersinia pestis* and is still endemic in natural foci of Asia, Africa, and America in rural areas (19). The affected population is mostly poor and is living under deplorable hygienic conditions. Due to the high lethality of plague a rapid and reliable identification of the organism is crucial, but medical services and laboratory facilities are very scarce in the endemic regions of Africa and Central Asia.
The validation of diagnostic assays for infectious diseases like plague can be demanding because of very limited access to clinical samples and isolates. None of the previously published real-time PCR assays for diagnosing plague had been clinically validated so far.
In Madagascar a relevant number of cases is reported each year and a good surveillance system based on the well equipped laboratory facility at the Institut Pasteur in the capital Antananarivo is in place. In a retrospective clinical study we evaluated real-time PCR assays by testing lymph node aspirates from 149 patients with a clinical diagnosis of bubonic plague. In this study results of real-time PCR assays targeting the virulence plasmids pPCP1 (*pla*), and pMT1 (*caf1* and *Ymt*) were compared with an F1-antigen immunochromatographic test (ICT) and cultivation of the organism. Out of the 149 samples infection with *Y. pestis* was confirmed by culture in 47 patients while ICT was positive in 88 patients including all culture proven cases. The most efficient real-time PCR assay was the 5´-nuclease assay targeting *pla* being positive in 120 cases. It can therefore be recommended as diagnostic tool for establishing a presumptive diagnosis when bubonic plague is clinically suspected (32).
Assays for targets on the chromosome and on the second *Y. pestis* specific plasmid were included because strains lacking one of the specific plasmids occur naturally and can also be highly pathogenic (13; 51).
The evolution and phylogenetic analysis of *Y. pestis* has been studied with MLVA and Clustered Regularly Interspaced Short Palindromic Repeats (CRISPR) (8; 24). These genotyping tools can also be used to trace a particular isolate and to determine its geographic origin. VNTRs will facilitate to distinguish between infections caused by attacks and naturally occurring plague infections. Isolates from human cases can be linked now effectively with isolates from environmental sources (25). A genetic match with environmental isolates was found in four out of nine human cases.

Whole-genome characterization of *Y. pestis* strains revealed dozens of SNPs per strain that differ relative to a reference genome and can be used for forensic microbiological investigations in the future (9).

6.3 Glanders and melioidosis

Burkholderia (B.) mallei is a gram-negative bacterium causing glanders and farcy in horses, donkeys, and mules (solipeds) and has been classified by the CDC as a priority category B biological agent.

Glanders in horses presents with pneumonia, purulent nasal discharge, and poor general condition, whereas farcy is a chronic cutaneous disease with massively enlarged lymph vessels ("farcy-pipes") and nodules developing into ulcers. Equines are the only known reservoir for sporadic infections in humans. Humans develop a clinical picture resembling melioidosis which is caused by the closely related bacterium *B. pseudomallei*.

In 2004, an outbreak of glanders in horses was reported to the Office International des Epizooties by the United Arab Emirates. In addition to cultivation and phenotypical identification a new real-time PCR assay was developed for the specific identification of *B. mallei*, which detected the bacteria in tissues of two horses (42).

B. pseudomallei is the etiologic agent of melioidosis, a tropical disease that is highly endemic in Southeast Asia and Northern Australia. *B. pseudomallei* is a facultative intracellular, opportunistic pathogen that can be acquired by inhalation or by contact of skin lesions with contaminated soil or water. The clinical presentation of melioidosis is variable including subclinical infection, cutaneous lesions, fulminate septicaemia and rapidly progressing pneumonia. Identification of the pathogen and specific antimicrobial therapy are critical, because *B. pseudomallei* is resistant to ampicillin and broad- and expanded-spectrum cephalosporines due to the production of a beta-lactamase.

Real-time PCR assays have been developed as rapid identification tools, but several assays were evaluated with strain collections and spiked samples only (30; 40; 41; 43). In fatal septicaemia the amount of bacterial DNA that can be extracted from blood is high enough to be detectable using real-time PCR (38), but a study in Thailand has shown that this diagnostic tool may be of little clinical value when compared with conventional diagnostic approaches (5). MLST analyses have shown that strains from Thailand and Australia can be discriminated and that some sequence types found in environmental samples are underrepresented among clinical isolates thus indicating that they may be less pathogenic for humans (12; 48). However, VNTR typing did not reproduce this geographic discrimination, but proved to have a higher resolving power that can be used to analyse outbreaks for microbial forensic purposes (11; 45).

6.4 Tularemia

Francisella (F.) tularensis is a biological agent of category A and the causative agent of tularemia. The subspecies *F. tularensis* subsp. *holarctica* can be found in many regions of the northern hemisphere, but the subspecies *F. tularensis* subsp. *tularensis* occurs only in North America. Surprisingly, isolates of *F. tularensis* subsp. *tularensis* were recovered repeatedly from fleas and mites captured in the region of the Danube river basin, close to Bratislava in Slovakia (17). This was extremely unusual and warranted further investigations. Multiple-locus variable-number tandem repeat analysis has been developed to elucidate the worldwide genetic relationships among *F. tularensis* isolates and to distinguish natural outbreaks from intentional (terrorist) dissemination (20). The two Slovakian isolates clustered with the highly pathogenic laboratory strain Schu4. The isolate FSC198 was finally sequenced completely and found to be almost identical to the laboratory strain Schu4 (6). A comparison of mutation patterns of an isolate propagated from Schu4 *in vitro* (FSC043) and FSC198 indicated that FSC198 diverged from its progenitor Schu4 and has subsequently passed life-cycles in a natural environment (36). This is a remarkable example for a microbial forensic investigation that also demonstrates how much effort is needed to elucidate the potential origin of an isolate and under which conditions it may have propagated.

In the above mentioned study it was not possible to clarify the phylogeographic expansion of *F. tularensis* completely (20). This can be explained by the low genetic diversity of *F. tularensis* subsp. *holarctica* and the limited number of *Francisella* strains available from certain geographic regions. Local inconsistencies in the genetic relationship were found and attributed to homoplasy effects. Recently, the phylogeography of *F. tularensis* was further investigated using SNP analysis and insertion/deletion events (INDELS) (39; 49). This is a promising straight forward approach that can be used to analyze the relationship of closely related strains. Outbreaks on a local scale can be investigated and the work load of sequencing of relevant gene loci is acceptable and affordable.

7. Animal pathogens and agroterrorism

"Agroterrorism is the deliberate tampering with and/or contamination of the food supply with the intent of adversely affecting the social, economic, physical and psychological well-being of society" (23). Agroterrorism carries less risk for the terrorist, could be carried out more covertly, and does not require sophisticated methodology for weaponization (53). Important vulnerabilities are intensive production practices, increased susceptibility of immunologically naïve animal populations, and rapid and fast movement of animals and their products over long distances (7). Attacks can result in disastrous economic losses due to eradication measures (mass culling), international trade embargos, loss of jobs, increased consumer costs, and may even cause difficulties in sustaining the food supply (26).

8. Quality assurance

Quality assurance is required to verify whether practices and test results are providing reliable and relevant information and quality control can verify whether test conditions are functioning appropriately to yield reproducible results. The Scientific Working Group on Microbial Genetics and Forensics has developed *Quality Assurance Guidelines for Laboratories Performing Microbial Forensic Work* to provide a framework for laboratories that carry out microbial forensic analysis (3).

9. Reporting and surveillance systems

The Global Early Warning and Response System for Major Animal Diseases, including Zoonoses (GLEWS) is the combined effort of WHO, FAO, and OIE. For zoonotic events, alerts of animal outbreaks can provide direct early warning so that human surveillance could be enhanced and preventive action taken.

10. Limitations

Crops, rangeland and forests can also be targets of biological attacks. However, the field of plant pathogen forensics is beyond the scope of this chapter. The interested reader can be referred to a comprehensive review written by Fletcher et al. (14).
Profiling of forensic soil samples by determining the bacterial content may provide valuable information, but depends on several factors such as heterogeneity within a habitat, distance of collection sites, and time (15; 28).

11. Conclusion

Microbial forensics is a young scientific discipline and probably only few scientists and institutions are aware of the methodological and quality assurance requirements. Epidemiological tools can be used to trace strains and to clarify the chain of infection, but typing systems have to be especially evaluated for forensic purposes. Classical microbiological techniques are indispensable, but most recent developments including very rapid whole genome sequencing complement the polyphasic approach needed for diagnostics and typing. Only large collections of strains from all over the world and high quality sequence data will provide the basis for meaningful results in microbial forensic investigations. International and interdisciplinary cooperation will improve our capabilities to rapidly identify the agents, elucidate the source, and provide these results as evidence in court.

12. Acknowledgment

The authors thank Lisa Sprague, Helmut Hotzel and Sascha Rommeiss for reading the manuscript and valuable discussions.

13. References

[1] Banaschak, S., M. Werwein, B. Brinkmann, and I. Hauber. 2000. Human immunodeficiency virus type 1 infection after sexual abuse: value of nucleic acid sequence analysis in identifying the offender. Clin Infect Dis 31 :1098-100.
[2] Budowle, B., S. E. Schutzer, J. P. Burans, D. J. Beecher, T. A. Cebula, R. Chakraborty, W. T. Cobb, J. Fletcher, M. L. Hale, R. B. Harris, M. A. Heitkamp, F. P. Keller, C. Kuske, J. E. Leclerc, B. L. Marrone, T. S. McKenna, S. A. Morse, L. L. Rodriguez, N. B. Valentine, and J. Yadev. 2006. Quality sample collection, handling, and preservation for an effective microbial forensics program. Appl Environ Microbiol 72:6431-8.
[3] Budowle, B., S. E. Schutzer, A. Einseln, L. C. Kelley, A. C. Walsh, J. A. Smith, B. L. Marrone, J. Robertson, and J. Campos. 2003. Public health. Building microbial forensics as a response to bioterrorism. Science 301:1852-3.
[4] Chanteau, S., L. Rahalison, L. Ralafiarisoa, J. Foulon, M. Ratsitorahina, L. Ratsifasoamanana, E. Carniel, and F. Nato. 2003. Development and testing of a rapid diagnostic test for bubonic and pneumonic plague. Lancet 361:211-6.

[5] Chantratita, N., V. Wuthiekanun, D. Limmathurotsakul, A. Thanwisai, W. Chantratita, N. P. Day, and S. J. Peacock. 2007. Prospective clinical evaluation of the accuracy of 16S rRNA real-time PCR assay for the diagnosis of melioidosis. Am J Trop Med Hyg 77:814-7.

[6] Chaudhuri, R. R., C. P. Ren, L. Desmond, G. A. Vincent, N. J. Silman, J. K. Brehm, M. J. Elmore, M. J. Hudson, M. Forsman, K. E. Isherwood, D. Gurycova, N. P. Minton, R. W. Titball, M. J. Pallen, and R. Vipond. 2007. Genome sequencing shows that European isolates of *Francisella tularensis* subspecies *tularensis* are almost identical to US laboratory strain Schu S4. PLoS One 2:e352.

[7] Crutchley, T. M., J. B. Rodgers, H. P. Whiteside Jr, M. Vanier, and T. E. Terndrup. 2007. Agroterrorism: where are we in the ongoing war on terrorism? J Food Prot 70:791-804.

[8] Cui, Y., Y. Li, O. Gorge, M. E. Platonov, Y. Yan, Z. Guo, C. Pourcel, S. V. Dentovskaya, S. V. Balakhonov, X. Wang, Y. Song, A. P. Anisimov, G. Vergnaud, and R. Yang. 2008. Insight into microevolution of *Yersinia pestis* by clustered regularly interspaced short palindromic repeats. PLoS One 3:e2652.

[9] Cummings, C. A., C. A. Bormann Chung, R. Fang, M. Barker, P. Brzoska, P. C. Williamson, J. Beaudry, M. Matthews, J. Schupp, D. M. Wagner, D. Birdsell, A. J. Vogler, M. R. Furtado, P. Keim, and B. Budowle. 2010. Accurate, rapid and high-throughput detection of strain-specific polymorphisms in *Bacillus anthracis* and *Yersinia pestis* by next-generation sequencing. Investig Genet 1:5.

[10] Cummings, C. A. and D. A. Relman. 2002. Genomics and microbiology. Microbial forensics--"cross-examining pathogens". Science 296:1976-9.

[11] Currie, B. J., A. Haslem, T. Pearson, H. Hornstra, B. Leadem, M. Mayo, D. Gal, L. Ward, D. Godoy, B. G. Spratt, and P. Keim. 2009. Identification of melioidosis outbreak by multilocus variable number tandem repeat analysis. Emerg Infect Dis 15:169-74.

[12] Currie, B. J., A. D. Thomas, D. Godoy, D. A. Dance, A. C. Cheng, L. Ward, M. Mayo, T. L. Pitt, and B. G. Spratt. 2007. Australian and Thai isolates of *Burkholderia pseudomallei* are distinct by multilocus sequence typing: revision of a case of mistaken identity. J Clin Microbiol 45:3828-9.

[13] Filippov, A. A., N. S. Solodovnikov, L. M. Kookleva, and O. A. Protsenko. 1990. Plasmid content in *Yersinia pestis* strains of different origin. FEMS Microbiol Lett 55:45-8.

[14] Fletcher, J., C. Bender, B. Budowle, W. T. Cobb, S. E. Gold, C. A. Ishimaru, D. Luster, U. Melcher, R. Murch, H. Scherm, R. C. Seem, J. L. Sherwood, B. W. Sobral, and S. A. Tolin. 2006. Plant pathogen forensics: capabilities, needs, and recommendations. Microbiol Mol Biol Rev 70:450-71.

[15] Foran, D. R. and J. E. Starrs. 2004. In search of the Boston Strangler: genetic evidence from the exhumation of Mary Sullivan. Med Sci Law 44:47-54.

[16] Gonzalez-Candelas, F., M. A. Bracho, and A. Moya. 2003. Molecular epidemiology and forensic genetics: application to a hepatitis C virus transmission event at a hemodialysis unit. J Infect Dis 187:352-8.

[17] Gurycova, D. 1998. First isolation of *Francisella tularensis* subsp. *tularensis* in Europe. Eur J Epidemiol 14:797-802.
[18] Hoffmaster, A. R., C. C. Fitzgerald, E. Ribot, L. W. Mayer, and T. Popovic. 2002. Molecular subtyping of *Bacillus anthracis* and the 2001 bioterrorism-associated anthrax outbreak, United States. Emerg Infect Dis 8:1111-6.
[19] Inglesby, T. V., D. T. Dennis, D. A. Henderson, J. G. Bartlett, M. S. Ascher, E. Eitzen, A. D. Fine, A. M. Friedlander, J. Hauer, J. F. Koerner, M. Layton, J. McDade, M. T. Osterholm, T. O'Toole, G. Parker, T. M. Perl, P. K. Russell, M. Schoch-Spana, and K. Tonat. 2000. Plague as a biological weapon: medical and public health management. Working Group on Civilian Biodefense. JAMA 283:2281-90.
[20] Johansson, A., J. Farlow, P. Larsson, M. Dukerich, E. Chambers, M. Bystrom, J. Fox, M. Chu, M. Forsman, A. Sjostedt, and P. Keim. 2004. Worldwide genetic relationships among *Francisella tularensis* isolates determined by multiple-locus variable-number tandem repeat analysis. J Bacteriol 186:5808-18.
[21] Jones, S. W., M. E. Dobson, S. C. Francesconi, R. Schoske, and R. Crawford. 2005. DNA assays for detection, identification, and individualization of select agent microorganisms. Croat Med J 46:522-9.
[22] Keim, P., L. B. Price, A. M. Klevytska, K. L. Smith, J. M. Schupp, R. Okinaka, P. J. Jackson, and M. E. Hugh-Jones. 2000. Multiple-locus variable-number tandem repeat analysis reveals genetic relationships within *Bacillus anthracis*. J Bacteriol 182:2928-36.
[23] Levin, J., K. Gilmore, T. Nalbone, and S. Shepherd. 2005. Agroterrorism workshop: engaging community preparedness. J Agromedicine 10:7-15.
[24] Li, Y., Y. Cui, Y. Hauck, M. E. Platonov, E. Dai, Y. Song, Z. Guo, C. Pourcel, S. V. Dentovskaya, A. P. Anisimov, R. Yang, and G. Vergnaud. 2009. Genotyping and phylogenetic analysis of *Yersinia pestis* by MLVA: insights into the worldwide expansion of Central Asia plague foci. PLoS One 4:e6000.
[25] Lowell, J. L., D. M. Wagner, B. Atshabar, M. F. Antolin, A. J. Vogler, P. Keim, M. C. Chu, and K. L. Gage. 2005. Identifying sources of human exposure to plague. J Clin Microbiol 43:650-6.
[26] McEwen, S. A., T. M. Wilson, D. A. Ashford, E. D. Heegaard, and B. Kournikakis. 2006. Microbial forensics for natural and intentional incidents of infectious disease involving animals. Rev Sci Tech 25:329-39.
[27] McEwen, S. A., T. M. Wilson, D. A. Ashford, E. D. Heegaard, and B. Kournikakis. 2006. Microbial forensics for natural and intentional incidents of infectious disease involving animals. Rev Sci Tech 25:329-39.
[28] Meyers, M. S. and D. R. Foran. 2008. Spatial and temporal influences on bacterial profiling of forensic soil samples. J Forensic Sci 53:652-60.
[29] Mizanbayeva, S., H. L. Smits, K. Zhalilova, T. H. Abdoel, S. Kozakov, K. S. Ospanov, P. H. Elzer, and J. T. Douglas. 2009. The evaluation of a user-friendly lateral flow assay for the serodiagnosis of human brucellosis in Kazakhstan. Diagn Microbiol Infect Dis 65:14-20.
[30] Novak, R. T., M. B. Glass, J. E. Gee, D. Gal, M. J. Mayo, B. J. Currie, and P. P. Wilkins. 2006. Development and evaluation of a real-time PCR assay targeting

the type III secretion system of *Burkholderia pseudomallei*. J Clin Microbiol 44:85-90.

[31] Popovic, T. and M. Glass. 2003. Laboratory aspects of bioterrorism-related anthrax--from identification to molecular subtyping to microbial forensics. Croat Med J 44:336-41.

[32] Riehm, J. M., L. Rahalison, H. C. Scholz, B. Thoma, M. Pfeffer, L. M. Razanakoto, S. Al Dahouk, H. Neubauer, and H. Tomaso. 2010. Detection of *Yersinia pestis* using real-time PCR in patients with suspected bubonic plague. Mol Cell Probes .

[33] Rotz, L. D., A. S. Khan, S. R. Lillibridge, S. M. Ostroff, and J. M. Hughes. 2002. Public health assessment of potential biological terrorism agents. Emerg Infect Dis 8:225-30.

[34] Schutzer, S. E., B. Budowle, and R. M. Atlas. 2005. Biocrimes, microbial forensics, and the physician. PLoS Med 2:e337.

[35] Sinclair, R., S. A. Boone, D. Greenberg, P. Keim, and C. P. Gerba. 2008. Persistence of category A select agents in the environment. Appl Environ Microbiol 74:555-63.

[36] Sjodin, A., K. Svensson, M. Lindgren, M. Forsman, and P. Larsson. 2010. Whole-genome sequencing reveals distinct mutational patterns in closely related laboratory and naturally propagated *Francisella tularensis* strains. PLoS One 5:e11556.

[37] Splettstoesser, W., V. Guglielmo-Viret, E. Seibold, and P. Thullier. 2010. Evaluation of an immunochromatographic test for rapid and reliable serodiagnosis of human tularemia and detection of *Francisella tularensis*-specific antibodies in sera from different mammalian species. J Clin Microbiol 48:1629-34.

[38] Supaprom, C., D. Wang, C. Leelayuwat, W. Thaewpia, W. Susaengrat, V. Koh, E. E. Ooi, G. Lertmemongkolchai, and Y. Liu. 2007. Development of real-time PCR assays and evaluation of their potential use for rapid detection of *Burkholderia pseudomallei* in clinical blood specimens. J Clin Microbiol 45:2894-901.

[39] Svensson, K., M. Granberg, L. Karlsson, V. Neubauerova, M. Forsman, and A. Johansson. 2009. A real-time PCR array for hierarchical identification of *Francisella* isolates. PLoS One 4:e8360.

[40] Thibault, F. M., E. Valade, and D. R. Vidal. 2004. Identification and discrimination of *Burkholderia pseudomallei*, *B. mallei*, and *B. thailandensis* by real-time PCR targeting type III secretion system genes. J Clin Microbiol 42:5871-4.

[41] Tomaso, H., T. L. Pitt, O. Landt, S. Al Dahouk, H. C. Scholz, E. C. Reisinger, L. D. Sprague, I. Rathmann, and H. Neubauer. 2005. Rapid presumptive identification of *Burkholderia pseudomallei* with real-time PCR assays using fluorescent hybridization probes. Mol Cell Probes 19:9-20.

[42] Tomaso, H., H. C. Scholz, S. Al Dahouk, M. Eickhoff, T. M. Treu, R. Wernery, U. Wernery, and H. Neubauer. 2006. Development of a 5'-nuclease real-time PCR assay targeting fliP for the rapid identification of *Burkholderia mallei* in clinical samples. Clin Chem 52:307-10.

[43] Tomaso, H., H. C. Scholz, S. Al Dahouk, T. L. Pitt, T. M. Treu, and H. Neubauer. 2004. Development of 5' nuclease real-time PCR assays for the rapid identification of the *Burkholderia mallei/ Burkholderia pseudomallei* complex. Diagn Mol Pathol 13:247-53.

[44] Tomaso, H., P. Thullier, E. Seibold, V. Guglielmo, A. Buckendahl, L. Rahalison, H. Neubauer, H. C. Scholz, and W. D. Splettstoesser. 2007. Comparison of hand-held test kits, immunofluorescence microscopy, enzyme-linked immunosorbent assay, and flow cytometric analysis for rapid presumptive identification of *Yersinia pestis*. J Clin Microbiol 45:3404-7.

[45] U'Ren, J. M., J. M. Schupp, T. Pearson, H. Hornstra, C. L. Friedman, K. L. Smith, R. R. Daugherty, S. D. Rhoton, B. Leadem, S. Georgia, M. Cardon, L. Y. Huynh, D. DeShazer, S. P. Harvey, R. Robison, D. Gal, M. J. Mayo, D. Wagner, B. J. Currie, and P. Keim. 2007. Tandem repeat regions within the *Burkholderia pseudomallei* genome and their application for high resolution genotyping. BMC Microbiol 7:23.

[46] van Belkum, A., P. T. Tassios, L. Dijkshoorn, S. Haeggman, B. Cookson, N. K. Fry, V. Fussing, J. Green, E. Feil, P. Gerner-Smidt, S. Brisse, and M. Struelens. 2007. Guidelines for the validation and application of typing methods for use in bacterial epidemiology. Clin Microbiol Infect 13 Suppl 3:1-46.

[47] Van Ert, M. N., W. R. Easterday, T. S. Simonson, J. M. U'Ren, T. Pearson, L. J. Kenefic, J. D. Busch, L. Y. Huynh, M. Dukerich, C. B. Trim, J. Beaudry, A. Welty-Bernard, T. Read, C. M. Fraser, J. Ravel, and P. Keim. 2007. Strain-specific single-nucleotide polymorphism assays for the *Bacillus anthracis* Ames strain. J Clin Microbiol 45:47-53.

[48] Vesaratchavest, M., S. Tumapa, N. P. Day, V. Wuthiekanun, W. Chierakul, M. T. Holden, N. J. White, B. J. Currie, B. G. Spratt, E. J. Feil, and S. J. Peacock. 2006. Non-random distribution of *Burkholderia pseudomallei* clones in relation to geographical location and virulence. J Clin Microbiol 44 :2553-7.

[49] Vogler, A. J., D. Birdsell, L. B. Price, J. R. Bowers, S. M. Beckstrom-Sternberg, R. K. Auerbach, J. S. Beckstrom-Sternberg, A. Johansson, A. Clare, J. L. Buchhagen, J. M. Petersen, T. Pearson, J. Vaissaire, M. P. Dempsey, P. Foxall, D. M. Engelthaler, D. M. Wagner, and P. Keim. 2009. Phylogeography of *Francisella tularensis*: global expansion of a highly fit clone. J Bacteriol 191:2474-84.

[50] Welch, T. J., W. F. Fricke, P. F. McDermott, D. G. White, M. L. Rosso, D. A. Rasko, M. K. Mammel, M. Eppinger, M. J. Rosovitz, D. Wagner, L. Rahalison, J. E. Leclerc, J. M. Hinshaw, L. E. Lindler, T. A. Cebula, E. Carniel, and J. Ravel. 2007. Multiple antimicrobial resistance in plague: an emerging public health risk. PLoS One 2:e309.

[51] Williams, J. E., D. N. Harrison, T. J. Quan, J. L. Mullins, A. M. Barnes, and D. C. Cavanaugh. 1978. Atypical plague bacilli isolated from rodents, fleas, and man. Am J Public Health 68:262-4.

[52] Wilmoth, B. A., M. C. Chu, and T. J. Quan. 1996. Identification of *Yersinia pestis* by BBL Crystal Enteric/Nonfermenter Identification System. J Clin Microbiol 34:2829-30.

[53] Wilson, T. M., D. A. Gregg, D. J. King, D. L. Noah, L. E. Perkins, D. E. Swayne, and W. Inskeep 2nd. 2001. Agroterrorism, biological crimes, and biowarfare targeting animal agriculture. The clinical, pathologic, diagnostic, and epidemiologic features of some important animal diseases. Clin Lab Med 21:549-91.

14

Advanced Medical Imaging and Reverse Engineering Technologies in Craniometric Study

Supakit Rooppakhun[1], Nattapon Chantarapanich[2] and Kriskrai Sitthiseripratip[3]
[1]School of Mechanical Engineering, Suranaree University of Technology
[2]Institute of Biomedical Engineering, Prince of Songkla University
[3]National Metal and Materials Technology Center (MTEC)
Thailand

1. Introduction

In crime scenes and accidents, the standard operating protocols for personal identification is not difficult when the entire body is found. As a result, the investigators can directly collect the sample of the decrease such as facial photograph, DNA, fingerprint and dental record in order to compare to possible relatives or with ante-mortem profile (De Valck, 2006). However, the investigators are not always lucky. In severe accidents such aircraft crashes, only little information of the decrease is available, the skin and soft tissue may be completely burnt out and the skeleton can be broken into small pieces due to the impact. The skeleton examination in historical sites by archaeologists presents even more complication. The archaeologists need not only to identify general aspects of the skeleton, for instant age, sex, cause of death, stature and race, but also to estimate the period of death and the possibility to discover the particular person that might be significant in the history.
Several techniques have been applied to assist the identification of the decrease ranging from the simplest technique which may acquire the evidence from the personal belonging until using the advance scientific techniques. These techniques can be generally categorized into two methods, invasive and non-invasive. The invasive method includes biochemical analysis, microscopy, accelerator mass spectrometry radiocarbon dating (with standard C-14), ancient DNA analysis, histology and endoscope whereas the non-invasive technique involved the aid of engineering technologies such as radiographic analysis and computed tomography (CT) examination.
From 1975 - 2005, the archaeological researches had been increasingly conducted by means of non-invasive techniques which 112 of 245 researches have applied the non-invasive technique and the trend of investigation gradually moved from invasive to non-invasive examinations (Zweifel, et al., 2009). The first non-invasive technique has been presented to the public in 1896 which the radiographic analysis was used to examine the ibis mummy in Belgium (Van Tiggelen, 2004). Soon after that, archaeologist realized the importance of radiological technique and applied broadly to examine great numbers of mummy (Dedouit, et al., 2010; Friedrich, et al., 2010; Recheis, et al., 1999; Zweifel, et al., 2009). One main

advantage of radiography includes the ability to access general aspects of mummy without releasing the bandages which may be destroyed important features or contaminated. In the early 1900s, another non-invasive medical examination device, computed tomography scanner, has been invented by Alessandro Vallebona, but the technology has remained unpopular until the 1970s which modern era of computed tomography scanner began (Hill, 2009). Not too long, computed tomography scanner became an effective tool in examination the autopsy. The computed tomography generally relies on medical imaging processing combined with reverse engineering principles which the object is captured the profile and presented the virtual three-dimensional models in computer. With these advanced features, the perspective of archaeology and forensic medicine has changed into three-dimensional aspect. Consequently, The two-dimensional radiographic image occlusion and the problem such uncertainty from bias of investigator in direct measurements are eliminated.

Apart from the advantages of computed tomography in forensic medicine, it also becomes an effective clinical diagnosis device in many hospitals. The use of three-dimensional model allows the surgeon to examine the abnormality of organs in any configurations which the two-dimensional technique may be inaccessible. Moreover, the three-dimensional models can be used to simulate the surgical operation prior surgery (Fürnstahl, et al., 2010), subsequently reduce operating time and increase safety of patients. Alternative uses of computed tomography include morphometric study (Chantarapanich, et al., 2008; Mahaisavariya, et al., 2002) and the evaluation the risk of implant usage (Mahaisavariya, et al., 2004; Sitthiseripratip, et al., 2003)

The purpose of this chapter is to present and discuss the medical imaging and reverse engineering techniques by means of demonstrating the application in craniometric study. Obviously, recent craniometric studies have been employed by two-dimensional techniques or direct measurement (Steyn & Işcan, 1997; Deshmukh & Devershi, 2006; Dayal, et al, 2008; Sangvichien, et al., 2008; Matamala, et al, 2009) such as the use of spreading caliper, sliding vernier calliper, mandibulometer and standard flexible steel tape. The diverse mentioned measurement techniques reflect the lack of engineering aids which the current trend in forensic medicine need the advanced technologies to provide the accurate measurements. Therefore, the scope of demonstration includes the brief detail of reverse engineering as to provide for who may not familiar with, data acquisition technique using computed tomography scanner, measurement of skull anatomical parameters and sex determination method based on logistic function. By this way of demonstration, the overview of forensic medicine by aid of advance medical imaging and reverse engineering is obtained.

2. Reverse engineering

Reverse engineering has been widely applied several years in clinical fields and forensic medicine (Aamodt, et al., 1999; Aghayev, et al., 2008; Fürnstahl, et al., 2010). Initially, reverse engineering was first used in free-form product designs which the conventional "Forward Engineering" has limited drawing functions and time consumption. Product design based on "Forward Engineering", the process involves turning the conceptual product design to physical product whereas reverse engineering is inversed (Zhou & Xi, 2002).

The process of reverse engineering involves turning the physical product back to the virtual models (normally three-dimension) (Li, et al., 2002; Várady, et al., 1997). From the three-dimensional virtual models, the conceptual design can be obtained. Reverse engineering can be described as two phases which are digitization and reconstruction phase, as summarized in Fig. 1. The digitization phase involves the data acquisition of the physical model using various types of scanner. The initial geometry from the scanner is then obtained in three forms, point clouds, polygon model and series of image depending on the acquisition technique of each scanner. In the reconstruction phase, the obtained data is processed in order to reconstruct the three-dimensional model. with "At this step, the elimination of noise data and filtering of unnecessary data may also be performed. For the production phases, it may be added as a final step in reverse engineering. This phase employs various manufacturing processes to fabricate the three-dimensional virtual model. However, this phase may not be mandatory, because sometime the geometry is only stored in database without any further processing.

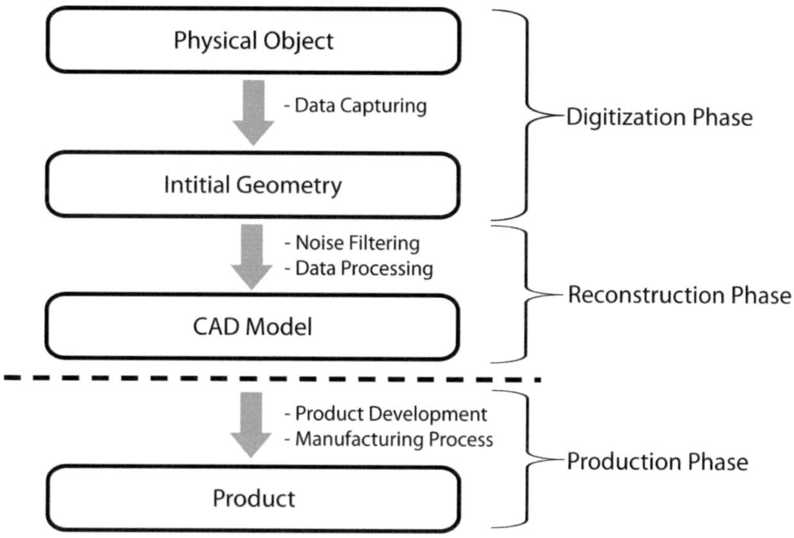

Fig. 1. Diagram of reverse engineering process.

The digitization methods can be categorized into two approaches which are tactile approach (contact method) and non-contact approach (Li, et al., 2002; Várady, et al., 1997). For tactile approach, the device contacts to the physical object directly whereas the non-contact approach uses the medium in digitization instead without contact of device.

The characteristic of tactile approach is relatively simple. Touch probe is used in conjunction with robotic mechanism such as coordinate measurement machine (CMM), articulated arm or computer numerical control (CNC) devices to determine the position of the object (Cartesian coordinate). The accuracy is considered to be a main advantage of tactile approach, nevertheless the digitization process is quite slow and difficult to digitize complex geometry. A wide range of object can be applied with this approach regardless of color, shininess and transparency, this approach is not appropriate for deformable materials.

In non-contact approach, the medium is used to measure the physical object using the principle of reflection or penetration. Laser beam and white light are medium sources commonly found in many three-dimensional scanners and they rely on the principle of reflection. The medium travels from the generator to the object before reflects and transmits to the receiver unit. The determination of geometry can be processed using at least one two-

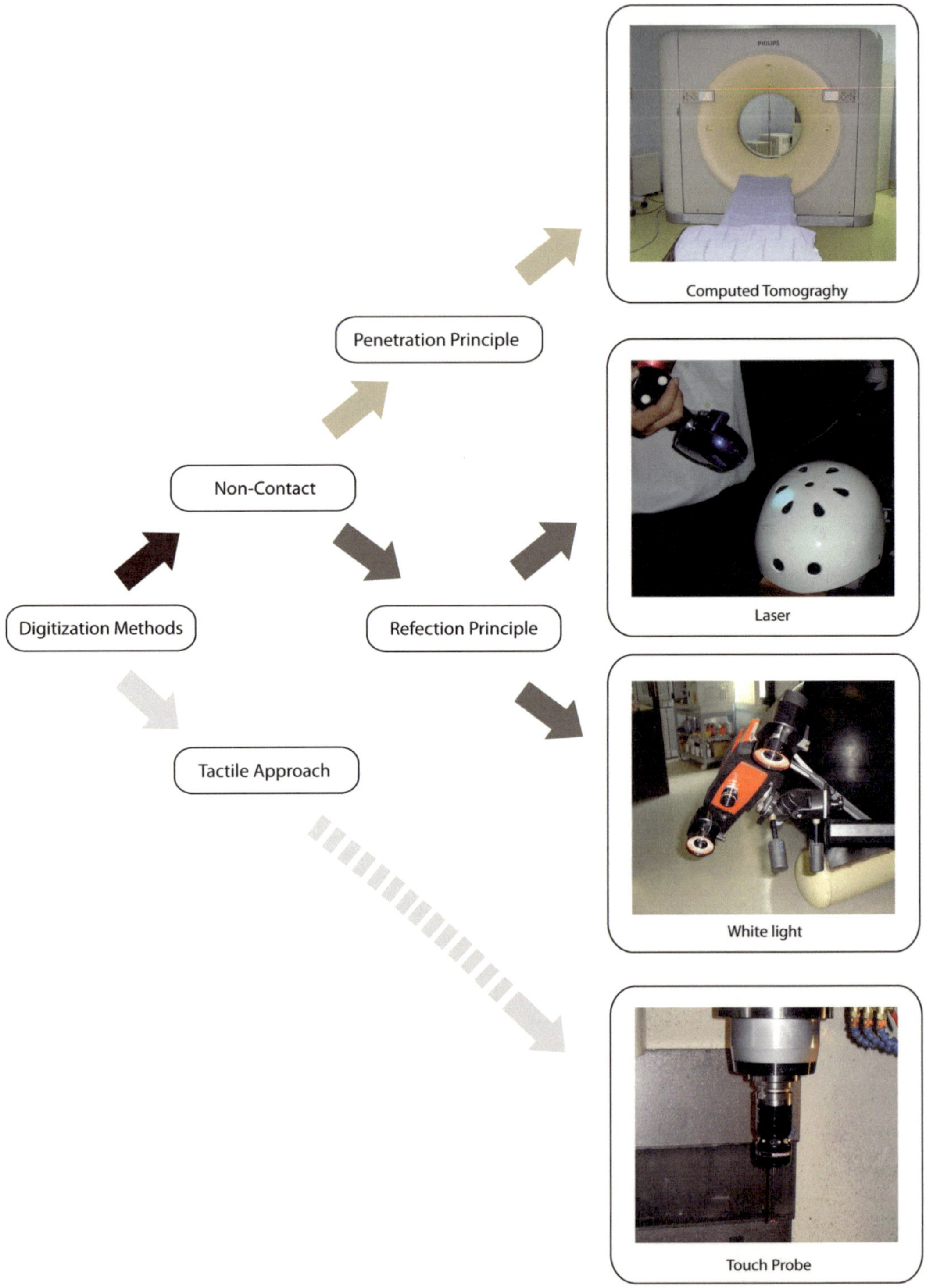

Fig. 2. Digitization Methods.

dimensional images combined with some optical parameters such as reflection angle, distance and time of flight. The initial geometry is presented in form of cloud point or of polygon model. Use of laser beam and white light has advantage in fast digitization and continuous data, but too shiny and transparent object present complication.

Even the laser beam and white light systems are applied in many forensic studies (Park, et al., 2006; Thali, et al., 2003; Vanezis, et al., 2000), but probably, the most efficient system for forensic studies is the use of non-contact device based on principle of penetration. This system uses the medium that can go though the object to capture both internal and external geometries. The most popular device is computed tomography scanner which involves the use of X-ray.

The digitization process initializes the transmission of the X-ray through the object. A set of data acquisitions is performed with the constant interval throughout entire object which subsequently give a series of slice image (Hounsfield, 1980). Each slice contains the information of object's position and the value of Hounsfield unit (HU). The density of object is proportional to the Hounsfield value. The higher Hounsfield value indicates high-density object such as enameled and cortical bone whereas the lower Hounsfield value indicates low-density object such as cancellous bone, fat and soft tissue. Various Hounsfield values of various substances are given in Table 1. In order to reconstruct the three-dimensional model, the optimal Hounsfield values must be selected (threshold). After that the threshold regions of each slice are combined to construct the volumetric model.

For the computed tomography device, the speed of digitization and ability to examine the internal topology are considered to be superior, but the artifact (noise data) caused by metallic structure is drawback.

Substances	**Hounsfield values**
Air	-1000
Fat	-70 to -90
Water	0
Tissue	+20 to +35
Blood Volume	Approx. +40
Bone	+900

Table 1. Hounsfield values of various substances. (Hounsfield, 1980)

3. Data acquisition of skull

Specimen of 104 dry cadaveric skulls donated by the Department of Anatomy, Faculty of Medicine, Khon Kaen University, Thailand is used to demonstrate the application of advanced medical imaging and reverse engineering technologies in craniometric study. The cadaver includes 63 males with average age of 55.16 years (standard deviation 18.38 years) and 41 females with average age of 49.00 years (standard deviation 17.94 years). The age rages from 17–81 years at the time of death. The skulls are placed in acrylic box with a set of four. The reverse engineering technique by means of spiral computed tomography scanner (Siemens AG, Germany) is used to capture the profile of each skull as shown in Fig. 3. The data acquisition protocol is axial scan with tube voltage of 120 kV and tube current of 100 mA. The digitization is performed with 1.5-mm slice thickness and the reconstruction is done at 1-mm thickness. Each slice contains the volumetric data that represent the density and position (contour) of the skull. The computed tomography images are then processed with medical image processing software (Mimics, Materialise NV, Belgium). To begin the reconstruction of three-dimensional model, a proper Hounsfield value (normally +900 for bone structure) is selected. After that, the threshold regions are used to calculate the complete topology of three-dimensional skull. The reconstruction process of skull model is illustrated in Fig. 4.

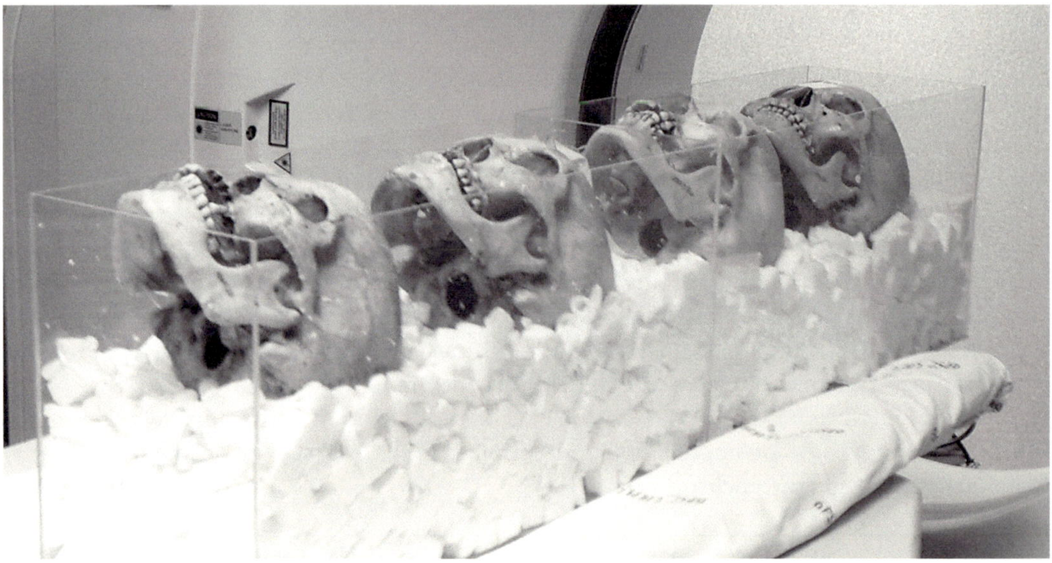

Fig. 3. A set of skull during data acquisition using computed tomography scanner.

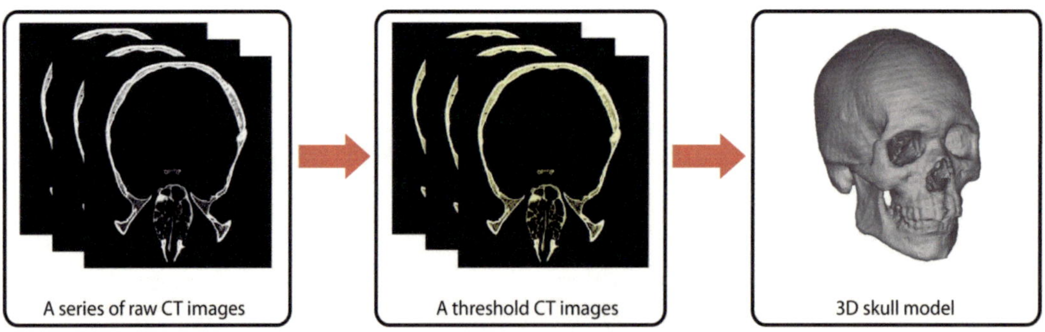

Fig. 4. Three-dimensional model reconstruction.

4. Three-dimensional computerized craniometric study

The anatomical landmarks in craniometric study are categorized in to median and bilateral landmarks (Rooppakhun, et al., 2010). The median landmarks are approximately located on sagittal plane. Each of them has only one location. There are 13 median landmarks which the specific definitions can be described as follows:

- *Glabella (GL)* - the most anterior point of frontal bone between supraorbital in the sagittal plane.
- *Bregma (BR)* - the crossing of the coronal and sagittal sutures on the top of the skull.
- *Opisthocranium (OPC)* - the most posterior point in midline of inion bone which length of the skull is maximum when measure from Galbella point.
- *Nasion (NA)* - the intersection point of the internasal and frontonasal sutures in the sagittal plane.
- *Opistion (OPS)* - the most posterior midsagittal point on the posterior margin of the foramen magnum.
- *Basion (BA)* - the most anterior point of the great foramen magnum in the sagittal plane.
- *Orale (OR)* - the midpoint on the intersection of posterior alveolar sockets rim of the cavities of two upper central incisors.
- *Prosthion (PR)* - the lowest, most anterior point on the alveolar portion of the premaxilla, in the median plane, between the upper central incisors.
- *Staphylion (STA)* - point in the medial line (interpalatal suture) of the posterior part of the hard palate where it is crossed by a line drawn tangent to the curves of the posterior margins of the palate.
- *Nasospinale (NAS)* - the lowest point of lower anterior nasal aperture in mid-sagittal plane.
- *Gnathion (GN)* - The midpoint on the lower border of the mandible in the sagittal plane.
- *Pogonion (PG)* - The most projecting point of the chin in the standard sagittal plane.
- *Infradentale (ID)* - The anterior superior point on the mandible at its labial contact between mandibular central incisors.

For the bilateral landmarks, each of them is located on both sides of skull. There are 17 bilateral landmarks which the specific definitions can be described as follows:

- *Euryon (EU)* - the lateral point on either side of the greatest transverse diameter of the skull.
- *Staphanion (ST)* - the intersection of the superior temporal line and the coronal suture.
- *Frontotemporale (FT)* - the most anterior point on either side of temporal crest of the minimum transverse breadth of frontal bone.
- *Bolton (BO)* - The superior point of the curvature between occipital condyle and posterior margin of foramen magnum.
- *Orbitale (ORB)* - the most inferior point of each infraorbital rim .
- *Ectoconchion (EC)* - the most lateral point on each orbital's margin where a line running parallel to upper orbital border cut the lateral orbital margin.
- *Maxillo-frontale (MF)* - the intersection point on anterior lacrimal crest and fronto-maxillary sutures.
- *Supraorbitale (SOR)* - the most superior point of each superior orbital rim.
- *Zygonion (ZG)* - The most lateral point on the outline of each zygomatic arch.
- *Zygomaxillare (ZM)* - The most interior point on each zygomatico-maxillary sutures.
- *Nasal (NS)* - The most lateral point on each nasal's margin where maximum nasal breadth.
- *Endomolare (ENM)* - the most medial point of internal curvature surface of alveolar ridge corresponding to second molar tooth.
- *Coronion (CO)* - The most superior point on each coroniod process.

- *Condylion superior (CS)* - the most superior point on each mandibular condyle.
- *Conlylion laterale (CDL)* - the most lateral point on each mandibular condyle.
- *Gonion (GO)* - the point at each mandibular angle that is defined by dropping a perpendicular from the intersection point of the tangent lines to the posterior margin of the mandibular vertical ramus and inferior margin of the mandibular body or horizontal ramus.
- *Laterla infradentale (LID)* - the midpoint of a line tangent to the outer margins of the cavities of the lateral incisor of each lower canine teeth.

In order to better understand the previous described definitions, every landmark is also illustrated in Fig. 5.

Each of the three-dimensional models of skull is used to determine the anatomical landmark according to previous description. Only one investigator locate the entire landmarks in every skull to avoid uncertainty of intra-observer. The anatomical landmarks are then used to obtain 40 craniometric parameters as shown in Table 2. The measurements are interpreted using statistical analysis and reported in form of average values and standard deviation regarding to gender. In order to distinguish craniometric parameters of each gender, an unpaired t-test is utilized for analysis. A p-value < 0.05 is a significant level that used to determine the difference. In addition, the linear regression and the correlation coefficient are also used for the pair-wise tests.

As also shown in Table 2, the craniometric parameters of male are larger than female. Thirty-one of forty parameters show the statistical significant differences among both genders, especially, Maximum cranial breadth, Facial length, Orbital height-left, Orbital height-right, Palatal breadth, Bicoronion breadth, Bizygometic breadth, Maxillary breadth, Upper facial height, Orbital breadth-left, Orbital breadth-Right, Nasal height, Bicondylar breath, Bi-gonion breadth, Coronion height-left, Coronion height-right, Mandibular body length-left, Mandibular body length-right, Maximum mandibular length-left and Maximum mandibular length-right which present the p-value $<< 0.001$. For Maximum cranial breadth, Facial length, Orbital height-left, Orbital height-right, Palatal breadth, Bicoronion breadth are considered to be relatively different as the p-value < 0.01. The parameters such Ramus height-left, Ramus height-right, Symphysic height shows some degrees of significance. In addition, nine parameters do not present the statistical differences which are Maximum frontal breadth, Anterior inter-orbital breadth, Nasal breadth, Palatal length, Mandibular angle-left, Mandibular angle-right, Notch length-left, Notch length-right, and Symphysic breadth.

From the pair-wise tests, the correlations of craniometric parameters are different among male and female population. Table 3 and Table 4 show the sample of correlations of craniometric parameters which correlation coefficient (r) are above 0.500. In both populations, the bilateral anatomy presents some degrees of correlation which can be signified the facial symmetry. The linear regression equations are considered to be useful to predict the craniometric parameters in forensic medicine. For example, the defected skull usually miss some landmarks, the use of known craniometric parameters can be used to determine the missing parameters. However, it should be noticed that the obtained missing parameters may not be always precise. The possibility of being can only be determined, but the accuracy strongly depends on the correlation coefficient. The regression scatters plot and 95% interval bands of some pair-wise tests are plotted in Fig. 6 and Fig. 7.

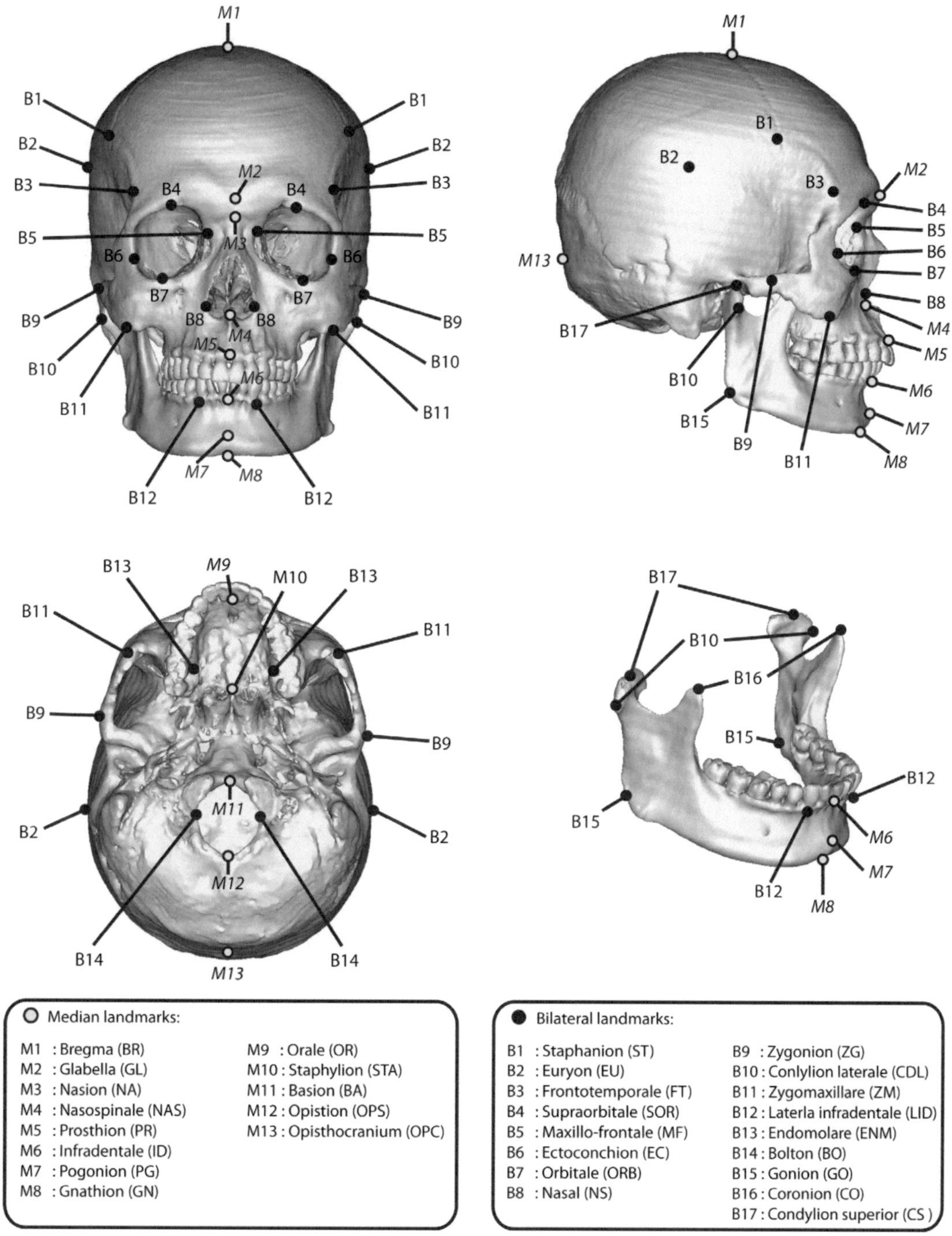

Fig. 5. The anatomical landmarks of skull.

Craniometric Parameter	Landmark	Average (S.D.)		p-value
		Male	Female	
Maximum cranial length	GL-OPC	173.6 (5.2)	165.4 (6.4)	<< 0.001
Maximum cranial breadth	EU_L-EU_R	144.9 (5.6)	141.2 (5.5)	0.001361
Maximum frontal breadth	ST_L -ST_R	115.8 (6.7)	113.3 (6.7)	0.070663
Minimum frontal breadth	FT_L-FT_R	94.9 (5.1)	91.4 (4.9)	0.000584
Basion-brema height	BA-BR	138.6 (4.8)	132.4 (5.2)	<< 0.001
Nasion-basion length	NA-BA	101.8 (4.0)	96.0 (3.4)	<< 0.001
Foramen magnum length	BA-OPC	36.7 (2.1)	34.5 (2.4)	0.000006
Foramen magnum breadth	BO_L-BO_R	30.5 (2.1)	28.9 (1.8)	0.000051
Nasion-bregma length	NA-BR	112.9 (4.2)	107.3 (6.0)	0.000002
Facial length	BA-PR	96.1 (5.4)	92.9 (5.5)	0.004704
Bi-orbital breadth	EC_L-EC_R	97.4 (3.8)	94.0 (3.8)	0.000024
Bi-zygometic breadth	ZG_L-ZG_R	133.7 (5.1)	127.7 (5.2)	<< 0.001
Maxillary breadth	ZM_L-ZM_R	104.5 (5.3)	99.1 (4.9)	0.000001
Upper facial height	NA-PR	70.3 (4.2)	66.2 (4.6)	0.000019
Orbital breadth-left	EC_L-MF_L	41.2 (2.2)	39.6 (2.4)	0.000743
Orbital breadth-right	EC_R-MF_R	41.5 (2.0)	39.8 (2.0)	0.000044
Orbital height-left	ORB_L-SOR_L	36.2 (2.3)	34.7 (2.5)	0.002714
Orbital height-right	ORB_R-SOR_R	36.3 (2.5)	34.9 (2.1)	0.004341
Anterior inter-orbital breadth	MF_L-MF_R	21.0 (2.2)	20.7 (2.4)	0.497642
Nasal breadth	NS_L-NS_R	27.0 (2.2)	26.8 (2.2)	0.632101
Nasal height	NA-NAS	52.7 (3.0)	49.6 (3.1)	0.000003
Palatal length	OR-STA	42.6 (4.2)	42.6 (4.4)	0.952028
Palatal breadth	ENM_L-ENM_R	39.1 (3.1)	37.6 (2.4)	0.006430
Bi-coronion breadth	CO_L-CO_R	98.6 (5.2)	94.3 (5.8)	0.002652
Bi-condylar breadth	CDL_L-CDL_R	123.1 (5.2)	118.7 (5.1)	0.000870
Bi-gonion breadth	GO_L-GO_R	99.1 (6.3)	92.8 (6.2)	0.000113
Coronion height-left	CO_L-GO_L	62.3 (4.9)	57.2 (4.8)	0.000065
Coronion height-right	CO_R-GO_R	62.83 (5.2)	57.5 (4.8)	0.000043
Mandibular angle-left*	CS_L-GO_L-GN	112.4 (5.1)	113.9 (6.4)	0.298443
Mandibular angle-right*	CS_R-GO_R-GN	112.4 (5.5)	112.8 (5.6)	0.759332
Mandibular body length-left	GO_L-PG	92.0 (4.8)	87.0 (4.9)	0.000083
Mandibular body length-right	GO_R-PG	92.5 (4.9)	87.6 (5.0)	0.000128
Maximum mandibular length-left	CS_L-PG	119.8 (6.1)	114.6 (5.1)	0.000383
Maximum mandibular length-right	CS_R-PG	120.6 (6.1)	115.0 (5.0)	0.000079
Notch length-left	CO_L-CS_L	35.3 (2.7)	34.1 (4.2)	0.202213
Notch length-right	CO_R-CS_R	35.1 (2.7)	33.7 (4.0)	0.105663
Ramus height-left	CS_L-GO_L	58.2 (5.0)	55.2 (4.5)	0.010815
Ramus height-right	CS_R-GO_R	58.3 (4.6)	55.3 (4.7)	0.010342
Symphysic breadth	LID_L-LID_R	23.1 (6.0)	23.7 (6.0)	0.689146
Symphysic height	GN-ID	31.6 (3.5)	26.5 (3.1)	0.011128

Table 2. Average values of craniometric parameters regarding to gender derived from 104 skulls (63-males and 41-females), (Unit: millimeter, *degree).

Craniometric Parameter (x vs. y)	Regression (Correlation, r)
Maximum mandibular length-left vs. -right	y = 0.916x + 10.470 (0.920)
Mandibular angle-left vs. -right	y = 0.976x + 2.630 (0.904)
Mandibular body length-left vs. -right	y = 0.883x + 11.227 (0.860)
Coronion height-left vs. -right	y = 0.908x + 6.233 (0.858)
Orbital height-left vs. -right	y = 0.875x + 4.561 (0.835)
Orbital breadth-left vs. -right	y = 0.741x + 10.969 (0.835)
Ramus height-left vs. -right	y = 0.724x + 16.146 (0.835)
Notch length-left vs. -right	y = 0.761x + 8.239 (0.770)
Bi-orbital breadth vs. Orbital breadth-left	y = 0.400x + 2.283 (0.685)
Bi-zygometic breadth vs. Bi-orbital breadth	y = 0.473x + 34.210 (0.643)
Upper facial height vs. Symphysic height	y = 0.485x – 2.733 (0.636)
Maximun cranial breadth vs. Bi-zygometic breadth	y = 0.109x + 17.063 (0.626)
Basion-brema heigth vs. Nasion-bregma length	y = 0.516x + 41.339 (0.594)
Nasal height vs. Upper facial height	y = 0.840x + 25.980 (0.592)
Palatal length vs. Facial length	y = 0.734x + 64.806 (0.570)
Nasion-basion length vs. Bi-coronion breadth	y = 0.730x + 24.429 (0.533)
Bi-condylar breadth vs. Bi-zygometic breadth	y = 0.528x + 67.980 (0.570)

Table 3. The correlation of craniometric parameters of Thai male population.

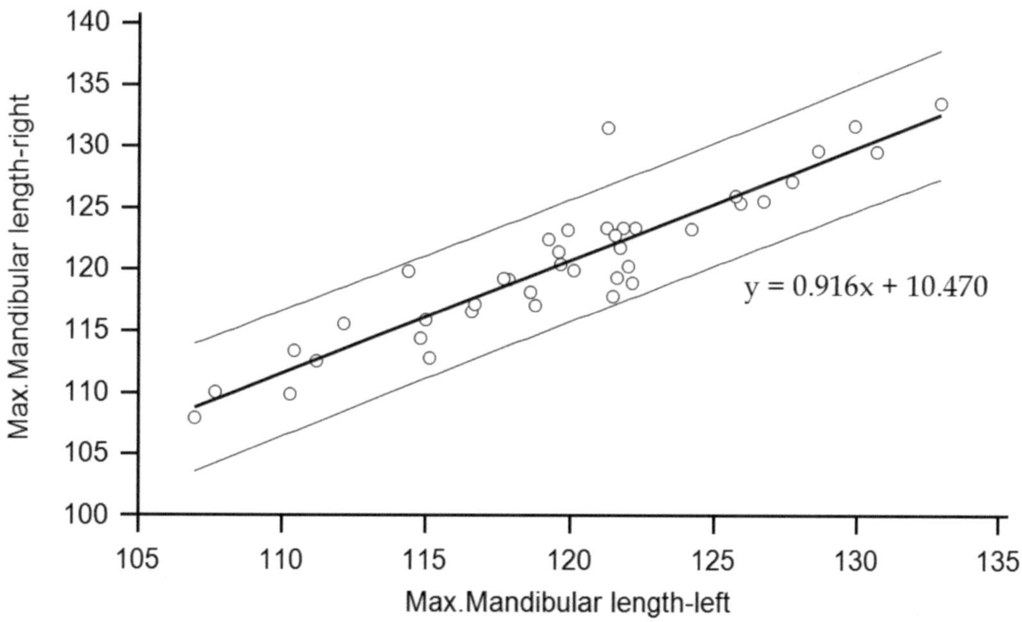

Fig. 6. The linear regression scatters plot and 95% interval bands of Maximum mandibular length-left (x) vs. Maximum mandibular length –right (y) (Unit: Millimeter).

Craniometric Parameter (x vs. y)	Regression (Correlation, r)
Mandibular body length-left vs. -right	y = 0.930x + 6.626 (0.922)
Maximun mandibular length-left vs. -right	y = 0.883x + 13.821 (0.904)
Coronion height-left vs. -right	y = 0.889x + 6.599 (0.895)
Notch length-left vs. -right	y = 0.831x + 5.335 (0.880)
Ramus height-left vs. -right	y = 0.912x + 4.958 (0.871)
Orbital breadth-left vs. -right	y = 0.693x + 12.370 (0.849)
Orbital height-left vs. -right	y = 0.728x + 9.680 (0.839)
Mandibular angle-left vs. -right	y = 0.737x + 28.837 (0.832)
Upper facial height vs. Nasal height	y = 0.522x + 15.065 (0.765)
Bi-orbital breadth vs. Orbital breadth-left	y = 0.478x - 5.357 (0.759)
Minimun frontal breadth vs. Maximum frontal breadth	y = 0.997x + 22.127 (0.723)
Maximun cranial breadth vs. Bi-zygometic breadth	y = 0.624x + 39.615 (0.662)
Symphysic height vs. Upper facial height	y = 0.784x + 42.987 (0.641)
Facial length vs. Palatal length	y = 0.507x - 4.481 (0.637)
Maxillary breadth vs. Bi-orbital breadth	y = 0.474x + 46.949 (0.609)
Anterior interorbital breadth vs. Bi-coronion breadth	y = 1.638x + 60.166 (0.590)
Maximum cranial length vs. Nasion-basion length	y = 0.314x + 43.994 (0.584)

Table 4. The correlation of craniometric parameters of Thai female population.

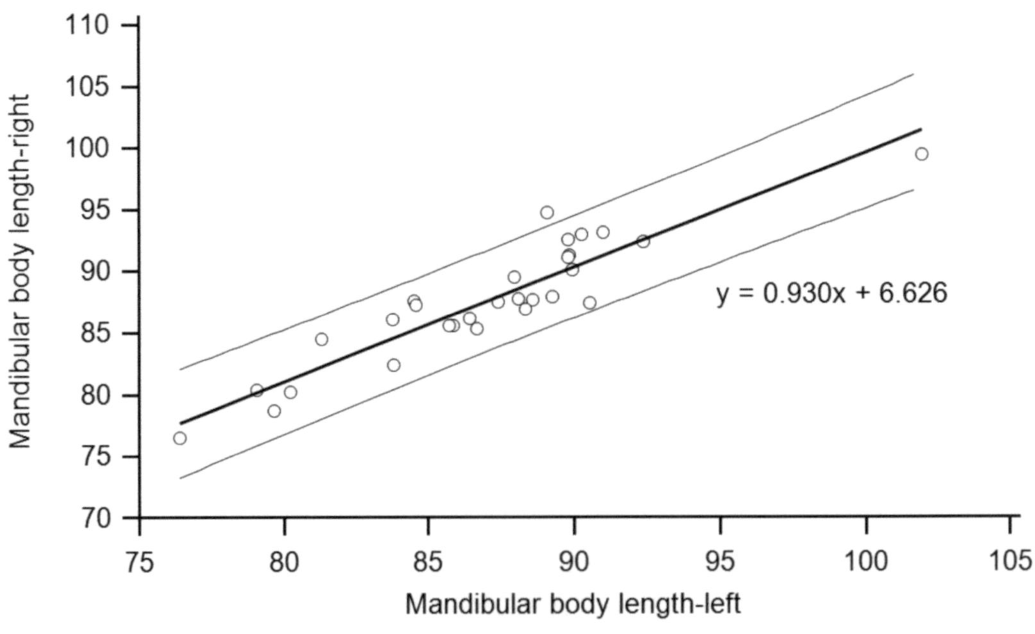

Fig. 7. The linear regression scatters plot and 95% interval bands of Mandibular body length -left (x) vs. Mandibular body length -right (y) (Unit: Millimeter).

5. Sex determination using logistic regression analysis

The determination of sex from skeleton is one of the critical components in forensic medicine as well as archaeology. The determination can be interpreted based on the average data from craniometric parameters of certain population. The accuracy of sex determination depends on several factors which one of them is osteological elements. Various osteological elements have been used to predict sex of skeleton which includes femur (Yaşar Işcan & Shihai, 1995), tibia (Steyn & Işcan, 1997), pelvis (Durić, et al., 2005), skull (King, et al., 1998) , humerus (Işcan, et al., 1998; Robinson & Bidmos, 2009), hyoid (Mukhopadhyay, 2010), talus (Murphy, 2002a) and calcaneus (Murphy, 2002b). However, among aforementioned elements, the best for prediction is pelvis, follow by skull and long bone (Durić, et al., 2005, Işcan, 2005). Rather than osteological element, population variation and method of data processing (data acquisition and statistical analysis) are also among important factors.

Logistic regression analysis is a method to analysis multi-variate analysis which aims to predict the probability of occurrence of an event under consideration by fitting the raw data using to a logit function logistic curve. The advantage of logistic regression is less of parameter restrictions than discriminant analysis and regression analysis. The output from the logistic regression analysis can only be "Yes" or "No" which normally designated as "0" and "1", respectively.

Basically, logistic regression function (Z) is written in form of

$$Z = \beta_0 + \beta_1 x_1 + \beta_2 x_2 + \beta_3 x_3 + \beta_4 x_4 + \ldots + \beta_n x_n + \beta_{n+1} x_{n+1} \quad (1)$$

where β_0 is called intercept and β_1, β_2, β_3 ,β_4, ...,β_n and β_{n+1} are regression coefficients of x_1, x_2, x_3, x_4, ...,x_n and x_{n+1} variable, respectively. From the following logistic model of Z, the probability of event (P.E.) under consideration can be calculate through

$$P.E. = e^Z / (1 + e^Z) \quad (2)$$

In equation (2) e is a natural logarithm, its value is approximately 2.71828.

The probability of event varies from "0" to "1". The near "1" value means the independent variables influences the probability of event whereas the value close to "0" means the independent variables have little effect to probability of event.

In this study, a binary logistic regression using forward stepwise is applied to determine sex based on average data of craniometric parameters in previous section. The fitting process excludes the measurement with high co-linearity. The probability from logistic regression function, "0" indicates male whereas "1" indicates female, respectively. All statistical analysis is preformed using statistic commercial software (SPSS, SPSSTM Inc, United States of America).

There are three logistic regression models used in sex prediction. *Model A* uses only cranial parameters whereas *Model B* uses only mandibular parameters. *Model C* uses combination of cranial and mandibular parameters. From the analysis, the coefficient (β), standard error of means and significant value are reported as shown in Table 5 to Table 7.

For *Model A*, there are four significant predictors ($p < 0.05$) in mandible parameters which are Nasion-basion length, Palatal length, Upper facial height and Maxillary breadth. The function is as follows:

Craniometric Parameter	Coefficient (β)	Standard error of mean (S.E.)	Significant level
Intercept	76.340	15.9577	0.00000
Nasion-basion length	-0.387	0.0984	0.00008
Palatal length	0.362	0.1238	0.00349
Upper facial height	-0.497	0.1608	0.00199
Maxillary breadth	-0.197	0.0708	0.00530

Table 5. Logistic response model using logistic regression analysis of *Model A*.

Craniometric Parameter	Coefficient (β)	Standard error of mean (S.E.)	Significant level
Intercept	70.589	18.7774	0.00017
Bi-gonion breadth	-0.184	0.0631	0.00347
Coronion height-left	-0.310	0.1042	0.00289
Mandibular angle-right	-0.208	0.0812	0.01033
Mandibular body length-right	-0.125	0.0888	0.15810

Table 6. Logistic response model using logistic regression analysis of *Model B*.

Craniometric Parameter	Coefficient (β)	Standard error of mean (S.E.)	Significant level
Intercept	88.202	24.4335	0.00031
Coronion height-left	-0.276	0.1242	0.02614
Nasion-basion length	-0.596	0.1741	0.00062
Palatal length	0.581	0.2032	0.00422
Upper facial height	-0.567	0.2186	0.00956

Table 7. Logistic response model using logistic regression analysis of *Model C*.

$$Z = 76.340 - 0.387(NA\text{-}BA) + 0.362(OR\text{-}STA) - 0.497(NA\text{-}PR) - 0.197(ZM_L\text{-}ZM_R) \quad (3)$$

where

NA-BA = Nasion-basion length (unit: millimeter)

OR-STA = Palatal length (unit: millimeter)

NA-PR = Upper facial height (unit: millimeter)

ZM_L-ZM_R = Maxillary breadth (unit: millimeter)

For *Model B*, there are four significant predictors ($p < 0.05$) in mandibular parameters which are Bigonion breadth, Coronion height-left, Mandibular angle-right and Mandibular body length-right. The function is as follows:

$$Z = 70.589 - 0.184(GO_L\text{-}GO_R) - 0.310(CO_L\text{-}GO_L) - 0.208(CS_R\text{-}GO_R\text{-}GN) - 0.125(GO_R\text{-}PG) \quad (4)$$

where

GO_L-GO_R = Bi-gonion breadth (unit: millimeter)

CO_L-GO_L = Coronion height-left (unit: millimeter)

CS_R-GO_R-GN = Mandibular angle-right (unit: degree)

GO_R-PG = Mandibular body length-right (unit: millimeter)

For *Model C*, there are four significant predictors in cranial and mandibular parameters ($p < 0.05$) which are Coronion height-left, Nasion-basion length, Palatal length, and Upper facial height. The function is as follows:

$$Z = 88.202 - 0.276(CO_L\text{-}GO_L) - 0.596(NA\text{-}BA) + 0.581(OR\text{-}STA) - 0.567(NA\text{-}PR) \quad (5)$$

where
CO_L-GO_L = Coronion height-left (unit: millimeter)
NA-BA = Nasion-basion length (unit: millimeter)
OR-STA = Palatal length (unit: millimeter)
NA-PR = Upper facial height (unit: millimeter)
The set of skulls are tested according to logistic regression models (*Model A, Model B and Model C*) to evaluate the accuracy as reported in Table 8.

Model	Male	Female	Overall
Model A	92.1	90.2	91.3
Model B	85.0	86.2	85.5
Model C	95.0	93.1	94.2

Table 8. Accuracy of each logistic model (percentage).

The logistic regression analysis revealed that 4 of 21 cranial parameters and 4 of 11 mandibular parameters are significant predictors ($p < 0.05$). The Basion-nasion length and Bigonion breadth are the most dimorphic of the cranial and mandibular measurement, respectively. For the best prediction model, *Model C* which includes both cranial and mandibular parameters is recommended.
In order to predict the gender by the parameters in *Model C*, the probability of being female can be calculated using equation (2) whereas the probability of being male is then inversed (1-P).
The accuracies from *Model C* of the present study are compared to previous studies on sexual dimorphism using the skull of some previous studies based on South African white, South African black, Indian and Thai population. Table 9 shows a comparison of measurement techniques and average accuracies obtained from the present study and previous studies which derived from many populations.
To the best of author's knowledge, there is only one study (Sangvichien, et al., 2007) that determine the sex of skull based on logistic function using on four parameters which as Nasion-basion length, Maximum breadth of the cranium, Facial height, and Bi-zygometic breadth. This presented the accuracy 88.8% for overall sex classification and 82.9% and 92.1% among females and males, respectively.
From the table, it reveals that the present study yields higher accuracies than the many previous studies. Therefore, the *Model C* presents in this study can be used to determine the gender of skeleton for intact skull in forensics and archaeology. However, in order to ensure the effectiveness of logistic regression, three skulls with known gender from Thammasat University Hospital, Thammasat University, Thailand are used to test the concept. The skull No.1 and skull No. 3 are adult males whereas the skull No. 2 is adult female.

Based on logistic regression Model C which is consider to be the best model for sex prediction in Thais' skull , Coronion height-left, nasion-basion length, palatal length, upper facial height are measured and predicted the gender. As shown in Table 10, all cases are predicted the gender correctly (3/3). Hence, the determination of sex based on the Model C of logistic regression is considered to be accurate.

Population	Measurement Technique	Statistical Analysis Method	Average Accuracies
South African White (Steyn & Işcan, 1997) • 44 males • 47 females	Direct measurement	Discriminant function	80% - 86%
South African black (Franklin, et al, 2005) • 182 males • 150 females	3D tactile digitizer	Discriminant function	75% - 80%
Indian (Deshmukh & Devershi, 2006) • 40 males • 34 females	Direct measurement	Discriminant function	85% - 90%
Thai (Sangvichien, et al., 2007) • 66 males • 35 males	Direct measurement	Logistic function	83% - 92%
South African black (Dayal, et al, 2008) • 60 males • 60 males	Direct measurement	Discriminant function	80% - 85%
Combination (Matamala, et al, 2009) • 149 males • 77 males	Direct measurement	Discriminant function	82%
Thai (Present study) • 63 males • 41 males	Three-dimensional CAD Model	Logistic function	93% - 95%

Table 9. Comparison on methods of data assessment and statistical analysis among different studies.

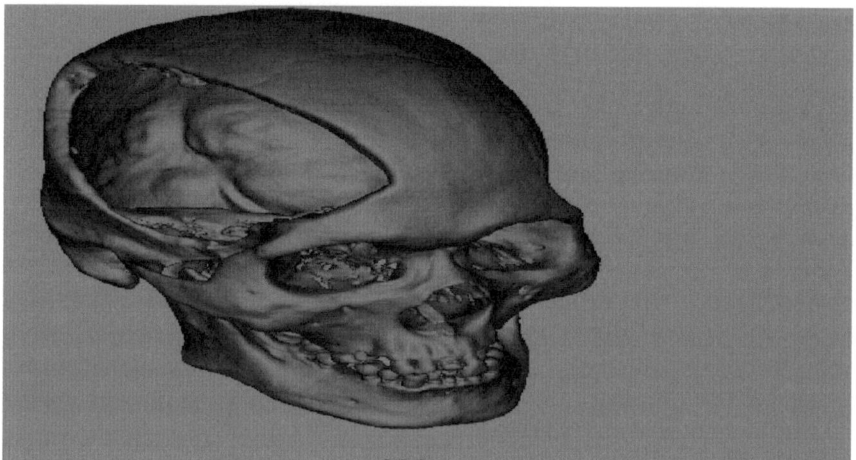

Fig. 8. The reconstruction of skull fragment (A) intact (B) intact with reconstruction unit.

Craniometric Parameter	**Skull No.1**	**Skull No.2**	**Skull No.3**
Intercept	88.202	88.202	88.202
Coronion height-left	69.63	53.12	72.09
Nasion-basion length	105.07	95.24	101.06
Palatal length	58.50	45.82	55.17
Upper facial height	76.91	72.26	71.81
Regression Analysis (Z)	-3.26	2.43	-0.59
Probability of event (P.E.)	0.037	0.919	0.357
Prediction Gender	male	female	male
Exact Gender	male	female	male
Result	correct	correct	correct

Table 10. Craniometric measurement and sex prediction.

6. Outlook

Since there is possibility to find skull as fragment bone in forensics and archaeology, then the assessment of necessary craniometric parameters becomes complex. Although the missing craniometric parameters can be predicted using correlation as shown in Table 3 and Table 4, but some correlation coefficients among these craniometric parameters are mostly inferior. With low correlation coefficient, the equation may not be an appropriate solution to determine those missing craniometric parameters.

As a result, a purposed alternative is to reconstruct defected skull surface based on the mirror surface topology of normal side with aids of Computer Aided Design technique as shown in Fig. 8. In fact, this technique is a standard protocol for implant design in cranial reconstruction (Müller, et al., 2003). The purposed alternative relies on the discovery that the symmetric between left and right of bilateral craniometric parameters as presented in Table 2. However, this concept should be further investigated to ensure the usability.

7. Conclusion

This study presents advantages of using advance medical imaging and reverse engineering through computed tomography scanner to reconstruct the three-dimensional model of skulls. This is very useful to analyze and measure craniometric parameters based on virtual model. Generally, in forensic medicine and archaeological researches, the study relies on direct measurement and other two-dimensional techniques which may not be accurate. The measurement errors can be influenced by human error, instrumental error, image magnification and image occlusion. The advantage of three-dimensional computed tomography technique includes the analysis of specimen without destruction or damage of specimens as well as the ability to analyze the specimens in configuration which the conventional technique cannot provide. Comparing to the other reverse engineering technologies, computed tomography presents the superior ability in accessing the internal geometry which the other tools find the difficulty in data capturing.

In the craniometric analysis, the medians and bilateral landmarks are accessed. From the analysis, the result reveals that Thai male presents the craniometric parameters greater than Thai female, especially, Maximum cranial breadth, Facial length, Orbital height-left, Orbital height-right, Palatal breadth, Bicoronion breadth, Bizygometic breadth, Maxillary breadth, Upper facial height, Orbital breadth-left, Orbital breadth-Right, Nasal height, Bicondylar breath, Bi-gonion breadth, Coronion height-left, Coronion height-right, Mandibular body length-left, Mandibular body length-right, Maximum mandibular length-left and Maximum mandibular length-right. In both populations, the bilateral anatomy presents some degrees of correlation which may be concluded the facial symmetry.

Logistic regression is used to derive functions for sex determination based on average numerical values which obtained from craniometric parameters. Three models are purposed, *Model A* is based on cranial parameters, *Model B* is based on mandible parameters and *Model C* is based on both cranial and mandibular parameters. From the result, *Model C* provides the best accuracy among other models which is 94.2%. The prediction equation relies on four parameters which are Coronion height-left, Nasion-basion length, Palatal length, and Upper facial height which subsequently produce logistic regression as in equation (5).

As seen in Table 9, our study yields higher accuracies than other previous studies. This is due to two main factors, the accurate landmark identification by the three-dimensional technique and developing logistic regression function from difference sample.

In addition, the authors suggest that the techniques described in this chapter which includes data acquisition, three-dimensional computerized craniometric study and sex determination based on logistic regression function can effectively be applied to the other osteological elements in specific race.

8. Acknowledgment

The research is supported the funding and facilities in part by the National Metal and Material Technology Center (MTEC), National Science and Technology Development Agency (NSTDA) of Thailand and Suranaree University of Technology, Thailand. In addition, the authors are grateful to Department of Anatomy, Faculty of Medicine, Khon Kaen University, Thailand for providing cadaveric skull specimens.

9. References

Aamodt, A., Kvistad, K. A., Andersen, E., Lund-Larsen, J., Eine, J., Benum, P. & Husby, O. S. (1999). Determination of the Hounsfield value for CT-based design of custom femoral stems. *J Bone Joint Surg [Br]*, Vol. 81(1), pp. 143-147

Aghayev, E., Staub, L., Dirnhofer, R., Ambrose, T., Jackowski, C., Yen, K., Bolliger, S., Christe, A., Roeder, C., Aebi, M. & Thali, M. J. (2008). Virtopsy - The concept of a centralized database in forensic medicine for analysis and comparison of radiological and autopsy data. *J Forensic Leg Med*, Vol. 15(3), pp. 135-140

Chantarapanich, N., Sitthiseripratip, K., Mahaisavariya, B., Wongcumchang, M. & Siribodhi, P. (2008). 3D geometrical assessment of femoral curvature: A reverse engineering technique. *J Med Assoc Thai*, Vol.91(9), pp. 1377-1381

Dayal, M. R., Spocter, M. A. & Bidmos, M. A. (2008). An assessment of sex using the skull of black South Africans by discriminant function analysis. *HOMO*, Vol.59(3), pp.209-221

De Valck, E. (2006). Major incident response: Collecting ante-mortem data. *Forensic Sci Int*, Vol. 159(1), pp. S15-S19

Dedouit, F., Géraut, A., Baranov, V., Ludes, B., Rougé, D., Telmon, N. & Crubézy, E. (2010). Virtual and macroscopical studies of mummies-Differences or complementarity? Report of a natural frozen Siberian mummy. *Forensic Sci Int*, Vol. 200(1-3), pp.e7-e13

Deshmukh, A. & Devershi, D. (2006). Comparison of Cranial Sex Determination by Univariate and Multivariate Analysis. *J Anat Soc*, Vol. 55(2), pp. 48-51

Durić, M., Rakočević, Z. & Donić, D. (2005). The reliability of sex determination of skeletons from forensic context in the Balkans. *Forensic Sci Int*, Vol. 147 (2-3 SPEC.ISS.), pp. 159-164

Franklin, D., Freedman, L. & Milne, N. (2005). Sexual dimorphism and discriminant function sexing in indigenous South African crania. *HOMO*, Vol. 55(3), pp. 213-228

Friedrich, K. M., Nemec, S., Czerny, C., Fischer, H., Plischke, S., Gahleitner, A., Viola, T. B., Imhof, H., Seidler, H. & Guillen, S. (2010). The story of 12 Chachapoyan mummies through multidetector computed tomography. *Eur J Radiol*, Vol. 76(2), pp. 143-150

Fürnstahl, P., Székely, G., Gerber, C., Hodler, J., Snedeker, J. G. & Harders, M. (2010). Computer assisted reconstruction of complex proximal humerus fractures for preoperative planning. *Med Image Anal*, doi:10.1016/j.media.2010.07.012

Hill, C. R. (2009). Early days of scanning: Pioneers and sleepwalkers. *Radiography*, Vol. 15(SUPPL.1), pp. e15-e22

Hounsfield, G. N. (1980). Computed medical imaging. *Science*, Vol. 210(4465), pp. 22-28

Işcan, M. Y. (2005). Forensic anthropology of sex and body size. *Forensic Sci Int*, Vol. 147 (2-3 SPEC.ISS.), pp. 107-112

Işcan, M. Y., Loth, S. R., King, C. A., Shihai, D. & Yoshino, M. (1998). Sexual dimorphism in the humerus: A comparative analysis of Chinese, Japanese and Thais. *Forensic Sci Int*, Vol. 98(1-2), pp. 17-29

King, C. A., Işcan, M. Y. & Loth, S. R. (1998). Metric and comparative analysis of sexual dimorphism in the Thai femur. *J Forensic Sci*, Vol. 43(5), pp. 954-958

Li, L., Schemenauer, N., Peng, X., Zeng, Y. & Gu, P. (2002). A reverse engineering system for rapid manufacturing of complex objects. *Robot CIM-Int Manuf*, Vol. 18(1), pp. 53-67

Mahaisavariya, B., Sitthiseripratip, K., Oris, P., Chaichanasiri, E. & Suwanprateeb, J. (2004). Fit-and-fill analysis of trochanteric gamma nail for the Thai proximal femur: A virtual simulation study. *J Med Assoc Thai*, Vol. 87(11), pp. 1315-1320

Mahaisavariya, B., Sitthiseripratip, K., Tongdee, T., Bohez, E. L. J., Vander Sloten, J. & Oris, P. (2002). Morphological study of the proximal femur: A new method of geometrical assessment using 3-dimensional reverse engineering. *Med Eng Phys*, Vol. 24(9), pp. 617-622

Matamala, D. A. Z., Galdames, I. C. S. & Smith, R. L. (2009). Sexual dimorphism determination from the lineal dimensions of skulls. *Int. J Morphol*, 27(1), 133-137

Mukhopadhyay, P. P. (2010). Morphometric features and sexual dimorphism of adult hyoid bone: A population specific study with forensic implications. *J Forensic Leg Med*, Vol. 17(6), pp. 321-324

Müller, A., Krishnan, K. G., Uhl, E. & Mast, G. (2003). The application of rapid prototyping techniques in cranial reconstruction and preoperative planning in neurosurgery. *The Journal of craniofacial surgery*, Vol. 14(6), pp. 899-914

Murphy, A. M. C. (2002b). The talus: Sex assessment of prehistoric New Zealand Polynesian skeletal remains. *Forensic Sci Int*, Vol. 128(3), pp. 155-158

Murphy, A. M. C. (2002a). The calcaneus: Sex assessment of prehistoric New Zealand Polynesian skeletal remains. *Forensic Sci Int*, Vol. 129(3), pp. 205-208

Park, H. K., Chung, J. W. & Kho, H. S. (2006). Use of hand-held laser scanning in the assessment of craniometry. *Forensic Sci Int*, Vol. 160(2-3), pp. 200-206

Recheis, W., Weber, G. W., Schäfer, K., Knapp, R., Seidler, H. & Zur Nedden, D. (1999). Virtual reality and anthropology. *Eur J Radiol*, Vol. 31(2), pp. 88-96

Robinson, M. S. & Bidmos, M. A. (2009). The skull and humerus in the determination of sex: Reliability of discriminant function equations. *Forensic Sci Int*, Vol. 186(1-3), pp. 86.e1-86.e5

Rooppakhun, S., Piyasin, S., Vatanapatimakul, N., Kaewprom, Y. & Sitthiseripratip, K. (2010). Craniometric study of Thai skull based on three-dimensional computed tomography (CT) data. *J Med Assoc Thai*, Vol. 93(1), pp. 90-98

Sangvichien, S., Boonkaew, K., Chuncharunee, A., Komoltri, C., Piyawinitwong, S., Wongsawut, A. & Namwongsa, S. (2007). Sex Determination in Thai Skulls by Using Craniometry: Multiple Logistic Regression Analysis. *Siriraj Med J*, Vol. 59(5), pp. 216-221

Sangvichien, S., Boonkaew, K., Chuncharunee, A., Komoltri, C., Udom, C. & Chandee, T. (2008). Accuracy of Cranial and Mandible Morphological Traits for Sex Determination in Thais. *Siriraj Med J*, Vol. 60(5), pp. 240-243

Sitthiseripratip, K., Van Oosterwyck, H., Vander Sloten, J., Mahaisavariya, B., Bohez, E. L. J., Suwanprateeb, J., Van Audekercke, R. & Oris, P. (2003). Finite element study of trochanteric gamma nail for trochanteric fracture. *Med Eng Phys*, Vol. 25(2), pp. 99-106

Steyn, M. & Işcan, M. Y. (1997). Sex determination from the femur and tibia in South African whites. *Forensic Sci Int*, Vol. 90(1-2), pp. 111-119

Thali, M. J., Braun, M. & Dirnhofer, R. (2003). Optical 3D surface digitizing in forensic medicine: 3D documentation of skin and bone injuries. *Forensic Sci Int*, Vol.137(2-3), pp. 203-208

Van Tiggelen, R. 2004. Ancient Egypt and radiology, a future for the past! *Nucl Instrum Meth B*, Vol. 226(1-2), pp. 10-14

Vanezis, P., Vanezis, M., McCombe, G. & Niblett, T. (2000). Facial reconstruction using 3-D computer graphics. *Forensic Sci Int*, Vol. 108(2), pp. 81-95

Várady, T., Martin, R. R. & Cox, J. (1997). Reverse engineering of geometric models - An introduction. *CAD*, Vol. 29(4), pp. 255-268

Yaşar Işcan, M. & Shihai, D. (1995). Sexual dimorphism in the Chinese femur. *Forensic Sci Int*, Vol. 74(1-2), pp. 79-87

Zhou, X. & Xi, F. (2002). Automated laser scanning system for reverse engineering and inspection. *Int J Mach Tool Manu*, Vol. 42(8), pp. 889-897

Zweifel, L., Büni, T. & Rühli, F. J. (2009). Evidence-based palaeopathology: Meta-analysis of PubMed-listed scientific studies on ancient Egyptian mummies. *HOMO*, Vol. 60(5), pp. 405-427

15

House Dust Mites, Other Domestic Mites and Forensic Medicine

Solarz Krzysztof
Medical University of Silesia in Katowice
Poland

1. Introduction

Many species of mites are the sources of potent allergens that sensitize and induce IgE-mediated allergic reactions in humans. Most of the mite allergens are proteins, and the allergic response mechanism to these allergens is the same as it is for allergens from other sources such as plant pollens, molds and foods (Arlian, 2002). Mites occurring in house dust, besides the ticks (Acari: Ixodida), are one of the most medically important group of mites. In total at least 150 species of mites have been found in dwellings, including plant parasites, animal parasites, predatory mites, oribatid mites and storage mites. But the most abundant mites in house dust are members of the family Pyroglyphidae (Astigmatina) (Wharton, 1976; Arlian, 2001; Arlian et al., 2002; Solarz, 2010). The three mite species, most often and most abundant found in house dust throughout the world, are *Dermatophagoides pteronyssinus*, *D. farinae* and *Euroglyphus maynei* (Arlian, 2001; Colloff, 2009; Pope et al., 1993). The house dust mites now constitute the most dangerous pests of temperate climate countries, causing both significant loss of human life and immense waste of resources. These mites are the major sources of indoor inhalant allergens facilitating both the sensitization of atopic subjects and asthmatic attacks in patients (Pope et al., 1993; Arlian, 2002; Colloff, 2009). For the first time, Voorhorst et al. reported that house dust contained mites of the genus *Dermatophagoides* and suggested that these were the source of the house dust allergen (Voorhorst et al., 1969). Therefore they are studied recently as causing atopic diseases in humans, known in medicine as house-dust-mite allergy or house-dust-mite atopy (Wharton, 1976; Van Bronswijk, 1981; Platts-Mills et al., 1992; Pope, 1993; Arlian, 2001; Colloff, 2009). These diseases are atopic asthma, atopic dermatitis (eczema) and allergic rhinitis, keratoconjunctivitis or oculorhinitis (Arlian & Platts-Mills, 2001; Arlian et al., 2008; Colloff, 2009). Many-faceted studies of house dust mites of the Pyroglyphidae family have been continued since 1964 in many countries of the world, including the surveys on their taxonomy and fauna, biology and ecology, epidemiology, allergenicity and control. To date, only 15 species were found in house-dust samples: *Dermatophagoides pteronyssinus, D. farinae, D. evansi, D. microceras, D. siboney, D. neotropicalis, Hirstia domicola, H. chelidonis, Malayoglyphus intermedius, M. carmelitus, Sturnophagoides brasiliensis, Hughesiella africana, Hu. valerioi, Euroglyphus maynei* and *Gymnoglyphus longior*. The house dust mites have been reported from human dwellings and a wide variety of other habitats associated with man and his environment, both indoor and outdoor (Van Bronswijk 1981; Fain et al., 1990; Solarz & Solarz, 1996; Arlian, 2002; Solarz, 2003; Solarz et al., 2007; Colloff, 2009; Perotti et al., 2009).

Most often they are found in habitats intimately associated with man, such as beds, bed linen, couches, sofas, other upholstery furnitures, clothing, curtains, window stills, floors and carpets (Van Bronswijk, 1981; Fain et al., 1990; Mehl, 1998; Colloff, 2009; Arlian & Platts-Mills, 2001; Arlian, 2002; Solarz, 2001a, b, 2004a, 2010). These domestic environments are very important locations for forensic investigations, but this richness of mite diversity has not been exploited by forensic investigators (Perotti et al., 2009). Next chapters are focused on the mites in a variety of indoor habitats. The natural sources of allergenic mites in dwellings or stores are still not quiet known (Solarz et al, 2007). The possible sources of these mites in house dust are nests of synanthropic birds and stored products (Hughes, 1976; van Bronswijk, 1981; Fain et al., 1990). In Poland, the knowledge of their occurrence in house dust is still poor and the number of faunistic surveys on dust acarofauna is anywhere from ten to twenty. So, exists indispensability of these surveys in Poland, especially in Upper Silesian region, where air vitiation may to have stimulating influence to sensitization of human beings with house dust allergens. It is also commonly known that certain industrial dusts may cause chronic lung diseases in occupational populations, including also coal workers (Solarz & Solarz, 1996). It cannot be excluded that apart from coal dust itself, certain constituents of biological origin may also contribute to the pathogenic effect. Our previous results reveal the occurrence of allergenic mites in samples of dust and debris from coal-mines of the Upper Silesian region (Solarz & Solarz, 1996; Solarz, 2003). Thus they should all be regarded as a potential source of mite allergens in this environment. Our studies suggest also that the allergenic mites belonging to Acaridae, Glycyphagidae, Pyroglyphidae and Tetranychidae should be considered as occupational risk factors contributing to the occurrence of respiratory and dermal diseases among workers of ZOO gardens (Solarz et al., 2004a, b). As the occurrence and concentration of mites in samples from different places may vary to a considerable extent, further studies are highly desirable. An understanding of the seasonal dynamics, as well as environmental factors influencing mite populations, can be exploited in mite control. Most studies on house dust mites within dwellings have traditionally sampled beds, carpets and upholstered furniture as the 3 main types of the indoor microhabitats of these mites. House-dust-mite species have been recovered from animal and human carcasses and only recently they are being studied for their potential as forensic indicators (Baker, 2009; Braig and Perotti, 2009; OConnor, 2009; Solarz, 2009). The usability of domestic mites in forensic investigations is dependent on a thorough knowledge of their diversity and abundance in a variety of indoor environments. The ubiquity of mites means that there are many situations in which human beings and different objects associated with crime are exposed to these arachnids (Perotti et al., 2009). This chapter gives a faunistic review of the pyroglyphid mites that have actually been recorded in Southern Poland, in dwellings (beds, carpeted and non-carpeted floors, upholstery furniture, desks, walls), hospitals, libraries, and other workplaces and/or public places, in heaps of litter soiled with communal wastes near fences, houses and public buildings. There are no detailed differential diagnoses and identification keys to the pyroglyphid dust mites and other domestic mites, especially for the juvenile stages. Therefore, an acarological diagnostics in forensic studies may be difficult. The taxonomic relationships and number of valid species within the family Pyroglyphidae are not established to date. The measurements and analysis of variation between individuals, populations, species and genera is fundamental to the study of systematic, ecology and evolution, and has numerous applications in the medical, veterinary and agricultural sciences, including the forensic medicine. Therefore, this chapter presents also results of morphological studies, including most medically important taxa of mites, especially genera from the families Pyroglyphidae (*Dermatophagoides, Euroglyphus, Gymnoglyphus, Sturnophagoides*), Acaridae (*Acarus, Tyrophagus*), Glycyphagidae (*Glycyphagus, Lepidoglyphus, Gohieria*) and Chortoglyphidae (*Chortoglyphus*). I obtained most mite specimens from house dust samples, bird nests, farming environments, and from research collections in the United States, UK and Belgium. Own detailed descriptions of all species examined, differential diagnoses and identification keys are presented. Results suggest that the current division of the subfamilies of the family Pyroglyphidae should be revised. These results are compared with published studies with the aim of outlining and examining the weaknesses of the approach. It is commonly known, that more detailed descriptions of mites in different indoor situations are very important for forensic investigations (Perotti et al., 2009).

2. Recent studies on the house-dust-mite acarofauna in Poland

The study was carried out from July 2007 to December 2009. During this period 1875 house dust samples were collected from flats and one-family homes at different localities in Poland (Silesian Province, Malopolskie Province, Swietokrzyskie Province); 1053 (56.16%) samples were positive for mites. A total of 15,698 mites were isolated and 18 species were identified, including 5 species from the family Pyroglyphidae (house dust mites). Among them *Dermatophagoides pteronyssinus* was predominant (6,870 specimens; 43.8% of the total count), followed by *D. farinae* (6,553 ones; 41.7%). The second species was predominant in Czestochowa (88.3%), Katowice (91.9%), Sosnowiec (89.4%), Chorzow (94.8%), Tychy (59.4-92.8%), Bytom (50.9%) and generally in Upper Silesia (55.8-87.61%), whereas *D. pteronyssinus* dominated in old buildings in Chorzow and Sosnowiec (60.31%), Bytom (52.7%) and vicinity (68.4%), in old buildings in Upper Silesia (49.6%), in Upper Silesian dwellings of allergic patients (70.8%), in Cracow (centre of the city; 50.83%), one-family homes in Zywiec and vicinity (90.3%), Miechow and vicinity (43.8%), Swietokrzyskie Province (mainly Staszow, Sedziszow and vicinity, Skarzysko-Kamienna; 41.9%) and Bielsko-Biala vicinity (76.51%). Another pyroglyphid mites, *E. maynei, G. longior* and *H. chelidonis*, occurred in very small numbers (190, 1 and 6 specimens, respectively). Highest mite densities per gram of dust were noted in one-family homes. *D. pteronyssinus* was more abundant per gram of dust mainly in the one-family houses on agricultural or subagricultural settlements, especially in bed mattresses, whereas *D. farinae* in samples from the remaining indoor places examined, and especially from dwellings in urban regions. Generally, the highest dust mite concentrations were usually found in dust from beds, upholstery furniture and carpeted floors. An influence of some abiotic indoor factors on the mite prevalence in the examined dwellings were analysed separately in relation to samples of bed dust, floor dust and dust from upholstery furniture. The density of mites was influenced mainly by the type of heating, temperature, relative humidity, type of sleeping accommodation, type of floor or furniture, age of building, type of building, number of inhabitants and weight of samples. Mean relative humidities were 59.7%, 60.4% and 72.0% for samplings of dust from the Upper Silesian dwellings, from other urban localities and from agricultural or subagricultural settlements, alternatively. In hospitals a total of 80 samples were examined, always from two sites - floor and patient's mattresses. Mites (209 specimens) were isolated from 44 samples (55%). The most abundant mites were members of the family Pyroglyphidae, which formed 99.01%of the total count. *D. farinae* was predominant (66.5% of all mites collected), followed by *D. pteronyssinus* (32.1%). The former species was more frequent in samples from floors than from patients' beds, whereas *D. pteronyssinus* was collected more frequently from beds than from floors. *D. farinae* was distinctly more abundant per 1 gram of dust (arithmetic mean 19.8) than *D. pteronyssinus* (7.7), whereas alive mites were slightly more numerous in populations of the second species (5.4 vs. 5.3). Populations of both species were dominated by adult mites. The density of mites was influenced mainly by the type of mattress, number of patients and relative humidity. The research has revealed differences in the occurrence and abundance of both species of house dust mites between hospitals examined and between particular places within the same hospital. Moreover, the study suggests that the house dust mites and other mites, including also some allergenic taxa, should be considered as occupational risk factors contributing to the occurrence of respiratory and dermal diseases among patients and different workers of hospitals. Most probably, these mites are introduced into hospitals by humans from their houses and/or flats. House dust mite prevalence was also studied in the rooms of a tertiary care hospital in Knurow (Upper Silesia). A total of 60 samples were examined, always from two sites - from floors and patient's beds. Only 10 samples were positive for mites (16,67%) and only 19 mites were isolated; among them the most abundant ones were pyroglyphids (16 specimens; 84.21% of the total count), two species of the family - *D. farinae* (12 specimens) and *D. pteronyssinus* (4 ones). The first species was more abundant per gram of dust (mean number 34.9) than *D. pteronyssinus* (27.0). Main sources of mites in libraries and drug-stores are shelves, upholstery chairs and carpeted floors, whereas in offices carpeted floors and upholstery furniture. Although beds are commonly known as the main indoor places of mite occurrence, they were however - besides the dwellings - more abundant in libraries than in hospitals. The highest numbers of *D. farinae* per gram of dust were found in samples of dust from book-shelves and carpets. *D. farinae* was the dominant constituting approximately 575 of mites collected. It is possible that older books, and also book-shelves and carpets contain significant quantities of skin scales or dander from the readers or library workers (librarians) which skin scales serve as suitable food for pyroglyphid mites. These data confirm the results of several acarologists of small numbers of mites in hospitals, offices, hotel rooms and other social buildings or public places, suggesting that the environment in these places is unsuitable for the mite growth. Repeated routine cleaning practices as well as maintenance of low relative humidity could in part explain the small abundance of mites in public places/buildings. This research, as well as some other studies, has revealed differences in the occurrence and prevalence of different species of domestic mites between geographical areas and between dwellings within the same geographical area, between particular places within the same dwelling, and between the seasons of the year. This knowledge may be very useful in the forensic medicine. Moreover, the study suggests that the house dust mites and other domestic mites, including also some allergenic or parasitic taxa, should be considered as occupational risk factors contributing to the occurrence of respiratory and dermal diseases among librarians, barkers, cleaners, different workers of hospitals, drug-stores, airports, offices, and many other occupational categories. Exposure to indoor allergens, especially dust mites has been recognized as a risk factor for sensitization and allergy symptoms that in extreme conditions could develop into asthma (Spiewak et al., 1995).

3. Species composition of the house-dust-mite acarofauna

Pyroglyphid mites usually make up 60-90% of the house dust acarofauna in temperate climate regions throughout the world (Van Bronwijk 1981; Fain et al., 1990; Colloff, 2009), also in Poland (Solarz, 2010). In the case of mite density, the number of mites per gram of dust may range from a few to 16,000 or more, although the results of the surveys are difficult to compare and evaluate because of the lack of standardization of both dust collecting methods and reporting procedures. It has been shown, however, that occurrence and abundance of house dust mites may vary in particular topographical regions and are associated to a large degree with the climate of a region, and especially with outdoor and indoor humidity (Korsgaard, 1998; Mumcuoglu, 1976; Mumcuoglu et al., 1999; Colloff, 2009). Ratios of numbers of the particular pyroglyphid dust mite species, especially between *D. pteronyssinus* and *D. farinae*, are different in separate regions of the world (Fain et al., 1990; Mumcuoglu, et al. 1999). Decisive factors influencing their occurrence and abundance are mainly relative humidity and temperature of both outdoor and indoor air (Solarz, 2001 a, b). It is commonly known that the optimal temperature is higher (25-30 °C) and optimal humidity lower (50-75 %RH) for *D. farinae* than for *D. pteronyssinus*. The former species appear to survive better in dryer habitats than the latter, whereas lower temperature (15-20 °C) and higher humidity (75-80 %RH) favours *D. pteronyssinus* in mixed laboratory cultures (Arlian et al., 1998). Within the wide zone of temperate climate *D. pteronyssinus* is the most common and dominant species in more damp areas, at the seaside or in lowlands, which have a more humid climate. *D. farinae,* however, is more common and abundant in areas with a dry continental climate (intercontinental and alpine regions) (Voorhorst et al., 1969; Fain et al., 1990; Colloff, 2009; Solarz, 2001a, b, 2010). In Europe, most abundant mite populations were usually collected from bed mattresses (Van Bronswijk, 1981; Fain et al., 1990; Hallas & Korsgaard, 1997; Horak et al., 1996; Solarz, 2006). In previous surveys (Solarz, 1998) of house-dust-mite fauna in dust samples from dwellings and hospitals located in Sosnowiec and Katowice (Upper Silesia), the dominance of the Pyroglyphidae was demonstrated (Solarz, 2001 a, b). Approximately 63.5% of the total mite population belonged to this family. Most abundant were the following members of Pyroglyphidae - *D. pteronyssinus* (29% of the total mite population), *D. farinae* (25.5%) and *E. maynei* (6.0%). Unidentified *Dermatophagoides* spp. formed 3% of mites isolated from the samples examined. As indicated by the results of other previous surveys in Poland, *D. pteronyssinus* was found to be the dominant species in Warsaw, Poznan, and two Upper Silesian cities-towns Katowice and Sosnowiec (Horak et al., 1996; Solarz, 1998). As demonstrated by the more direct investigations of the house dust samples from dwellings (in Katowice, Sosnowiec, Myslowice, Chorzow, Tarnowskie Gory, Bytom, Zabrze, Gliwice, Dabrowa Gornicza and Ogrodzieniec), libraries (in Sosnowiec), institutes (in Katowice) and hospitals (in Katowice and Sosnowiec), the dominance of Pyroglyphidae was more significant than previously (Solarz, 1998, 2001a, b). About 89.2% of the total mite population from dwellings constituted the following members of this family - *D. pteronyssinus* (45.1%), *D. farinae* (40.2%), *E. maynei* (2.6%), *G. longior* (0.05%) and unidentified *Dermatophagoides* (1.24%). A total of 31 species of mites from 15 families were identified, of which 18 species belonged to Astigmatina, 3 to Prostigmata, 3 to Oribatida sensu lato and 7 to Mesostigmata. The fauna of house dust mites was therefore rather differentiated in this region. This was particularly apparent in dwellings, where 49 combinations of species composition in collected mite populations were observed. This study has clearly established that mite species in beds and other sleeping accommodations are different from the mite species on bedroom floors. The pyroglyphid mites were most abundant in samples from beds and upholstery furniture whereas floors were dominated with the non-pyroglyphid mites. A total of 402 samples were analysed: 238

samples from dwellings, 122 samples from hospitals, 14 from libraries and 28 from institutes. Mites were present in 51.3%, 50.0%, 21.3% and 17.9% of dust samples from dwellings, libraries, hospitals and institutes, respectively. Generally, they were found in 160 samples (39.8% of the total count). The majority of mites (96.0 %) were found in samples from the dwellings, especially in dust from upholstery furniture, couches, sofas and beds. Altogether, the pyroglyphid mites constituted 89.2%, 78.9% and 57.5% of a total population of mites collected from dwellings, libraries and hospitals, respectively, but were not found in institutes. In total, *D. pteronyssinus* was the most dominant, especially in libraries and hospitals, however in dwellings *D. farinae* was more abundant per 1 gram of dust than the former species. Another pyroglyphid mite, *E. maynei*, occurred in very small numbers (Solarz, 1998, 2001a, b). Mites of families Glycyphagidae, Chortoglyphidae and Acaridae are considered to be much more sensitive to desiccation than pyroglyphids (Van Bronswijk, 1981; Fain et al., 1990; Hallas & Korsgaard, 1997). It has also been suggested that some domestic mite species thrive in very damp conditions; this group include domestic acarids, glycyphagids (*L. destructor, G. domesticus*) and cheyletids (*Cheyletus* spp). Therefore, the presence and abundance of these mite species can be used as an indicator of humid environments (Fain et al., 1990; Solarz, 1998, 2003). The relatively low frequency of mites in a total of samples from dwellings examined and relatively lower abundance of glycyphagids, acarids, cheyletids and *E. maynei* mites is clear, taking into account the aforementioned values of indoor relative humidity observed in these dwellings (Fain et al., 1990; Solarz, 1998, 2003). In general, these mites are not as abundant or frequent in Europe as in the Tropics (Fain et al., 1990; Puerta et al., 1993; Mehl, 1998; Mumcuoglu et al., 1999; da Silva et al., 2001; Colloff, 2009). The mean concentration of mites in examined samples and mite frequency was at the lower end of the published range for more humid regions (Van Bronswijk, 1981; Fain et al., 1990; Mumcuoglu, et al. 1999; Colloff, 2009) and was comparable with some European results from France, Denmark and Holland (Van Bronswijk, 1981; Fain et al., 1990; Harving et al., 1993) and with other results from Poland (Horak et al., 1996; Racewicz, 2001).

4. Acarofauna of the synanthropic outdoor sites

The occurrence of allergenic mites (pyroglyphid house-dust mites, acarid and glycyphagid storage mites and others) in synanthropic outdoor sites in a densely populated urban area was investigated. Litter soiled with communal wastes was sampled. 80.5% of the total population was formed by allergenic mites. These mites (11 species) belong to Acaridae and Winterschmidtiidae. Among the astigmatic mites two acarids were dominant: *Tyrophagus silvester* and *T. longior* (28.7% and 25.1% of all mites respectively), with the latter being the most frequent (44.2% of all samples). The age structures of the two species versus relative humidity were investigated. The correlations between the age structures of *T. silvester, T. longior, T. molitor* and *T. similis* were statistically analysed. The most important allergenic mites from Pyroglyphidae (house dust mites) or Glycyphagidae (stored food mites) were not found. However, allergenic mites from Tarsonemidae – important for house dust, and Acaridae – reported from food stores, were presented numerously in the samples, which bring us to the conclusion that litter can be an important source of invasion of the mites into dwellings or food stores.

5. Allergenic mites as the occupational and/or environmental risk factors

Many species of mites that humans come in contact with, besides the house dust mites or storage mites, induce allergic reactions. These include some species of spider mites (e.g., the 2-spotted spider mite *Tetranychus urticae* and *Panonychus ulmi*), which are common pests in orchards, greenhouses, and gardens. These mites were recently proved to induce IgE-mediated reactions (Arlian, 2001, 2002; Solarz, 2004a, 2006). It should come as no surprise to learn that chigger mites (larvae of Trombiculidae), ticks (Ixodida) and other species of ectoparasitic mites (Mesostigmata) of fowl, pigeons, other birds, mice, guinea pigs, and other mammals and some predaceous mites sensitize and induce allergic reactions in human (Arlian and Platts-Mills, 2001). Many species of stored-product mites occur in both residential and occupational environments and in processed foods and can cause allergic disease. In addition, humans may contact or be exposed to predaceous mites and parasitic mites of plants and animals that are also the sources of allergens that induce allergic disease.

5.1 Storage mites

The stored-product mites, especially several species from the families Acaridae, Glycyphagidae and Chortoglyphidae (Acari: Astigmatina), are commonly found in different stored food products, hay, straw, granaries, barns and other farming and occupational environments, as well as in samples of house dust. The most abundant and most often reported are *Acarus siro, A. farris* and *Tyrophagus putrescentiae* from Acaridae, *Lepidoglyphus destructor, Glycyphagus domesticus* and *Gohieria fusca* from Glycyphagidae and *Chortoglyphus arcuatus* from Chortoglyphidae (Hughes, 1976; Franz et al., 1997; Mehl, 1998; Baker, 1999; Müsken et al., 2000; Solarz, 2011; Solarz et al., 1997, 2004b). These mites are also the source of clinically important allergens and the cause of occupational allergies (known as an allergy to storage mites) among farmers, grain-storage workers and other agricultural workers (van Hage-Hamsten & Johansson, 1998; Morgan & Arlian, 2006; Fernández-Caldas et al., 2007). The greatest exposure to storage mites usually occurs in an occupational and/or rural setting where allergies to these mites are of major importance (van Hage-Hamsten et al., 1992; van Hage-Hamsten & Johansson, 1998; Arlian, 2001, 2002; Stejskal & Hubert, 2008). Many species of storage mites are found in processed foods (flour, boxed baking mixes such as cakes, pancakes, and beignets); in stored hay, grain and straw; in dust in grain and hay storage and livestock feeding facilities. Exposure to storage mite allergens can be by ingestion or by inhalation. Several studies report anaphylactic reactions after patients consumed beignets, cakes, pancakes, pizza, pasta, cornmeal cakes, and bread made from ingredients contaminated with mites. The importance of storage mites as ingested or aeroallergens in the urban population has not been studied extensively. The greatest exposure to storage mites usually occurs in an occupational setting where allergies to storage mites are of major importance. Kronqvist et al. (2000) reported that 12% of 440 farmers tested were sensitive to the storage mites *Acarus siro, L. destructor, T. putrescentiae,* and *Glycyphagus domesticus.* Similar sensitivities to storage mites have been reported for farmers in Scotland and USA (Arlian et al., 1997; Arlian, 2002). Important storage mite species in occupational settings are *L. destructor, G. domesticus, A. siro, T. putrescentiae, Tyrophagus longior, Aleuroglyphus ovatus, Suidasia medanensis, Chortoglyphus arcuatus,* and *Carpoglyphus* sp. Sensitization to the storage mite *T. putrescentiae* is present in the urban population of Upper Silesia in similar proportions as to pyroglyphid house-dust mites (*Dermatophagoides* spp.) (Szilman et al., 2004). Testing with storage mites should be considered routine allergological diagnostic procedure. In other words it is necessary to establish methods for identification and quantification of mites in the Upper Silesia (Szilman et al., 2004).

5.2 Other mites inducing allergic reactions

Many species of mites that humans come in contact with, besides those found in house dust, induce allergic reactions. These include the citrus red mite (*Panonychus citri*) and the two-spotted spider mite (*Tetranychus urticae*), which are common pests of apple orchards. Mites are ubiquitous and thrive in many diverse environments. Thus humans contact many species of mites and their products in their daily lives. The role of these less-known mites in causing allergic disease is not yet known. Phytophagous mites of fruit trees, vegetable crops, and yard, greenhouse, and house plants can cause allergic disease in at-risk populations. A study of 725 Korean farmers working in apple orchards found that 23.2% and 21.2% were sensitive based on skin tests to the two-spotted spider mite (*T. urticae*) and the European red mite (*Panonychus ulmi*), respectively. In this study population, the prevalence of sensitivity to these mites was greater than it was to the house dust mites, *D. farinae* and *D. pteronyssinus* (Kim et al., 1999; Arlian, 2002; Solarz 2003, 2004a, 2006). Another study by this group found that skin tests of 14.2% of 1055 children living around citrus orchards were positive to *P. citri* (Lee et al., 2000). Multiple erythematous papules accompanied by severe pruritus were observed in humans bitten by the mites *Pyemotes tritici* (Pyemotidae), *Dermanyssus gallinae* (Dermanysidae), *Ornithonyssus bacoti* (Macronyssidae) and *Andrlaelaps casalis* (Laelapidae) in Israel (Rosen et al., 2002). The mite *Hemisarcoptes cooremani*, a parasite of scale insects that is commonly found in orchards, yards, and gardens, was discovered to induce IgE-mediated reactions (Arlian et al., 1999). *Hemisarcoptes cooremani* that feeds on scale insects that parasitize trees and shrubs in orchards, yards, and gardens can induce allergic diseases. Immunoblotting of extracts of this mite showed that they contain 16- and 19-kDa proteins that bound IgE in the serum of an exposed and symptomatic individual (Arlian et al., 1999). It should come as no surprise to learn that chigger mites (Trombiculidae), ticks (Ixodida) and other species of ectoparasitic mites (Mesostigmata) of fowl, pigeons, other birds, mice, guinea pigs, and other mammals and some predaceous mites either sensitize or induce allergic reactions in human as well (Arlian & Platts-Mills, 2001). The saliva of ticks (Ixodida) contains immunogenic proteins that can induce IgE-mediated reactions while they feed; cases of anaphylactic reactions from a tick bite have been reported (Arlian, 2002). Predaceous mites such as *Phytoseiulus persimilis* and *Amblyseius cucumeris*, that feed on spider mites and larvae of thrips, respectively, can sensitize greenhouse workers (Kronqvist et al., 2000). This raises the possibility that predaceous mites, used for biological control of pest species in fields and orchards, may be important sources of allergens for gardeners, farmers, and people living around fields and orchards (Arlian, 2002). Molecules from the human itch mite (*Sarcoptes scabiei var. hominis*), which burrow in the stratum corneum of the skin, induce IgE production and an IgE-mediated reaction in some parasitized human hosts (Arlian, 2002; Arlian & Platts-Mills, 2001). Many of these immunogens are cross-reactive with antigens of the house dust mites *D. farinae* and *D. pteronyssinus*. Capability of other parasitic mites, such as follicle mites (*Demodex folliculorum, Demodex brevis*), red chicken mites (*Dermanyssus gallinae*), rat mites (*Ornithonyssus bacoti*) and sheep scab mites (*Psoroptes ovis*), inducing IgE reactions in humans needs to be investigated (Arlian, 2002).

6. Identification diagnoses to mites of the families Acaridae, Glycyphagidae, Chortoglyphidae and Pyroglyphidae in taxonomic order

The measurements and analysis of variation between individuals, populations, species and genera (or subfamilies), is fundamental to the study of systematics, ecology and evolution, and has numerous applications in the agricultural, veterinary and medical sciences (Klimov & OConnor, 2009; Dabert et al., 2010), including the forensic medicine (Perotti, 2009a). In forensic acarology it is necessary to produce the data that clearly demonstrate how mites can contribute to investigations (Perotti et al., 2009). Therefore, a following priority is to provide more user and friendly identification aids, such as differential diagnoses and/or keys for different groups of synanthropic or semisynanthropic mites, including the domestic and storage mites (Baker, 1999; Colloff, 1998; 2009; Desch, 2009; Perotti et al., 2009; Solarz, 2011).

6.1 Family: Acaridae

6.1.1 Genus: *Acarus* L.

Differential diagnosis: In both sexes: solenidion sigma 1 on genu I at least 3 times as long as sigma 2 (Fig. 1A); setae *v e* less than half the length of setae *v i* ; setae *v e* arising near the anterior angles of the dorsal propodosomal sclerite or slightly posterior; ventral apex of tarsus I with proral (*p, q*) and unguinal (*u, v*) setae as thin, not short, stout spines; setae *c 1* and *d 2* short; setae *sc e* about equal in length to *sc i* (Fig. 1B); seta *sc x* generally expanded basally and thickly pectinate (Figs 1B, 2). In males: legs I enlarged; femur I with a stout ventral apophysis or process (seta *vF*) (Fig. 1); ventral side of genu I with small thickenings of cuticle; lateral arms of the penis support diverge posteriorly. In females: characteristic structure of reproductive system, with chitinised depression in body wall, external opening of expansible tube of bursa copulatrix, chitinised bell-shaped structure leading into receptaculum seminis and two armed flame-like chitinised opening to thin-walled oviduct; claws of female never bifid.

6.1.1.1 *Acarus siro* L.

Differential diagnosis: In both sexes: setae *sc e* slightly shorter than *sc i*; setae *d 1* intermediate in length between *c 1* and *e 1*, never more than 3 times longer than *c 1*; seta *sc x* expanded basally and thickly pectinate; solenidion omega 1 on tarsi I and II long, recumbent and the angle between the dorsal surface of the tarsus and the anterior face of the solenidion rarely exceeds 45 degrees (generally about 30). In males: tarsus II of male with seta *s* large, about equal in length to length of empodial claw; ventro-posterior margin of this seta concave, claw tip directed backwards; seta *sc x* expanded basally and thickly pectinate (Fig. 2); lateral arms of the penis support diverge posteriorly; penis (aedeagus) as an arc-shaped tube with a blunt end. In females: tarsi I-II with seta *s* large, about equal in length to length of empodial claw (Fig. 3); ventro-posterior margin of the seta concave, claw tip directed backwards; setae more sparsely pectinate as that of the male; bursa copulatrix opens into a narrow expansible tube which joins a sclerotized bell-shaped structure; setae *ps 3* are twice and *ps 2* almost four times the lengths of *ad 3*, *ad 2* and *ad 1*; vulva characteristic, positioned between *coxae* III and IV. Hypopi: mobile form; gnathosomal remnant with well developed solenidia; posterior ventral attachment organ (sucker plate) well developed, with 8 distinct suckers; legs well developed, with normally formed setae and solenidia; scapular setae relatively long; length of *sc i* greater than distance between alveoli; hysterosomal setae *c 1, d 1, d 2* and *e 1* long, extending beyond base of next most posterior seta; *sc i* about 1.5 times length of *c 1* and 1.2 times length of *d 1*; setae *c 1* and *d 1* about 3 times longer than *h 1*; bases of genital setae and flanking pair of coxal suckers almost in line, distance between base of sucker and base of seta is less than width of setal base.

6.1.1.2 *Acarus farris* (Oudemans)

Differential diagnosis: In both sexes: setae *sc e* about equal in length to *sc i*; setae *d 1* intermediate in length between *c 1* and *e 1*, never more than 3 times longer than *c 1*; most dorsal setae short, setae *d 1* and *e 1* not extending to base of next posterior seta; solenidion omega 1 of tarsus II short, compact, with sides expanding gradually from the base, then narrowing to an indistinct neck before expanding into a terminal head, width of widest part of head equal to width of widest part of shaft; the angle between anterior margin of the solenidion and the dorsal surface of the tarsus II is nearer to 90 degrees than 45 degrees. In males: tarsus II of male with seta *s* slender, about 1/2-2/3 the length of empodial claw and points anteriorly; ventro-posterior margin of the seta convex, seta tip directed forward. In females: tarsi I-II with seta *s* slender, about half to two-thirds the length of empodial claw; ventro-posterior margin of seta convex, seta tip directed forward; setae *ad 3*, *ad 2* and *ad 1* almost equal in length, *ps 3* about 1/3 and *ps 2* about twice as long; vulva as in *A. siro*. Hypopi: hysterosomal setae *c 1*, *d 1*, *d 2* and *e 1* appreciably shorter than scapulars, and not extending to bases of next most posterior setae; setae *sc i* at least 2 times length of *c 1* and *d 1*; setae *c 1* and *d 1* about equal in length to *h 1*; bases of genital setae just forward of coxal sucker bases; distance between base of sucker and base of seta about equal to width of setal base.

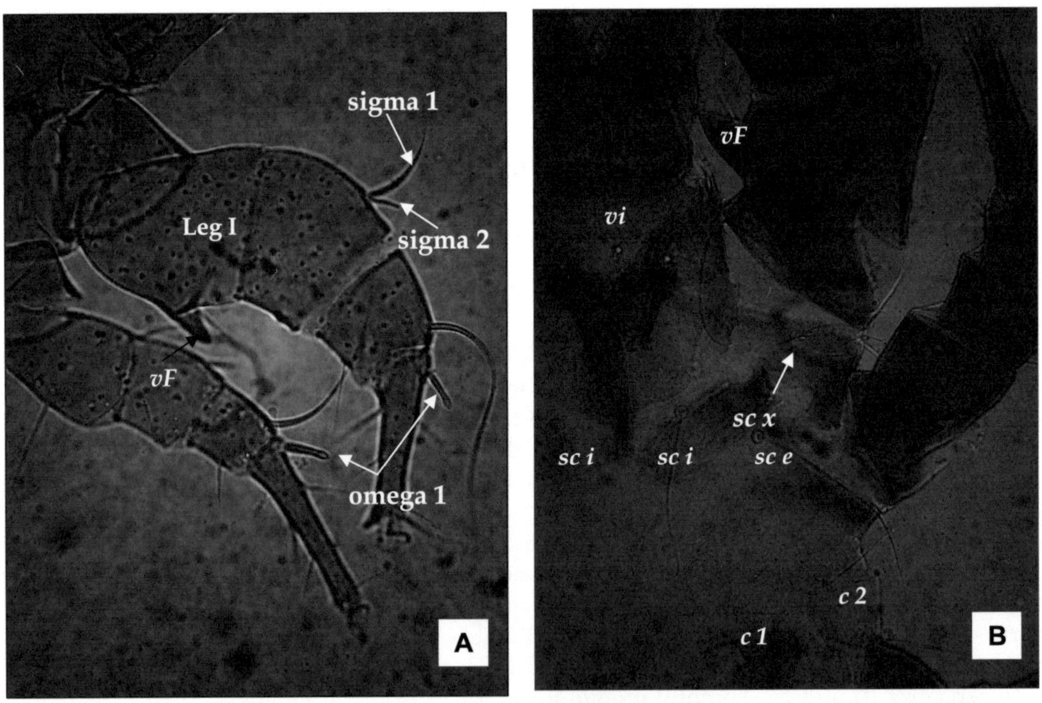

Fig. 1. *Acarus* sp. - A. *Acarus immobilis*, male: legs I and II; B. *Acarus nidicolous*, male in dorsal aspect: seta *vF* on femur I, shape of supracoxal seta (*sc x*) and propodosomal chaetotaxy; key: solenidia omega 1 on tarsi I and II; solenidia sigma 1 and 2 on genu I; *vF* = seta *vF* on femur I; *sc x* = supracoxal seta; external (*sc e*) and internal (*sc i*) scapular setae; dorsal setae *c 1* and *c 2*.

6.1.1.3 *Acarus immobilis* Griffiths

Differential diagnosis: In both sexes: setae *sc e* about equal in length to *sc i*; setae *d 1* intermediate in length between *c 1* and *e 1*, never more than three times longer than *c 1*; most dorsal setae short, setae *d 1* and *e 1* not extending to base of next posterior seta; tarsus II with solenidion omega1 with sides almost parallel, expanding into a distinct egg-shaped terminal head which is wider than widest part of shaft (Fig. 1A); the angle between the dorsal surface of the tarsus and the anterior face of the solenidion generally about 45-50 degrees. In males: tarsus II with seta *s* slender, about half the length of empodial claw; ventro-posterior margin of the seta convex, seta tip directed forward. In females: tarsi I-II with seta *s* slender; ventro-posterior margin of the seta convex, seta tip directed forward. Hypopi: inert forms; legs short (in dorso-ventral mounts tarsi of legs I and II are the only segments completely visible); setae very reduced or absent; gnathosoma rudimentary, flagelliform bristles (solenidia) not present; posterior ventral attachment organ rudimentary, with at most one pair of well-developed suckers on sucker plate, the central pair of suckers vestigial, anterior peripheral pair moderately well developed; all setae on tarsus III and IV shorter than length of tarsus, spine-like, never leaf-shaped; solenidion omega 1 on tarsus I long, at least twice the length of empodial claw.

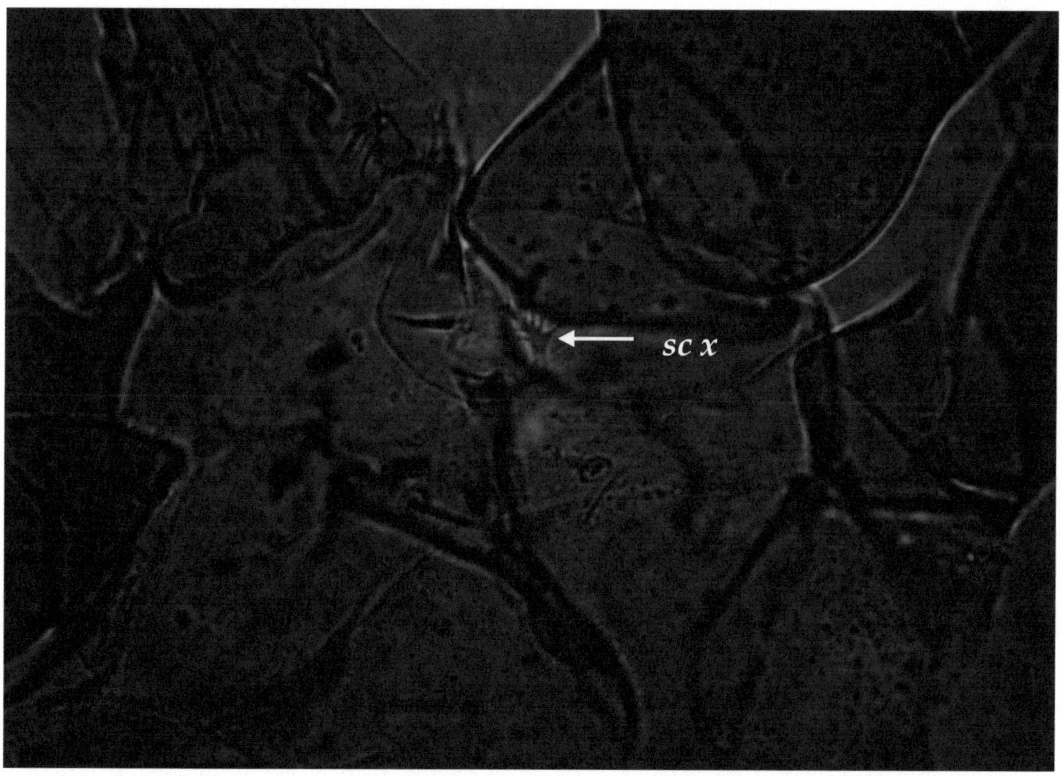

Fig. 2. *Acarus siro* – male, dorsal aspect: supracoxal seta; key: *sc x* = supracoxal seta.

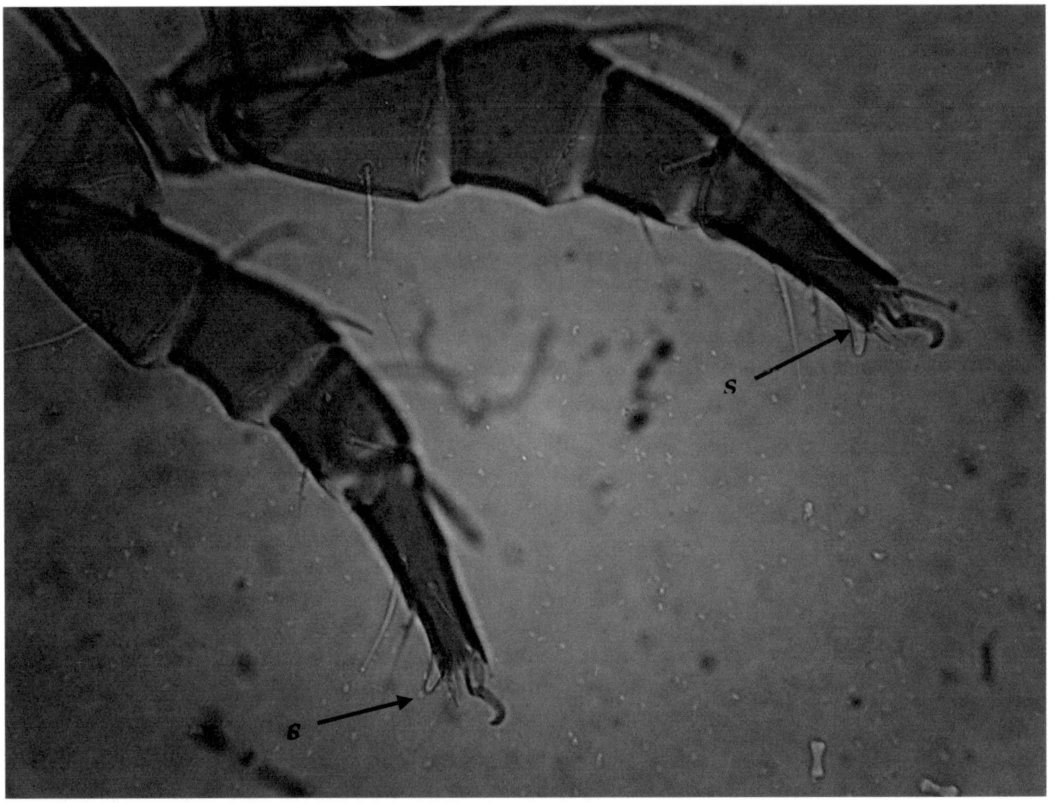

Fig. 3. *Acarus siro* – female, legs I and II; key: s = seta (spine) *s*.

6.1.2 Genus: *Tyrophagus* Oudemans

Differential diagnosis: In both sexes: setae *v e* distinctly barbed, relatively long, longer than the length of the genu I and usually positioned near anterior lateral corners of propodosomal shield; setae *v e* at almost the same level as *v i* and curve downwards; setae *sc i* longer than *sc e*; setae *c 1* and *d 2* usually almost equal in length, and shorter than *e 1* and *h 1*; the dorsal terminal seta *e* on tarsi I needle-shaped; presence of 5 ventral setae on tarsi I, of which the three central ones are thickened; solenidion sigma 1 on tibia I always less than three times as long as sigma 2; ventral apex of tarsi with proral and unguinal setae usually in the form of short, stout spines, occasionally one or both pairs strongly reduced or absent; tarsi I-II more than twice as long as basal width; proral setae thinner than unguinal setae but similar in length; Grandjean's organ finger-like. In males: without modifications of leg I; legs I not enlarged and the femur does not bear a ventral apophysis.

6.1.2.1 *Tyrophagus putrescentiae* (Schrank) (Fig. 4)

Differential diagnosis: In both sexes: anterior margins of propodosomal shield with pigmented spots (corneae); coxal plate II with a sinuous posterior margin so that the plate narrows sharply along the distal 1/3; tarsi I and II with solenidion omega 1 terminating in a distinctly expanded tip; distal 2/3 of solenidion omega 1 on tarsi I widened. In females: genital seta *g* longer than vulva; paraproctal setae *ad 1* much shorter than *ad 2*; setae *ad 2* distinctly longer than anal slit; internal spermathecal apparatus large, base of spermatheca expanded, flat, spermathecal duct with distinct constriction about halfway along length; proximal part of spermathecal duct gradually widened. In males: aedeagus shorter (<20μm), S-shaped with two deep curves, one at base, the other in apical third; distal 1/3 of aedeagus curved at an angle of about 75-100° to its median part; tarsal copulatory suckers on tarsus IV equidistant from the base and apex of the segment; setae *ps 2* more than 1.8-2 times longer than the anal slit.

6.1.2.2 *Tyrophagus longior* (Gervais)

Differential diagnosis: In both sexes: anterior margins of propodosomal sclerite without pigmented spots *(corneae)*; supracoxal seta (*sc x*) thin, not expanded basally, pectination variable; setae *d 2* short, at most only slightly longer than *c 1*; setae *d 1* about 1.3-2 times as long as *c 1* and *d 2*; tarsi I-II with solenidion omega 1 long, slender, tapering toward tip; tip pointed and not expanded apically. In males: supracoxal seta (*sc x*) thin, with short lateral barbs of about equal lengt; the lateral sclerites supporting the penis (*aedeagus*) turned inwards; aedeagus straight only slightly curved distally and shaped like the spout of a teapot; aedeagus long, slender and tapering towards its free end; tarsus IV longer than the combined length of the genu and tibia; both tarsal copulatory suckers positioned nearer to the base of tarsus than the apex. In females: anterior margins of propodosomal sclerite without pigmented spots (*corneae*); internal spermathecal apparatus large, spermathecal duct moderate or large, base of spermatheca moderately long or very wide, distinctly wider than spermathecal duct; setae *ad 2* considerably longer than *ad 3, ps 3, ps 2* and *ad 1*.

6.2 Family: Glycyphagidae

6.2.1 Genus: *Lepidoglyphus* Zachvatkin

Differential diagnosis: In both sexes: setae *v e* absent; setae *v i* long and barbed, extend well beyond the tips of chelicerae; scapular setae arranged in a trapezoid or rectangle; gnathosoma at anterior apex of the body; prodorsal sclerite crista metopica absent; seta *sc x* slender, much branched; trochanteres I-II not surrounded basally by large, thickened apodemes (as in the genus *Xenocaster*); with pectinate subtarsal scales on all tarsi; on genu I solenidion sigma 2 more than 3 times longer than solenidion sigma 1; setae *la, ra, ba* on tarsus I arise in the distal third of the tarsus. In males: penis (*aedeagus*) posterior to coxal epimera I and positioned between coxae II and III and with anterior end marked by a triangular plate. In females: epigynium not fused to coxal apodemes I; vulva positioned between coxae II and III.

6.2.1.1 *Lepidoglyphus destructor* (Schrank)

Differential diagnosis: In both sexes: ventral seta *nG* of genua III not widened to form a pectinate scale; solenidion sigma on genu II not thickened. In males: without modifications of leg I; on genu I sigma 2 more than 4 times longer than sigma 1; ventral setae *kT* on tibiae III and IV does not arise from the edge of the arthrodial membrane. In females: setae *4 a* arises behind the posterior edge of the genital opening; anus terminal; 2 pairs of setae (*ad 3, ps 3*) inserted on either side of its anterior end. Hypopi: inactive, oval colourless, with reduced legs, rudiment of the genital slit and apodemes I and II feebly sclerotized; enclosed within the protonymphal cuticle.

6.2.2 Genus: *Glycyphagus* Hering

Differential diagnosis: In both sexes: without a subtarsal pectinate scale on all tarsi; usually with a prodorsal sclerite crista metopica; seta *sc x* more robust, forked and branched;

solenidion sigma 2 on genu I is more than twice as long as solenidia sigma 1 and omega 1; 2 ventral setae present on tibiae I and II; genital opening lies between coxae II and III.

6.2.2.1 *Glycyphagus domesticus* (De Geer)

Differential diagnosis: In both sexes: crista metopica extends from the base of the chelicerae to level of the anterior scapular setae (= *sc i*) (Fig. 5A); setae *v i* inserted almost in the middle of the crista metopica; setae *d 1* arising almost at the same

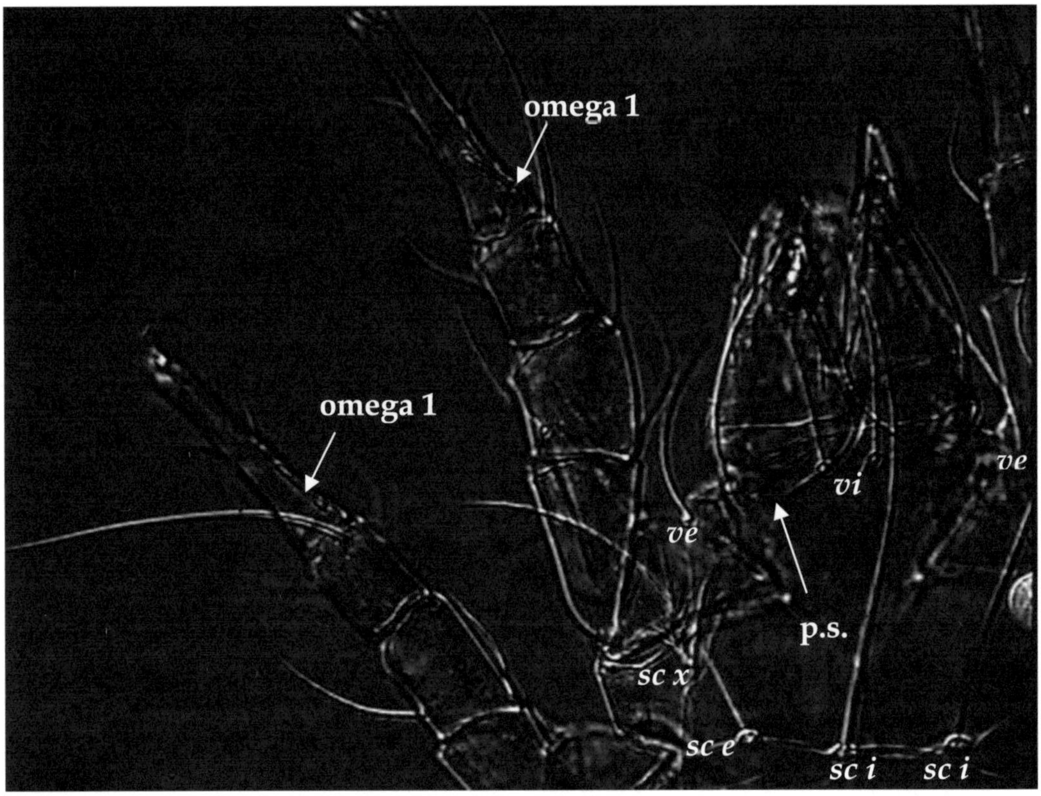

Fig. 4. *Tyrophagus putrescentiae* – legs I and II and dorsal propodosomal chaetotaxy; key: solenidia omega 1 on tarsi I and II; *sc x* = supracoxal seta; external (*v e*) and internal (*v i*) vertical setae; external (*sc e*) and internal (*sc i*) scapular setae.

level as *e 1*; the subtarsal seta is replaced on all the legs by a pectinate seta *wa* arising from the middle of the tarsus; setae *la*, *ba* and *ra* arise between the base of *wa* and the apex of the tarsus; solenidion omega 1 on tarsus I as a slender rod longer than omega 1 on tarsus II; solenidion omega 2 is relatively long and about half the length of solenidion omega 1 and much longer than the famulus epsilon; on genu I solenidion sigma 1 is less than half the length of sigma 2 and about the same length as omega 1. In males: with normal setae on tibiae I and II; on tibiae III and IV seta *kT* is well removed from the distal edge of the segment. In females: genital opening extends to the posterior edge of acetabula III and it is shorter than the distance separating it from the anterior end of the anus; setae *4a* inserted just behind the hind end of the genital opening; 2 pairs of setae (*ad 3*, *ps 3*) lie on either side of the anterior end of the anal slit; a tubular bursa copulatrix projects from the hind margin of the opisthosoma; setae *d 1* arising almost at the same level as *e 1*; distal setae (*la, ra, ba, wa*) on tarsus I more widely spaced. Hypopi: oval body, white in colour, with small bud-like gnathosoma, enclosed in protonymphal cuticle without reticulations.

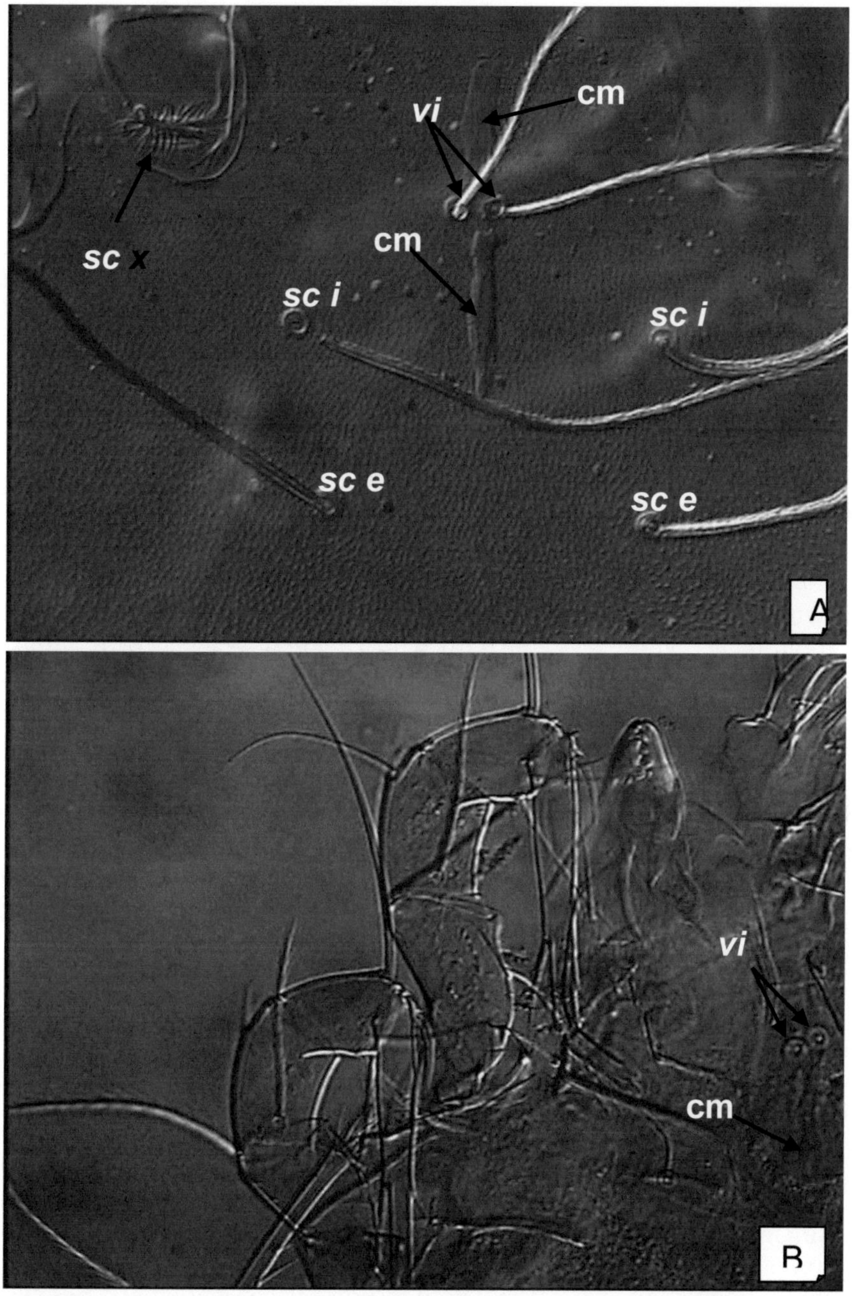

Fig. 5. *Glycyphagus* spp., females, dorsal aspects – shape of *crista metopica*: A. *G. domesticus*; B. *G. privatus*; key: cm = *crista metopica*; *v i* = internal vertical setae *sc i* = internal scapular setae; *sc e* = external scapular setae; *sc x* = supracoxal seta.

6.2.2.2 *Glycyphagus privatus* Oudemans (Syn.: *G. cadaverum* Schrank)

Differential diagnosis: In both sexes: setae *v i* inserted almost at the anterior end of the crista metopica (Fig. 5B); setae *d 1* arising anterior to *e 1* and on the same level as *c 1*; solenidion omega 2 on tarsus I very short, the same length as the famulus; solenidion sigma 1 on genu I shorter than in *G. domesticus*, much shorter than omega 1; seta *sc x* forked and branched. In females: genital opening (*vulva*) longer than in *G. domesticus*, extending as far back as the posterior edge of acetabula IV and longer than the distance between it and the anus. In males: with normal setae on tibiae I and II.

6.2.3 Genus: *Gohieria* Oudemans; *Gohieria fusca* (Oudemans)

Differential diagnosis: In both sexes: propodosoma without a division into 2 planes and extended forward and overhangs the gnathosoma; chelicerae with 1 seta; cuticle evenly sclerotized, pitted deeply tanned, pinkish-brown and ornamented with fine setae; ornamentation not in the form of small triangular microtrichae; no distinct propodonotal sclerite (or crista metopica) present; lateral body setae of both sexes not arising from tubercles; lamellae absent; setae *v i* and *sc x* pectinate, the remaining setae of the idiosoma only slightly serrated; setae *v i* situated almost on the apex of the propodosoma (only slightly more posterior); setae *v e* much more posterior, positioned almost in the same transverse line as setae *sc x*; seate *sc i*, *sc e* and *c 2* on a level with one another; legs short and massive, distinctly ridged; apodemes of all legs slender and unite to surround the genital opening; empodial claws present; tibiae and genua distinctly ridged especially in females; genua and femora freely articulated on all legs, distal edges of genua and femora expanded, femora without large ventral keel; tibiae I-II with 2 ventral setae; genu III with solenidion sigma present; solenidion phi on tibia I unusually long. In males: pretarsi expanded basally and arising ventrally on tarsal apex; legs III and IV with long pretarsi and noticeably bent; genitalia relatively simple, aedeagus anteriorly directed, positioned between coxal fields IV; body form of males similar to females, sexual dimorphism slight. In females: legs more slender than in males, the longitudinal ridges better developed; setae on tarsus I spaced out along the segment instead of being concentrated at the distal end; genital papillae everting in posterior region of oviporus (vulva); female oviporus region elongate, parallel sided; coxal apodemes I fusing separately with epigynium; ventral seta of femur I nude, without barbs.

6.3 Family: Chortoglyphidae

6.3.1 Genus: *Chortoglyphus* Berlese; *Chortoglyphus arcuatus* (Troupeau)

Differential diagnosis: In both sexes: chelicerae chelate, conspicuous; idiosoma oval and not divided into propodosoma and hysterosoma; body cuticle smooth and shining, without striations and microtrichae; discrete propodosomal sclerite absent; body setae short and nearly all smooth; genital papillae normal in form, strongly enlarged and reduced; solenidion omega 1 on tarsus I formed as a long curved rod arising close to a small solenidion omega 2; tarsus I with seta *wa* enlarged to form a stout spine and *ba* as a thin seta; only 1 solenidion sigma on genu I; tibiae I-II with dorsal solenidion and 0-2 ventral setae; legs ventrally positioned; praetarsi fleshy with inserted claws; empodial claws simple; anus positioned near posterior margin of body; both sexes with empodial claws simple or absent; ventral subcapitulum without external ridges; discrete coxal apodemes III and sometimes IV absent. In females: vulva (*oviporus*) longitudinal with genital valves fused to body anteriorly, free posteriorly, and situated between coxae III and IV; genital papillae always associated with genital opening; 5 pairs of setae in anal region. In males: aedeagus long, situated between coxae I and II; adanal suckers conspicuous; 2 pairs of setae in anal region; tarsal suckers present on tarsi IV; legs III similar to legs IV.

6.4 Family: Pyroglyphidae

6.4.1 Subfamily Pyroglyphinae

Differential diagnosis: In both sexes: setae *v i* absent; tegmen well developed; cuticle from slightly to strongly sclerotized; striations either relatively thick, irregular and well spaced, or completely lacking; the median area separating the epimera I punctate; idiosomal setae variable, either all very thin and very short, or with some setae (*sc e, h 2* and *h 3*) very long and strong. In females: cuticle lacking projections as in the genus *Glycyphagus;* setae *sc i* never very strong and long; ventral surface of tarsi I and II without projections; cuticle variable; epigynium distinctly separated from epimera I; tarsi III and IV lacking apical spines (except in *Weelawadjia* which presents these spines); posterior lip of the vulva always punctate; posterior vulvar lip generally fairly long and in some species incised in its anterior angle. In males: cuticle variable - slightly or strongly sclerotized; striations either present but irregular, thick and well spaced, or absent; setae *sc i* never very strong and very long; tarsi IV normal (not very short); legs III variable; femora III lacking a spur; tarsi IV always without a bifid or trifid subapicoventral spine; tarsi III with or without the subapicoventral spine; adanal copulatory suckers either present or lacking; tarsal copulatory suckers (on tarsi IV) either present or (generally) replaced by thin and short setae; setae *sc e* either long and strong (genera *Weelawadjia* and *Campephilocoptes*) or short and thin (other genera); tarsi III lacking an apical forked spine.

6.4.1.1 Genus: *Euroglyphus* Fain; *Euroglyphus maynei* (Cooreman)

Differential diagnosis: In both sexes: tegmen well developed, triangular with rounded apex (not bifid in the male as figured in the typical description); cuticle slightly sclerotized with rather well formed striations or folds; hysteronotum with in a median shield with poorly distinct margins; anterior legs lacking chitinous membranes; chaetotaxy reduced: trochanterals I-III, tibials IV, genital anterior setae (*3 b*) and anal external (*ps 2*) setae are lacking; tarsi III with 5 setae; tarsi IV with 3 setae; dorsal setae very thin and short; setae *h 3* very thin and short (maximum length 50 µm); setae *h 2* short (not exceeding 30 µm) and very thin; genu I with one solenidion. In males: tegmen with rounded, unforked apex; dorsal setae variable; opisthosoma slightly but regularly narrowed backwards; anus more posterior (anal suckers situated at 25 µm from the posterior margin of the body); posterior margin of the body straight and wide with 2 very small paramedian lobes; adanal suckers well developed; tarsi IV lacking suckers. In females: setae *sc e* thin and short (maximum 50 µm); no chitinous pouches at the bases of legs II; tegmen either triangular and prominent but with apex rounded and not forked or poorly developed, rounded with a small median notch; posterior lip of vulva punctate and short, not covering the vulvar slit; anterior angle of posterior vulvar lip not incised; tegmen triangular with rounded, not incised apex; hysteronotum striated with a median shield; copulatory vestibule ovoid, strongly sclerotized and opaque; tarsi I-IV without apical processes nor spines.

6.4.1.2 Genus: *Gymnoglyphus* Fain

Differential diagnosis: In both sexes: tegmen is triangular with bifid apex and the chaetotaxy is not reduced: the setae trochanterals I-III, tibials IV, setae *ps 2* and *3 b* are present; the tarsi

III and IV bear 6 and 5 setae, respectively. In males: adanal suckers well developed; dorsal setae short and thin; setae *h 3* and *h 2* very thin and short (maximum length 50 µm); tegmen deeply incised at apex; opisthosoma strongly narrowed backwards; anus more anterior (adanal suckers at 40 µm from posterior margin of body); posterior margin of body (idiosoma, opisthosoma) narrower, concave in the middle and with 2 small but well distinct paramedian lobes; chaetotaxy normal (trochanteral setae I-III, tibial IV setae, *ps 2* and *3 b* setae present). In females: setae *sc e* thin and short (maximum 50 µm); setae *h 2* and *h 3* short or very short (less than 50 µm) and thin; no chitinous pouches at bases of legs II; tegmen triangular, prominent with apex forked; posterior vulvar lip very long; anteriorly and completely covering the vulvar slit, its anterior angle not incised; opening of bursa copulatrix situated near the posterior extremity of anus and followed by a small ovoid strongly sclerotized pouch (vestibule); dorsum with thick striations and a small median opisthosomal (opisthonotal) shield; epimera I free.

6.4.1.2.1 *Gymnoglyphus longior* (Trouessart)

Differential diagnosis: posterior region of opisthonotum not punctate; setae *ps 3* situated at the junction of the anterior third and the posterior two thirds of the anus; setae *h 2* 20-25 µm long; idiosoma 280-290 µm long.

6.4.1.2.2 *Gymnoglyphus osu* Fain et Johnston

Differential diagnosis: only the female of this species is known; posterior region of dorsum (opisthonotum) punctate; setae *a i* situated close to the anterior angle of the anus; setae *h 2* 40-50 µm long; larger species; idiosoma 328-345 µm long; smaller length of the solenidia of tibiae I and II.

6.4.2 Subfamily: Dermatophagoidinae

Differential diagnosis: In both sexes: setae *v i* absent; tegmen absent; cuticle lacking projections as in the genus *Glycyphagus;* cuticle soft, with well-developed striations; striations generally very thin and set close together, only rarely of the striated-punctate type (*Sturnophagoides*); the area separating epimera I exceptionally punctate; setae *sc e* strong and long (except in the genus *Malayoglyphus* where they are short or very short); setae *h 2* and *h 3* long. In females: setae *sc i* never very strong and long; ventral surface of tarsi I and II without projections; epigynium distinctly separated from epimera I; tarsi III and IV lacking apical spines; cuticle soft and finely striated; hysteronotal shield present only in *Sturnophagoides;* posterior lip of vulva (vulvar lip) soft and striated, not punctate and not incised anteriorly (except in *Sturnophagoides* where this lip is punctate, either partly or completely, and incised anteriorly. In males: cuticle soft and striated; setae *sc i* never very strong and very long; tarsi IV normal (not very short); legs III variable; femora III lacking a spur; tarsi IV always without a bifid or trifid subapicoventral spine; tarsi III with or without the subapicoventral spine; adanal copulatory suckers present; tarsal copulatory suckers (on tarsi IV) present (except in *Malayoglyphus*); tarsi III with an apico-ventral forkate spine (except in *Malayoglyphus* and *Sturnophagoides*, where this spine is lacking).

6.4.2.1 Genus: *Sturnophagoides* Fain

Differential diagnosis: In both sexes: striations of the cuticle punctate and more or less sclerotized over a part or all of the body; the region between epimera I completely punctate; setae *sc e*, *h 2* and *h 3* long or very long; setae *c p* very short.

In females: dorsum with a median hysteronotal shield (absent in the other genera of *Dermatophagoidinae*); cuticle striated-punctate over a large part or all of the body; posterior lip of vulva long, punctate (either partially or completely) and incised in its anterior angle (as in some Pyroglyphinae). In males: perianal chitinous frame not denticulate; legs III and IV less unequal; the legs III a maximum of 1.6 times as long as IV; tarsi III either with a subapical conical unforked spine and 5 thin setae or with all setae simple; tarsi IV with 2 small tarsal copulatory suckers; adanal copulatory suckers well developed; legs III distinctly stronger and longer than legs IV; at least tarsus I with an apical process; setae *sc e* strong and long (minimum 110 µm).

6.4.2.1.1 *Sturnophagoides brasiliensis* Fain

In females: small species; idiosoma 246-262 µm long; posterior lip of vulva punctate only in its lateral parts; hysteronotal shield situated inside setae *e 1;* striations behind the hysteronotal shield distinctly thickened, more punctate and more spaced than on other parts of the body; solenidia of genua I very short (10 and 4 µm). In males: idiosoma 175-185 µm long; perianal chitinous frame narrow, oval in shape; tarsi III with an apical curved process, but lacking a subapical spine.

6.4.2.1.2 *Sturnophagoides bakeri Fain*

Differential diagnosis: In females: larger species (idiosoma 390-420 µm long); posterior lip of vulva completely punctate; striations behind the hysteronotal shield not modified; setae *d 1* and *e 1* situated outside the hysteronotal shield; solenidia of genua I 30-35 and 6 µm long, respectively. In males: idiosoma 270-290 µm long; perianal chitinous frame wide, piriform (pear-shaped); tarsi III ending in a conical spine and a curved apical process; hysteronotal shield piriform passing hardly beyond setae *d 1* (heteromorphic males).

6.4.2.1.3 *Sturnophagoides petrochelidonis* Cuervo et Dusbabek

Differential diagnosis: In females: idiosoma 310-379 µm long; posterior lip of vulva completely punctate; striations behind the hysteronotal shield not modified; setae *d 1* and *e 1* situated on the margins of the hysteronotal shield. In males: idiosoma 245-272 µm long; perianal chitinous frame wide, piriform (pear-shaped); tarsi III ending in a conical spine and a curved apical process; hysteronotal shield rectangular, reaching setae *c 1* (heteromorphic males).

6.4.2.2 Genus: *Hirstia* Hull

Differential diagnosis: In both sexes: striations of the cuticle are finer and set closer together; striations are separated by less than 1 µm (at the level of setae *d 1*); more distinct reduction of legs IV compared to legs III. In females: hysteronotum striated, lacking a median shield; cuticle with non-punctate striations; cuticle between epimera I not punctate; posterior lip of vulva smaller and shorter and with anterior angle not incised; legs III distinctly longer (length of the four apical segments - tarsus-femur) and thicker than legs IV; the ratio of the lengths of legs IV / lengths of legs III = 1 : 1.4 (to 1.56); cuticle with very thin striations separated by less than 1 µm (at the level of setae *d 1*). In males: perianal chitinous frame finely denticulate inside; legs III much thicker than legs IV and from 1.8 to 1.9 times longer than the latter (length of the 4 apical segments); tarsi III bearing in their middle 2 strong conical spines (setae *w* and *r*).

6.4.2.2.1. *Hirstia chelidonis* Hull

Differential diagnosis: In both sexes: larger species. In females: idiosoma 395-426 µm long; posterior region of dorsum not punctate and not sclerotized; length of legs III 174 µm, legs

IV 118 μm (= length of 4 apical segments); length of tarsi I-IV = 40-43-66-48 μm. In males: idiosoma 321 to 345 μm long; tarsi I-IV = 33-39-51-24 μm long.

6.4.2.2.2. *Hirstia domicola* Fain, Oshima et van Bronswijk

Differential diagnosis: In females: idiosoma 298-310 μm long; posterior region of dorsum sclerotized and punctate mainly around the bases of setae *h 2* and *h 3;* legs III and IV - 123-129μm and 85-90 μm long, respectively (= length of 4 apical segments); tarsi I-IV = 40-43-66-48 μm long, respectively. In males: idiosoma 240 to 248 μm long; tarsi I-IV shorter, 22-27-32-18 μm long, respectively.

6.4.2.3 Genus: *Malayoglyphus* Fain, Cunnington et Spieksma

Differential diagnosis: In both sexes: short, thin shape of setae of the setae *sc e* ; the normal development of legs IV which are as long as legs III; the presence of only one solenidion on genu I. In females: hysteronotum striated, lacking a median shield; cuticle with non-punctate striations; cuticle between epimera I not punctate; posterior lip of vulva smaller and shorter and with anterior angle not incised; legs III and IV equal or subequal in length and in width; cuticle with dorsal striations more spaced (separated by 1.2 to 2.3 μm at level of setae *d 1*); setae *sc i* and *sc e* thin and short, either equal or suequal, or slightly unequal (*sc e* less than 35 μm long); epigynium poorly developed and slightly sclerotized; genu I with only one very short solenidion (5-6 μm). In males: perianal chitinous frame not denticulate; legs III and legs IV less unequal; the legs III a maximum of 1.6 times as long as legs IV; tarsi III with only thin setae (there is no forked spine on the apex of tarsus III as in *Dermatophagoides*) setae *sc e* thin and short (maximum 30 μm long); adanal copulatory suckers poorly developed (reduced); tarsi I and II without apical processes; legs III and IV subequal; tarsi IV without suckers; tarsus IV bears 3 thin setae and one rounded papilla which is a remnant of a sucker.

6.4.2.3.1 *Malayoglyphus intermedius* Fain, Cunnington et Spieksma

Differential diagnosis: In both sexes: smaller species. In females: idiosoma 218-243 μm long; setae *sc i* and *sc e* equal or subequal (about 12-15 μm long); posterior half of opisthonotum distinctly punctate and with thicker and more spaced striations than on other parts of the dorsum. In males: idiosoma 168 to 175 μm long; setae *sc e* and *sc i* equal or subequal (12-15 μm long); striations of the posterior half of hysteronotum thick, punctate and sclerotized.

6.4.2.3.2. *Malayoglyphus carmelitus* Spieksma

Differential diagnosis: In both sexes: larger species. In females: idiosoma 320-348 μm long; setae *sc e* distinctly longer (30-35 μm) than *sc i* (15 μm); punctation of posterior half of opisthonotum indistinct. In males: idiosoma 240 to 283 μm long; setae *sc e* distinctly longer (30 μm long) than setae *sc i* (15 μm); posterior half of hysteronotum with a large punctate and not striated shield.

6.4.2.4 Genus: *Dermatophagoides* Bogdanov

Differential diagnosis: In both sexes: cuticle with dorsal striations more spaced (separated by 1.2 to 2.3 μm at level of setae *d 1*); setae *sc i* and *sc e* very unequal; the *sc e* long and strong; genu I with 2 very unequal solenidia. In females: hysteronotum striated, lacking a median shield; cuticle with non-punctate striations; cuticle between epimera I not punctate; posterior lip of vulva smaller and shorter and with anterior angle not incised; legs III and IV equal or subequal in length and in width; setae *sc i* and *sc e* very unequal; the *sc e* long and strong; epigynium well developed and sclerotized. In males: perianal chitinous frame not denticulate; legs III distinctly stronger and longer than legs IV; but the legs III a maximum of

1.6 times as long as legs IV; tarsi III with a strong subapical forked (bifid) spine (seta *f*); setae *sc e* minimum 110 μm long; tarsi IV with two small copulatory tarsal suckers; adanal suckers well developed; at least tarsus I with an apical process.

6.4.2.4.1 The *Dermatophagoides pteronyssinus* group

Differential diagnosis: In females: median area comprized between setae *d 1* and *e 1* [= M area] completely striated longitudinally; opening of the bursa copulatrix situated on posterior margin of the body. In males: hysteronotal shield long, reaching forwards to setae *d 1* and/or further in front (anteriorly).

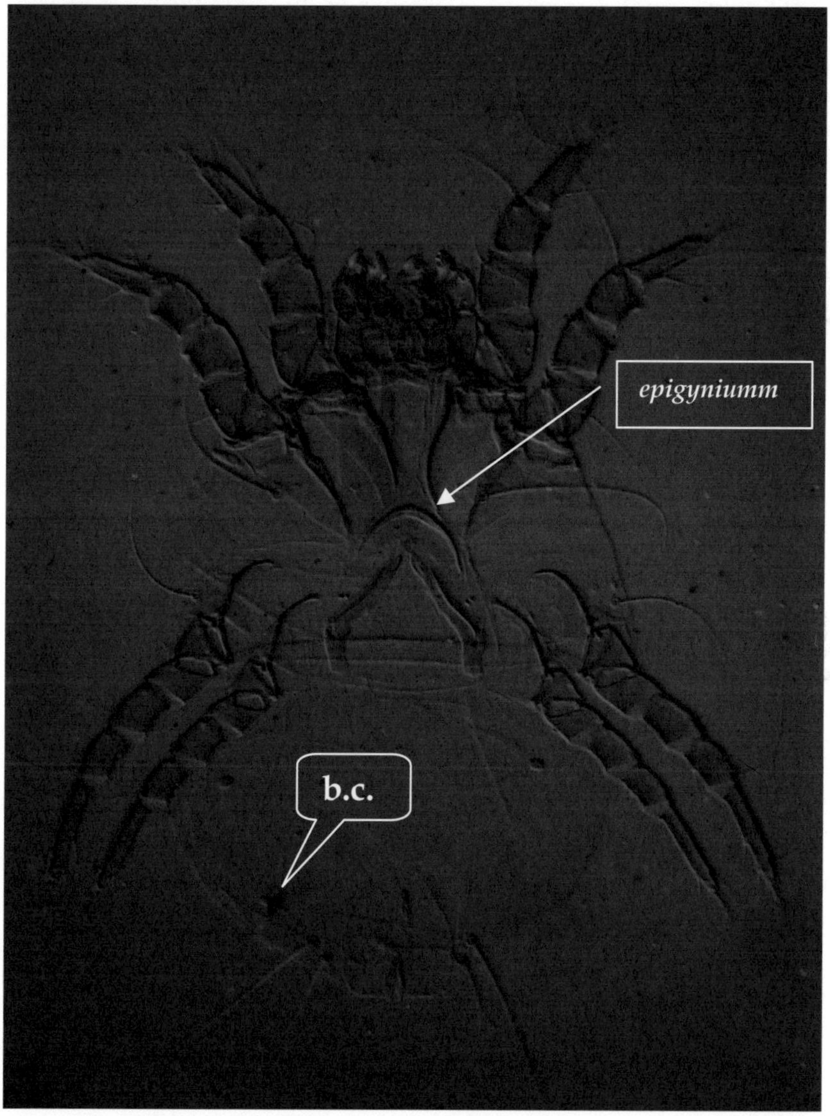

Fig. 6. *Dermatophagoides pteronyssinus*, female - ventral aspect; key: b.c. = sclerite surrounding an internal opening of *bursa copulatrix*; *epigynium* = anterior genital apodeme, pregenital sclerite.

6.4.2.4.1.1. *Dermatophagoides pteronyssinus* (Trouessart)

Differential diagnosis: In females (Fig. 6): bursa copulatrix very narrow, of uniform calibre and ending inside (proximally) in a daisy-like sclerite. In males: hysteronotal shield distinctly extending forward to beyond the bases of setae *d 1;* coxae II closed; adanal suckers 12 µm in diameter; males homeomorphic; epimera I free; tarsi I with 2 unequal apical processes (ongles); tarsus II with a small apical process; legs III 1.3 times thicker (at level of femur) and 1.46 times longer (length of 4 distal segments) than legs IV; setae *h 2* and *h 3* with bases poorly sclerotized; setae *cp* 80-90 µm long; setae *d 2* situated at 40 µm from the opening of the fat gland; the male differs from that of *D. evansi* mainly by: the dorsal shield is shorter and broader than in *D. evansi;* ratio width (at level of *d 1*) : length = 1 : 1.8-1.9 [whilst in *D. evansi* this ratio is 1 : 2.5]; legs III and IV are much less unequal than in *D. evansi.*

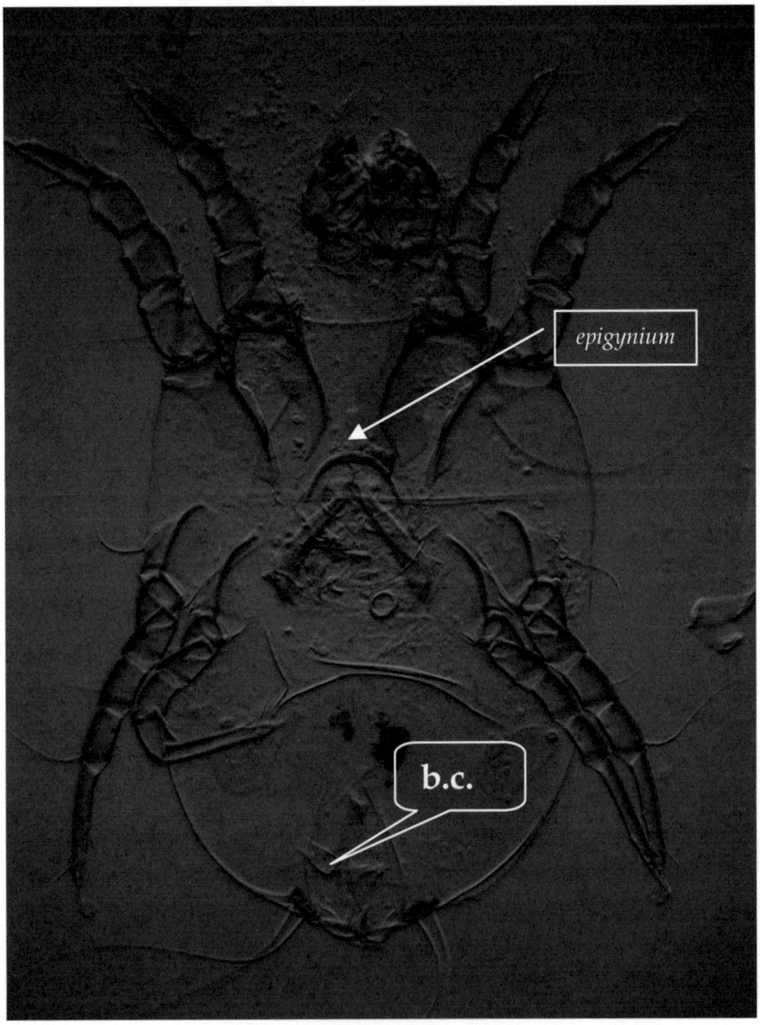

Fig. 7. *Dermatophagoides evansi,* female – ventral aspect; key: b.c. = sclerite surrounding an internal opening of *bursa copulatrix; epigynium* = anterior genital apodeme, pregenital sclerite.

6.4.2.4.1.2 *Dermatophagoides evansi* Fain, Hughes et Johnston

Differential diagnosis: In females (Fig. 7): bursa copulatrix strongly enlarged in its distal third and very narrow in its proximal two thirds (internal); spermatheca sclerotized and tulip-like. In males: hysteronotal shield distinctly extending forward to beyond the bases of setae *d 1;* coxae II closed; adanal suckers 12 μm in diameter; males homeomorphic; epimera I free; tarsi I with 2 unequal apical processes (ongles); tarsus II with a small

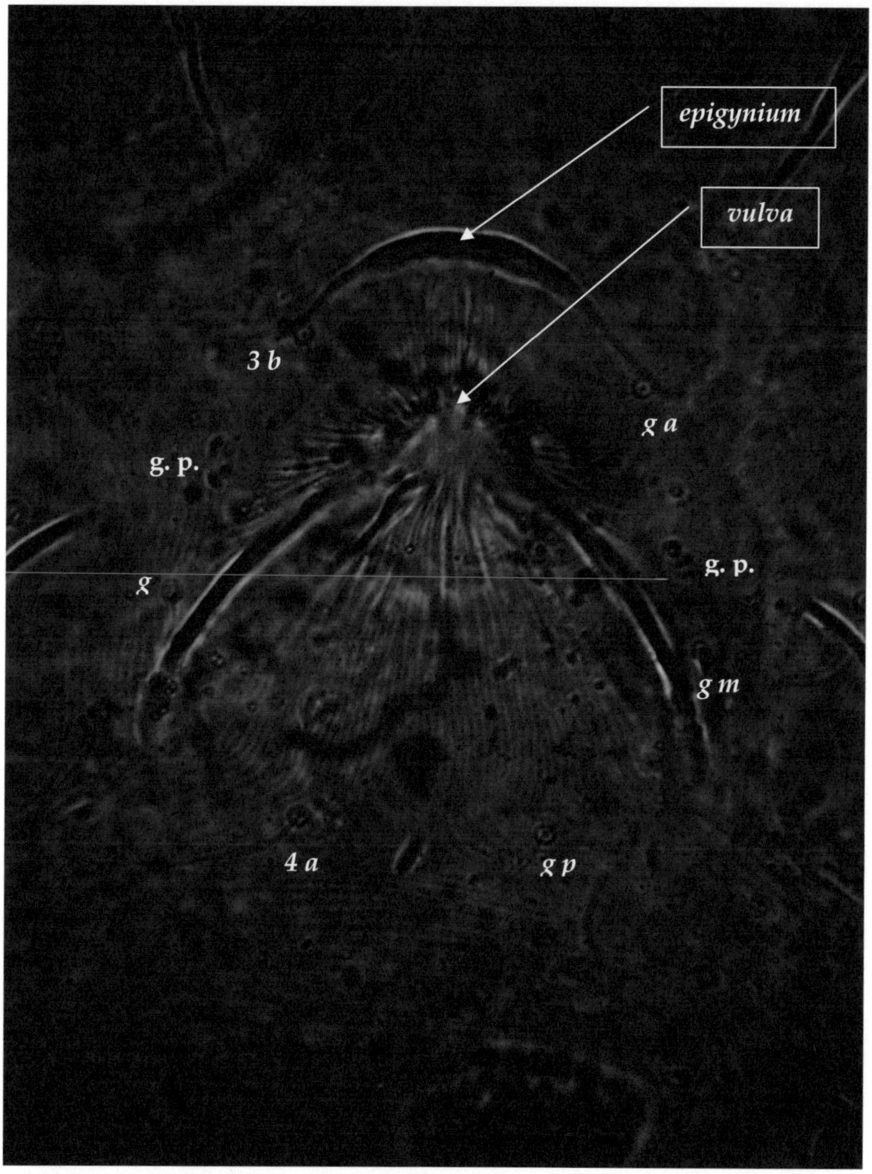

Fig. 8. *Dermatophagoides farinae*, female - ventral aspect, *vulva* and *epigynium* (anterior genital apodeme, pregenital sclerite); genital chaetotaxy: setae *3 b* (or genital anterior setae *g a*), genital setae *g* (or genital median setae *g m*), setae *4 a* (or genital posterior setae *g p*); g. p. = genital papillae.

apical process; legs III 1.8 times thicker (at level of femur) and 1.6 times longer (length of 4 distal segments) than legs IV; setae *h 2* and *h 3* with bases strongly sclerotized; setae *cp* 110 µm long; setae *d 2* situated at 55-65 µm from the opening of the fat gland; the male differs from that of *D. pteronyssinus* mainly by: the dorsal hysterosomal shield is longer and narrower; ratio width (at level of setae *d 1*) : length = 1 : 2.5 [whereas in *D. pteronyssinus* this ratio is 1.8 to 1.9]; legs III and IV are much more unequal than in *D. pteronyssinus.*

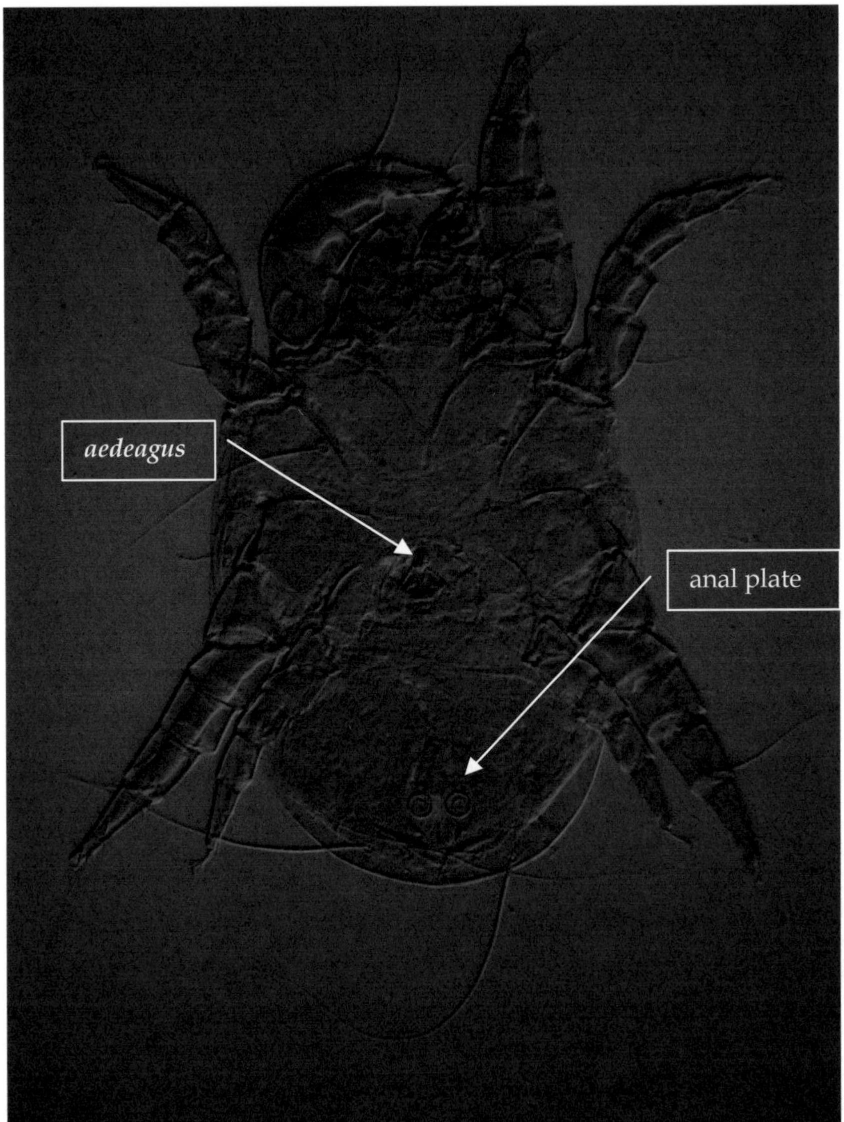

Fig. 9. *Dermatophagoides farinae*, heteromorphic male – ventral aspect.

6.4.2.4.2 The *Dermatophagoides farinae* group

Differential diagnosis: In females: striations of the posterior half of the area M only slightly convex; opening of the bursa situated ventrally on the side of the posterior third of the anus;

first part of the bursa forming (sometimes not) a sclerotized pocket (vestibule). In males: hysteronotal shield short, extending forwards to a point situated at equal distance from setae *d 1* and *e 1*; hysteronotal shield wider than long (in its middle); seta r on tarsus III is thin and situated basally; epimera I free in the homeomorphic male.

6.4.2.4.2.1 *Dermatophagoides siboney* **Dusbabek, Cuervo et Cruz**

Differential diagnosis: In both sexes: small species. In females: idiosoma 258-311 μm long; propodonotal shield approximately twice as long as wide. In males: small species; idiosoma 199-245 μm long; all known males are homeomorphic.

6.4.2.4.2.2 *Dermatophagoides farinae* Hughes

Differential diagnosis: In both sexes: larger species. In females: idiosoma 395 to 435 μm long; propodonotal shield approximately 1.4 times as long as wide; vestibule of bursa well sclerotized and shaped like a calabash pipe; beyond this vestibule the bursa is not expanded; tarsus I generally with well developed curved process (ongle); epigynium crescent-shaped (Fig. 8). In males: idiosoma 285-345 μm long; males either homeomorphic with epimera I free (and normal first legs) or heteromorphic with epimera I fused to form a V or Y (and enlarged I legs) (Fig. 9).

6.4.2.4.2.3. *Dermatophagoides microceras* Griffiths et Cunnington

Differential diagnosis: In females: idiosoma 395 to 435 μm long; propodonotal shield approximately 1.4 times as long as wide; vestibule of bursa lacking, the bursa opens at the bottom of a non-sclerotized depression of the tegumen; the first part of the bursa proper is slightly dilated and distinctly sclerotized; apical process of tarsus I generally very small or lacking. In males: idiosoma 285-345 μm long; males either homeomorphic with epimera I free (and normal first legs) or heteromorphic with epimera I fused to form a V or Y (and enlarged I legs).

7. Phylogenetic reconstructions of the Pyroglyphidae

The family Pyroglyphidae presently consists of 47 species and 20 genera, whose species are associated with birds, mammals or house dust and stored products (Mumcuoglu et al., 1976; Fain et al., 1990; Evans, 1992; Colloff, 2009; Krantz and Walter, 2009; Solarz, 2004b, 2011). The majority of these species are nidicolous, with bird associates outnumbering mammal associates. They are associated with many avian groups, but most of them are nidicoles of Passeriformes. These mites feed on animal detritus and/or dander in the nests and have given rise to several more typically parasitic taxa (Fain et al., 1990). The Pyroglyphidae are small mites, whitish in colour; the length of idiosoma of adults ranges from 168 μm (*Malayoglyphus intermedius*) to 585 μm (*Onychalges longitarsus*). The idiosoma is generally oval in shape with parallel sides, and broadly rounded anterior and posterior margins. The degree of the cuticle sclerotization is variable; in some subfamilies or genera it is almost completely sclerotized, without true striations, whereas in others the cuticle is soft and striated, in which case the dorsal shields are more poorly developed. Morphology and biology of the pyroglyphids seems to indicate that the free-living forms have evolved from obligate parasitic ancestors (OConnor, 1982; Woolley, 1988). These mites morphologically show some characters of parasitic Psoroptidia, particularly a regression of legs IV (especially in males), dorsal shields (mainly the hysterosomal), copulatory suckers (vestigial or reduced, in the shape of small sclerotized rings), tarsal claws (only in the form of a small median axis). On the other hand, it has been suggested by Fain (Fain et al. 1990) that in the Pyroglyphidae the regression of the organs has preceeded the invasion of the host as if there were a preadaptation. This regression involves also an idiosomal and leg chaetotaxy. Pyroglyphids have 8 setae on tarsi I and on II, and 1 seta on each of tibiae I and II, whereas in the Acaridae there are 13 and 12 tarsal setae on tarsi I and II, respectively, and 2 tibial setae on tibiae I and II. Vertical setae are generally absent; thus, the scapular setae (*sc e* and *sc i*) are the first pair, most anteriorly located. The absence of setae *v e* is the typical feature of the Pyroglyphidae; whereas setae *v i* occur only in the members of the genus *Paralgopsis* (subfamily Paralgopsinae). The external scapulars (*sc e*) are longer, more or less, as the internal setae (*sc i*). Female have only 2 pairs of adanal setae (*ps 2* and *ps 3*), whereas females of the family Acaridae have 5-6 pairs of anal/adanal setae. Phylogeny basically means, the history of the tribe. Reconstructing a phylogeny is similar to compiling a genealogic tree in that both indicate the degree of relatedness between the members of the tribe, or other taxon. However, the family tree is based on known fact and documentary evidence, whereas a phylogeny is only ever, at best, an hypothesis of the most likely evolutionary history of the taxon (Colloff, 1998). There has been no detailed phylogenetic revision of the family Pyroglyphidae to date. In opinion of Colloff (1998), the host relationships of pyroglyphid mites with birds indicate that the two subfamilies which contain species found in house dust, the Pyroglyphinae and Dermatophagoidinae, are the most widespread geographically and the most species-rich. They are associated with a higher diversity of avian taxa than the other subfamilies, that do not contain the house-dust-mite species (Colloff, 1998). Indeed, the Pyroglyphidae probably form a link between the free living and parasitic Astigmatina. It was also shown that some pyroglyphids are able to adopt a parasitic mode of life and feeding (Fain et al., 1990; Proctor, 2003; Dabert et al., 2010). But mites of this family are perhaps best known as the house dust mites, because of their occurrence in human dwellings. Main sources of the mite allergens in dwellings usually are beds, couches or sofas in bedrooms and couches or sofas in living-rooms (family rooms). New dwellings might be colonized via mite-infested furniture, by humans, on skin, clothing, or by their pets (Hewitt et al., 1973; Hoeven et al., 1992; Perotti et al., 2009) The natural sources of allergenic mites in stores are still not quiet known (Hallas & Iversen, 1996; Solarz et al., 2007; Hallas, 2010). Possible sources of these mites in farming environments are also the nests of synanthropic birds (Hughes, 1976; Wharton, 1976; van Bronswijk, 1981; Fain et al., 1990; Solarz et al., 1999). On the other hand, it has been suggested that the majority of the mite population is brought from the cultivated field into the stores, and that the open field is the main source of storage-mite populations (Hallas & Iversen, 1996), whereas the bird nests are less important (Solarz, 2003).

Indoor acarofauna depends on the people living and working in these buildings. Different indoor environments are very important places for forensic investigations, but the richness of mite biodiversity, phylogenetic relationships between different groups of domestic mites and their associations with potential hosts has not been exploited by forensic investigators. Summarizing it should be stressed that knowledge about occurrence of particular species of parasitic and/or synanthropic mites on man or in human environment as well as the correct identification of mites colonising dead body are very important factors in forensic investigations of past human activity (Perotti, 2009b; Braig & Perotti, 2009; Perotti & Braig, 2009; OConnor, 2009; Turner, 2009; Solarz, 2009; Desch, 2009; Baker, 2009, Proctor, 2009).

8. Domestic mites and forensic medicine. Final remarks

More than 100 species of mites from over 60 families were collected from animal carcases, and approximately 75 mite species from over 20 families from human corpses (Braig & Perotti, 2009), including also the astigmatid mite taxa. Within the Astigmatina were involved some domestic mite species such as *Acarus siro, A. farris, A. immobilis, Tyrophagus longior, T. putrescentiae, Tyrolichus casei, Caloglyphus berlesei, Rhizoglyphus echinopus, Lardoglyphus* spp. and *Lepidoglyphus destructor*. Among them from human carcases were noted *Myianoetus diadematus* (mass population), *C. berlesei* (many), *A. siro* (common), *A. immobilis* (common), *T. longior* (abundant), *T. putrescentiae* (common and abundant) and *L. destructor* (very rare) (Braig & Perotti, 2009). *Tyrophagus longior* is particularly active at lower temperatures. This mite is almost always associated with dry cheese and/or meat. It was known to feed on the fatty acids and soapy substances containing ammonia that form on carcasses during dry decomposition (Perotti et al., 2009). In 1878 these mites were found in the mummified body of a newborn baby girl in Paris and they were studied by Mégnin. He estimated and identified approximately 2.4 million specimens of *T. longior* in this material (Perotti, 2009). In a more recent case reported from Germany a child corpse found in a basement was also associated with a mass populations of *Myianoetus diadematus, A. immobilis* and *T. putrescentiae* (OConnor, 2009; Braig & Perotti, 2009). Mites originating from outdoor environments can also be useful trace evidence and give accurate evidence about movements or transportation of a body (Perotti et al., 2009). Many mite species arrive at a carcase via phoresy on insects. The phoresy is often taxon specific (Braig and Perotti, 2009). Phoretic hypopi (heteromorphic deutonymphs) are known in *Acarus farris, A. siro, Caloglyphus berlesei, Rhizoglyphus echinopus* and *Myianoetus diadematus.* Summarizing, it should be stressed that the astigmatid mites have played little role in the field of forensic medicine to date (OConnor, 2009). Domestic mites have not yet been explored in forensic investigations, but there is every reason for doing this. Dust mites and other domestic mites are globally present, yet species composition may vary between seasons, between dwellings and even places within a single indoor environment (e.g., beds vs. floors, floors vs. upholstery furniture, or dust from a book shelve vs. a librarian's desk) (Solarz, 2009). Subtle differences in the house-dust-mite acarofauna between sites may yield valuable information, for instance as indicator of time and circumtances of death (Solarz 2009; Perotti, 2009).

9. Acknowledgements

The morphological studies received support from the Synthesys Projects BE-TAF-5061 and BE-TAF- 557 which were financed by the European Community Research Infrastructure Action. This work was also supported in part by the Medical University of Silesia in Katowice through grant number KNW-1-029/P/1/0.

10. References

Arlian, L.G. (2001). Dust mites: Update on their allergens and control. *Current Allergy and Asthma Reports*, Vol.1, No.6, (November 2001), pp. 581-586, ISSN 1529-7322

Arlian, L.G. (2002). Arthropod allergens and human health. *Annual Review of Entomology*, Vol.47, (January 2002), pp. 395-433, ISSN 0066-4170

Arlian, L.G. & Platts-Mills, T.A.E. (2001). The biology of dust mites and the remediation of mite allergens in allergic disease. *Journal of Allergy and Clinical Immunology*, Vol.107, No.3, (March 2001), pp. 406-413, ISSN 00917-6749

Arlian, L.G.; Morgan, M.S. & Houck, M.A. (1999). Allergenicity of the mite *Hemisarcoptes cooremani*. *Annals of Allergy, Asthma and Immunology*, Vol.83, No.6, (December 1999), pp. 529-532, ISSN 1081-1206

Arlian, L.G.; Morgan, M. S. & Neal, J. S. (2002). Dust mite allergens: ecology and distribution. *Current Allergy and Asthma Reports*, Vol.2, No.5, (September 2002), pp. 401-41, ISSN 1529-7322

Arlian, L.G.; Morgan, M.S. & Peterson, K.T. (2008). House dust and storage mite extracts influence skin keratinocyte and fibroblast function. *International Archives of Allergy and Immunology*, Vol.145, No.1, (December 2007), pp. 33-42, ISSN 1018-2438

Arlian, L.G.; Vyszenski-Moher, D.A.L.; Ahmed, S.G. & Estes, S.A. (1991). Cross-antigenicity between the scabies mite, *Sarcoptes scabiei*, and the house dust mite, *Dermatophagoides pteronyssinus*. *Journal of Investigational Dermatology*, Vol.96, No.3, (March 1991), pp. 349-354, ISSN 0022-202X

Arlian, L.G.; Vyszenski-Moher, D. L.; Johansson, S.G.O. & van Hage-Hamsten, M. (1997). Allergenic characterization of *Tyrophagus putrescentiae* using sera from occupationally exposed farmers. *Annals of Allergy, Asthma and Immunology*, Vol.79, No.6, (December 1997), pp. 525-529, ISSN1081-1206

Arlian, L.G.; Confer, P.D.; Rapp, C.M.; Vyszenski-Moher, D.A.L. & Chang, J.S.C. (1998). Population dynamics of the house dust mites *Dermatophagoides farinae, D. pteronyssinus*, and *Euroglyphus maynei* (Acari: Pyroglyphidae) at specific relative humidities. *Journal of Medical Entomology*, Vol.35, No.1, (January 1998), pp. 46-53, ISSN 0022-2585

Baker, A.S. (1999). *Mites and ticks of domesic animals. An identification guide and information source*. The Stationery Office, ISBN 0 11 310049 3, London, UK

Baker, A.S. (2009). Acari in archeology. *Experimental and Applied Acarology*, Vol.49, No.1-2, (September-October 2009), pp. 147-160, 45-84, ISSN 0168-8162

Braig, H.R. & Perotti, M.A. (2009). Carcasses and mites. *Experimental and Applied Acarology*, Vol.49, No.1-2, (September- October 2009), pp. 45-84, ISSN 0168-8162

Bronswijk, J.E.M.H., van (1981). *House dust biology (for allergists, acarologists and mycologists)*. N.I.B. Publishers, ISBN 90 275 3501 9, Zoelmond, The Netherlands

Colloff, M.J. (1998). Taxonomy and identification of dust mites. *Allergy*, Vol.53, No.Suppl.48, (December 1998), pp. 7-12, ISSN 0105-4538

Colloff, M.J. (2009). *Dust mites*. Springer Science + Business Media B.V., ISBN 978-90-481-2223-3, Dordrecht, The Netherlands

Dabert, M.; Witalinski, W.; Kazmierski, A.; Olszanowski, Z. & Dabert, J. (2010). Molecular phylogeny of acariform mites (Acari, Arachnida): Strong conflict between phylogenetic signal and long-branch attraction artifacts. *Molecular Phylogenetics and Evolution*, Vol.56, No.1, (July 2010), pp. 222-241, ISSN 1055-7903

Desch, C.E. (2009). Human hair follicle mites and forensic acarology. *Experimental and Applied Acarology*, Vol.49, No.1-2, (September-October 2009), pp. 143-146, ISSN 0168-8162

Evans, G.O. (1992). *Principles of Acarology*. CABI, ISBN 0 851 98-822-9, Wallingford, UK

Fain, A.; Guerin, B. & Hart, B.J. (1990). *Mites and allergic disease*. Allerbio, ISBN 90-71868-12-5, Varennes en Argonne, France

Fernández-Caldas, E. ; Iraola, V. & Carnés, J. (2007). Molecular and biochemical properties of storage mites (except *Blomia* species). *Protein and Peptide Letters*, Vol.14, No.10, (October 2007), pp. 954-959, ISSN 0929-8665

Franz, J.T.; Masuch, G.; Müsken, H. & Bergmann, K.C. (1997). Mite fauna of German farms. *Allergy*, Vol.52, No.12, (December 1997), pp. 1233-1237, ISSN 0105-4538

Hage-Hamsten, M. van & Johansson, S.G.O. (1998). Clinical and immunologic aspects of storage mite allergy. *Allergy*, Vol.53, No. Suppl.48, (December 1998), pp. 49-53, ISSN 0105-4538

Hage-Hamsten, M. van; Scheynius, A.; Harfast, B.; Wiren, A. & Johansson, S.G.O. (1992). Localization of allergens in the domestic mite *Lepidoglyphus destructor*. *Clinical and Experimental Allergy*, Vol.22, No.2, (February 1992), pp.251-256, ISSN 1365-2222

Hallas, T.E. (2010). House-dust mites in our homes are a contamination from outdoor sources. *Medical Hypotheses*, Vol.74, No.5, (May 2010), pp. 777–779, ISSN 0306-9677

Hallas, T.E. & Iversen, M. (1996). Sources of exposure to storage mites in the farming environment. *Annals of Agricultural and Environmental Medicine*, Vol.3, No.1, pp. 9-12, ISSN 1232-1966

Hallas, T. E. & Korsgaard, J. (1997). Systematic variations in the appearance of house-dust mites (*Dermatophagoides* spp.), house mites (*Glycyphagus domesticus*) and of *Tarsonemus* sp. in dust samples from dwellings. *Revista Española de Alergologia e Immunologia Clinica*, Vol.12, No.4, (Junio 1997), pp. 173-177, ISSN 0214-2139

Harving, H.; Korsgaard, J. & Dahl, R. (1993). House-dust mites and associated environmental conditions in Danish homes. *Allergy*, Vol.48, No2., (February 1993), pp. 106–109, ISSN 0105-4538

Hewitt, M.; Barrow, G.I.; Miller, D.C.; Turk, F. & Turk, S. (1973). Mites in the personal environment and their role in skin disorders. *British Journal of Dermatology*, Vol.89, No.4, (October 1973), pp. 401-409, ISSN 0007-0963

Hoeven, W.A.D. van der; de Boer, R. & Bruin, J. (1992) The colonisation of new houses by house dust mites (Acari: Pyroglyphidae). *Experimental and Applied Acarology*, Vol.16, No.1-2, (November 1992), pp. 75-84, ISSN 0168-8162

Horak, B.; Dutkiewicz, J. & Solarz, K. (1996). Microflora and acarofauna of bed dust from homes in Upper Silesia, Poland. *Annals of Allergy, Asthma, and Immunology*, Vol.76, No.1, (January 1996), pp. 41-50, ISSN 1081-1206

Hughes, A.M. (1976). *The mites of stored food and houses*. H.M.S.O., ISBN 0 11 240909 1, London, UK

Kim, Y.K.; Lee, M.H.; Jee, Y.K.; Hong, S.C.; Bae, J.M.; Chang, Y.S.; Jung, J.W.; Lee, B.J.; Son, J.W.; Cho, S.H.; Min, K.U. & Kim, Y.Y. (1999). Spider mite allergy in apple-cultivating farmers: European red mite (*Panonychus ulmi*) and two-spotted spider mite (*Tetranychus urticae*) may be important allergens in the development of work-related asthma and rhinitis symptoms. *Journal of Allergy and Clinical Immunology*, Vol.104, No.6, (December 1999), pp. 1285-1292, ISSN 00917-6749

Klimov, P.B. & OConnor, B.M. (2009). Conservation of the name Tyrophagus putrescentiae, a medically and economically important mite species (Acari: Acaridae). *International Journal of Acarology*, Vol.35, No.2, (01 April 2009), pp. 95-114, ISSN 0164-7954

Korsgaard, J. (1998). Epidemiology of house-dust mites. *Allergy*, Vol.53, No.Suppl.48, (December 1998), pp. 36-40, ISSN 0105-4538

Krantz, G.W. & Walter, D.E. (2009). A manual of acarology. Third edition. Texas Tech. University Press, ISBN 978-0-89672- 620-8, Lubbock, USA

Kronqvist, M.; Johansson, E.; Magnusson, C.G.M.; Olsson, S.; Eriksson, T.L.J.; Gafvelin, G. & van Hage-Hamsten, M. (2000). Skin prick test and serological analysis with recombinant group 2 allergens of the dust mites *L. destructor* and *T. putrescentiae*. *Clinical and Experimental Allergy*, Vol.30, No.5, (May 2000), pp. 670-676, ISSN 1365-2222

Lee, M.H.; Cho, S.H.; Park, H.S.; Bahn, J.W.; Lee, B.J.; Son, J.W.; Kim, Y.K.; Koh, Y.Y.; Min, K.U. & Kim, Y.Y. (2000). Citrus red mite (*Panonychus citri*) is a common sensitizing allergen among children living around citrus orchards. *Annals of Allergy, Asthma and Immunology*, Vol.85, No.3, (September 2000), pp. 200-204, ISSN 1081-1206

Mehl, R. (1998). Occurrence of mites in Norway and the rest of Scandinavia. *Allergy*, Vol.53, No. Suppl.48, (December 1998), pp. 28-35, ISSN 0105-4538

Morgan, M.S. & Arlian, L.G. (2006). Enzymatic activity in extracts of allergy-causing astigmatid mites. *Journal of Medical Entomology*, Vol.43, No.6, (November 2006), pp. 1200-1207, ISSN 1938-2928

Mumcuoglu, Y. (1976). House dust mites in Switzerland. I. Distribution and taxonomy. *Journal of Medical Entomology,* Vol.13, No.3, (8 December 1976), pp. 361-373, ISSN 0022-2585

Mumcuoglu, K.Y.; Gat, Z.; Horowitz, T.; Miller, J.; Bartana, R.; Benzvi, A. & Naparstek, Y. 1999. Abundance of house dust mites in relation to climate in contrasting agricultural settlements in Israel. *Medical and Veterinary Entomology*, Vol.13, No.3, (September 1999), pp. 252-258; 0269-283X

Müsken, H.; Franz, J.T.; Wahl, R.; Paap, A.; Cromwell, O.; Masuch, G. & Bergmann, K.C. (2000). Sensitization to different mite species in German farmers: clinical aspects. *Journal of Investigational Allergology and Clinical Immunology,* Vol.10, No.6, (November-December 2000), pp. 346-351, ISSN 1018-9068

OConnor, B.M. (1982). Evolutionary ecology of astigmatid mites. *Annual Review of Entomology*, Vol.27, (January 1982), pp. 385-409, ISSN 0066-4170

OConnor, B.M. (2009). Astigmatid mites (Acari: Sarcoptiformes) of forensic interest. *Experimental and Applied Acarology,* Vol.49, No. 1-2, (September-October 2009), pp. 125-133, ISSN 0168-8162

Perotti, M.A. (2009a). Preface. *Experimental and Applied Acarology,* Vol.49, No. 1-2, (September-October 2009), pp. 1-2, ISSN 0168-8162

Perotti, M.A. (2009b). Mégnin re-analysed: the case of the newborn baby girl, Paris, 1878. *Experimental and Applied Acarology,* Vol.49, No. 1-2, (September-October 2009), pp. 37-44, ISSN 0168-8162

Perotti, M.A. & Braig, H.R. (2009). Phoretic mites associated with animal and human decomposition. *Experimental and Applied Acarology,* Vol.49, No. 1-2, (September-October 2009), pp. 85-124, ISSN 0168-8162

Perotti, M.A.; Goff, M.L.; Baker, A.S.; Turner, B.D. & Braig, H. R. (2009). Forensic acarology: an introduction. *Experimental and Applied Acarology,* Vol.49, No. 1-2, (September-October 2009), pp. 3-13, ISSN 0168-8162

Platts-Mills, T.A.E.; Thomas, W.R.; Aalberse, R.C.; Vervloet, D. and Chapman, M.D. (1992). Dust mite allergens and asthma: Report of a Second International Workshop. *Journal of Allergy and Clinical Immunology,* Vol.89, No.5, (May 1992), pp. 1046-1060, ISSN 00917-6749

Pope, A.M., Patterson, R., Burge, H., 1993. *Indoor allergens. Assessing and controlling adverse health effects.* National Academy Press, ISBN0-309-04831-1, Washington, USA

Proctor, H.C. (2003). Feather mites (Acari: Astigmata): Ecology, behavior, and evolution. *Annual Review of Entomology*, Vol.48, (January 2003), pp. 185-209, ISSN 0066-4170

Proctor, H.C. (2009). Can freshwater mites act as forensic tools? *Experimental and Applied Acarology*, Vol.49, No.1-2, (September-October 2009), pp. 161-165, 45-84, ISSN 0168-8162

Puerta, L.; Fernández-Caldas, E.; Lockey, R.F. & Caraballo, L. (1993). Mite allergy in the tropics: Sensitization to six domestic mite species in Cartagena, Colombia. *Journal of Investigational Allergology and Clinical Immunology*, Vol.3, No.4, (July-August 1993), pp. 198-204, ISSN 1018-9068

Racewicz, M. (2001). House dust mites (Acari: Pyroglyphidae) in the cities of Gdańsk and Gdynia (Northern Poland). *Annals of Agricultural and Environmental Medicine*, Vol.8, No.1, pp. 33-38, ISSN 1232-1966

Rosen, S.; Yeruham, I. & Braverman, Y. (2002). Dermatitis in humans associated with the mites *Pyemotes tritici*, *Deramnyssus gallinae*, *Ornithonyssus bacoti* and *Androlaelaps casalis* in Israel. *Medical and Veterinary Entomology*, Vol.16, No.4, (December 2002), pp. 442-444, 0269-283X

Silva da Ezequiel, O.; Gazêta, G.S.; Amorim, M. & Serra-Freire, N.M. (2001). Evaluation of the acarofauna of the domiciliary ecosystem in Juiz de Fora, State of Minas Gerais, Brazil. *Memórias do Instituto Oswaldo Cruz*, Vol.96, No.7, (October 2001), pp. 911-916, ISSN 00740276

Solarz, K. (1998). The allergenic acarofauna of house dust from dwellings, hospitals, libraries and institutes in Upper Silesia (Poland). *Annals of Agricultural and Environmental Medicine*, Vol. 5, No.1, pp. 73-85, ISSN 1232-1966

Solarz, K. (2001a). Risk of exposure to house dust pyroglyphid mites in Poland. *Annals of Agricultural and Environmental Medicine*, Vol.8, No.1, pp. 11-24, ISSN 1232-1966

Solarz, K. (2001b). Pyroglyphidae (Acari : Astigmata) in Poland. Distribution, biology, population ecology and epidemiology. *Acta Zoologica Cracoviensia*, Vol.44, No.4, pp. 435-528, ISSN 0065-1710

Solarz, K. (2003). Pyroglyphidae (Acari: Acaridida) in Poland: distribution, biology, population ecology and epidemiology. Risk of exposure to house dust pyroglyphid mites in Poland. *Annales Academiae Medicae Silesiensis*, Suppl.82, pp. 1-244, ISSN 0208-5607

Solarz, K. (2004a). Distribution and ecology of allergenic mites in Poland. *Phytophaga*, Vol.14, pp. 675-694, ISSN 0393-8131

Solarz, K. (2004b). Revision of immature stages of mites from the family Pyroglyphidae. *Annales Academiae Medicae Silesiensis*, Suppl.52, pp. 1-300, ISSN 0208-5607

Solarz, K. (2006). Allergenic mites in habitats associated with man. *Biological Letters*, Vol.43, No.2, pp. 299-306, ISSN 1644- 7700

Solarz, K. (2009). Indoor mites and forensic acarology. *Experimental and Applied Acarology*, Vol.49, No. 1-2, (September- October 2009), pp. 135-142, ISSN 0168-8162

Solarz, K. (2010). Temporal changes in the composition of house-dust-mite fauna in Poland. *Acta Zoologica Cracoviensia*, Vol.53B, No.1-2, pp. 39-64, ISSN 1895-3131

Solarz, K. (2011). *Domestic and storage mites. An identification guide and diagnoses of taxa.* Medical University of Silesia in Katowice, Advert Studio, ISBN 978-83-7509-161-8, Ruda Slaska, Poland

Solarz, K. & Solarz, D. (1996). The allergenic mites in coal-mine dust from coal mines in Upper Silesia (Poland). *Annals of Agricultural and Environmental Medicine*, Vol.3, No.1, pp. 49-55, ISSN 1232-1966

Solarz, K.; Szilman, P. & Szilman, E. (1997). Preliminary study on the occurrence and species composition of astigmatic mites (Acari: Astigmata) in samples of dust, debris and residues from farming environments in Poland. *Annals of Agricultural and Environmental Medicine,* Vol.4, No.2, pp. 249-252, ISSN 1232-1966

Solarz, K.; Szilman, P. & Szilman, E. (1999). Allergenic mites associated with bird nests in Poland (Astigmata: Pyroglyphidae, Acaridae, Glycyphagidae), In: *Ecology and Evolution of the Acari,* J. Bruin, L.P.S. Van der Geest & M.W. Sabelis, [Eds], 651-656, Kluwer Academic Publishers, ISSN 1438-4639, Dordrecht, The Netherlands

Solarz, K.; Szilman, P. & Szilman, E. (2004a). Occupational exposure to Allergenic Mites in a Polish ZOO. *Annals of Agricultural and Environmental Medicine,* Vol.11, No.1, pp. 1–7, ISSN 1232-1966

Solarz, K.; Senczuk, L.; Maniurka, H.; Cichecka, E. & Peszke, M. (2007). Comparisons of the allergenic mite prevalence in dwellings and certain outdoor environments of the Upper Silesia (southwest Poland). *International Journal of Hygiene and Environmental Health,* Vol.210, No.6, (3 December 2007), pp. 715-724, ISSN 1438-4639

Solarz, K.; Szilman, P.; Szilman, E.; Krzak, M. & Jagła, A. (2004b). Some allergenic species of astigmatid mites (Acari, Acaridida) from different synanthropic environments in southern Poland. *Acta Zoologica Cracoviensia,* Vol.47, No. 3-4, pp. 125-145, ISSN 0065-1710

Spiewak, R.; Bozek, A.; Solarz, K.; Maslowski, T. & Brewczynski, P.Z. (1995). Das Prurigo-Asthma Syndrom infolge beruflicher Exposition gegen Mehlallergene [Occupational prurigo-asthma syndrome caused by exposure to flour allergens]. *Allergologie,* Vol.18, No.3, pp. 102-106, ISSN 0344-5062

Stejskal, V & Hubert, J. (2008). Risk of occupational allergy to stored grain arthropods and false pest-risk perception in Czech grain stores. *Annals of Agricultural and Environmental Medicine,* Vol.15, No.1, (June 2008), pp. 29-35, ISSN 1232- 1966

Szilman, E.; Szilman, P.; Solarz, K.; Brewczyński, P. & Sieroń, A.L. (2004). Sensitization to the storage mite *Tyrophagus putrescentiae* in urban population of Upper Silesia (Poland). *Wiadomosci Parazytologiczne,* Vol.50, No.3, pp. 471-476, ISSN 0043-5163

Turner, B. (2009). Forensic entomology: a template for forensic acarology? *Experimental and Applied Acarology,* Vol.49, No. 1-2, (September-October 2009), pp. 15-20, ISSN 0168-8162

Voorhorst, R.; Spieksma, F.T.M. & Varekamp, H. (1969). *House-dust atopy and the house-dust mite Dermatophagoides pteronyssinus Trouessart, 1897).* Stafleu's Scientific Publishing Co., Leiden, The Netherlands

Wharton, G.W. (1976). House dust mites. *Journal of Medical Entomology,* Vol.12, No.6, (20 February 1976), pp. 577-621, ISSN 0022-2585

Wooley, T.A. (1988). Acarology: mites and human welfare. John Wiley and Sons, Inc., ISBN 0-471-04168-8, New York, USA

16

Types and Subtypes of the Posterior Part of the Cerebral Arterial Circle in Human Adult Cadavers

Ljiljana Vasović[1], Milena Trandafilović[2], Ivan Jovanović[1], Slađana Ugrenović[1], Slobodan Vlajković[1] and Jovan Stojanović[3]
University of Niš,
[1-3]Faculty of Medicine,
[1]Department of Anatomy,
[3]Institute of Forensic Medicine
Serbia

1. Introduction

The main cerebral distribution center of 15-20% blood flow from the cardiac output is the cerebral arterial circle or circle of Willis, a nonagon of collateral vessels on the human brain base.

At about 4 mm stage of the embryo, the primitive internal carotid arteries, which develop as cranial extensions of the paired dorsal aorta, are formed. Paired longitudinal neural arteries appear along the hindbrain and coalesce to form the basilar trunk at the 7- to 12-mm stage. The caudal division of the primitive internal carotid artery anastomoses with ipsilateral neural artery and becomes the posterior communicating artery. At the 40-mm stage the posterior cerebral arteries are as extensions of the posterior communicating arteries. The vertebrobasilar system develops and thus participates in the supply of the posterior cerebral artery through the segment between the basilar artery and the post-communicating part of the posterior cerebral artery. In that phase, the component vessels of the circle of Willis all have the same caliber (Silver & Wilkins, 1991).

The posterior cerebral artery originates from the basilar bifurcation within the interpeduncular cistern. From its origin the artery curves superior to the corresponding oculomotor nerve in relation to the antero-medial portion of the cerebral peduncle and joins ipsilateral posterior communicating artery (Yasargil, 1984).

The posterior communicating artery takes origin from the infero-lateral wall of the cerebral part of the internal carotid artery. It is encased in a sleeve of arachnoid along the course from the carotid cistern to the piercing of the interpeduncular cistern and junction with posterior cerebral artery (Yasargil, 1984).

Topographically, the circle of Willis is divided on anterior and posterior parts. The anterior part composes five vascular components - bilateral cerebral parts of internal carotid arteries (communicating and choroid subparts) and the pre-communicating part of anterior cerebral arteries interconnected by the anterior communicating artery; the posterior part composes four vascular components. As a rule, the posterior part of the circle of Willis is normal as it is formed with posterior communicating artery and the pre-communicating part of the posterior cerebral artery on both sides, where the left and right pre-communicating parts of the posterior cerebral arteries have normal calibres which are larger in relation to posterior communicating arteries, as well as that posterior communicating arteries are not hypoplastic (Saeki & Rhoton, 1977). In the fetal period, the posterior circle part develops into one of three variants: an adult configuration, a transitional configuration or a fetal configuration (Silver & Wilkins, 1991).

It has been assumed that the arrangement of the arteries at the base of the brain is symmetrical and that the architecture of the circle of Willis provides a structural basis for free anastomotic flow (Riggs & Rupp, 1963). The collateral potential of the circle of Willis is believed to be dependent with the presence and size of its component vessels, which vary among normal individuals. The anterior communicating artery and posterior communicating arteries are designated as primary collateral pathways (Hartkamp et al., 1999). The integrity of the circle of Willis may be critical because anomalies and hypoplasia of the circle of Willis are frequent (Merkkola et al., 2006). Anomalies found in a pattern of the posterior part of the circle of Willis result due to persistence of vessels that normally disappear or disappearance of normal vessels (Vasović, 2004; Kapoor et al., 2008; Vasović et al., 2010). Although the association of variations and aneurysms had been used as an argument in favor of a congenital theory of aneurismal development, it should be interpreted in terms of the hemodynamic stress caused by variations (Kayembe et al., 1984). However, a significantly higher percentage of complete posterior circle configurations were demonstrated on magnetic resonance angiograms in some patients rather than in the controlled subjects (Hartkamp et al., 1999). The size and patency of primary collateral pathways may be risk factors for cerebral infarction in patients with severe stenosis or occlusion of a carotid artery (Schomer et al., 1994).

The purpose of the present morphologic study is to obtain wider, more precise and more detailed information about the relationship between caliber variations in the posterior part of the circle of Willis forming different (sub) types of its posterior part, as well as to compare those results with previous literature data.

2. Material and methods

Examination was carried out on the brains of human adult cadavers, during the period between 2006 and 2010. Approval was granted by the Research Ethics Committee (No. 01-9068-1) of the Faculty of Medicine of Niš. All subjects had died from natural or violent death and were candidates for autopsy for medico-legal reasons in Institute of Forensic Medicine of Niš, Serbia. The brain base with blood vessels was photographed on each cadaver; the ventral side of the brainstem and diencephalon was specially zoomed. Each case was recorded as the schematic drawing in the workbook. External morphology (calibre of the arteries, possible abnormalities) was inspected using magnifying glass. We used only cases with complete Willis' circle (Figure 1). These circles originated from 110 cadavers of both sexes (62 male and 48 female) and of different ages (from 20 to 95). The numbers of cadavers in each age deciles were as follows: 2nd decade, two cadavers; 3rd decade, three cadavers; 4th decade, seven cadavers; 5th decade, 16 cadavers; 6th decade, six cadavers; 7th decade, 23 cadavers; 8th decade, 35 cadavers, 9th decade, 17 cadavers; and 10th decade, one cadaver.

Only one cadaver had cerebral infarction, while the others were on autopsy because of cardiac, respiratory, incidental and other causes of no cerebral pathology.
Measurement of the outer diameter of the pre-communicating part of the posterior cerebral artery and the posterior communicating artery of both sides, as well basilar bifurcation angle was performed using ImageJ (http://rsb.info.nih.gov/ij/index.html). Statistical analysis of quantitative data is performed with PASW statistical software SPSS version 15. According to Kamath (1981), values of ≤ 0.5 and 1.0 mm for the posterior communicating and pre-communicating part of the posterior cerebral arteries are respectively used as hypoplastic calibers.

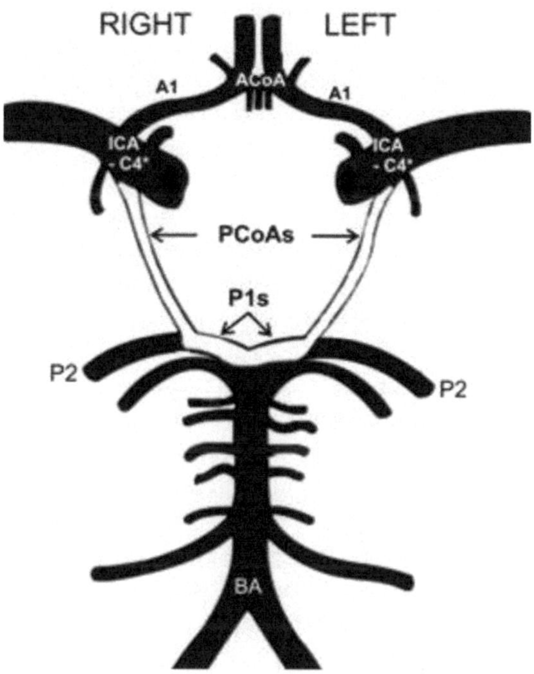

Fig. 1. Diagram of vessels of the carotid and vertebrobasilar systems. Vascular components of the circle of Willis (choroids and communicating subparts of the cerebral part of the internal carotid artery, ICA-C4*; pre-communicating part of the anterior cerebral artery, A1; anterior communicating artery, ACoA; posterior communicating artery, PCoA; pre-communicating part of the posterior cerebral artery, P1), and some of other arteries of the vertebrobasilar system (post-communicating part of the posterior cerebral artery, P2; basilar artery, BA) are marked. Vessels (PCoAs and P1s) of the circle posterior part are white colored.

Form of types and subtypes of the posterior part of 110 circles of Willis follows their previous description in human fetuses (Vasović et al., 2008a). Bilateral fetal or FF-type is characterized with the larger diameter of the posterior communicating arteries in relation to the pre-communicating part of the posterior cerebral arteries (normal or hypoplastic); bilateral adult or AA-type is characterized with bilaterally larger diameter of the pre-communicating part of the posterior cerebral arteries in relation to the posterior

communicating arteries (normal or hypoplastic); bilateral transitory or TT-type is characterized with the same diameter (normal or hypoplastic) of the pre-communicating part of the posterior cerebral artery and the posterior communicating artery on both sides; the fetal-transitory or transitory-fetal type (FT/TF) is characterized with the same size of the posterior communicating and pre-communicating part of the posterior cerebral artery on one side and the larger posterior communicating artery in relation to the pre-communicating part of the posterior cerebral artery on the right or left side; the adult-transitory or transitory-adult type (AT/TA) is characterized with the same size of the posterior communicating artery and pre-communicating part of the posterior cerebral artery on one side and the larger pre-communicating part of the posterior cerebral artery in relation to the posterior communicating artery on the right or left side; the adult-fetal or fetal-adult type (AF/FA) is characterized with the larger diameter of the pre-communicating part of the posterior cerebral artery in relation to the posterior communicating artery and the larger diameter of the posterior communicating artery in relation to the pre-communicating part of the posterior cerebral artery on the right or left side. Subtypes with the ideal caliber relations are marked with zero in the subscript. The mark of every next subtype retains the first letters of the basic type but in the subscript contains Arabic numerals starting from number 1. To differentiate the side of the TT, FF, and AA subtypes in schemes, we emphasize that the numeral in the subscript designates right side and the numeral with the apostrophe designates left side (as the images in the mirror). To differentiate the side on FT/TF, AT/TA, and AF/FA schemes, we emphasize that the first letter in the designation marks right-sided origin, and the second marks left-sided origin of arteries. The lines of different thicknesses and broken lines on the schemes of the circle posterior part show the difference in the caliber size, independently from whether the caliber of an artery was normal and/or (slightly) hypoplastic or hyperplastic.
Macroscopic visualization of atheromatous plaques in vessels' wall of the circle of Willis is graduated according to personal proposes (grade 0 – without atheromatous changes; grade 1 - atheromatous plaques at vessels bifurcations; grade 2 - atheromatous plaques at bifurcations and up to half vessels length; grade 3 – islands or diffuse atheromatous plaques).

3. Results

Basic statistic analysis of calibres of the pre-communicating part of the posterior cerebral artery and posterior communicating artery on both sides in the circle of Willis of human cadavers of different ages and genders is presented in Table 1.
The least caliber of the pre-communicating parts of the right and left posterior cerebral arteries (0.89 and 0.80 mm) is found in a 75-year-old female and a 42-year-old male, while their largest caliber (3.69 and 3.60 mm) is found in 47-year-old and 80-year-old males. The least caliber of the right and left posterior communicating arteries (0.30 and 0.45 mm) is found in a 44-year-old and in a 64-year-old woman, while the largest caliber (2.86 and 3.31 mm) is found in 80-year old woman. Average values of the caliber and the standard deviations for right and left pre-communicating part of the posterior cerebral artery are 2.17 (±0.58) mm and 2.29 (±0.48) mm, as well 1.19 (±0.54) mm and 1.22 (±0.57) mm for the right and left posterior communicating artery, respectively (Table 1).

		Total			
Parameter	Age	Right PCA-P1	Left PCA-P1	Right PCoA	Left PCoA
Mean	65.59	2.17	2.20	1.19	1.22
SE	1.66	0.06	0.05	0.06	0.06
Median	71	2.17	2.21	1.05	1.03
Mode	78	2.50	2.43	0.98	1.43
SD	17.62	0.58	0.48	0.54	0.57
Range	75	2.80	2.80	2.60	2.86
Minimum	20	0.89	0.80	0.30	0.45
Maximum	95	3.69	3.60	2.90	3.31
CI (95.0%)	3.28	0.12	0.10	0.11	0.12
		Male			
Mean	63.12	2.26	2.22	1.22	1.23
SE	2.30	0.08	0.07	0.07	0.07
Median	70	2.24	2.28	1.16	1.06
Mode	70	2.50	2.29	1.35	1.43
SD	18.71	0.58	0.50	0.54	0.51
Range	70	2.75	2.63	2.40	2.84
Minimum	20	0.94	0.80	0.50	0.47
Maximum	90	3.69	3.43	2.90	3.31
CI (95.0%)	4.60	0.16	0.14	0.15	0.14
		Female			
Mean	69.06	2.04	2.17	1.15	1.21
SE	2.26	0.09	0.08	0.09	0.11
Median	74	1.95	2.13	1.00	0.99
Mode	78	1.81	1.84	0.98	0.71
SD	15.49	0.56	0.46	0.55	0.64
Range	68	2.04	2.33	2.47	2.41
Minimum	27	0.89	1.27	0.30	0.45
Maximum	95	2.93	3.60	2.77	2.86
CI (95.0%)	4.55	0.19	0.15	0.18	0.21

Table 1. Statistical parameters of caliber values of the pre-communicating part (P1) of the posterior cerebral artery (PCA) and posterior communicating artery (PCoA) on both sides in the posterior circle part of human cadavers

We established four (two symmetric and two asymmetric) types. The incidences of types in adult specimens are as follow: 8 cases (7.27%) of the FF-type (four subtypes), 75 cases (68.18%) of the AA-type (six subtypes), 15 cases (13.63%) of the AF-type (four subtypes) and 12 cases (10.91%) of the AT-type (three subtypes). Sequences of same or special subtypes in fetal and adult specimens are compared and showed in Table 2.

FETAL CASES* - SUBTYPES -		ADULT CASES** - SUBTYPES -	
Mark	%	Mark	%
TTo	17.95		
TT1/TT1'			
FFo	10.10	FFo	7.27
FF1 / FF1'		FF1 / FF1'	
		FF2'	
		FF4'	
AAo	32.55	AAo	68.18
AA1/ AA1'		AA1 / AA1'	
AA2/ AA2'		AA2 / AA2'	
AA3'		AA3 / AA3'	
AA4		AA4 / AA4'	
		AA5 / AA5'	
FTo / TFo	5.95		
FT2			
AFo/FAo	19.55	AFo/FAo	13.63
AF1/FA1			
AF3/FA3			
AF4/FA4		FA4	
		AF5 / FA5	
FA6			
AF7		AF7	
AF8			
ATo/TAo	13.85	ATo/TAo	10.91
AT1		AT1	
AT2/TA2			
AT3/TA3		AT3/TA3	

Table 2. Sequences of subtypes of the posterior part of fetal and adult circles of Willis.

Special subtypes are in gray rows;
*Vasović et al. (2008a);
**recent findings.

It is obvious that an incidence of bilateral adult type dominates (68.18%) and that the cases of bilateral transitory and fetal-transitory types as well some subtypes of bilateral fetal and adult types are missing; an unilateral adult configuration is associated with fetal or transitory configuration in about 25% of these adult cases; there is the least incidence (7.27) of bilateral fetal configuration in relation to other three patterns of posterior circle part (Table 2).

Distribution of cases of corresponding subtypes according to causes of death in female and male adults cadavers is showed in Table 3. A presence of atheromatous plaques in carotid and vertebrobasilar systems on the brain base is noted according to age and graduated independently from cause of death (Table 4).

Types / Subtypes		N	Myocardial infarction	Cardiorespiratory arrest	Polytrauma	Intoxication	Singular cases of no cerebral pathology	Cerebral pathology
			(females + males)					
AA	AA_0	29	3 + 0	5 + 2	2 + 5	2 + 2	3 + 4	0 + 1
	$AA_1/AA_{1'}$	7		0 + 1	2 + 2	0 + 1	0 + 1	
	$AA_2/AA_{2'}$	27	1 + 4	3 + 3	1 + 6	0 + 1	5 + 3	
	$AA_3/AA_{3'}$	2	0 + 1		0 + 1			
	$AA_4/AA_{4'}$	7	0 + 3		1 + 2		1 + 0	
	$AA_5/AA_{5'}$	3	1 + 0	1 + 1				
FF	FF_0	3	0 + 1		1 + 0		1 + 0	
	$FF_1/FF_{1'}$	3		1 + 1	0 + 1			
	$FF_{2'}$	1				0 + 1		
	$FF_{4'}$	1		1 + 0				
AF/FA	AF_0/FA_0	8	1 + 3		0 + 2		2 + 0	
	FA_4	1	0 + 1					
	AF_5/FA_5	5	1 + 0	1 + 1			2 + 0	
	AF_7	1	0 + 1					
AT/TA	AT_0/TA_0	8	0 + 1		1 + 2	0 + 1	2 + 1	
	AT_1	1				0 + 1		
	AT_3/TA_3	3	1 + 0	1 + 0		1 + 0		

Table 3. Sex distribution of number of cases of the posterior circle subtypes according to causes of death

Atheromatous changes (grade 1) were first visualized in a 34-years old male (AA2 subtype), as well as, in five cases (one in FF2' , two in AAo and two in AA2 subtype) of the fifth decade of life. Atheromatous changes of grades 2 and 3 were first visualized in 42-years old and 47-years old males, respectively. Incidences of atheromatous changes are as follow: Grade 1: Five (2 females and 3 males) or 62.5% of the FF-type cases; 24 (8 females and 16 males) or 32% of the AA-type cases; four (2 females and 2 males) or 26.6% of the AF/FA-type cases, and two (males) or 16.6% of the AT/TA-type cases. Grade 2: Two (female and male) or 25% of the FF-type cases; 26 (12 females and 14 males) or 34.6% of the AA-type cases; three (two females and one male) or 20% of the AF/FA-type cases, and two (males) or 16.6% of the AT/TA-type cases. Grade 3: One (male) or 12.5% of the FF-type cases; four (two females and two males) or 5.3% of the AA-type cases; four (two females and two males) or 26.6% of the AF/FA-type cases, and one (female) or 8.3% of the AT/TA-type cases. There are 21 (9 females and 12 males) or 28% of the AA-type cases from the 20th to 78th year, then four (two females and two males) or 26.6% of the AF/FA-type cases from the 28th to 54th year, and seven (two females and five males) or 58.3% of the AF/FA-type cases from the 35th to 82nd year without atheromatous changes.

Diagrams and appropriate pictures are showed at Figures 2-5. General incidences of types and/or subtypes are compared with other literature data in Table 5.

Types	Subtypes		Grade 0	Grade 1	Grade 2	Grade 3	N
FF	FF_0	f		78		80	2
		m		84			1
	$FF_1/FF_{1'}$	f		75			1
		m		79	70		2
	$FF_{2'}$	f					0
		m		41			1
	$FF_{4'}$	f			79		1
		m					0
AA	AA_0	f	27,34,58,67	46,72,85	68,74,75,80,95	71,87	15
		m	20, 37,45,47,50,60,75	45,52,81,83	70,86	70	14
	$AA_1/AA_{1'}$	f	34,43				2
		m	70	69	78,80,90		5
	$AA_2/AA_{2'}$	f	44,44,61	45,71,82	65,74,76,80		10
		m	23,51,78	34,43,54,61,70,79,81	68,69,72,77,78,79,82		17
	$AA_3/AA_{3'}$	f					0
		m		63,65			2
	$AA_4/AA_{4'}$	f		79	64		2
		m	20	80,84	70	85	5
	$AA_5/AA_{5'}$	f		64	85		2
		m			42		1
AF/FA	AF_0/FA_0	f	45,54			81	3
		m	28,42	80	74	82	5
	FA_4	f					0
		m		89			1
	AF_5/FA_5	f		68,70	78	78	4
		m				47	1
	AF_7	f					0
		m			74		1
AT/TA	AT_0/TA_0	f	82	78	72		3
		m	39,50,76,80			61	5
	AT_1	f					0
		m	35				1
	AT_3/TA_3	f	40	73	67		3
		m					0

Table 4. Graduation of atheromatosis according to gender (female - f and male - m) and age

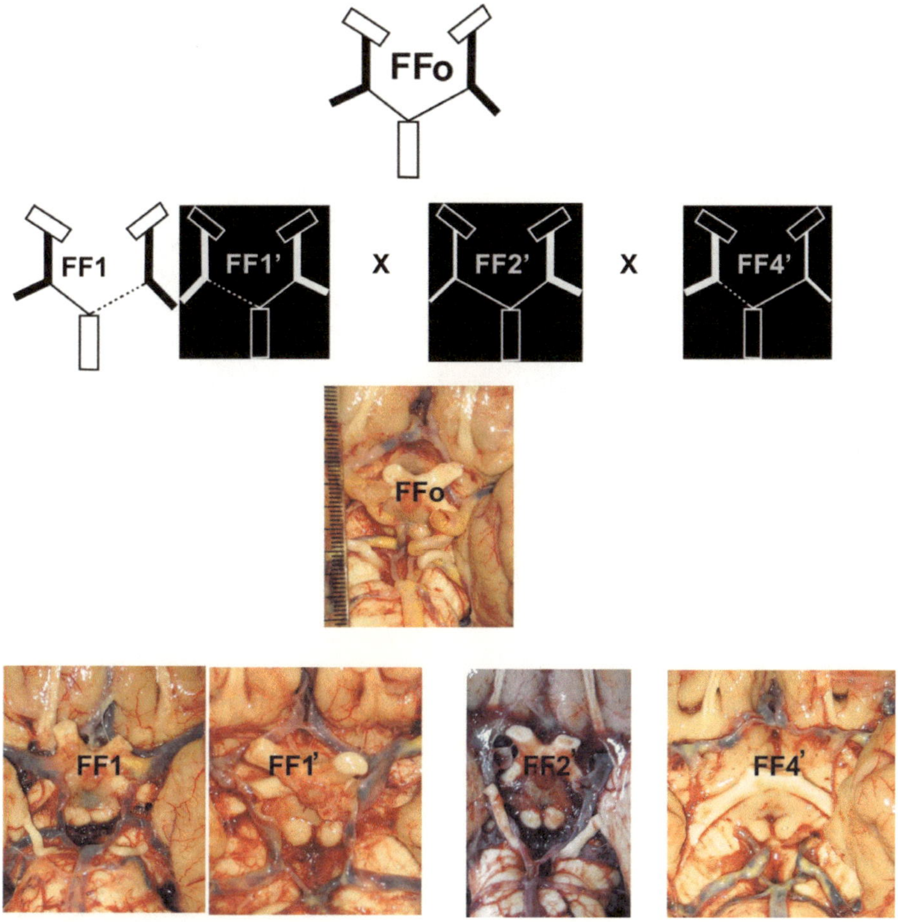

Fig. 2. Diagrams and corresponding photos of subtypes of the bilateral fetal (FF) type.

Right or left posterior communicating artery, rPCoA or lPCoA; right or left pre-communicating part of the posterior cerebral artery, rP1 or lP1.
FFo (rPCoA > rP1 = lP1 < lPCoA ^ lPCoA = rPCoA): 3 cases (37.5%).
FF1/FF1' (lP1 < rP1 < rPCoA = lPCoA) or (rP1 < lP1 < lPCoA = rPCoA): 3 cases (37.5%).
FF2' (lP1 = rP1 < rPCoA < lPCoA): 1 case.
FF4' (rP1 < lP1 < lPCoA < rPCoA): 1 case. Note: PCoAs are accidentally broken.

In FF-type, more frequent are the cases where calibers of paired posterior communicating arteries and pre-communicating parts of the posterior cerebral arteries are equaled, respectively with larger caliber of posterior communicating arteries (FFo-subtype), as well as the cases with same relationship of posterior communicating arteries and caliber difference of pre-communicating parts of the posterior cerebral arteries (FF1/FF1'subtype).

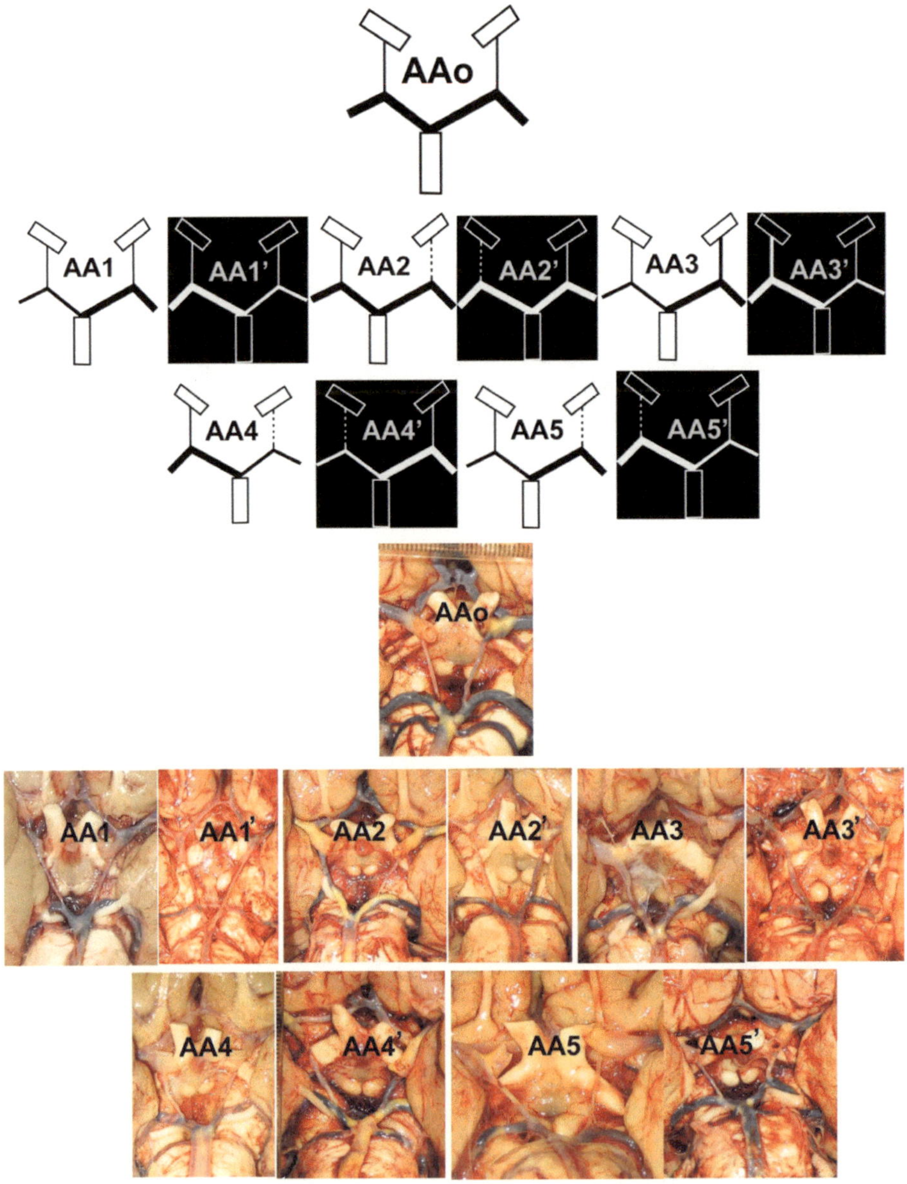

Fig. 3. Diagrams and corresponding photos of subtypes of the bilateral adult (AA) type.

Right or left posterior communicating artery, rPCoA or lPCoA; right or left pre communicating part of the posterior cerebral artery, rP1 or lP1.
AAo (rPCoA < rP1 = lP1 > lPCoA ^ lPCoA = rPCoA): 29 cases (38.6%).
AA1/AA1′ (lPCoA = rPCoA < rP1 < lP1) or (rPCoA = lPCoA < lP1 < rP1): 7 cases (9.3%).
AA2/AA2′ (lPCoA < rPCoA < rP1 = lP1) or (rPCoA < lPCoA < lP1 = rP1): 27 cases (36%).
AA3/AA3′ (rPCoA < rP1 = lPCoA < lP1) or (lPCoA < rPCoA = lP1 < rP1): 2 cases.
Note: left PCoA is accidentally broken in AA3 subtype.
AA4/AA4′ (lPCoA < rPCoA < lP1 < rP1) or (rPCoA < lPCoA < lP1 < rP1): 7 cases (9.3%).
AA5/AA5′ (lPCoA < rPCoA < rP1 < lP1) or (rPCoA < lPCoA < lP1 < rP1): 3 cases.

In AA-type, more frequent are the cases where calibers of paired pre-communicating parts of posterior cerebral arteries are equaled and larger in relation to equaled caliber of posterior communicating arteries (AAo-subtype), as well as the cases with same relationship of posterior cerebral arteries and caliber difference of posterior communicating arteries (AA2/AA2′ subtype). Cases of two subtypes (AA1/AA1′ and AA4/AA4′) have same frequency (9.3%), while cases of AA3/AA3′ (2/75) and AA5/AA5′ (3/75) have the least frequency.

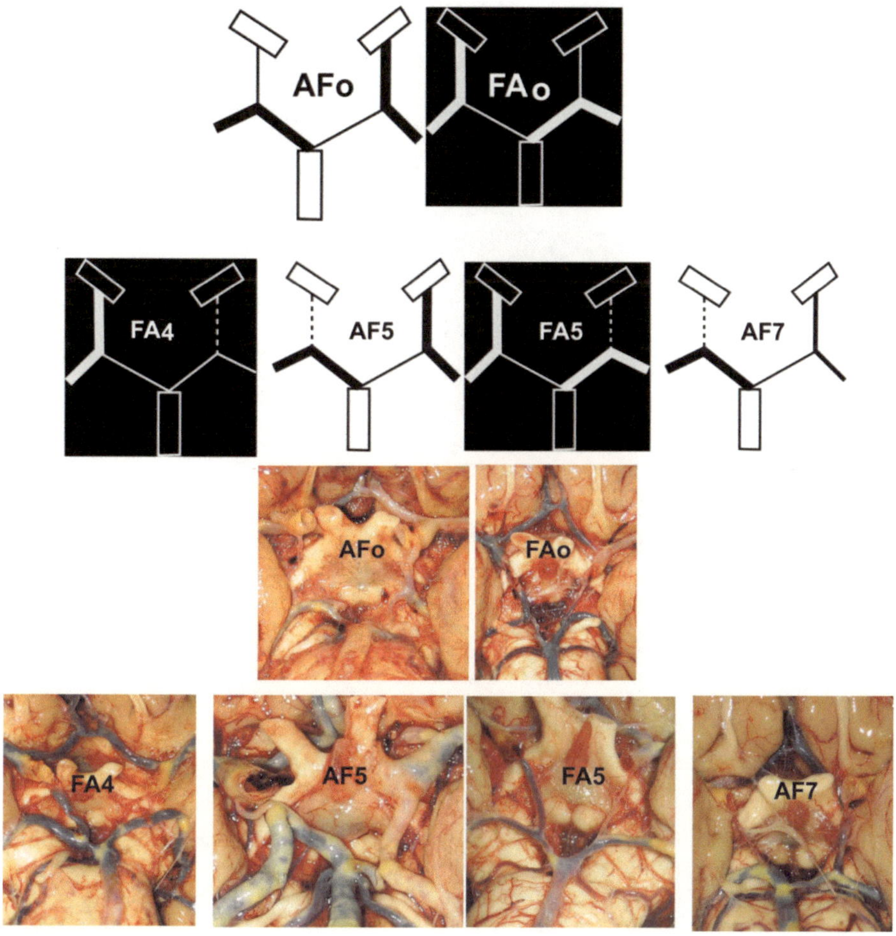

Fig. 4. Diagrams and corresponding photos of subtypes of the adult-fetal or fetal-adult (AF/FA) type.

Right or left posterior communicating artery, rPCoA or lPCoA; right or left pre communicating part of the posterior cerebral artery, rP1 or lP1.
AFo/FAo (rP1 > rPCoA = lP1 < lPCoA ^ lPCoA = rP1) or (rPCoA > rP1 = lPCoA < lP1 ^ lP1 = rPCoA): 8 cases (53.3%).
Note: rPCoA and lP1 are accidentally broken in AFo.
FA4 (lPCoA < lP1 = rP1 < rPCoA ^ lPCoA < rPCoA): 1 case.
AF5/FA5 (lPCoA = rP1 > lP1 > rPCoA) or (rPCoA = lP1 > rP1 > lPCoA): 5 cases (33.3%).
AF7 (rP1 > lP1 > lPCoA > rPCoA): 1 case.

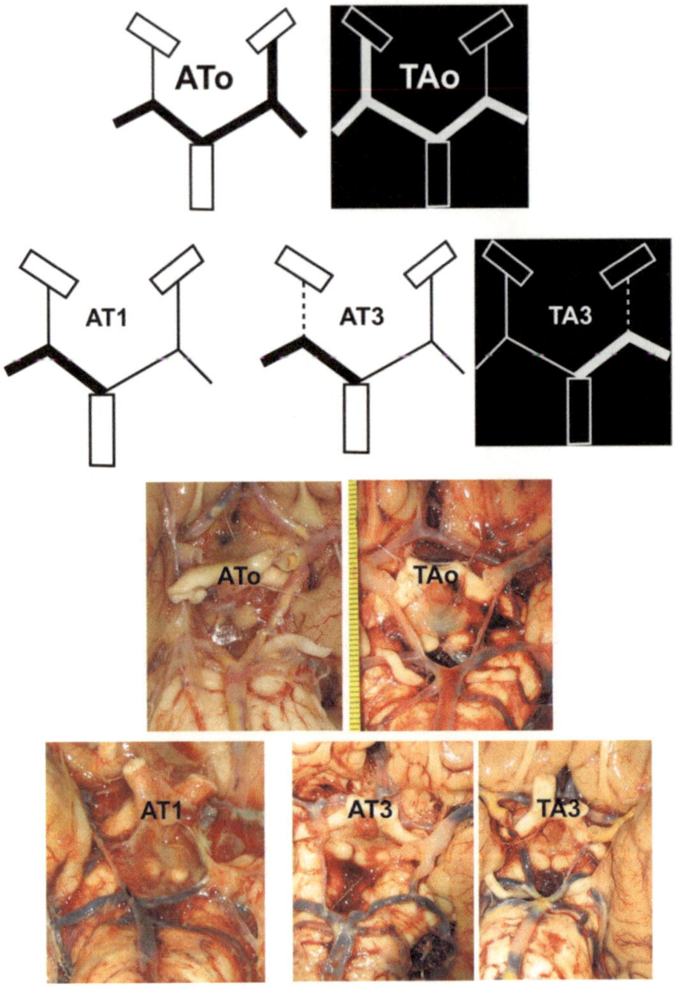

Fig. 5. Diagrams and corresponding photos of subtypes of the adult-transitory or transitory-adult (AT/TA) type.

Right or left posterior communicating artery, rPCoA or lPCoA; right or left pre-communicating part of the posterior cerebral artery, rP1 or lP1.
ATo/TAo (rPCoA < rP1 = lP1 = lPCoA) or (rP1 = rPCoA = lPCoA < lP1): 8 cases (66.6%).
Note: rPCoA and lP1 are accidentally broken.
AT1 (rP1 > lP1 = lPCoA = rPCoA): 1 case.
AT3/TA3 (rP1 > lP1 = lPCoA > rPCoA) or (lP1 > rP1 = rPCoA > lPCoA): 3 cases (25%).
Note: Left PCoA origin is infundibular.

In AF/FA-type, more frequent are the cases where calibers of the posterior communicating artery and pre-communicating part of the posterior cerebral artery are equaled on opposite sides (AFo/FAo subtype), as well as cases with same caliber of the left or right posterior communicating artery and pre-communicating part of the posterior cerebral artery on corresponding opposite side simultaneously with larger caliber of the left or right pre-communicating part of the posterior cerebral artery in relation to opposite posterior communicating artery (AF5/FA5 subtype). Cases of two subtypes (FA4 and AF7) are singular.

In AT/TA-type, more frequent are the cases where calibers of the left or right posterior communicating artery and pre-communicating part of both posterior cerebral arteries are equaled and larger in relation to opposite posterior communicating artery (ATo/TAo subtype), as well cases where the left or right pre-communicating part of posterior cerebral artery is larger than corresponding opposite pre-communicating part of posterior cerebral artery and posterior communicating artery, simultaneously with their larger caliber than ipsilateral posterior communicating artery (AT3/TA3 subtype).

AUTHORS	N	COUNTRY	AGE*	METHOD	TYPES OF POSTERIOR PART OF THE CIRCLE OF WILLIS (%)										
					BILAT ADULT (AA)	BILAT FETAL (FF)	BILAT TRANSIT (TT)	ADULT-FETAL (AF)	ADULT-TRANSIT (AT)	UNILAT ADULT	UNILAT FETAL	UNILAT TRANSIT	UNKNOWNED UNILATERAL OR BILATERAL		
													Adult	Fetal	Transitory
Riggs and Rupp (1963)	994	USA	ADULTS	AUTOPSY	72.8	5.6	5.4	≈16							
Saeki and Rhoton (1977)	50	USA	ADULTS	AUTOPSY	60	2		8			20				
Zeal and Rhoton (1978)	25	USA	ADULTS	AUTOPSY									58	40	20
Zada et al. (2007)	271	USA	ANEURYSMATIC SERIE	RETROSPECTIVE REVIEW		10					11				
Kayembe et al. (1984)	44	Japan	ADULTS	AUTOPSY		9.1					6.8				
	148		ANEURYSMATIC AND CONTROL SERIES			6					8.3				
Tanaka et al. (2006)	117	Japan	20-29	MRI	≈95										
Chen et al. (2004)	111	China	<40	MRA	27.9	5.4		≈9							
	396		>40		10.6	6		≈4							
Sahni et al. (2007)	45	India	CHILDREN	AUTOPSY							6.6				
	280		ADULTS			0.3					6.8				
Krishnamurthy et al. (2008)	89	India	ADULTS	AUTOPSY		2.2									
Pai et al. (2007)	25	India	40-84	AUTOPSY									78	10	12
Poudel and Bhattarai (2010)	35	Nepal	ADULTS	AUTOPSY	91.4	8.6									
De Silva et al. (2010)	225	Sri Lanka	ADULTS	AUTOPSY	88	1.3	0.8			8.8	6.1	2.6			
Efekhtar et al. (2006)	102	Iran	15-75 (male)	AUTOPSY							26 (right)				
											28 (left)				
Songur et al. (2008)	110	Turkey	17-58	AUTOPSY									35.4		
Al-Hussain et al. (2001)	50	Jordan	20-55	AUTOPSY									77	15	8
Alawad et al. (2009)	143	Sudan	40-65	MRA	97.5										
Malamateniou et al. (2009)	94	UK	INFANTS (PRETERM-AT-TERM AND TERM-BORN)	MRA		25.5	≈8								
Van Overbeeke et al. (1991)	100	Netherlands	ADULTS	AUTOPSY									84	14	2
Hartkamp et al. (1999)	175	Netherlands	PATIENTS	MRA		54	1			8					
			CONTROLS			25	8			14					
Yasargil (1984)	200	Switzerland	ADULTS	AUTOPSY									67.5	24.5	8
Gabrovsky (2002)	35	Bulgaria		AUTOPSY										41.4	11.4
Papantchev et al. (2007)	99	Bulgaria	ADULTS	AUTOPSY										30.4	9.1
RECENT STUDY	110	Serbia	20-95	AUTOPSY	68.18	7.27		13.63	10.91						

Table 5. Incidences of (sub) types of the circle posterior part in human specimens in same and/or different countries on four continents.

Thicker black lines separate corresponding continents;
N (number of investigated specimens);
*population group or years.

There are about 65% of hypoplastic posterior communicating arteries (≤0.5 mm + 1SD) in AA type; about one half of the cases are bilateral. There is about 44% of unilaterally hypoplastic posterior communicating artery in AF/FA and AT/TA types with relatively more frequency on the left side. Generally, about 60% of hypoplastic posterior communicating arteries are in adults after 65. There are 6.6% of bilaterally and about 14% of unilaterally hypoplasia of the pre-communicating part of the posterior cerebral artery (≤1 mm + 1SD) in FF, AF/FA and AT/TA types, respectively.

There is significant correlation ($R=0.51$, $p<0.01$) between right and left pre-communicating parts of the posterior cerebral arteries calibers, between the right pre-communicating part of the posterior cerebral artery and left posterior communicating artery caliber ($R=0.39$, $p<0.01$) and between right and left posterior communicating arteries caliber ($R=0.44$, $p<0.01$) in AA type. In AF type, significant correlation is present between right pre-communicating part of the posterior cerebral artery and left posterior communicating artery caliber ($R=0.76$, p<0.01). Significant correlation is present between right pre-communicating part of the posterior cerebral artery and right posterior communicating artery (R=-0.87, p=0.012) and left posterior communicating artery (R=0.87, p=0.011) caliber, as well as, right and left posterior communicating artery caliber (R=0.86, p=0.013) in AT type of cases. Correlations between calibers of right and left pre-communicating parts of the posterior cerebral arteries, as well as, right and left posterior communicating arteries of AA and corresponding arteries of both AF and AT types are not statistically significant (Fig. 6).

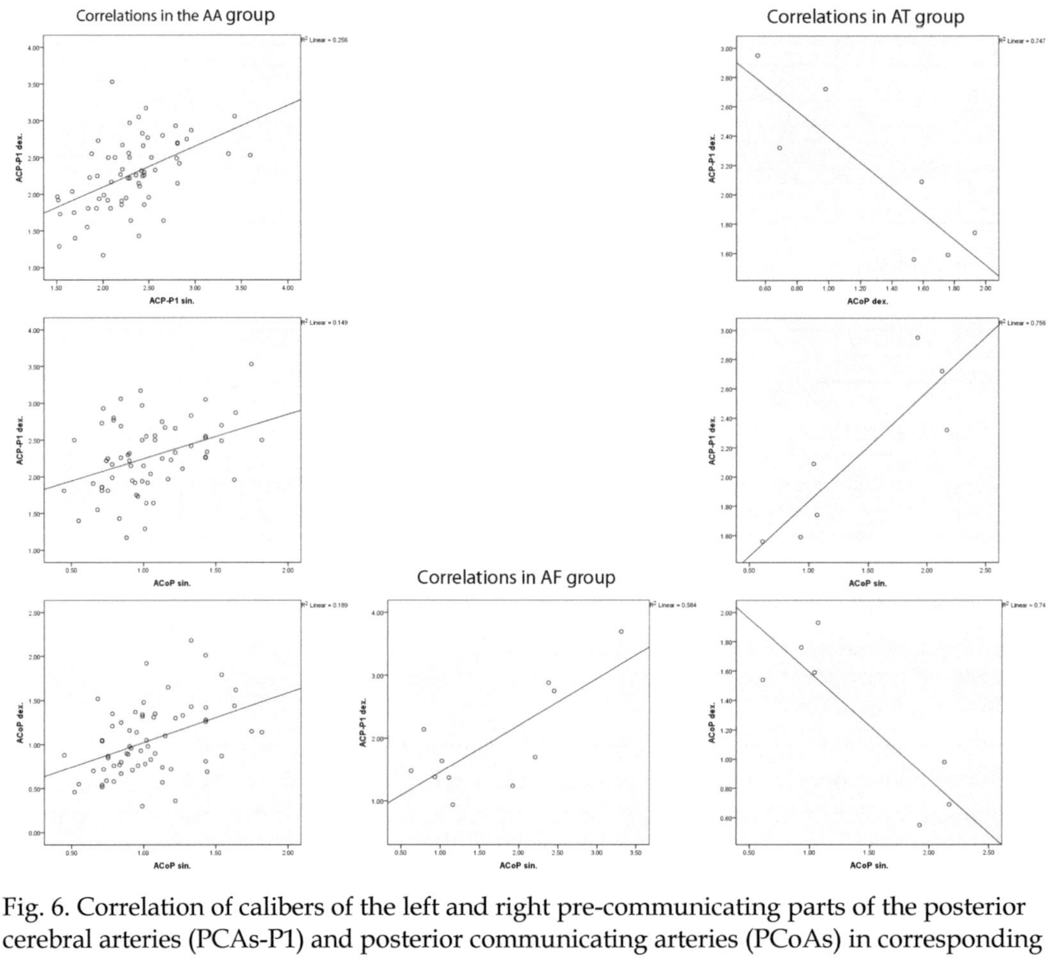

Fig. 6. Correlation of calibers of the left and right pre-communicating parts of the posterior cerebral arteries (PCAs-P1) and posterior communicating arteries (PCoAs) in corresponding type (group) of the circle posterior part

In our specimens, basilar bifurcation angle ranges from 63.4-168.1° (111.9°) in AA type and from 37.8-154.6° (96.6°) in FF type, as well from 67.3-142.2° (111.6°) and from 71.4-161.1° (128.4°) in AT/TA and AF/FA types, respectively; in average, it is 109.68° (Fig. 7). We found only one case of the basilar aneurysm originating from an obtuse basilar bifurcation angle in AAo subtype.

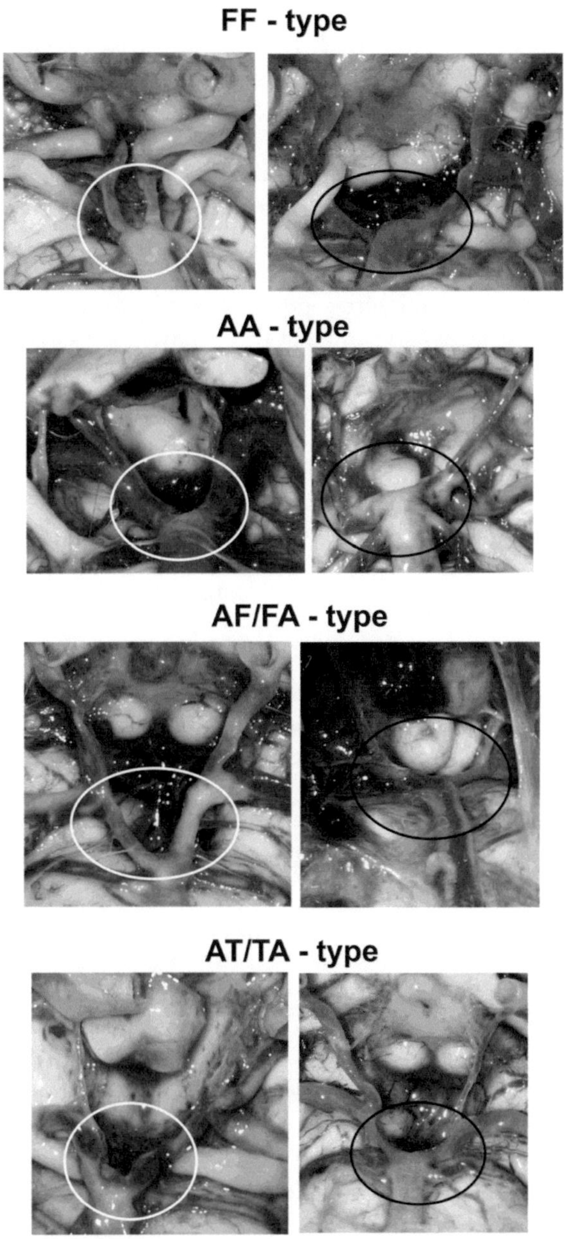

Fig. 7. The basilar bifurcation angle in corresponding type of the posterior circle part. The least and the greatest angle are encircled by white and black lines.

4. Discussion

We selected 110 circles of Willis according to the presence of four vascular components (posterior communicating and pre-communicating parts of the posterior cerebral arteries) in the circle posterior part. The "typical" circle of Willis was defined with respect to its components as a closed circuit in which fluid may circulate from any entrance point back to the same point with all vessels more than 1 mm in external diameter and with no excess vessels (Kayembe et al., 1984). Variable five vascular components in the circle posterior part are previous described in fetuses and adults (Vasović, 2004; Vasović et al., 2010). Many authors wide world have studied about the length, diameter and anomalies in the origin of vascular components of the circle of Willis and found that the parameters in different geographical limits were different. However Efekhtar et al. (2006) concluded that there is no evidence that the distributions of the variations of the circle of Willis varied in different populations. Our selection of authors in Table 5 had the aim to check previous data. Different incidences of types of the circle posterior part are obvious as from continent to continent, as from the city to city in same country. Many years ago, Kayembe et al. (1984) found that the incidence of variations in the circle of Willis was significantly higher in the aneurysm series than in the control. Hartcamp et al. (1999) noted that several factors may explain a significantly higher percentage of entirely complete circle anterior or posterior configurations in different patients, including population selection, adaptation of circle morphology and improved detection of vessels with increased flow on magnetic resonance angiograms. Recently, in a study of volume flow rates of the basilar and bilateral internal carotid arteries in 125 healthy volunteers, Tanaka et al. (2006) found that the relative contribution of each of the proximal arteries correlated significantly with variations in the circle of Willis.

Average diameter of the posterior cerebral artery was seen to be 1.7 mm (Krishnamurthy et al., 2008) or 1.8 mm (Chen et al., 2004) on both sides, or 2.76 mm on the right and 2.5 mm on the left side (Pai et al., 2007), as well 1.83 mm on the right and 1.88 mm on the left side (Songur et al., 2008). Many years ago, Kamath (1981) noted that average diameter of the posterior cerebral artery was 2.1 mm on the right and 2.2 mm on the left side. Similar to these data, average diameter of the pre-communicating part of the posterior cerebral artery were 2.17 mm on the right and 2.20 mm on the left in our specimens. We found the least caliber of the pre-communicating parts of the right and left posterior cerebral arteries in a 75-year-old female and a 42-year-old male, as well the largest caliber in 47-year-old and 80-year-old males, respectively. Average diameter of the posterior communicating artery was seen to be 1.5 mm on the right and 1.4 mm on the left side (Kamath, 1981). The diameter of the posterior communicating artery varied from hypoplastic (less than 0.5 mm) to 4 mm (fetal circulation) on the right side (average 1.25 mm) and 0.5 mm to 3 mm (average 1.12 mm) on the left side (Pai et al., 2007). In our specimens, average diameter of this artery was similar on both sides (1.22 mm on the right and 1.23 mm on the left). We found the least caliber of posterior communicating arteries in 44-year-old and in a 64-year-old woman, respectively, while the largest caliber in 80-year old woman, too. However, values of calibers of these vascular components in our study were in the function of forming basic types and their subtypes of the posterior circle part.

Al-Hussain et al. (2001) noted a possibility that the circle of Willis may have different configurations of the posterior bifurcation of the posterior communicating artery on both sides. In that case, two primary visual areas of the same individual may receive their blood from different sources; one from the basilar artery through the pre-communicating segment (adult configuration) and the other from the internal carotid artery through the posterior communicating artery (fetal configuration).

Because of many anatomical variations of the circle of Willis, its classification into clearly arranged groups is hardly possible. Urbanski et al. (2008) divided arterial variations into three groups in regard to the possible impact on the cerebral cross-perfusion. In the first group, there was only one location of hypoplasia or aplasia within the circle of Willis. In the second group, the abnormalities existed within the posterior pre-communicating or communicating arteries. In the third group, the pathologies were found in both anterior and posterior vascular components of the circle of Willis. According to Saeki & Rhoton (1977) the posterior part of the circle of Willis is normal if the posterior communicating arteries are not hypoplastic. However, we include those arteries during formation different subtypes because of no cerebral cause of death, oldest of cadavers and the presence of posterior communicating side branches. In continuation of the study on fetuses (Vasović et al., 2008a), we accepted a classification of the circle posterior part into bilateral adult (AA-), fetal (FF-) and transitory (TT-) types and their three combinations. We presented incidences of some patterns of the circle part in Table 5. According to the fact that many authors have noted incidence of one of three configurations (adult or fetal or transitory) without data about unilateral or bilateral pattern (Zeal & Rhoton, 1978; Al-Houssain et al., 2001; Gabrovsky, 2002; Pai et al., 2007; Papantchev et al., 2007; Songur et al., 2008), complete comparison is difficult. We calculated the percentages of different configurations according to diameters of the vessels, and presented in Table 5. We found four (two symmetric and two asymmetric) types and labeled with initial letters of their marks, opposite to the authors listing in Table 5. As early as seven weeks after conception, a preliminary form of the circle of Willis is present with approximately equal diameters of all vessels. As fetal growth occurs, the relative sizes of the various components of the circle of Willis change significantly to assume the eventual adult morphology (Cuchiara & Detre, 2007). Adult configurations occur in the majority of circles of Willis through further fetal and newborn life (Van Overbeeke et al., 1991), as well in majority of other and our study of adults, except in the studies of Chen et al. (2004) and Songur et al. (2008). No sexual prevalence or prevalence for the right or left side of the adult or fetal configuration was noted in a study of complete circles of Willis of 53 brains taken from fetuses and neonates aged 12 to 60 weeks after conception (Van Overbeeke et al., 1991). The preterm infants born after 30 weeks' gestation age have more significantly increased prevalence in the bilateral fetal-type origin of the posterior cerebral artery (83.3%) than those infants born before 30 weeks (Malamateniou et al., 2009). We found bilateral adult and fetal (AA and FF) types in 68.18% and 7.27%, respectively, while De Silva et al. (2010) noted in 88.8% and 1.3%, respectively in Sri Lankan population. Hendrikse et al. (2005) cited literature data that in the circle posterior part, the variant type with a unilateral fetal-type posterior cerebral artery is present on up to 25% of angiograms, and a bilateral fetal-type posterior cerebral artery present on up to 10% of angiograms. Zada et al. (2008) noted that the overall incidence of the fetal-type posterior circulation has been reported to occur in 4 to 29% of patients, whereas bilaterally occurring fetal posterior cerebral arteries have been reported to occur in 1 to 9% of patients. We also found unilateral adult configuration associated with opposite fetal (AF/FA) or transitory pattern (AT/TA) in 13.63% and 10.91%, respectively. A central hypothesis is that the circle of Willis anomalies correlates with alterations in cerebral hemodynamic. Songur et al. (2008) described that cerebral blood flow was in direct proportion to vessel diameter and thus there is more blood flow in larger vessels. In addition, a large posterior communicating artery may protect against watershed infarction in patients with ipsilateral occlusion of the internal carotid artery, while a very small or absent ipsilateral posterior communicating artery increases the risk of a watershed infarction in these patients (Schomer et al., 1994). The patients with fetal type could be more prone to develop vascular insufficiency (Van Raamt et al., 2006) or internal carotid-posterior communicating aneurysms (Zada et al., 2008). According to De Silva et al. (2010), fetal configuration has been reported in adults at 4% to 46% on the basis of anatomical and angiographic studies, and a higher percentage of on the basis of anatomical studies has been reported in older fetuses and newborns: 35% and 56%, while only a minority of circles showed a transitional configuration, 14% and 20%, respectively. In our adult cases there was not bilateral transitory configuration as in other studies of infants or adults (Riggs & Rupp, 1963; Hartkamp et al., 1999; Malamateniou et al., 2009, De Silva et al., 2010) or fetuses (Van Overbeeke et al., 1991; Vasović et al., 2008a; De Silva et al., 2010).

Anastomotic flow between carotid and basilar arteries is limited when one or both posterior communicating arteries are hypoplastic, while effective circulation across the circle and between its anterior and posterior components is restricted when both anterior and posterior anastomotic stems are hypoplastic, as well similar limitation of collateral flow results when all component stems of the circle are hypoplastic (Riggs and Rupp, 1963). The resistance to flow across the posterior communicating artery is greater than across the anterior communicating artery, because the posterior communicating artery is usually a longer vessel (Hartkamp et al., 1999). Arteries of less than 1 mm diameter were considered abnormal, barring the communicating arteries, where less than 0.5 mm diameter was considered abnormal (Kamath, 1981; Pai et al., 2007). The relative importance of the caliber values of the brain arteries have thus been assessed, although no clear consensus is found among reports. One of limitations is also potential minor changes in the diameter of the vessels during time (Efekhtar et al., 2006). Hypoplastic vessels were defined to be those with external diameters less than 0.8 mm (Hartkamp et al., 1999; Chen et al., 2004) or 1.0 mm (Schomer et al., 1994; Gabrovsky, 2002; Efekhtar et al., 2006; Tanaka et al., 2006). When taking into account only static anatomic observations, Merkkola et al. (2006) hypothesized that the circulation to the left hemisphere would be sufficient in the majority of patients when using a threshold of 0.5 mm. The results of Hoksbergen et al. (2000) indicate that the threshold diameter for collateral function of the posterior communicating artery lies between 0.4 and 0.6 mm. This threshold diameter might be used in future studies evaluating the influence of its collateral ability in symmetric or asymmetric circle posterior part. The most common anatomic variation in the group without vascular-related abnormalities was the absence or hypoplasia of the posterior communicating artery (Malamateniou et al., 2009). Dysregulation of cerebral blood flow may allow relative ischemia to develop in the setting of increased metabolic demand related to neuronal hyper excitability, may trigger cortical spreading depression, and may predispose individuals to ischemic lesions and stroke (Cucchiara and Detre, 2008).

The study of Sahni et al. (2007) was conducted on brains of 280 adults and 45 children. The hypoplastic posterior communicating artery on the right side was present in 2 children and 17 adults, whereas on left side, it was seen in 1 child and 6 adults; bilateral hypoplastic posterior communicating artery was observed in 4 children and 17 adults. Fetal type on the right side was observed in 2 children and 12 adults, whereas on the left side, it was in 1 child and in 7 adults; bilaterally, it was found to be present only in 1 adult male. In the literature it was also noted that absence/hypoplasia of the posterior communicating artery was more common in preterm boys than in girls, while absence/hypoplasia of the pre-communicating part of the posterior cerebral artery occurred twice as often in term-born girls than in boys (Malamateniou et al., 2009). In a study of 1000 brains, the pre-communicating part of the posterior cerebral artery was hypoplastic in 10.6% and the posterior communicating artery in 16.4% of cases (Kapoor et al., 2008). There are about 65% of hypoplastic posterior communicating arteries in bilateral adult (AA) group, and about 44% of unilaterally hypoplastic posterior communicating artery in asymmetric groups with relative more frequency on the left side in our study. Generally, about 60% of hypoplastic posterior communicating arteries are in adults aging after 65. There are 6.6% of bilaterally and about 14% of unilaterally hypoplasia of the pre-communicating part of the posterior cerebral artery in bilateral fetal (FF), adult-fetal (AF/FA) and adult-transitory groups (AT/TA), respectively. We evidenced percentile of hypoplastic pre-communicating part of the posterior cerebral and posterior communicating arteries in corresponding type and subtype, while other authors presented it as general data, except of Gabrowsky (2002). He noted that the mean diameter of the adult and fetal types of the posterior communicating artery was 1.28 and 2.33 mm, respectively. He also found that a reduction of the diameter from the anterior to the posterior third of this artery in both configurations and more frequently for the hypoplastic (51%), than for the adult type (37%). A hypoplasia of the right posterior communicating artery in 16% and left posterior communicating artery in 11%, as well of both arteries in 33% of males were seen (Efekhtar et al., 2006). Incidence of a hypoplastic pre-communicating segment of the posterior cerebral artery, according to Tanaka et al. (2006), ranges from 4% to 14% of subjects. However, a hypoplasia of the pre-communicating segment of the posterior cerebral artery and posterior communicating artery was 1% and 33%, respectively (Al-Houssain et al., 2001). A hypoplasia of the posterior cerebral artery also was noted in 2.1% on the right and in 1.4% on the left side (Alawad et al., 2009).

Since a significant inverse relationship existed between the diameters of ipsilateral posterior cerebral and posterior communicating arteries, as well as a smaller posterior communicating artery on the left would be associated with a larger posterior cerebral artery on that side (Kamath, 1981). In our study there was significant correlation between right and left pre-communicating parts of the posterior cerebral arteries calibers, between the right pre-communicating part of the posterior cerebral artery and left posterior communicating artery caliber, and between right and left posterior communicating arteries caliber in AA group. In AF group, significant correlation is present between right pre-communicating part of the posterior cerebral artery and left posterior communicating artery caliber. It was also present between right pre-communicating part of the posterior cerebral artery and right posterior communicating artery and left posterior communicating artery caliber, as well as, right and left posterior communicating artery caliber in AT group of cases.

Atheromatous changes (grade 1) were first visualized in a 34-years old male (AA2 subtype) and in five cases (one in FF2' , two in AAo and two in AA2 subtype) of the fifth decade of life. We did not visualize atheromatous changes in 21 adults (9 female and 12 male) of the fifth decade and older. Atheromatous changes of grades 2 and 3 were first visualized in 42 and 47-years old males, respectively, as well as in females of the seventh decade of life (Table 4). Ravensbergen et al. (1998) noted that a strong argument for the (causal) relationship between hemodynamics and atherosclerosis can be found if variations of the geometry result in changes of the location of the atheromatous lesions, which correspond to the changes of the flow force distribution. Songur et al. (2008) established atheromatous plaques in the basilar artery in 30% of cases. We visualized these plaques particularly for every type. Very interesting findings were that atheromatous changes of Grade 1 and 3 were the most frequent in FF (62.5) and AF/FA (26.6%) types, while the least frequency was observed both in AT/TA (16.6%) and AA- (5.3%) types. Atheromatous changes of grade1 for male gender were more frequent in AA type; a relation was 2:1.

In our adult specimens, basilar bifurcation angle ranged from 37.8-168.1°, in average, it was 109.68°. The average basilar angle in adults was 109 degrees and ranged between 30 and 180 degrees in a study of Caruso et al. (1990). The average basilar bifurcation angle of 98 patients aging from 12 to 78 years was determined to be 117.7° (30.93°–172.2°) (Żurada et al., 2008). During a study of fetal specimens, this angle ranged from 35 to 175 degrees (Vasović et al., 2008b). Żurada et al. (2008) described three types of the basilar bifurcation angle in which a type "T" is with an angle greater than 145°, a type "Y" with an angle being equal or less than 145° but greater than 100° and a type "V" for angles less than 100°. Ingebrigsten et al. (2004) hypothesized that normal bifurcations of cerebral arteries beyond the circle of Willis would follow optimality principles of minimum work and that the presence of aneurysms would be associated with deviations from optimum bifurcation geometry. We found only one case of basilar tip aneurysm arising from an obtuse basilar bifurcation angle. However Valleé et al. (2003) showed two basilar apex aneurysms originating from bifurcation angles of about 90 degrees and 180 degrees.

We presented six AA-subtypes of the AA-type, four subtypes of the FF-type, three subtypes of the AT/TA-type and four subtypes of the AF/FA-type of the posterior part of the circle of Willis. Van Raamt et al. (2006) proposed to define a partial fetal-type posterior circle of Willis, in which a small pre-communicating part between the basilar artery and the post-communicating part of the posterior cerebral artery is present, and a full fetal-type posterior circle of Willis, in which the pre-communicating part is absent. Besides our study confirms a domination of bilateral adult configuration of the circle posterior part as other authors, we are the first who classified and marked posterior circle subtypes, as well as new subtypes, which missing in fetal status (Vasović, 2004). We found some similar schemes of (sub) types in Riggs' paper (Riggs & Rupp, 1963) and Yasargil's book (Yasargil, 1984); however, we can not do precise comparison with them. It is difficult confirm that some subtypes of the posterior circle part is a feature of Serbian population. This study offers a possibility to evaluate that angioarchitecture in different health population groups or in patients with or without cerebral pathology wide our or other countries, especially if proposed (sub) types of the circle posterior part many authors could be accept.

5. Acknowledgment

Contract grant sponsor: Ministry of Science and Technological Development of Republic of Serbia (No: 41018 and 175092).

6. References

Alawad, A.H.M.; Hussein, M.A. & Hassan, M.A. (2009). Morphology and Normal Variations of the Cerebral Arterial Circle "of Willis" in Khartoum Diagnostic Centre. *Khartoum Medical Journal*, Vol.2, No.2, (May 2009), pp. 215–219, ISSN 0491-4481

Al-Hussain, S.M.; Shoter, A.M. & Bataina, Z.M. (2001). Circle of Willis in Adults. *Saudi Medical Journal,* Vol.22, No.10, (October 2001), pp. 895-898, ISSN 0379-5284

Caruso, G.; Vincentelli, F.; Guidecelli, G.; Grisoli, F.; Xu, T. & Gouaze, A. (1990). Perforating Branches of the Basilar Bifurcation. *Journal of Neurosurgery,* Vol.73, No.2, (August 1990), pp. 259–265, ISSN 0022-3085

Chen, H-W.; Yen, P-S.; Lee, C-C.; Chen, C-C.; Chang, P-Y.; Lee, S-K.; Lee, W-H.; Ling, C-M. & Chou, A.S-M. (2004). Magnetic Resonance Angiographic Evaluation of Circle of Willis in General Population: A Morphologic Study in 507 Cases. *Chinese Journal of Radiology,* Vol.29, No.5, (October 2004), pp. 223-229, ISSN 1018-8940

Cucchiara, B. & Detre. J. (2008). Migraine and Circle of Willis Anomalies. *Medical Hypotheses,* Vol.70, No.4, (January 2008), pp. 860–865, ISSN 0306-9877

De Silva, K.R.D.; Silva, R.; De Silva, C.; Gunasekera, W.S.L. & Jayesekera, P.D.R.W. (2010). Comparison of the Configuration of the Posterior Bifurcation of the Posterior Communicating Artery between Fetal and Adult Brains: A Study of a Sri Lankan Population. *Annals of Indian Academy of Neurology,* Vol.13, No.3, (October 2010), pp.198-201, ISSN 0972-2327

Eftekhar, B.; Dadmehr, M.; Ansari, S.; Ghodsi, M.; Nazparvar, B. & Ketabchi, E. (June 2006). Are the Distributions of Variations of Circle of Willis Different in Different Populations? - Results of an Anatomical Study and Review of Literature, In: *BMC Neurology,* 24.06.2006, Available from
http://www.ncbi.nlm.nih.gov/pmc/articles/PMC1543654/

Gabrovsky, N. (2002). Microanatomical Bases for Intraoperative Division of the Posterior Communicating Artery. *Acta Neurochirurgica,* Vol.144, No.11, (November 2002), pp.1205-1211, ISSN 0001-6268

Hartkamp, M.J.; Van der Grond, J.; Van Everdingen, K.J.; Hillen, B. & Mali, W.P.T.M. (1999). Circle of Willis Collateral Flow Investigated by Magnetic Resonance Angiography. *Stroke,* Vol.30, No.12, (September 1999), pp.2671-2678, ISSN 0039-2499

Hendrikse, J.; Van Raamt, A.F.; Van der Graaf, J.; Mali, W.P.T.M. & Van der Grond, J. (2005). Distribution of Cerebral Blood Flow in the Circle of Willis. *Radiology,* Vol.235, No.1, (April 2005), pp.184-189, ISSN 0033-8419

Hoksbergen, A.W.J.; Fülesdi, B.; Legemate, D.A, & Csiba, L. (2000). Collateral Configuration of the Circle of Willis Transcranial Color-Coded Duplex Ultrasonography and Comparison with Postmortem Anatomy. *Stroke,* 2000; Vol.31, No.6, (June 2000), pp. 1346-1351, ISSN 0039-2499

Ingebrigtsen, T.; Morgan, M.K.; Faulder, K.; Ingebrigtsen, L.; Sparr, T. & Schirmer, H. (2004). Bifurcation Geometry and the Presence of Cerebral Artery Aneurysms. *Journal of Neurosurgery,* Vol.101, No.1, (July 2004), pp. 108–113, ISSN 0022- 3085

Kamath, S. (1981). Observations on the Length and Diameter of Vessels Forming the Circle of Willis. *Journal of Anatomy,* 1981; Vol.133, No.3, (October 1981), pp. 419-423, ISSN 0021-8782

Kapoor, K.; Singh, B. & Dewan, L.I.J. (2008). Variations in the Configuration of the Circle of Willis. *Anatomical Science International,* Vol.83, No.2, (June 2008), pp. 96–106, ISSN 1447-6959

Kayembe, K.N.; Sasahara, M. & Hazama, F. (1984). Cerebral Aneurysms and Variations in the Circle of Willis. *Stroke,* Vol.15, No.5, (September-October 1984), pp. 846-850, ISSN 0039-2499

Krishnamurthy, A.; Nayak, S.R.; Kumar, C.G.; Jetti, R.; Prabhu, L.V.; Ranade, A.V. & Rai, R. (2008). Morphometry of Posterior Cerebral Artery: Embryological and Clinical Significance. *Romanian Journal of Morphology and Embryology*, Vol.49,No.1, (January 2008), pp. 43–45, ISSN 1220-0522

Malamateniou, C.; Adams, M.E.; Srinivasan. L.; Allsop, J.N.; Counsell, S.J.; Cowan, F.M.; Hajnal, J.V. & Rutherford, M.A. (2009). The Anatomic Variations of the Circle of Willis in Preterm-at-Term and Term-Born Infants: An MR Angiography Study at 3T. *AJNR American Journal of Neuroradiology*, Vol.30, No.10, (November-December 2009), pp.1955– 1962, ISSN 0195-6108

Merkkola, P.; Tulla, H.; Ronkainen, A.; Soppi,, V.; Oksala, A.; Koivisto, T. & Hippeläinen, M. (2006). Incomplete Circle of Willis and Right Axillary Artery Perfusion. *The Annals of Thoracic Surgery*, Vol.82, No.1, (July 2006), pp.74–80, ISSN 0003-4975

Pai, B.S.; Varma, R.G.; Kulkarni, R.N.; Nirmala, S.; Manjunath, L.C. & Rakshith, S. (2007). Microsurgical Anatomy of the Posterior Circulation. *Neurology India*, Vol.55, No.1, (November 2006), pp. 31-41, ISSN 0028-3886

Papantchev, V.; Hristov, S.; Todorova, D.; Naydenov, E.; Paloff, A.; Nikolov, D.; Tschirkov, A. & Ovtscharoff, W. (2007). Some Variations of the Circle of Willis, Important for Cerebral Protection in Aortic Surgery — A Study in Eastern Europeans. *European Journal of Cardio-thoracic Surgery*, Vol.31, No.6, (June 2007), pp. 982-989, ISSN 1010-7940

Poudel, P.P. & Bhattarai, C. (Jun 2010). Anomalous Formation of the Circulus Arteriosus and its Clinico-anatomical Significance, In: *Nepal Medical College Journal: NMCJ*, 01.06.2010, Available from
http://www.nmcth.edu/nmcj_articles_pdf/volume_wise/nmcj_vol12_no2_june2010/p_paudel.pdf

Ravensbergen, J.; Ravensbergen, J.W.; Krijger, J.K.B.; Hillen B. & Hoogstraten, H. W. (1998). Localizing Role of Hemodynamics in Atherosclerosis in Several Human Vertebrobasilar Junction Geometries. *Arteriosclerosis, Thrombosis, and Vascular Biology*, Vol.18; No. 5, (May 1998), pp.708-716, ISSN 1524-4636

Riggs, H.E. & Rupp, C. (1963). Variation in Form of Circle of Willis. *Archives of Neurology*, Vol.8, No.1, (January 1963), pp. 8-14,ISSN 0003-9942

Saeki, N. & Rhoton, A.L. (1977). Microsurgical Anatomy of the Upper Basilar Artery and the Posterior Circle of Willis. *Journal of Neurosurgery*, Vol.46, No.5, (May 1977), pp. 563-578, ISSN 0022-3085

Sahni, D.; Jit, I. & Lal, V. (2007). Variations and Anomalies of the Posterior Communicating Artery in Northwest Indian Brains. *Surgical Neurology*, Vol.68, No.4, (October 2007), pp. 449-453, ISSN 0035-6336

Schomer, D.F.; Marks, M.P.; Steinberg, G.K.; Johnstone, I.M.; Boothroyd, D.B.; Ross, M.R.; Pelc, N.J. & Enzmann, D.R. (1994). The Anatomy of the Posterior Communicating Artery as a Risk Factor for Ischemic Cerebral Infarction. *The New England Journal of Medicine*, Vol.330, No.22, (June 1994), pp.1565-1570, ISSN 0028-4793

Silver, J.M. & Wilkins, R.H. (1991). Arterial Embryology, In: Persistent Embryonic Intracranial and Extracranial Vessels, In: *Neurosurgery Update II: Vascular, Spinal, Pediatric, and Functional Neurosurgery*, R.H. Wilkins, S.S. Rengachary, (Eds),50-51, McGraw-Hill, Health Professions Divisions, ISBN 9780070798298, New York, USA

Songur, A.; Gonul, Y.; Ozen, O.A.; Kucuker, H.; Uzun, I.; Bas, O. & Toktas, M. (2008). Variations in the Intracranial Vertebrobasilar System. *Surgical and Radiologic Anatomy*, Vol.30, No.3, (May 2008), pp. 257-264, ISSN 0930-1038

Tanaka, H.; Fujita, N.; Enoki, T.; Matsumoto, K.; Watanabe, Y.; Murase, K. & Nakamura, H. (2006). Relationship between Variations in the Circle of Willis and Flow Rates in Internal Carotid and Basilar Arteries Determined by Means of Magnetic Resonance Imaging with Semiautomated Lumen Segmentation: Reference Data from 125 Healthy Volunteers. *AJNR American Journal of Neuroradiology*, Vol.27, No.8, (September 2006), pp. 1770 -1775, ISSN 0195-6108

Urbanski, P.P.; Lenos, A.; Blume, J.C.; Ziegler, V.; Griewing, B.; Schmitt, R.; Diegeler, & Dinkel, M. (2008). Does Anatomical Completeness of the circle of Willis Correlate with Sufficient Cross-perfusion during Unilateral Cerebral Perfusion? *European Journal of Cardio-thoracic Surgery*, Vol.33, No.3, (December 2007), pp. 402-408, ISSN 1010-7940

Van Overbeeke, J.J.; Hillen, B. & Tulleken, C.A.F. (1991). A Comparative Study of the Circle of Willis in Fetal and Adult Life. The Configuration of the Posterior Bifurcation of the Posterior Communicating Artery. *Journal of Anatomy*, Vol.176,No.1, (June 1991), pp. 45-54, ISSN 0021-8782

Vallee, J-N.; Aymard, A.; Vicaut, E.; Reis, M. & Merland, J-J. (2003). Endovascular Treatment of Basilar Tip Aneurysms with Guglielmi Detachable Coils: Predictors of Immediate and Long-term Results with Multivariate Analysis– 6-year Experience. *Radiology*, Vol.226, No.3, (March 2003), pp. 867–879, ISSN 0033-8419

Van Raamt, A.F.; Mali, W.P.T.M.; Van Laar, P.J. & Van der Graaf, Y. (2006). The Fetal Variant of the Circle of Willis and Its Influence on the Cerebral Collateral Circulation. *Cerebrovascular Disease*, Vol.22, No.4, (Jun 2006), pp. 217-224, ISSN 1015-9770

Vasović, L.P. (2004). The Tenth Vascular Component in a Rare Form of the Cerebral Arterial Circle of Fetuses. *Cells Tissues Organs*, Vol. 178, No.4, (November 2004), pp. 231-238, ISSN 1422-6405

Vasović, L.P.; Jovanović, I.D.; Ugrenović, S.Z. & Andjelković, Z.P. (2008a). Normal Subtypes of the Posterior Part of the Cerebral Arterial Circle in Human Fetuses. *Surgical Neurology*, Vol.70, No.3, (September 2008), pp. 287–294, ISSN 0035-6336

Vasović, L.; Jovanović, I.; Ugrenović, S.; Stojanov, D. & Radovanović, Z. (2008b). Basilar Bifurcation: A Comparison of Prenatal and Postnatal Cases. *Neuroanatomy*, Vol.7, (December 2008), pp. 66-71, ISSN 1303-1783

Vasović, L.; Trandafilović, M.; Jovanović, I.; Antović, A.; Stojanović, J.; Zdravković, M. & Milić M. (June 2010). An Excess

Vessel in the Posterior Part of the Human Cerebral Arterial Circle (CAC): A Case Series, In: *BioMedCentral Neurology*, 23.06.2010, Available from http://www.ncbi.nlm.nih.gov/pmc/articles/PMC2909942/

Yasargil, M.G. (1984). Intracranial Arteries, In: Operative Anatomy, In: Microneurosurgery Vol I, M.G. Yasargil, (Ed.), 54-158, Thieme, ISBN: 3136448014, Sttutgart-New York, Germany-USA

Zada, G.; Breault, J.B.A.; Liu, C.Y.; Khalessi, A.A.; Larsen, D.W.; Teitelbaum, G.P. & Giannotta, S.L. (2008). Internal Carotid Artery Aneurysms Occurring At the Origin of Fetal Variant Posterior Cerebral Arteries: Surgical and Endovascular Experience. *Neurosurgery*, Vol.63, Suppl.1, (July 2008), pp. 55-62, ISSN 0148-396X

Zeal, A.A. & Rhoton, A.L. (1978). Microsurgical Anatomy of the Posterior Cerebral Artery. *Journal of Neurosurgery*, Vol.48, No.4, (April 1978), pp. 534-559 ISSN 0022-3085

Żurada, A., Gielecki, J.S.; Baron, J.; Zawiliński, J. & Kozlowska H. (2008). Interactive 3D stereoscopic digital-image analysis of the basilar artery bifurcation. *Clinical Anatomy*, Vol.21, No.2, (March 2008), pp. 127-137, ISSN 0897-3806